THE HOME ENCYCLOPEDIA *of* HERBAL MEDICINE

Natural Remedies
for Emerging *and*
Drug-Resistant Infections

THE HOME ENCYCLOPEDIA *of* HERBAL MEDICINE

*More Than 200
Make-at-Home Remedies

Stephen Harrod Buhner

RODALE

This book is intended as a reference volume only, not as a medical manual. The information given here is designed to help you make informed decisions about your health. It is not intended as a substitute for any treatment that may have been prescribed by your doctor. If you suspect that you have a medical problem, we urge you to seek competent medical help.

Mention of specific companies, organizations, or authorities in this book does not imply endorsement by the author or publisher, nor does mention of specific companies, organizations, or authorities imply that they endorse this book, its author, or the publisher.

Internet addresses and telephone numbers given in this book were accurate at the time it went to press.

Exclusive direct mail edition published by Rodale Inc. in May 2014 by arrangement with Storey Publishing, 210 Mass MoCa Way, North Adams, MA 01247. *Herbal Antibiotics* (2012) and *Herbal Antivirals* (2013) were originally published by Storey Publishing.

Printed in the United States of America
Rodale Inc. makes every effort to use acid-free ♾, recycled paper ♻.

Library of Congress Cataloging-in-Publication Data is on file with the direct mail publisher.

ISBN 978-1-62336-392-5

2 4 6 8 10 9 7 5 3 direct mail hardcover

RODALE

We inspire and enable people to improve their lives and the world around them.
For more of our products, visit rodalestore.com or call 800-848-4375.

For David Hoffmann,
who began it all

CONTENTS

Symptom Finder.......viii

Prologue: Rise of the Superbugs....... 1

Chapter 1: The End of Antibiotics....... 7

Chapter 2: The Resistant Organisms, the Diseases They Cause, and How to Treat Them....... 39

Chapter 3: Emerging Viruses: What We Are Facing....... 79

Chapter 4: Common Viral Illnesses and How to Treat Them....... 96

Chapter 5: About Herbal Medicines.......179

Chapter 6: The Materia Medica....... 189

Chapter 7: The First Line of Defense: Strengthening the Immune System....... 458

Chapter 8: A Handbook of Herbal Medicine Making....... 535

Chapter 9: An Herbal Formulary....... 581

Sources of Supply....... 599

Endnotes....... 601

Index....... 608

SYMPTOM FINDER

Page references in **bold** denote recipes.

A

Abdominal pain, causes, 58, 69, 101, 163

Abdominal pain, remedies, 452

Abrasion, remedies, 552

Abscess, remedies, 215, 238, 274, 305, 361, 363–64, 381, 452

Aches and pains, causes, 72, 101, 132, 163

Aches and pains, remedies, 405, 444, 489

Acne, remedies, 263, 266

Agitation, causes, 132

Altitude sickness, remedies, 517, 531

Anemia, causes, 59, 77, 158

Anemia, remedies, 209, 220, 224, 226–28, 473, 531

Anxiety, remedies, 153, 325, 441, 466, 517, 533

Appetite loss, causes, 157, 158, 160, 162

Appetite loss, remedies, 286, 306, 444, 473, 488, 515

Arthritis, causes, 61

Arthritis, remedies, 63, 148, 150, 202, 237, 274, 277, 286, 327, 343, 349–50, 381, 400, 412, 436, 466, 485, 491, 501, 517, 522

Ascites, remedies, 287

Asthma, remedies, 215–17, 226, 229, 296, 306, 412, 434, 444, 488–89, 492, 522

Ataxia, causes, 142

Athlete's foot, remedies, **573**

B

Bacteremia, causes, 51, 53, 54, 59, 61, 64, 70, 73

Bacteremia, remedies, 47, 51, 54–55, 60, 63, 65, 71, 74

Behavior changes, causes, 132, 134, 142

Bladder problems, remedies, 434

Bleeding, causes, 156, 158, 161

Bleeding, remedies, 215–17, 239, 287, 323, 413

Blisters, causes, 157, 158–60, 162

Blisters, remedies, 168

Boils, causes, 53

Boils, remedies, 217, 237, 274, 361, 399

Bone disease, remedies, 348, 351, 405

Brain fog, remedies, 465, 485, 509, 526

Bronchitis, causes, 61, 78

Bronchitis, remedies, 78, 217, 226, 238–39, 278, 296, 300, 306, 327, 364, 412, 434, 441, 492, 517, 522, 524

Burns/burn infections, causes, 67

Burns/burn infections, remedies, 68–69, 237, 274, 290, 292–96, 306, 439, 500

C

Cancer, remedies, 154, 204, 209, 215, 225, 238, 246, 255, 273, 278, 279, 299, 306–7, 315, 319, 324, 327–28, 350, 364, 378, 381–82, 398, 406, 436–37, 453, 473–74, 485, 488, 493, 524, 534

Canker sores, remedies, 274

Cardiopulmonary edema, causes, 157

Cavities, remedies, 226, 500

Cellulitis, causes, 61

Cellulitis, remedies, 63

Chills, remedies, 226, 238, 322, 401, 405, 441

Cholangitis, causes, 59

Cholangitis, remedies, 60

Chronic obstructive pulmonary disease (COPD), remedies, 287, 492–93

Cognition problems, remedies, 147, 153

Cold aversion, remedies, 489

Colds, causes, 129

Colds, remedies, 117, 129–30, 215, 218, 237–39, 287, 290, 322, **335**, 349, 379, 405–7, 440–41, 443–44, 460, 471, 473, 488, 495–96, 501–3, 531, 550, **551**, 563

Cold sores, causes, 158–60

Colic, remedies, 200, 216–17, 349, 444

Colitis, causes, 155

Colitis, remedies, 238, 273, 366

Collagen problems, remedies, 277, 496, 503

Coma, causes, 132, 142, 155, 157, 160

Concentration problems, remedies, 517, 533

Confusion, causes, 132, 142, 160

Confusion, remedies, 485

Congestion, remedies, 287

Conjunctivitis, causes, 61, 70, 128

Conjunctivitis, remedies, 63, 224, 226, 292, 300, 305–6, 375, 380–81

Consciousness loss, remedies, 380

Constipation, remedies, 226, 349, 452, 453

Convulsions, causes, 77, 132, 139–40

Convulsions, remedies, 140, 238, 287, 319, 323, 325

Cough, causes, 101, 129, 132, 156

Cough, remedies, **125–26**, 128, 201, 217, 226, 237–39, 274, 286–87, 295, 305–6, 322–23, 364, 405, 412, 434–36, 441, 444, 485, 488–89, 531, **551**

Cramps, causes, 69, 72

Cramps, remedies, 178, 217, 432, 441, 444, 501

Crohn's disease, remedies, 576

Croup, causes, 129

D

Dandruff, remedies, 216, 295

Debility, remedies, 215, 217, 221, 385, 405, 434, 465, 507–9, 522, 526

Dehydration, causes, 72, 74, 163

Delirium, remedies, 399

Dementia, remedies, 147, 151, 334

Depression, remedies, 147, 153, 217, 221, 253, 326, 447, 466, 509, 526, 531, 533

Dermatitis, remedies, 435

Diabetes, remedies, 204, 220, 229, 237, 241, 280, 286, 473, 488, 492, 523

Diarrhea, causes, 24–25, 26, 50, 58, 64, 69, 74, 101, 155, 157, 163

Diarrhea, remedies, 25, 47, 50, 65, 168, 177–78, 200–201, 209, 215–17, 224, 226–28, 233, 237–39, 254, 263–64, 273, 276, 279, 287, 306, 319, 322–23, 349, 361, 363, 366, 434–35, 441, 444–45, 452–53, 473, 579, **580**

Digestion problems, remedies, 286, 444, 452

Diptheria, remedies, 496, 501

Disorientation, causes, 132

Diverticulitis, causes, 51

Diverticulitis, remedies, 51

Dizziness, remedies, 254, 485, 517, 523

Dreaming frequently, remedies, 515

Dropsy, remedies, 274, 286, 287, 344, 347, 349

Dysentery, remedies, 47, 200–201, 209, 215–17, 224, 226–28, 233, 263–64, 267, 273–74, 276, 279, 280, 319, 323, 328, 361, 363–64, 399, 412, 422, 452

Dyspepsia, remedies, 217, 254, 444

Dysphagia, remedies, 436, 453

Dyspnea, remedies, 364

Dysuria, remedies, 399

E

Earache, causes, 157

Earache, remedies, 238, 363–64, 452

Ear infection, causes, 24, 54, 61, 67

Ear infection, remedies, 63, 69, 237, 273, 364, 366, 563, **564**, **578–79**

Eczema, remedies, 206, 209, 215, 217, 274, 287, 399

Edema, remedies, 226, 228, 239, 325, 344, 348, 364, 473

Encephalitis, causes, 72, 130–43, 155, 157, 158, 160, 162

Encephalitis, remedies, 137–38, 139–40, 143–54, 164, 169, 173, 311, 319, 326, 338, 379–81, 389, 400, 426, 469, 485

Endocarditis, causes, 51, 61, 70, 73

Endocarditis, remedies, 51

Epiglottitis, causes, 61

Epiglottitis, remedies, 63

Erectile dysfunction, remedies, 488–89

Eye infection, remedies, 206, 209, 215, 224–25, 226, 231, 273, 328, 361, 363

Eye pain, causes, 156

Eye problems, causes, 61, 101, 128, 158–59

Eye problems, remedies, 63, 71, 173, 222, 322

F

Fasciitis, causes, 55

Fasciitis, remedies, 54–55

Fatigue, causes, 101, 154, 157, 158, 160, 169

Fatigue, remedies, 402, 473, 475, 485, 488, 494, 509, 511, 517, 518, 522, 526, 531, 533

Fever, causes, 53, 58, 69, 72, 77, 101, 124, 128, 132, 134, 141, 142, 154, 156, 157, 158, 160, 162, 163

Fever, remedies, 124, 165, 169, 200–202, 204, 209, 215–17, 224, 226, 238, 241, 243, 253–54, 273–74, 286, 306, 319, 322–23, 331, 334, 349, 379, 396, 399–401, 400, 405, 413, 434–35, 441, 444, 452, 500, 579

Fever blisters, causes, 158–60

Flatulence, remedies, 444

Flu (influenza), causes, 96–114

Flu (influenza), remedies, 104, 107–11, 113, 114–28, 215, 218, 237–39, 287, 290, 322, 326–27, 331, **335**, 341–43, 345–46, 351–52, 360, 374–75, 379, 380, 385, 389, 396–97, 399–400, 405, 406–7, 407, 412, 440–41, 443, 448, 460, 471, 473, 488, 491, 495–96, 501–3, 505, 516, 526, 531, 550, **551**, 563

G

Gallbladder problems, remedies, 273

Gangrene, remedies, 292, 296, 452

Gastrointestinal (GI) problems, causes, 54, 58, 67, 72, 155, 157, 162–63, 176, 238

Gastrointestinal (GI) problems, remedies, 55, 68, 164, 176–78, 200, 215, 224, 226, 243, 253, 259, 273–74, 280, 291, 299, 319, 322, 366, 375, 380, 432, 434, 452, 470, 501, 531

Genital infections, remedies, 361

Gingivitis, remedies, 291–92

Glomerulonephritis, causes, 54

Glomerulonephritis, remedies, 54

Gynecological infections, remedies, 274, 279

H

Hangover, remedies, 237

Headache, causes, 77, 101, 125, 132, 134, 141, 156, 157, 160, 163

Headache, remedies, 125, 215, 226, 237–38, 254, 305, 323, 349, 379, 399, 441, 444

Hearing problems, causes, 155

Heart disease, remedies, 238, 322, 452, 469, 474–75, 493, 515, 517, 522

Hemoptysis, remedies, 323, 380

Hemorrhage, remedies, 226, 287

Hemorrhoids, remedies, 215–17, 226, 238, 574

Hernia, remedies, 200, 452

Hiccups, remedies, 323

Hoarseness, remedies, 434, 452

Hypertension, remedies, 241, 323, 325–26, 328, 522, 524

Hypothermia, causes, 134, 156

Hysteria, remedies, 215, 253, 323

I

Immune system problems, remedies, 461–534, **476**

Impetigo, remedies, 209, 290, 300

Impotence, remedies, 215, 489, 493, 531

Indigestion, remedies, 215, 322, 444, 452, 577

Inflammation, causes, 50, 97, 101, 103, 106–7, 109, 111, 140–41, 156, 160, 162

Inflammation, remedies, 50, 144, 147, 148–51, 152, 153, 165–67, 201–2, 225, 228, 238–39, 241, 273–74, 283, 297, 305–6, 311, 319, 327, 334, 343–44, 348–50, 364, 377, 379–81, 398–400, 405–6, 411, 434, 436, 441, 444–45, 453–54, 467, 475, 485, 489–91, 505–6, **554–55**, 577

Irritability, remedies, 319, 532

Irritable bowel syndrome, remedies, 238, 576

Itching, remedies, 217, 238, 399

J

Jaundice, causes, 158

Jaundice, remedies, 200, 218, 226, 237–38, 254, 273–74, 323, 349, 399, 488

Joint disease, remedies, 348, 350

Joint pain, causes, 156

Joint pain, remedies, 202, 217, 238, 452

K

Keratitis, causes, 159

Keratitis, remedies, 474

Kidney problems, causes, 54, 58–59, 65, 72

Kidney problems, remedies, 54, 215–18, 237, 274, 283, 287–88, 319, 322, 346, 348, 361, 364–65, 485, 488–89, 492–93, 514, 518, 522

L

Laryngitis, remedies, 375, 379, 434

Leg numbness, causes, 155

Leg numbness, remedies, 473

Lethargy, causes, 134, 163

Libido problems, remedies, 485, 488–89, 493, 532

Liver problems, causes, 77, 155, 158

Liver problems, remedies, 20, 170, 216, 218, 220–21, 238, 243, 254, 273–74, 286–88, 319, 323, 328, 343, 344, 346, 348–50, 375, 398, 411–13, 434–36, 440, 452, 475, 488, 515, 518, 522–24

Lymph node enlargement/tenderness, causes, 154, 156, 158, 159–60, 162, 411–13

Lymph node enlargement/tenderness, remedies, 399

M

Malaise, causes, 58, 72, 77, 132, 157, 158, 162

Malaria, causes, 25–26

Malaria, remedies, 194, 197, 200–203, 209, 215, 218–19, 226, 228–29, 231, 233, 237, 240, 242, 244–45, 248–49, 251–54, 256–58, 274, 405–6

Mastitis, remedies, 553

Memory problems, remedies, 147, 325–26, 445, 453, 465, 466, 467, 475, 492, 518, 524, 532

Meningitis, causes, 51, 54, 59, 61, 64, 70, 73, 128, 134, 141, 157, 158, 159–60

Meningitis, remedies, 47, 51–52, 55, 60, 63, 65, 71, 74, 169, 173, 319, 327, 328, 375, 379, 400, 485

Menstrual irregularities, remedies, 273–74, 286

Mental dysfunction, causes, 134, 160

Mental dysfunction, remedies, 517, 523, 532–33

Mouth infection, causes, 76

Mouth infection, remedies, 77, 273–74, 432, 452

Mouth sores, remedies, 226, 237, 267, 413, 435, 495, 500, 502, 531

Movement disorders, causes, 132, 134, 142

Movement disorders, remedies, 151, 323, 334

Mucous membrane problems, remedies, 233, 239, 266, 273, 381, 434, 501–5

Muscle problems, causes, 77, 154, 156

Muscle problems, remedies, 202, 523

Myelitis, causes, 132, 155

N

Nasal problems, 444

Nausea, causes, 156, 160, 163

Nausea, remedies, 441, 443, 445

Neck stiffness, causes, 134, 142, 160

Nerve problems/pain, causes, 158, 159, 161–62

Nerve problems/pain, remedies, 172–73, 175–76, 452, 522–23

Nervous exhaustion, remedies, 465

Nervous problems, remedies, 216–17, 253–54, 323

Night sweats, remedies, 274

Nocturia, remedies, 485

Nosebleeds, remedies, 215

Numbness, causes, 155, 161

Numbness, remedies, 348, 473

O

Osteomyelitis, causes, 61, 64, 70

Osteomyelitis, remedies, 63, 65, 71

P

Pain, causes, 58, 72, 77, 101, 156, 162, 163, 174

Pain, remedies, 149, 168, 172–73, 175–76, 217, 220–21, 239, 273–74, 274, 322, 344, 348–49, 405–6, 435, 436, 439, 441, 454, 466, 506, 507, 522–23

Palpitations, remedies, 434

Pap smear abnormality, remedies, 497, **575**

Paralysis, causes, 132, 134, 139–40, 157

Paralysis, remedies, 140, 201, 216, 473

Parasites, remedies, **548**

Peritonitis, causes, 59

Peritonitis, remedies, 60

Personality alterations, causes, 132, 134

Petechiae, causes, 140, 158

Phonophobia, causes, 134

Photophobia, causes, 132, 134, 142, 159–60

Pneumonia, causes, 24, 53, 54, 57, 59, 61, 64, 66, 67, 70, 72, 73, 101, 106, 110, 128–29, 155, 156

Pneumonia, remedies, 54–55, 57, 60, 63, 65, 67, 71, 74, 78, 164, 238, 305, 319, 323, 364, 366, 375, 380, 385, 389, 396, 400, 405, 407, 485, 534

Pneumonitis, causes, 158

Prostate problems, remedies, 153–54, 488

Psoriasis, remedies, 287

Psychosis/delirium, causes, 141

Pulmonary problems, remedies, 78, 286–87, 300, 327, 349, 361, 363–66, 375, 381, 396, 413, 434, 452

R

Rashes, causes, 53, 134, 156, 157, 386

Rashes, remedies, 209, 237, 400, 500, **554–55**

Respiratory infections, causes, 52, 61, 64, 70, 128–29, 238–39, 434

Respiratory infections, remedies, 52–53, 65, 128–29, 209, 217, 219, 224, 226, 233, 243, 273, 286, 290, 295–96, 319, 343, 361, 375, 432, 441, 470, 485, 488, 495, 500, 501, 516, 531

Restlessness, remedies, 399

Rheumatism, remedies, 200, 202, 215–17, 226, 237, 344, 348–50, 364, 436, 452, 465, 501, 507

Rhinitis, remedies, 296

S

Seborrheic dermatitis, remedies, 290, 295

Seizures, causes, 132, 139, 142, 155, 160

Seizures, remedies, 221, 226, 238, 319, 334, 347, 349, 452–53

Sepsis/septicemia, causes, 53, 59, 61, 66, 67, 69, 72

Sepsis/septicemia, remedies, 47, 58, 60, 66, 68, 70, 73, 495–96, 501–3

Sexually transmitted diseases, causes, 25, 61, 65

Sexually transmitted diseases, remedies, 63, 65, 197, 200, 215–17, 226, 274, 286–87, 295, 363–64, 412

Sexual problems, remedies, 485, 488–89, 493, 531

Shivering, causes, 77

Shivering, remedies, 216

Shortness of breath, remedies, 473

Sinus infections, causes, 54, 61, 78

Sinus infections, remedies, 78, 217, 296, 301, 364, **566**

Skin infections, causes, 23, 42, 53, 54, 67

Skin infections, remedies, 47, 194, 206, 215, 222, 225, 259, 266, 273–74, 280, 287, 289, 292, 300–301, 304–5, 344, 349–50, 361, 363–64, 439, **552**, **570**, 572–73, **573**

Skin sores, causes, 158–60, 161–62

Skin sores, remedies, 172, **174**, 175–76, 217, 323, 364, 379–81, 399–400, 400, 434–36, 502

Sleepiness in daytime, remedies, 532

Sleep problems, remedies, 273, 311, 319, 321, 323–24, 452, 488, 515, 517, 522–23, 532–33

Soreness, remedies, 515

Sore throat, causes, 35, 54, 101, 129, 132, 156, 157, 158, 160, 170

Sore throat, remedies, 55, 117, 170, 226, 238–39, 267, 349, 375, 379–80, 400, 409, 434–35, 443, 495, 500, 502, 550

Spleen problems, causes, 77, 158

Spleen problems, remedies, 170, 226, 237, 274, 287, 411–13, 434, 473, 514, 516, 518

Sprains, remedies, 238, 349

Stings and bites, remedies, 200, 215, 217, 219, 226, 237–38, 240, 344, 364, 380, 452, 497, 500–501, 502

Stomachache, remedies, 218, 531

Stomach cramps, remedies, 441, 444, 501

Stress, remedies, 466, 517, 523, 532–33

Sunburn, remedies, 452, 552, 569

Swallowing difficulty, remedies, 238

Sweating, causes, 141, 156

Sweating, remedies, 274, 287, 473, 489

Swelling, remedies, 217, 238, 274, 344, 348, 363, 435, 500

Systemic infections, remedies, 47, 77, 197, 206, 209, 215, 224, 231, 233

T

Tennis elbow, remedies, 577

Throat infection, remedies, 273, 287

Tinnitus, remedies, 485, 489

Tonsilitis, remedies, 218, 238, 279, 327, 364, 375, 409, 495, 500, 501

Toothache, remedies, 215, 226, 238, 435, 452, 500

Tremors, causes, 132, 134, 141

Tremors, remedies, 323

Tuberculosis, causes, 25, 52–53

Tuberculosis, remedies, 197, 217, 219, 226, 286–88, 300, 305–6, 435, 465

U

Ulcers, causes, 155, 157

Ulcers, remedies, 201, 215, 220, 226, 237–39, 241, 273–74, 278, 287, 290–91, 294–96, 413, 432, 434–36, 473, 501, 522–23, 573–74, **574**, 576

Upper respiratory infections, causes, 97, 110, 128–29

Upper respiratory infections, remedies, 128–30, 200, 279, 280–81, 295, 305, 327, 368, 380, 389, 402, 470, **553**, 566

Urinary tract infections, causes, 24, 42, 51, 53, 57, 58–59, 64, 66, 67, 70, 76, 452

Urinary tract infections, remedies, 47, 51, 54, 58, 65, 66, 68, 70–71, 76, 197, 200–201, 204, 216–17, 224, 233, 238–39, 273–74, 273–75, 289, 299, 307, 319, 361, 501

V

Vaginal discharge, remedies, 273–74

Vaginal infections, causes, 76

Vaginal infections, remedies, 76, 173, 215, 217, 233, 239, 266–67, 279, 287, 300, 305–6, 505, 568, 574, **575**

Vertigo, causes, 141

Vision problems, causes, 132, 155, 159

Vision problems, remedies, 518

Vomiting, causes, 69, 77, 101, 141, 142, 156, 157, 160, 163

Vomiting, remedies, 444–45

W

Wasting, remedies, 473, 489

Weakness, causes, 132, 134, 155, 163

Weakness, remedies, 405, 473, 485, 489, 507, 509, 514–15

Wheezing, remedies, 217

Wound infections, causes, 23, 47, 53, 56–57, 64, 66, 67, 70, 73

Wound infections, remedies, 57, 65, 66, 68–69, 71, 74, 78, 194, 197, 206, 209, 215, 222, 224, 237–38, 243, 263, 267, 289–90, 292, 344, 497, 500, 502

Wounds, remedies, 200, 216, 222, 226, 290–91, 293–96, 298, 305–6, 322, 349–51, 354, 380, 497, 500, 501, 502, 505, 572–73, **573**

Y

Yeast infections, remedies, 266–67, 279, 505

It is naive to think we can win.
David Livermore, MD

PROLOGUE: RISE OF THE SUPERBUGS

In the late 1940s, the successes of Waksman and Schatz (streptomycin) and Duggar (tetracycline) led many to believe that bacterial infections were basically conquered. That conceit led to widespread misuse and outright abuse of antibacterial agents. Nonetheless, we still neither fully understand nor appreciate resistance to antibacterial agents. . . . Many important advances in the practice of medicine are actually at serious risk. Multidrug resistant bacteria are compromising our ability to perform what are now considered routine surgical procedures. . . . A ubiquitous phrase encountered in obituaries is "died from complications following surgery," but what is not well understood is that these "complications" are quite frequently multidrug resistant infections.

—Steven Projan, *Bacterial Resistance to Antimicrobials*

We have let our profligate use of antibiotics reshape the evolution of the microbial world and wrest any hope of safe management from us. . . . Resistance to antibiotics has spread to so many different, and such unanticipated types of bacteria, that the only fair appraisal is that we have succeeded in upsetting the balance of nature.

—Marc Lappé, *When Antibiotics Fail*

It serves little purpose merely to be scared by viruses. But it serves a good deal of purpose to understand them.

—Frank Ryan, MD, *Virus X: Tracking the New Killer Plagues*

It's hard to escape the realization that when it comes to bacterial disease, we are in trouble. Twenty years ago, when my interest was first stimulated by it, there might have been a newspaper article on antibiotic resistance or a resistant disease outbreak perhaps once a month. I come across them almost daily now. The headlines often look like this:

Hospital Continues to Limit Visitors as It Fights Superbugs

—*Ottawa Citizen,* December 21, 2010

Deadlier Than AIDS: Scientists Discover New STD That Kills Within Days

—Vangret, *Code World News,* January 29, 2014

Drug-Resistant TB Spreading Fast in Russia

—*The Business Standard,* January 27, 2014

NIH Reveals Battle with Outbreak of Dangerous Resistant *Klebsiella Pneumoniae* Bacteria

—*Daily Kos,* August 24, 2014

Dangerous MRSA Bacteria Expand into Communities

—Peter Eisler, *USA Today,* December 13, 2013

New "Superbugs" Raising Concerns Worldwide

—Rob Stein, *Washington Post,* October 11, 2010

The Spread of Superbugs

—Nicholas Kristof, *New York Times,* March 7, 2010

Report: Superbugs Killed Record Number

—UPI, May 23, 2008

Sometimes they take a more personal turn:

How American Healthcare Killed My Father: Q and A with David Goldhill

—Nick Gillespie, *Reason,* November 2, 2013

'The NHS Failed My Mum,' Says Distraught Daughter

—*Grantham Journal,* December 14, 2010

The 'Catalogue of Errors' That Cost This Father His Life

—Denis Campbell and Anushka Asthana, *The Guardian,* November 27, 2010

Superbug Ate My Arm: Woman's Terrifying Encounter with Flesh-Eating Bacteria in South Australia

—Penelope Debelle, *Adelaide Now,* November 8, 2013

The first sort of article (i.e., "Superbugs on the increase in care homes," Daniel Martin, *The Mail Online,* July 16, 2007) tends to focus on numbers and statistics and rarely reflects the human face of the problem. Such articles often end with a statement from a government or medical authority mentioning how new procedures are being instituted or that new antibiotics are just down the road a ways (they aren't). Nothing to be concerned about even though it sounds a bit scary, say the experts; we have it all in hand (they don't).

The second sort of piece, growing more common every year, presents the human face of the problem. These articles are rarely so blasé. This report, from an article by Sarah White, "The empowered patient," is representative. It recounts the story of Jeanine Thomas (who later began a "survivors of MRSA support group") and the moment when all those headlines changed from the theoretical to the very personal:

> Thomas' expertise in the MRSA patient perspective comes from her life-threatening battle with bacteria. In 2001, she was in critical condition after contracting MRSA [methicillin-resistant *Staphylococcus aureus*] following ankle surgery.
>
> "You're just living a normal life—never been sick, never been unhealthy, and all of a sudden you are fighting for your life. And this is happening to individuals every day," Thomas said.
>
> The infection went to her blood stream and bone marrow and caused septic shock and organ failure. After undergoing multiple surgeries including a bone-marrow transplant and a "never-ending cycle of antibiotics," she survived the ordeal.[1]

Thomas survived relatively intact. Some don't, losing limbs in a desperate bid to stop the infection from spreading and then living permanently debilitated lives. Others aren't even that "lucky."

Denis Campbell's and Anushka Asthana's article appeared in November 2010 in the English paper *The Guardian*. It describes the last few months of Frank Collinson's life.

> Ex-docker Frank Collinson, 72, was admitted to hospital following a fall in May 2009. When he went home days later he had cracked ribs and a skin infection. . . . Four months later he was dead. . . .
>
> Soon after arriving in Hull's main hospital, Collinson contracted the deadly superbug MRSA. Astonishingly, no health professional told his son, Gary. It was only by Googling the name of the drug being administered through a drip that Gary discovered that it was a strong antibiotic and that his father had the potentially fatal infection. "I went ballistic," he said.[2]

This is often how the personal face of the resistance epidemic emerges into someone's awareness. They, or a relative, go into the hospital for a minor procedure or for help after an accident, but what they find in the hospital is far worse than the trouble that sent them there in the first place.

> Devastated siblings still reeling from the death of their mother several months ago continue to push for answers on how she contracted a deadly superbug.
>
> Fiona Weatherstone and her four brothers were shocked when their 73-year-old mother, Sylvia Weatherstone, died at Lincoln County Hospital after being admitted for a simple pain-killing injection. . . .
>
> It was in January that Mrs. Weatherstone, formerly of Bristol Close, was admitted for a nerve root injection to numb pain in her back, caused by severe pressure on a nerve root.
>
> The following day, Mrs. Weatherstone's health began to deteriorate and tests were undertaken to find the source of an infection.
>
> Several days later, C. Diff [*Clostridium difficile*] was diagnosed and Mrs. Weatherstone later passed away after a month in hospital.[3]

In fact, other than factory farms, hospitals and doctors' offices are the primary breeding ground of superbugs. A simple injection or a minor surgery can now, fairly routinely, lead to months in the hospital, or loss of limb, or loss of life. It's a new world out there, or rather it's an old one that is letting us know there is a price to be paid for hubris.

For several decades now, I have been deeply interested in antibiotic resistance, the intelligence of bacteria, and the use of treatment approaches that are, ultimately, more elegant than pharmaceuticals. As you will soon read, plant-based medicines, unlike pharmaceuticals, don't cause resistance problems, they are much safer, *and* they are ecologically sound—they are biodegradable *and* renewable, which most pharmaceuticals are not.

My long-term interest in herbal antibacterials resulted in a very deep exploration of systemic herbal antibacterials for resistant infections. And during that exploration, many aspects of plant medicine not hitherto developed in the West began to reveal themselves (such as the importance of plant synergists).

In this exclusive, expanded edition, you will find not only everything you need to create your own herbal antibiotics, but also a similar exploration into the world of viruses, emerging and resistant viral diseases, and more ecologically responsible (and often more effective) forms of treatment. You will find information on some of the best broad-spectrum, systemic, antiviral herbs on Earth. As with herbal antibiotics, they are easy to use, easy to grow, and easy to make into medicines for yourself, your family, your patients. And they are very, very effective for emerging and resistant viral infections. For the plants themselves learned long ago, just as they did with bacteria, how to stop viruses from killing them. Plants can't run, but they sure can do chemistry.

The concept of herbal antibiotics as primary interventives has, over the past several decades, become common in cultures outside the Western industrialized nations. Medical systems in Africa, Asia, and South and Central America are turning away from pharmaceuticals as a first-line treatment for bacterial infections because of resistance problems and, most especially, because pharmaceutical corporations make a great deal too much money off the suffering of their populations. Cultures other than those in the West have realized that they just can't afford corporate greed any longer—*and* they are unwilling to let the poorer members of their populations die because of it. Researchers in cultures across the globe have found that plant antibacterials are often *more* effective than pharmaceuticals. So they are exploring which ones are most potent, which forms of preparation are most effective, and how best to grow them. Then they are traveling throughout their regions (especially in Africa), giving seeds to local villages, teaching them all they have learned, and letting them get on with their healing. There is no middleman raking off profits in the process. A new model of health care is coming into being—and it's about time.

It is my hope that this same kind of movement will begin in the treatment of viral diseases. (And in China, they are already years ahead of us; they *see* the writing on the wall.) We need a new paradigm of healing. We need new ways of thinking about viruses, their emergence, and their treatment—just as we have needed them about bacteria. (Even in the herbal communities in the West, our approaches to viral infections and viruses have been extremely shallow.) There is a lot we can do to create a more effective healing paradigm in our world, one that is ecologically sustainable while at the same time being more human friendly . . . if we step outside the box that our thinking has been trapped by.

I hope that you find the material in this book stimulating to your thinking. I hope that you begin, yourself, to add to this emerging paradigm of healing, one that is slowly extricating itself from the outmoded thinking of the past. We have a great opportunity to create something new, something that reflects more accurately the world around us, something that truly addresses the healing needs of the people who come to us.

I think the bacteria and viruses are going to be pretty insistent that we do so. And soon.

1

THE END OF ANTIBIOTICS

[Once] the germ theory of contagion finally caught on, it did so with a vengeance. Different types of bacteria were implicated in anthrax, gonorrhea, typhoid, and leprosy. Microbes, once amusing little anomalies, became demonized. . . . [They] became a virulent "other" to be destroyed.

—Lynn Margulis and Dorion Sagan, *What Is Life?*

It is worth considering that despite being smaller than one millionth of a meter long, microbes compromise fully 60 percent of the mass of life on the planet.

—Brad Spellberg, *Rising Plague*

There is a unique smell to hospitals, composed of equal parts illness, rubbing alcohol, fear, and hope. Few of us who have been in a hospital can forget that smell or the feelings it engenders. But underneath those memory-laden smells and feelings is the belief that in this place, this hospital, an army of men and women is fighting for our lives, working to bring us back from the brink of death. We have learned, been taught, know for a fact, that this army is winning the war against disease, that antibiotics have made an end to most bacterial diseases. It is a comforting belief. Unfortunately, what we "know" couldn't be more wrong.

Late in 1993, as *Newsweek*'s Sharon Begley reported, infectious disease specialist Dr. Cynthia Gilbert entered the room of a long-term kidney patient. Her face was set in the mask that physicians have used for centuries when coming to pass sentence on their patients. The man was not fooled; he took it in in a glance. "You're coming to tell me I'm dying," he said.

She paused, then nodded curtly. "There's just nothing we can do."

They each paused then. One contemplating the end of life, the other the failure of her craft and the loss that goes with it.

Dr. Gilbert took a deep, painful breath. "I'm sorry," she said.

The man said nothing; for what he was contemplating there were no words. His physician nodded sharply as if settling her mind. Then she turned and left him, facing once again the long hall filled with the smells of illness, rubbing alcohol, fear, and hope, and the questions for which she had no answer.

Her patient was going to die of something easily curable a few years earlier—an enterococcal bacterial infection. But this particular bacteria was now resistant to antibiotics; for 9 months she had tried every antibiotic in her arsenal. The man, weakened as he was by disease, could not fight off a bacteria impervious to pharmaceuticals. Several days later he succumbed to a massive infection of the blood and heart.

This outcome, inconceivable even a few decades earlier, is growing ever more common. Millions of people are contracting resistant infections every year in the United States, and hundreds of millions more are doing so around the globe. Increasingly, as the virulence and resistance of bacteria worsen, more of them are succumbing to formerly treatable diseases. Estimates of the dead and maimed rise every year with little hope in sight for their reduction.

The toll is mounting because the number of people infected by resistant bacteria is increasing, especially in places where the ill, the young or old, or the poor congregate, such as homeless shelters, inner cities, prisons, and child care centers. And the most dangerous place of all? Well, it's your average hospital. For there is no place else on Earth where so many sick people congregate. No place else where so many pathogenic bacteria congregate. And there is no place else where the bacteria will experience such a multiplicity of antibiotics.

We face an uncertain future, but it's not widely understood just how this has come to pass.

The Antibiotic Age

You probably haven't heard of Anne Miller; almost no one has. Nevertheless, when she died in 1999 at the age of 90, her obituary was published in the *New York Times*. Why did "the paper of record" publish the obituary of an obscure elderly woman? Well, because she was the first person to be saved by a very new, experimental drug—a drug that altered human history.

In March of 1942 Anne Sheafe Miller was in a hospital in New Haven, Connecticut, dying from pneumonia caused by a streptococcal infection. She was delirious, slipping in and out of consciousness, with a temperature near 107°F. Her doctors had tried everything they could think of, sulfa drugs and blood transfusions, and nothing had worked. But then someone remembered reading about a new, highly experimental drug. The doctors managed to get a small amount of it from a laboratory in New Jersey. Once they injected her with it, Anne's temperature dropped to near normal overnight. The next day she was no longer delirious, and within a few days she was sitting up, eating full meals, and chatting with her visitors. That moment changed our world. News of her miraculous recovery made headlines across the country. The pharmaceutical companies took note and began full production of the first "miracle" drug in existence. The drug? Penicillin.

In 1942 the world's entire supply of penicillin was a mere 32 liters (its weight? about 64 pounds). By 1949, 156,000 pounds a year of penicillin and a new antibiotic, streptomycin (isolated from common soil fungi), were being produced. By 1999—*in the United States alone*—this figure had grown to an incredible 40 million pounds a year of scores of antibiotics for people, livestock, research, and agricultural plants. Ten years later some *60 million pounds per year of antibiotics were being used in the United States* and scores of millions of pounds more by other countries around the world. Nearly 30 million pounds were being used in the United States solely on animals raised for human consumption. And those figures? That is *per year*. Year in, year out.

Epidemiologist and veterinarian Wendy Powell, of the Canadian Food Inspection Agency, comments that "in 1991, there were more than 50 penicillins, 70 cephalosporins, 12 tetracyclines, 8 aminoglycosides, 1 monobactam, 3 carbapenems, 9 macrolides, 2 new streptogramins, and 3 dihydrofolate reductase inhibitors" on the market.[1] Those numbers are even higher now.

Most people don't realize it, but—these antibiotics? They never go away.

Antibiotics, in their pure or metabolized states, form a significant part of hospital waste streams. They are excreted in their millions of pounds from the millions of patients who visit hospitals each year. Expired antibiotics (sold or unsold, in their millions of pounds) are simply thrown into the garbage. Antibacterials, as disinfectants, and antibiotic remnants from various treatments also enter the hospital waste streams. *All* of the antibiotics that hospitals buy end up, one way or another, in the environment, usually in wastewater streams. They travel to treatment plants and pass relatively unchanged into the world's water supplies.

American physicians outside of hospitals dispense an additional 260 million antibiotic prescriptions yearly, and those, too, are excreted into the environment. Adding to the antibiotic waste stream, pharmaceutical manufacturers discharge thousands of tons of spent mycelial and other antibiotic-related waste into the environment, much of it still containing antibiotic residues. Yearly, American factory farms dispense nearly 30 million pounds, or more, of antibiotics so that America's food animals—primarily pigs, cattle, and chickens—will survive overcrowding (low levels of antibiotics also stimulate weight gain, increasing revenue). The millions of gallons of their excrement is funneled into waste lagoons, from where it flows relatively unchanged into local ecosystems. Open-range farm animals (as well as millions of other domesticated animals—mostly dogs and cats) deposit their antibiotic-laden feces directly onto the ground. Ninety-seven percent of the antibiotic kanamycin passes unchanged through animal gastrointestinal (GI) tracts onto the surface of the soil.

In short, the American continent, like much of the world, is literally awash in antibiotics. And as physician and researcher Stuart Levy remarks, many of these antibiotics are not easily biodegradable. "They can remain intact in the environment unless they are destroyed by high temperatures or other physical damage such as ultraviolet light from the sun. As active antibiotics they continue to kill off susceptible bacteria with which they have contact."[2]

In an extremely short period of geologic time, the earth has been saturated with hundreds of millions of tons of nonbiodegradable, often biologically unique pharmaceuticals designed to kill bacteria. Many antibiotics (whose name literally means "against life") do not discriminate in their activity but kill broad groups of diverse bacteria whenever they are used. The worldwide environmental dumping over the past 65 years of such huge quantities of synthetic antibiotics has initiated the most pervasive impacts on the earth's bacterial underpinnings since oxygen-generating bacteria supplanted methanogens 2.5 billion years ago. It has, as Levy comments, "stimulated evolutionary changes that are unparalleled in recorded biologic history."[3] In the short run this means the emergence of unique pathogenic bacteria in human, animal, and agricultural crop populations. In the long run it means the emergence of infectious disease epidemics more deadly than *any* in human history.

The Limits of Antibiotics

Perhaps no technological advance has been more widely advertised and capitalized upon than the development of antibiotics. It is routinely lauded as one of the primary accomplishments of the application of science and modern medicine in Western culture—the success of the scientific method over the uninformed medicine of the past.

The excitement over the discovery and successful use of antibiotics in medicine was so strong in the late 1950s and early 1960s that many physicians, including my great-uncle Lee Burney, then surgeon general of the United States, and my grandfather David Cox, president of the Kentucky Medical Association, jointly proclaimed the end for all time of epidemic disease. A 1963 comment by the Australian physician Sir F. Macfarlane Burnet, a Nobel laureate, is typical. By the end of the twentieth century, he said, humanity would see the "virtual elimination of infectious disease as a significant factor in societal life."[4]

Seven years later, one of my great-uncle's successors, Surgeon General William Stewart, testified to Congress that "it was time to close the book on infectious diseases."[5] Smallpox was being eradicated, and polio vaccines were showing astonishing success in preventing infection in millions of people in the United States, Africa, and Europe. Tuberculosis and malaria, it was predicted, would be gone by the year 2000. With satisfaction David Moreau observed in an article in *Vogue* magazine that "the chemotherapeutic revolution [had] reduced nearly all non-viral disease to the significance of a bad cold."[6]

Hospital-acquired resistant infections, by conservative estimates, are now the fourth leading cause of death in the United States.

They couldn't have been more wrong.

In spite of Moreau's optimism, when his article appeared in 1976, infectious disease was already on the rise. By 1997 it had become so bad that three million people a year in the United States were being admitted to hospitals with difficult-to-treat, antibiotic-resistant bacterial infections. The Centers for Disease Control (CDC) estimated in 2002 that another 1.7 million were becoming infected while visiting hospitals and 100,000 were estimated to be dying after contracting a resistant infection in a hospital.

"To reiterate," says Brad Spellberg of the Infectious Diseases Society of America, "these people come into the hospital for a heart attack, or cancer, or trauma after a car accident, or to have elective surgery, or with some other medical problem and then ended up dying of infection that they picked up in the hospital. . . . The number of people who die from hospital-acquired infections is unquestionably much higher now, and is almost certainly more than 100,000 per year in the United States alone."[7]

This would make hospital-acquired resistant infections, by conservative estimates, the fourth leading cause of death in the United States. And that doesn't even include the death toll from infectious diseases in general, the same infectious diseases that were going to be eradicated by the year 2000. R. L. Berkelman and J. M. Hughes commented in 1993 in the *Annals of Internal Medicine* that "the stark reality is that infectious diseases are the leading cause of death worldwide and remain the leading cause of illness and death in the United States."[8] Pathologist and researcher Marc Lappé went even further, declaring in his book *When Antibiotics Fail,* "The period once euphemistically called the Age of Miracle Drugs is dead."[9]

The End of Miracle Drugs

Though penicillin was discovered in 1929, it was only with World War II that it was commercially developed, and it wasn't until after the war that its use became routine. Those were heady days. It seemed science could do anything. New antibiotics were being discovered daily; the arsenal of medicine seemed overwhelming. In the euphoria of the moment no one heeded the few voices raising concerns. Among them, ironically enough, was Alexander Fleming, the discoverer of penicillin. Dr. Fleming noted as early as 1929 in the *British Journal of Experimental Pathology* that numerous bacteria were already resistant to the drug he had discovered, and in a 1945 *New York Times* interview, he warned that improper use of penicillin would inevitably lead to the development of resistant bacteria. Fleming's observations were prescient. At the time of his interview just 14 percent of *Staphylococcus aureus* bacteria were resistant to penicillin; by 1953, as the use of penicillin became widespread, 64 percent to 80 percent of the bacteria had become resistant and resistance to tetracycline and erythromycin was also being reported. (In 1995 an incredible 95 percent of staph was resistant to penicillin.) By 1960 resistant staph had become the most common source of hospital-acquired infections worldwide. So physicians began to use methicillin, a *beta*-lactam antibiotic that they found to be effective against penicillin-resistant strains. Methicillin-resistant staph (MRSA) emerged within a year. The first severe outbreak in hospitals occurred in the United States in 1968—a mere 8 years later. Eventually MRSA strains resistant to all clinically available antibiotics except the glycopeptides (vancomycin and teicoplanin) emerged. And by 1999, 54 years after the commercial production of antibiotics, the first staph strain resistant to all clinical antibiotics had infected its first three people.

Originally limited to patients in hospitals (the primary breeding ground for such bacteria), by the 1970s resistant strains had begun appearing outside hospitals. Now they are common throughout the world's population. In 2002 I saw my first resistant staph infection outside a hospital setting. Now every month brings an e-mail or call from someone with another.

> The period once euphemistically called the Age of Miracle Drugs is dead.
> —*Marc Lappé*

This rate of resistance development was supposed to be impossible. Evolutionary biologists had insisted that evolution in bacteria (as in all species) could come only from spontaneous, usable mutations that occur with an extremely low frequency (from one out of every 10 million to one out of every 10 billion mutations) in each generation. That bacteria could generate significant resistance to antibiotics in only 35 years was considered impossible. That the human species could be facing the end of antibiotics only 60 years after their introduction was ludicrous. But in fact, bacteria are showing extremely sophisticated responses to the human "war" on disease.

The Rise of Bacterial Resistance

The thing that so many people missed, including my ancestors, is that *all* life on Earth is highly intelligent and very, very adaptable. Bacteria are the oldest forms of life on this planet, and they have learned very, very well how to respond to threats to their well-being. Among those threats are the thousands if not millions of antibacterial substances that have existed as long as life itself.

One of the crucial understandings that those early researchers ignored, though tremendously obvious now (only hubris could have hidden it so long), is that the world is filled with antibacterial substances, most produced by other bacteria, as well as fungi and plants. Bacteria, to survive, learned how to respond to those substances a very long time ago. Or as Steven Projan of Wyeth Research puts it, bacteria "are the oldest of living organisms and thus have been subject to three billion years of evolution in harsh environments and therefore have been selected to withstand chemical assault."[10]

What makes the problem even more egregious is that most of the antibiotics originally developed by human beings came from fungi, fungi that bacteria had encountered a very long time ago. Given those circumstances, *of course* there were going to be problems with our antibiotics. Perhaps, *perhaps*, if our antibiotic use had been restrained, the problems would have been minor. But it hasn't been; the amount of pure antibiotics being dumped into the environment is unprecedented in evolutionary history. And that has had tremendous impacts on the bacterial communities of Earth, and the bacteria have set about solving the problem they face very methodically. Just like us, they want

> The trend in the bacterial development of antibiotic resistance is not unlike the increasing resistance of agricultural pests to pesticides. In 1938, scientists knew of just seven insect and mite species that had acquired resistance to pesticides. By 1984 that figure had climbed to 447 and included most of the world's major pests. In response to heavier pesticide use and a wider variety of pesticides, pests have evolved sophisticated mechanisms for resisting the action of chemicals designed to kill them. Pesticides also kill the pests' natural enemies, much like antibiotics kill the natural enemies of harmful bacteria in the body.
>
> —*Michael Schmidt,* Beyond Antibiotics

to survive, and just like us, they are very adaptable. In fact, they are much more adaptable than we ever will be.

Developing Resistance

As soon as a bacterium encounters an antibiotic, it begins to generate possible responses. This takes time, usually a number of bacterial generations. But bacteria live a lot more quickly than we do; a new generation can occur every 20 minutes for many species. This is some 500,000 times faster than us. And during that quickened time scale, bacteria have found a lot of different ways to respond to our antibiotics.

Just like us, bacteria want to survive, and just like us, they are very adaptable.

ALTERED UPTAKE

Bacteria can decrease the amount of the antibiotic that gets inside them. Antimicrobials, in most instances, need to enter bacterial cells in order to kill them—they need to negotiate the cell envelope that surrounds the bacteria. Some do this by taking advantage of the normal influx of materials that must go into the bacterial cells daily in order for them to live. In other words, they sneak in by attaching themselves to nutrients of one sort or another or even appear to be a necessary nutrient so that the bacteria take them up.

To avoid this infiltration, the bacteria alter the permeability of their cell membranes, often by altering the structure of the doorways that let outside substances into the cell. This makes it harder, or impossible, for antibiotics to sneak in—essentially keeping the level of the drug below that needed to affect the bacteria.

TARGET MODIFICATION

Bacteria can alter their internal structure so that the intended target of the antibiotic won't be affected by it. As David Hooper at the Division of Infectious Diseases at Massachusetts General Hospital puts it, "Resistance by the general mechanisms of target modification can be brought about, however, by a remarkable variety of specific means, which have been exploited by different clinically important bacteria. The modification mechanism often results in an altered structure of the original drug target structure that binds the drug poorly or not at all."[11]

In other words, they change the structure of their bodies so specifically that the parts of themselves that would be affected by the antibiotics aren't. The antibiotic enters the cell, but it just doesn't do anything.

ANTIBIOTIC MODIFICATION

Bacteria can degrade or destroy the antibiotic, even if it gets inside them, by creating antibiotic-specific inactivation or disabling compounds—often these are enzymes such as extended-spectrum beta-lactamases (ESBLs). As Harry Taber of the New York Department of Health puts it, "It is not surprising to find, then, that antibiotic inactivating enzymes are found in the [cell] envelope: ß-lactamases and aminoglycoside-modifying enzymes are examples."[12]

The newest member of this group is NDM-1, New Delhi metallo-beta-lactamase. NDM-1 is a kind of ESBL but much more problematical than any known so far because it is potently active against carbapenem antibiotics, a class of beta-lactams that were previously resistant to ESBL deactivation. NDM-1 is carried on plasmids and transfers easily to a wide range of bacteria. "The frightening thing about this," says Timothy Walsh, a professor of microbiology and antibiotic resistance at Cardiff University in the UK, is that "it appears to be spreading fast."[13]

EFFLUX PUMPS

Bacteria can remove antibiotics from their cells as fast as the antibiotics enter them using something called an efflux pump. Essentially they create a kind of sump pump that will pump out exactly the things they want pumped out. There are a variety of efflux pumps in all bacteria, each coded for particular substances. Some efflux pumps act on only a single substance, while others (multidrug efflux pumps) can pump out a wide range of compounds. Often the compounds have very little in common with each other; no one yet understands why one pump can act on so many different kinds of substances.

But when one of those substances is identified by a bacterium, the pump kicks in, and the drug goes out. Researchers have commented that these "pumps can recognize and extrude positive-, negative-, or neutral-charged molecules, substances as hydrophobic as organic solvents and lipids, and compounds as hydrophilic as aminoglycoside antibiotics."[14]

Bacteria have, over long evolutionary time, created a wide range of pump types in order to protect themselves from the millions of antimicrobial substances that exist in the world. There are five main forms:

- The major facilitator superfamily (MFS)
- The APT-binding cassette superfamily (ABC)
- The small multidrug resistance family (SMR)
- The resistance-nodulation-cell division superfamily (RND)
- The multi-antimicrobial extrusion protein family (MATE)

Most Gram-positive bacteria use MFS as their primary efflux mechanism. Most Gram-negative bacteria use RND. These pumps have a wide variety of purposes, among them the protection of the organism from things like bile salts and stomach acids, which, in their own way, act much like antimicrobials on pathogenic bacteria.

SUPER ADAPTABILITY

Sometimes bacteria learn how to live and prosper in antimicrobial environments, such as the cleaning solutions in hospitals. As one journal article put it, "Contamination, mainly by Gram-negative bacteria, was found in 10 freshly prepared solutions and in 21 of 22 at discard."[15] Sometimes, they even learn to use the antibiotics for food.

Sharing Resistance

Once a bacterium develops a method for countering an antibiotic, it systematically begins to pass the knowledge on to other bacteria at an extremely rapid rate. Under the pressure of antibiotics, bacteria are interacting with as many other forms and numbers of bacteria as they can. In fact, bacteria are communicating across bacterial species lines, something they were never known to do before the advent of commercial antibiotics. The first thing they share is resistance information, and they do this in a number of different ways.

ENCODING PLASMIDS

Bacteria encode several different kinds of plasmids, essentially chromosome-independent DNA strands, each of which contains resistance information, and they pass these on to other bacteria. Plasmids are highly mobile genetic strands and are widely exchanged throughout the bacterial world. Aminoglycosides, for example, some of the most potent antibacterials known, were originally isolated from actinomycetes, a type of bacteria. Those bacteria created and used aminoglycosides themselves to kill invading or competing bacteria, but the aminoglycosides could also kill actinomycetes, so the actinomycetes also created something to deactivate aminoglycosides and they stored that information on plasmids inside themselves. *All* resistance to aminoglycosides worldwide, including in *Pseudomonas* and *Acinetobacter* organisms, has come from those ancient plasmids created by the actinomycetes. Once aminoglycosides began to be promiscuously prescribed by the medical community, the actinomycetes released the plasmids like a puff of dandelion seeds on the wind.

USING TRANSPOSONS AND INTEGRONS

Bacteria use transposons, unique movable segments of DNA that are a normal component of their genome. Sometimes called jumping genes, transposons easily move between chromosomes and plasmids. They are readily integrated into DNA structures, and when they are, the genetic makeup, and hence the physical form of the organism, is altered. Bacteria use transposons to transfer a significant amount of resistance information and often release them in free form into the environment to be taken up later by other bacteria.

They use integrons as well, a type of DNA sequence that integrates into the genome structure at specific sites. Integrons are especially active in the transfer of both resistance and virulence information.

USING VIRUSES

Bacterial viruses, or bacteriophages, also help transfer resistance information between different bacteria. It is now known that instead of making only copies of themselves when they reproduce, bacteriophages take up and make copies of host chromosome segments that contain resistance information, which are then transferred to newly infected bacteria. In other words, the viruses that infect bacteria (they get colds, too) teach them how to be resistant to antibiotics.

Bacteria can share resistance information directly or simply extrude it from their cells, allowing it to be picked up later by other roving bacteria. They often experiment, combining resistance information from multiple sources in unique ways that increase resistance, generate new resistance pathways, or even stimulate resistance to antibiotics that they have never encountered before. Even bacteria in hibernating or moribund states will share whatever information on resistance they have with any bacteria that encounter them. When bacteria take up any encoded information on resistance, they weave it into their own DNA, and this acquired resistance becomes a genetic trait that can be passed on to their descendants forever—distressingly Lamarckian. Researchers have noted that the rise of resistance over the past 50 years has had a one-to-one correlation to the production and use of antibiotics and that resistance mechanisms are not just passed on to other bacteria but are conserved within species.

Bacterial Learning

Antibiotics, ultimately and regrettably for us, have actions similar to pheromones; they act as chemical attractants and literally pull bacteria to them. Once in the presence of an antibiotic, a bacterium's learning rate immediately increases by several orders of magnitude.

Tetracycline, in even extremely low doses—in fact, especially in low doses—stimulates from 100 to 1,000 times the transfer, mobilization, and movement of transposons and plasmids. (Treatment of acne and fattening of industrial farm animals, by the way, generally involves low doses of tetracycline, often over years.) Wendy Powell comments that "this means that in times of stress, predicated by the presence of antibiotics, the antibiotics themselves promote the exchange of plasmids, which may contain resistance genes."[16]

Bacteria are not competing with each other for resources, but rather cooperating in the sharing of survival information.

The fairly recent discovery that *all* of the water supplies in the industrialized countries are contaminated with minute amounts of antibiotics (from their excretion into water supplies) means that bacteria everywhere are experiencing low doses of antibiotics *all the time*. This exposure is exponentially driving resistance learning; the more antibiotics that go into the water, the faster the bacteria learn.

What is more, as bacteria gain resistance, they pass that knowledge on to *all* forms of bacteria they meet. They are not competing with each other for resources, as standard evolutionary theory predicted, but rather promiscuously cooperating in the sharing of survival information. "More surprising," one research group commented, "is the apparent movement of genes, such as *tetQ* and *ermB* between members of the normal microflora of humans and animals, populations of bacteria that differ in species composition."[17] Anaerobic and aerobic, Gram-positive and Gram-negative, spirochetes and plasmodial parasites, all are exchanging resistance information—something that, prior to antibiotic usage, was never known to occur (and contributing to a growing recognition that nature may not be red in tooth and claw but much more mutualistic and interdependently connected than formerly supposed). The recognition, long delayed by incorrect assumptions about the nature of the genome, is now widespread—genetic structures in all organisms are not static but fluid, sometimes along a

How Smart Are Bacteria, Anyway?

After placing a single bacterial species in a nutrient solution containing sublethal doses of a newly developed and rare antibiotic, researchers found that within a short period of time the bacteria developed resistance to that antibiotic *and* to 12 other antibiotics that they had never before encountered—some of which were structurally dissimilar to the first. Stuart Levy observes, "It's almost as if bacteria strategically anticipate the confrontation of other drugs when they resist one."[18]

In essence, bacteria are anticipating the creation of antibiotics that people haven't even thought of yet. They are also teaching themselves how to become more virulent, how to make their diseases stronger, by sharing virulence factors among themselves through the same mechanisms they use to share resistance information. In fact, they are acting in concert so well in response to the human "war on disease" that it has led Levy to remark, "One begins to see bacteria, not as individual species, but as a vast array of interacting constituents of an integrated microbial world."[19] Former FDA commissioner Donald Kennedy echoes this, stating, "The evidence indicates that enteric microorganisms in animals and man, their R plasmids, and human pathogens form a linked ecosystem of their own in which action at any one point can affect every other."[20]

And wherever antibacterial use is high, bacterial congregation and rate of learning are also high. Heavy antibiotic usage in fact causes immediate bacterial congregation, rapid learning, and a subsequent cascade of resistance information throughout the microbial membrane, where it can be accessed at any time. Researcher J. Davies notes, "This gene pool [of resistance information] is readily accessible to bacteria when they are exposed to the strong selective pressures of antibiotic usage in hospitals, for veterinary and agricultural purposes, and as growth promotants in animal and poultry husbandry."[21]

Wherever antibiotics and overcrowded or ill animal life meet in large numbers, resistance cascades occur: nursing homes, day care centers, homeless shelters, prisons, inner cities, animal hospitals, and factory farming operations. But they aren't the worst. In spite of the apparent cleanliness of hospitals, the white coats, the quiet voices, the surety of purpose, the truth is that there is no place on Earth that contains more resistant bacteria.

wide range. Barbara McClintock, who early recognized the existence of transposons, noted in her 1983 Nobel lecture that the genome "is a highly sensitive organ of the cell, that in times of stress can initiate its own restructuring and renovation."[22] She noted as well that the instructions for how the genotype reassembled came from not only the organism but the environment itself. The greater the stress, the more fluid and specific the action of the genome in responding to it.

Research, new since the first edition of *Herbal Antibiotics,* has borne out McClintock's observations with a vengeance. The genome of an organism is stored in its DNA. It turns out that antibiotics often damage bacterial DNA through boosting production of free-radical oxygen molecules inside the bacteria. In other words, this highly flexible organ of the cell is partially corrupted by antibiotics. Once that occurs, the organism immediately begins repairing the damage. The bacteria begins to reweave the DNA, including the genomic structure encoded within it. Part of the data that informs those repair processes is the factors that caused the damage. So the bacteria literally restructure the genome in such a way as to counteract the damaging event. And since the damaging event *is* the antibiotic creation of free radicals, the bacteria develop resistance to *all* antibiotics that create free radicals.

The Spread of Resistant Disease

Resistant bacteria tend to specialize in the part of the body they infect. *Enterococcus, Pseudomonas, Staphylococcus,* and *Klebsiella* bacteria take advantage of surgical procedures to infect surgical wounds or patients' blood in hospitals.

It turns out that staph bacteria need the iron that occurs naturally in blood cells, and the organisms prefer one kind of blood—ours. Anyplace where human blood is widely available, staph organisms congregate in large numbers. *Staphylococcus* organisms are "the leading cause of pus-forming skin and soft tissue infections, the leading cause of infectious heart disease, the number one hospital acquired infection, and one of the four leading causes of food-borne illness."[23] And the organisms keep learning.

Effluent streams from cities, filled with excreted antibiotics and resistant staph organisms, flow into the seas surrounding cities. Resistant staph is endemic in all oceans abutting land masses—and the adjoining beaches. It also learned how to transmit itself from person to person during sex. Welcome to the newest STD.

Haemophilus, Pseudomonas, Staphylococcus, Klebsiella, and *Streptococcus* infect lung tissue, many times gaining access by hitching a ride on infected breathing tubes, oh-so-carefully inserted into patients by hospital staff. The bacteria cause pneumonia, often untreatable, in elderly patients in hospitals and nursing homes. Once known as the old person's friend (because it, relatively gently, eased the old into death), pneumonia was significantly reduced through antibiotic use but is now making a comeback as a leading cause of death in the elderly.

Pseudomonas and *Klebsiella,* traveling into urinary passageways on nurse-inserted catheters, initiate serious or intransigent urinary tract infections in many patients. They also gain entry into female nurses' urinary tracts through poor hygiene, where they rapidly mutate under the pressure of the free antibiotics dispensed to such hospital personnel. (Most nurses' and physicians' hands are covered in resistant bacteria whether they wash or not—hand disinfection and hand washing are not the same thing.)

> **Complete and total antibiotic resistance of the [staph] organism is inevitable at this point.**
> —*Eric Skaar*
> *Vanderbilt University*

Haemophilus and *Streptococcus* initiate serious ear infections (sometimes leading to meningitis) in pediatric wards, which multiple rounds of antibiotics often fail to cure. These organisms can also cause debilitating infections of the GI tract accompanied by severe, unremitting diarrhea. And they are not alone in this. One of the newer, more dangerous infectious organisms of the GI tract is *Clostridium difficile*. As the Infectious Diseases Society of America reports, "The rate of infections caused by *Clostridium difficile* in U.S. hospitals doubled between 2000 and 2003. Outbreaks of severe *C. difficile* disease among hospital patients and clusters of unusually severe *C. difficile* disease among previously low-risk patients have been reported from multiple states. Many of the changes in the behavior of this infection appear due to the spread of an epidemic strain of *C. difficile* with increased virulence and increased resistance to commonly used fluoroquinolone antimicrobials."[24]

According to the CDC, there were four times as many deaths from this disease in 2004 as there were in 1999. The organism has become so difficult to treat with antibiotics that Western doctors are turning to a new treatment: fecal transplants. Yes, you heard that right, they put someone else's poop into your bowel in hopes that a healthy bowel population might just reestablish itself. The new poop is fed into the body through a tube in the patient's nose. (This is *modern* medicine.)

The Return of Diseases Once Thought Cured

Tuberculosis (TB) is increasingly resistant and is spreading in inner cities, homeless shelters, and prisons. About two billion people worldwide are thought to have latent TB, about one in three people. Two hundred million of those will become infectious (15 million in the United States) while three million a year will die. About 80 percent of those infected show some signs of antibiotic resistance. Two percent, or 40 million people worldwide, currently have an untreatable, resistant strain. TB is, in fact, becoming so difficult to treat that older approaches, such as surgical removal of the diseased lung, are sometimes being utilized.

Gonorrhea has reemerged with a potent resistance it learned in brothels in Vietnam among prostitutes who were regularly given daily courses of antibiotics. It now causes 700,000 infections in the United States each year. Malaria, spread by mosquitoes and once considered only a disease of the tropics, kills one million people a year worldwide and is resistant to pharmaceuticals more than 85 percent of the time.

Cholera has also learned resistance to a number of antibiotics through improper dosing by physicians. Even more telling, it has learned resistance to the primary drug used to kill it in the wild—chlorine. Chlorine, though naturally present in the ecosystem, rarely exists in pure form. Generally, it is chemically bonded to something else, as in such things as table salt (sodium chloride). Industrial production is around 50 million pounds a year of chemically pure chlorine. It is used in products such as organochlorines (e.g., the PVCs used in medicine) and, commonly, in water supplies as an antimicrobial disinfectant. Both cholera and *E. coli* have developed resistance to chlorine as a result. This is dangerous in and of itself but more so because *E. coli*, exposed to such large numbers of antibiotics in the human GI tract, is one of the principal bacteria that learns resistance and passes it on. This information exchange is especially easy with other types of GI tract bacteria, especially if they are Gram-negative, which cholera is. In 2000, when the first documented outbreak of simultaneous infection by enterotoxigenic *E. coli* and cholera occurred in India, both were resistant organisms.

Cholera lives in water, usually near human settlements, in a quiescent state between epidemics. During these lulls cholera encounters not only chlorine but the scores of other antibiotics that flow in sublethal doses into nearly all water supplies on Earth. Resistance determinants are widely shared between multiple serotypes of cholera. Like all pathogenic bacteria, the resistance curve of cholera organisms is exponential. In 1992, only 35 percent of cholera O1 serotypes were resistant to ampicillin. By 1997, 100 percent were.

Cholera epidemics tend to emerge in human populations when the fecal content of waste streams from population centers is high. The organisms follow the effluent upstream, seeking its source. They usually find it.

Antimicrobial pressure has caused *E. coli*, not normally pathogenic, to also develop unexpected virulence capacities in such forms as the potentially deadly *E. coli* O157:H7. Epidemiologists now know, through genetic markers, that it was taught its virulence by *Shigella* bacteria. Researcher and physician Marguerite Neill, a specialist in infectious medicine, observes that judicious reflection on the meaning of this finding suggests a larger significance—that *E. coli* O157:H7 is a messenger, bringing an unwelcome message that "in mankind's battle to conquer infectious diseases, the opposing army is being replenished with fresh replacements."[25]

How Hospitals Create the Problem

Hospitals, where large numbers of pathogenic bacteria and antibiotics come into frequent contact, give bacteria the most opportunity to develop resistance *and* virulence. Researchers examining the effluent streams from hospitals have found them to contain exceptionally large numbers of resistant bacteria as well as large amounts of excreted antibiotics. These antibiotics and resistant bacteria flow into the environment and spread everywhere. As Julie Gerberding of the Centers for Disease Control comments, "Once restricted to hospitals, where seriously ill patients are exposed to constant infusions of drugs, these [resistant bacteria] are now being found in the community."[26]

The prodigious production of antibacterial soaps that end up going into the water are stimulating resistance among many classes of bacteria as well. Even though resistance dynamics were well understood long before antibacterial soaps were allowed on the market,

> The lesson from both our agricultural and medical experience is remarkable for its consistency: Ignoring the evolutionary attributes of biological systems can only be done at the peril of ecological catastrophe.
>
> —Marc Lappé, *When Antibiotics Fail*

under pressure from corporations they were still allowed in the United States. And like all other antibacterial substances, they have begun to confer unique forms of resistance on the planet's bacteria. The fear of microbes, so thoroughly leveraged by television advertising, has only hastened the resistance problem. The Centers for Disease Control and Prevention found that the average amount of the antibacterial component of such soaps, triclosan, increased in Americans' urine by 42 percent between 2003 and 2006. Studies have shown that the chemical encourages bacterial resistance and that it disrupts hormone levels in regular users. Triclosan is common in many toothpastes, in nearly all antibacterial soaps, and even on knives and cutting boards.

These circumstances have increased the rate of resistance in bacteria exponentially. In 1999, 95 percent of *E. coli* was susceptible to ciprofloxacin, but that had dropped to 60 percent by 2006; *Acinetobacter* susceptibility decreased by 70 percent in just 4 years; 36 percent of *Staphylococcus* organisms were resistant in 1992, but by 2003 64 percent were—the usual exponential learning curves. But these are only part of the story.

Factory Farms: The Story Gets Worse

The use of antibiotics by factory farms and wide antibiotic use by veterinarians for our pets has created a similar bacterial evolution in fast-forward. At least half, if not more, of all antibiotics used in the United States goes to huge factory farm operations. This has generated tremendously potent and quick resistance in a large range of bacteria. As reporter Brandon Keim comments, "Much of it is used to treat diseases spread by industrial husbandry practices, or simply to accelerate growth. As a result, farms have become giant petri dishes for superbugs, especially multidrug-resistant *Staphylococcus aureus* or MRSA, which kills 20,000 Americans every year—more than AIDS."[27]

Nicols Fox comments in her exposé of the problem in her book *Spoiled: The Dangerous Truth about a Food Chain Gone Haywire*:

> The conditions under which [farm animals were] raised presented all the conditions for infection and disease: the animals were closely confined; subjected to stress; often fed contaminated food and water; exposed to vectors (flies, mice, rats) that could carry contaminants from one flock to another; bedded on filth-collecting litter; and given antibiotics (which, ironically, made them more vulnerable to disease) to encourage growth as well as ward off other infections.... Every condition that predisposed the spread of disease from animal to human actually worsened. Farming became more intensive, slaughtering became more mechanical and faster, products were processed in even more massive lots, and distribution became wider.[28]

As with human diseases, pathogenic animal bacteria have specialized: *E. coli* O157:H7 in beef, *Salmonella* in chicken eggs, *Campylobacter* in chickens, *Listeria* in deli meat. (And there are others such as *Cyclospora, Cryptosporidium,* and *Yersinia.*) Like the resistant bacteria emerging from our hospitals, bacteria from factory farms spread quickly into the wider world. And while factory farm owners deny their practices have *anything* to do with the problem, the only place where antibiotic-resistant organisms genetically identical to those from factory farming operations don't yet seem to exist is in indigenous animals in the northern arctic regions.

One of the early pioneers in antibiotic resistance is Stuart Levy, a professor who runs the Levy Lab at the Center for Adaptation Genetics and Drug Resistance at Tufts University School of Medicine. To trace the flow into the environment of resistant bacteria from farming operations, he took six groups of chickens and placed them 50 to a cage. Four cages were in a barn, two just outside. Half the chickens received food containing subtherapeutic doses of oxytetracycline. The feces of all the chickens as well as the farm family living nearby and farm families in the neighborhood were examined weekly. Within 24 to 36 hours of eating the first batch of antibiotic-containing food, the feces of the dosed chickens showed *E. coli*–resistant bacteria. Soon the undosed chickens also showed *E. coli* that were resistant to tetracycline. But even more remarkable, by the end of 3 months, the *E. coli* of *all* chickens were also resistant to ampicillin, streptomycin, and sulfonamides *even though they had never been fed these drugs.* Still more startling: At the end of 5 months, the feces of the nearby farm family (who had had no contact with the chickens) contained *E. coli* resistant to tetracycline. By the sixth month their *E. coli* were also resistant to five other antibiotics. A similar but longer study in Germany found that this resistance eventually moved into the surrounding community—taking a little more than 2 years.

At least half, if not more, of all antibiotics used in the United States goes to huge factory farms.

Salmonella, which is now genetically lodged *in the ovaries* (and hence the eggs that come from them) of many agribusiness chickens, can survive refrigeration, boiling, basting, and frying. To kill salmonella bacteria, the egg must be fried hard or boiled for 9 minutes or longer. *Listeria* in deli meat can survive refrigeration. *E. coli* can now live in both orange juice and apple juice—two acidic mediums that previously killed it. And a recent study (2011) found that nearly 50 percent of all store-bought meat and poultry tested were contaminated with staph, and more than half the bacteria tested were resistant strains. Lance Price, the lead author of the study, remarked, "The fact that drug-resistant *S. aureus* was so prevalent, and likely came from the food animals themselves, is troubling."[29]

These food-borne bacteria are moving with greater frequency into the human food chain and human populations. There were more than 230 recalls by the U.S. FDA in 2012 for contamination from *Salmonella, Listeria, Clostridium, E. coli, Staphylococcus areus, Burkholdia cepacia,* and *Bacillus* organisms.

Recent research has found that one of the main vectors for the spread of resistant organisms into the general community is flies. At minimum, more than 30,000 flies will visit a poultry farming operation within any 6-week period. Researchers who studied groups of flies from such operations found them to be infected with exactly the same genetic variants of resistant bacteria as those found in the poultry wastes the flies were feeding on. This same phenomenon occurs at all large-animal factory farms, with both cattle and pigs.

The growth rate of resistance and virulence is so fast that 15 years ago Stuart Levy observed, "Some analysts warn of present-day scenarios in which infectious antibiotic-resistant bacteria devastate whole human populations.... This situation raises the staggering possibility that a time will come when antibiotics as a mode of therapy will only be a fact of historic interest."[30] To people such as David Livermore, MD, at the Antibiotic Resistance Monitoring and Reference Laboratory in London, it has now gone much further. "It is," he says, "naive to think we can win."[31]

In the first edition of *Herbal Antibiotics* I noted that bacteria are, in fact, learning resistance to new antibiotics in only a few years instead of the decades that it took previously. At the time of this writing, that span has lessened to 6 months to a year. As infectious disease specialist Brad Spellberg has commented, "Resistance is inevitable."

Resistance in the Ecosystem

Though resistance in the bacteria affecting people and farm animals has been the most publicized and studied, these bacteria are not confined to people or their food animals. They move freely in the ecosystem and among species. Newer research has found that seagulls, and other birds, not only humans, are spreading resistant bacteria throughout the world. As Dr. Jeffrey Fisher, in his book *The Plague Makers*, notes:

> The resistant bacteria that result from this reckless practice do not stay confined to the animals from which they develop. There are no "cow bacteria" or "pig bacteria" or "chicken bacteria." In terms of the microbial world, we humans along with the rest of the animal kingdom are part of one giant ecosystem. The same resistant bacteria that grow in the intestinal tract of a cow or pig can, and do, eventually end up in our bodies.[32]

This is especially true if antibiotics flow into water. This promotes the transmission of resistant traits throughout the environment because bacterial growth is high wherever water-related biofilms occur: on the surface of water, on stones in water, and in the sediment of ponds, rivers, and oceans. Antibiotics given to fish contact all these regions, as does the antibiotic-rich effluent from factory farms and human waste treatment facilities. Resistance transfers in these biofilm regions from domestic to wild bacteria, and it tends to persist in these natural ecosystems.

Researchers Christian Daughton and Thomas Ternes report that "a number of stream surveys documented the significant prevalence of native bacteria that display resistance to a wide array of antibiotics including vancomycin. Isolates from wild geese near Chicago, Illinois, are reported to be resistant to ampicillin, tetracycline, penicillin, and erythromycin."[33] Researchers have found 16 antibiotics commonly present in groundwater/surface waters that are detectable in the microgram-per-liter range. Some researchers report that these antibiotic compounds are showing genotoxicity; that is, they are affecting the integrity of genetic structures in other life-forms. Daughton and Ternes comment that this is indeed cause for concern, as the bacteria never seem to forget what has been done to them:

> Indeed, the rampant, widespread (and sometimes indiscriminate) use of antibiotics, coupled with their subsequent release into the environment, is the leading proposed cause of accelerated spreading resistance among bacterial pathogens, which is exacerbated by the fact that resistance is maintained even in the absence of continued selective pressure (an irreversible occurrence). Sufficiently high concentrations could also have acute effects on bacteria. Such exposures could easily lead to altered microbial community structures in nature and thereby affect the higher food chain.[34]

Salmon, catfish, and trout—all raised commercially—are heavily dosed with antibiotics and other drugs, which are often blended into their food. As the food gets wet, the antibiotics begin to leach into the water. Commercial salmon, unlike catfish and trout, are raised in the open sea in pens, speeding the flow of antibacterials throughout the oceans. Because of crowded conditions, the 55 million pounds of commercial U.S. salmon are frequently dosed with antibiotics for long periods of time—about 150 pounds of antibiotic per acre of salmon. Stuart Levy comments:

> Since they are deposited in the water, [antibiotics] can be picked up easily by other marine animals. Tetracycline is not rapidly degraded in fish. Thus, it is excreted in its active state in feces and deposited on the sea floor. Here, too, it remains relatively stable, out of direct sunlight, which can degrade it. Consequently, the ecological effect of this antibacterial agent in the sea is the same as it is in land animals: the long-term selection of resistant and multi-resistant bacteria in salmon and other marine life.[35]

Plant communities and soil are also exposed to direct antibiotic use, not just through effluent flows. To treat infections in mono-cropped fields, especially while attacking fire blight in apple and pear orchards, antibiotics such as streptomycin are sometimes sprayed in heavy doses directly on crops. In the United States, between 40,000 and 50,000 pounds of tetracycline and streptomycin are sprayed on fruit trees every year (1 pound of tetracycline will treat 450 people). This kills not only bacteria on the plants but all susceptible bacteria in the soil itself with cascading effects on soil integrity and health. While spraying allows potent doses of streptomycin to directly enter the ecosystem, other antibiotics, like oxytetracycline, are sometimes injected, much as they are with people, directly into larger plants' trunks and roots. Not surprisingly, resistant pathogenic plant bacteria have been found in soil and plant communities wherever such practices occur. The bacterial transposon developed by leaf blight during resistance acquisition has been found in seven wild bacterial species in the soil. All these bacteria now have resistance to the streptomycin normally produced by the soil fungi in the region. This same dynamic has also been found occurring in the soil under wheat plants. The application or spread of antibiotic effluents in the environment is promoting resistance impacts in natural soil communities among wild bacteria, thus interfering with the normal balance of the soil biota. Agricultural practices such as liming fields and industrial heavy-metal pollution have been found, as well, to increase the density of resistant pathogens in the soil. Researchers have also started to insert bacterial resistance factors directly into the genetic structure of some plants (e.g., sugar beets), and these resistance factors have also been found to move into ecosystem bacteria.

The immense production of antibacterial substances once found only in minute quantities in the environment—substances produced by soil fungi, bacteria, or plants to protect their territorial integrity—has begun to affect the life cycle of bacteria and thousands of other organisms in the ecosystem and subsequently is affecting the health of the soil and the planet itself.

We have, as Mark Lappé remarked in *The End of Antibiotics*, "let our profligate use of antibiotics reshape the evolution of the microbial world and wrest any hope of safe management from us."

Bacterial Partners

Bacteria are not our enemies, as some scientists have postulated, nor a dangerous life-form bent on sickening mankind, as so many television commercials would have us believe. They are our ancestors and we are very much alike; we both metabolize fats, vitamins, sugars, and proteins. Lynn Margulis comments succinctly, "The more balanced view of microbe as colleague and ancestor remains almost unexpressed. Our culture ignores the hard-won fact that these disease 'agents,' these 'germs,' also germinated all life. Our ancestors, the germs, were bacteria."[36] Bacteria are not germs but the germinators—and fabric—of all life on Earth. In declaring war on them, we declared war on the underlying living structure of the planet, on all life-forms we can see, on ourselves.

One of the few naturally sterile places on Earth is a woman's womb, and the gestation period prior to birth is the only time any human body is bacteria free. At birth, assuming it is a healthy one, the baby is immediately placed on the mother's chest near the nipple. As the first movements toward bonding are taking place, the bacteria that live on the mother's skin begin to colonize her baby's body. When the infant begins to nurse, the interior of the baby's intestinal tract is colonized—from the skin around the nipple and the milk itself—and these bacteria are crucially important. Nursing introduces lactobacilli and other bacteria such as *Bifidobacterium bifidus* into the intestinal tract of newborns. This has significant effects on their health. *Lactobacillus acidophilus* bacteria create important vitamins and nutrients such as B_1, B_2, B_3, B_{12}, and folate (B_9) in the intestinal tract. They help digest food, and they also secrete natural antibiotic substances such as acidophilin, various organic acids, and peroxides that help prevent bacterial infections.

One to two pounds of our adult body weight comes from our coevolutionary bacteria. The bacteria that colonize us as infants have an ancient, coevolutionary relationship with human beings; they are an integral part of our species' development and our body ecology. They are in fact our first line of defense against disease.

> In declaring war on bacteria, we declared war on the underlying living structure of the planet, on all life-forms we can see, on ourselves.

The skin of our bodies and the mucosal systems of our sinus passages and intestinal tracts are to bacteria much like fresh fertile black soil is to plants. Plow up the soil, disturbing the plants that grow there, and even if you don't plant anything, the soil will soon be covered with a profusion of new plant growth. The same thing occurs in our bodies if our bacterial ecology is disturbed, as it often is, by antibiotics.

Why We Need Bacteria

The bacteria that colonize our bodies are friendly, mutualistic bacteria. They take up all the space on and in our bodies on which bacteria can grow. By so doing, they leave no room for other, less benign bacteria to live. But the relationship goes beyond this. *All* of our coevolutionary bacteria generate antibiotic substances that kill off other, less friendly bacteria. The *Streptococcus* bacteria that normally live in our throats produce large quantities of antibacterial substances that are specifically active against the *Streptococcus pyogenes* bacteria that cause strep throat.

Regular exposure to pathogenic bacteria as we are growing teaches our bodies and our symbiotic bacteria how to respond most effectively to disease organisms. This produces much higher levels of health in later life. Research continually finds that children who are "protected" from bacteria by keeping them in exceptionally clean environments where they are constantly exposed to antibacterial soaps and wipes are not in fact healthier but much sicker overall than children not so protected. The constant exposure to a world filled with bacteria, the world out of which we emerged as a species, in fact stimulates the immune health of all of us as we grow. We actually *need* to come into contact with the microorganisms of the world to be healthy.

The truth is, we live in an ancient, healthy symbiosis with bacterial, viral, and microfaunal colonizers. Our bodies are much like the soil of the earth, covered inside and out with a broad diversity of microfauna providing an interdependent complex of support services. When we become ill, our symbiotic relationship with the healthy bacteria and other microfauna—our body ecology—is disturbed. The underlying factor that disrupts the body ecology is the illness, not the pathogenic bacteria that take advantage of it to occupy body sites. Antibiotics do not cure disease, they simply kill off opportunistic bacteria. Without the body's ability to restore a healthy ecology, people die anyway. More than any other disease, AIDS has taught us the limitations of antibiotics and the bacterial model of disease. Irrespective of the quantities of antibiotics used, when AIDS patients' bodies can no longer reestablish their internal ecology, they die. As Marc Lappé says, "It is the *body* which ultimately controls infections, not chemicals. Without underlying immunity, drugs are meaningless."[37] Ironically, as many public health historians now know, the major decreases in human mortality and disease proclaimed to be brought about by antibiotics were due more, in fact, to better public hygiene.

Because they kill off so much of the internal symbiotic microfauna along with pathogenic bacteria, antibiotics create significant changes in human microfaunal ecology and makeup. The appearance of many diseases new to humankind such as certain nutrient deficiencies, candida overgrowth, certain chronic infections, allergies, and chronic immune suppression are now being directly linked to the distorted internal landscape antibiotics cause. Marc Lappé comments:

> Lincomycin eliminates virtually all of the bacteria that require oxygen, while neomycin and kanamycin decrease the number of oxygen-requiring germs and gram-positive anaerobic ones, leading to overgrowth of *Candida albicans* and *Staphylococcus aureus*. Polymyxin can reduce native *E. coli* to the point of extinction, leaving the terrain open for staph and strep organisms. Erythromycin has a similar favorable effect on streptococci, while bacitracin and damycin, by contrast, appear to favor the growth of *Clostridium difficile*.[38]

And it is not just humans that have coevolutionary bacterial partners but all plant, insect, and animal life. When these other life-forms encounter antibiotics, their interior and exterior ecologies are disturbed as well.

If bacteria had not learned how to develop resistance, all life on Earth, including humans, would already have died. When we try to kill all disease organisms on this planet, ultimately, we are acting to kill ourselves.

The situation is dire and there are solutions, but they are not easy ones. As David Livermore has said, "A lot of modern medicine would become impossible if we lost our ability to treat infections."[39] Routine surgeries would no longer be routine but nearly impossible to perform safely. Infectious diseases would regularly become epidemic, sweeping through whole communities. The use of quarantine, rare now, would become common. Mortality among the old and the very young would rise tremendously. An entire world view, commonly accepted by most people in Western countries, would begin to crumble. It would be (medically speaking), for all practical purposes, 1928 again.

In the first edition of *Herbal Antibiotics*, I, as many others have done, urged people to give up using antibiotics unless there were a serious threat of death or disability if they did not. (I also thought real estate in Nevada might be a good investment.) More than a decade later, it is clear that antibiotics are not going to be used any less and in fact are being used at far greater rates than they were 15 years ago. The human species, as a group, has never really been known for doing the sensible thing before it is too late. We will stop using antibiotics only when they truly fail to work. And even then most of the people in the Western world will still try to hold on to them and our fatally flawed approach to bacterial disease.

But for those who clearly understand what the word "exponential" means, who want to truly empower themselves and their families and prepare for the time that is so quickly approaching us, there are options.

You can take control over your own health and health care. You can prepare. You can learn to use herbal medicines to heal yourself from disease. And you can learn what to do if you find that one day you need to know how to treat a resistant infection.

The rest of this book is designed to help you do just that.

2

THE RESISTANT ORGANISMS, THE DISEASES THEY CAUSE, AND HOW TO TREAT THEM

The significant problems we face cannot be solved at the same level of thinking we were at when we created them.

—**Albert Einstein**

Included among the Gram-positive pathogens are methicillin-resistant Staphylococcus aureus *and* S. epidermidis, *vancomycin-resistant* Enterococcus faecium *and* E. faecialis, *and the rapidly growing mycobacteria. In the past five years, however, no fewer than four novel agents have been approved that have clinical activity versus these bacteria. It is really among the multidrug-resistant Gram-negative bacteria that we find growing unmet medical need, and only a single new agent has been approved in well over a decade.*

—**Steven Projan, *Bacterial Resistance to Antimicrobials***

Many people believe that there will always be antibiotics and that if the ones we have now aren't working, others will be discovered that will work just as well, so no need to worry. The truth, unfortunately, is very different. There are virtually no new antibiotics in development, and there are unlikely to be. Pharmaceutical companies have almost completely given up the search for them. There are a number of reasons for this, the main one being, of course, financial.

In spite of cultural beliefs to the contrary, physicians can cure relatively few of the conditions that plague us. For high cholesterol they prescribe anticholesterol drugs, for arthritis anti-inflammatories, and so on. These drugs artificially alter the condition of the body, but they do not cure the underlying condition. In consequence, the drugs are often taken for decades; they are a never-ending source of money for the companies that make them. (And the profit of the top 12 pharmaceutical companies in the world in 2009? 100 *billion* dollars.)

Antibiotics, on the other hand, are too successful. They are used for a short period of time, the disease is eradicated, the patient cured. They are a victim of their own success. Brad Spellberg, author of *Rising Plague*, notes: "For many years now, leading members of the Infectious Diseases Society of America (IDSA) have been aware that antibiotics were no longer being developed by many pharmaceutical companies. Indeed, many pharmaceutical companies have actually completely eliminated their research and development programs for antibiotic drug discovery."[1] Stuart Levy, perhaps the foremost researcher on resistant organisms in the United States, comments that "the problem is the pharmaceutical industry has left the discovery field and so new antibiotics are not coming along."[2] He says, rather matter-of-factly, that it is just more profitable for the drug companies to develop medications for long-term conditions such as heart disease and arthritis than it is to find new antibiotics.

The money's not in the cure. The money's in the medicine.
—Comedian Chris Rock

Research by Spellberg's group found that between 1983 and 2008, investment in antibiotic research and development in the United States fell by 75 percent. His team found only five to seven new antibiotics in the pipeline, most expected to reach the market by 2012, and all of them just slightly altered versions of existing antibiotics.

And no, biotechnology companies are not doing any better. In 2004 all biotech companies combined had only one antibiotic in any kind of development stage. Worse, *every* one of the antibiotics expected to reach market by 2012 are for Gram-positive bacteria. There are *none* in any stage of development that can treat Gram-negative organisms, the fastest growing category of resistant pathogens. After 2012? That's it. There are none in any stage of development and no plans for any, a fact that shocks most people. They just don't believe that the drug companies would be so complacent—or that they would care so little. I mean, they are in the business of helping people . . . aren't they?

Resistance: An Exponential Growth Curve

There is a very old story—it's about greed actually, and just a little bit about mathematics—of a king and the man who saved his life. The king was very grateful and told the man he would reward him with anything he wished. The man told the king that the only thing he wanted was some rice. He then asked the king if he played chess. The king replied that yes, he did. So the man said he would like to use the chess board to determine the amount of rice with which he would be rewarded. He wanted the king to put one grain of rice on the first square, then two on the second, four on the next, and so on. The king said sure, that sounds like a good idea, and he told his councilors to arrange it. They came back a bit later and very hesitantly told the king that they couldn't do it. The king was pretty upset and asked why and was told that by the last square the man would receive more rice than existed in the entire kingdom. (I'm not sure, but I think the king beheaded the man who made the request—nobody likes a smart-ass.)

Bacterial resistance grows exponentially, just like those grains of rice. In practical terms that means we will be fine for a while (say from 1945 to 2014) because, as you can see, it takes a while to get into the big numbers. Welcome to big-number territory.

MRSA, once limited to the very young, the old, and the immuno-compromised, has not only emerged in the general community; it is now exceptionally virulent and infecting the healthiest population of all—young adults. As Spellberg comments, "The highly publicized outbreaks of MRSA infections are dwarfed by the enormous number of cases that occur every day across the United States and throughout the world. Overall, healthy children, adolescents, and teenagers have been particularly heavily hit by MRSA infections, and these cases had gone unheralded until very recently."[3]

Young people, completely healthy, begin to fall ill, enter emergency rooms, and are found to have out-of-control MRSA infections. After just a simple skin break, their arms swell with cellulitis, or the infection becomes systemic and infects the blood (bacteremia), the heart (endocarditis), spinal cord (myelitis), or bones (osteomyelitis). In 2007 the state of Virginia closed 21 high schools to try to stop an MRSA infection that had killed one student and sickened others.

The situation will only get worse. We are within 5 years of MRSA being completely untreatable by any antibiotics at all.

Thirty percent of all *E. coli* urinary tract infections are resistant to treatment, up from 5 percent 10 years ago. The resistance rate has increased fifty fold in the last decade. One of the more troubling resistance mechanisms in *E. coli* is what is called extended-spectrum beta-lactamase resistance, or ESBL. ESBL bacteria are highly virulent and strongly resistant to a class of antibiotics called beta-lactams, some of the most potent antibiotics still useful for Gram-negative bacteria. Beta-lactamase is an enzyme that the bacteria create and use to deactivate the antibiotics. *All* the bacteria in the Gram-negative family have begun acquiring that genetic resistance information. *E. coli* and *Klebsiella* are two of the forerunners.

ESBL resistance in *E. coli* in 1990 was only 3.6 percent; by 1993 it was 14.4 percent; by 1995 it was 25 percent in Europe and as high as 40 percent in France. The only antibiotic that until recently could still treat the ESBL-resistant strains of *Klebsiella* was carbapenem and a much older antibiotic, polymyxin, that is only partially effective and often causes severe kidney damage.

Fully resistant strains of *Klebsiella* have now become common and are often, like MRSA, referred to by an acronym, CRKP. It stands for carbapenem-resistant *Klebsiella pneumoniae*. It is virtually untreatable; 40 percent of those infected with it die. "These are very serious infections, hugely complicated by the fact that the treatment options are severely limited," is how Dr. Ajun Srinivasan of the Centers for Disease Control and Prevention puts it. The first isolated reports of CRKP occurred in 1999 in New Jersey. As of 2010, Srinivasan says, "we are seeing reports of this organism from all over the country."[4]

In March of 2010 a severe outbreak of CRKP occurred in Southern California followed by another in March of 2011 in Los Angeles. Another plagued a Denver hospital for 10 months in 2012. And another infected scores of patients in a hospital in Chicago, Illinois, in early 2014. Brad Spellberg, speaking from the Los Angeles Biomedical Research Institute near Torrance, California, commented, "In the next decade there isn't going to be anything that becomes available that's going to be able to treat these bacteria. . . . [There] is no current treatment for CRKP bacteria, and there might not be any in the future either."[5]

Neil Fishman, president of the Society for Healthcare Epidemiology of America, is more blunt: "We have lost our drug of last resort."[6]

Pan-resistant *Pseudomonas* and *Acinetobacter* are similarly dangerous. *Pseudomonas* has also begun to develop resistance to carbapenem antibiotics; the bacteria are now reliably treatable only by polymyxin. *Acinetobacter*, *E. coli*, and *Klebsiella* have also been promiscuously sharing a new plasmid, NDM-1, that confers resistance along a wide range of antibiotics, including carbapenem. "In many ways, this is it," says Timothy Walsh, a microbiologist and resistant bacteria specialist at Cardiff University in the UK. "There are no antibiotics in the pipeline that have activity against NDM-1-producing Enterobacteriaceae. We have a bleak window of maybe 10 years."[7]

Enterococcal organisms, once readily treatable, are so no longer. George Eliopoulos in the Division of Infectious Diseases at Beth Israel Deaconess Medical Center in Boston, Massachusetts, observes:

> Ominously, in recent years, enterococci resistant to multiple antimicrobial agents have become increasingly prevalent in the hospital environment. . . . More than half of these enterococcal isolates were resistant to tetracycline, levofloxacin, and quinupristin-dalfopristin; 28 percent were resistant to ampicillin; and approximately 20 percent were nonsusceptible to vancomycin. From ICUs in the United States, even higher rates of vancomycin resistance have been reported. . . . Vancomycin resistance genes originating in enterococci have now been found in several clinical isolates of *S. aureus*. This validates concerns expressed more than a decade ago that VRE may serve as a reservoir of genes that could confer upon staphylococci resistance to glycopeptides, the principal antibiotics [remaining] for treatment of infections caused by methicillin-resistant strains [MRSA].[8]

There are *no* new antibiotics being developed to treat these resistant strains. The most recent, tigecycline, entered the market in 2005. It is active against resistant forms of *Acinetobacter* but not resistant *Pseudomonas*. Only tigecycline and that rather dangerous older antibiotic, polymyxin, can now treat *Acinetobacter*, and polymyxin itself has begun to encounter resistant forms of the bacteria. But then, so has tigecycline.

As Spellberg comments, “If we did not have tigecycline, these infections would be essentially untreatable.” But as he continues, “tigecycline resistance spread within 2 years of the drug’s availability. Indeed, on a recent trip to visit a hospital on the East Coast, I was told that nearly all the hospital’s *Acinetobacter* is already fully resistant to tigecycline.”[9]

People who now enter hospitals, even for very minor treatments, are at serious risk of contracting untreatable infections. More than 70 percent of all pathogenic bacteria in hospitals are at least minimally resistant; the ones discussed herein are considerably more so, being resistant to most major groups of antimicrobials. As oncology nurse Sue Fischer says, “These kids come in for a short treatment and the next day they complain about a pain in their side and the next day they’re gone. We open them up and find their whole body shot through with resistant bacteria that have attacked nearly every organ. Nothing works to stop it and it happens as quick as that.”[10]

Resistant Microorganisms: The Specifics

There are 21 resistant pathogens on this list, and that doesn't count the various subspecies in each genus that are now resistant (at least 40, not including variants) or several others that are lurking out there on the horizon. The problem, as many epidemiologists have warned, is increasing exponentially and there is no end in sight.

Some of these organisms, such as methicillin-resistant *Staphylococcus aureus* (MRSA), are already causing significant problems in hospitals and communities throughout the world. Others, such as *Clostridium difficile*, are becoming increasingly widespread and dangerous. And still others, such as *Stenotrophomonas maltophilia*, are just beginning their run as resistant organisms.

Most of the resistant pathogens are either Gram-positive or Gram-negative bacteria—a list is included under the respective headings that follow; there are, in addition, one parasitic protist (the malarial parasite), one mold (aspergillus), and one yeast (candida) that have now become dangerously resistant. The parasitic protist is *Plasmodium falciparum*, which causes malaria; the mold is *Aspergillus* spp. (*A. fumigatus, A. flavus, A. terres*); the yeast is *Candida* spp. (*Candida albicans* is dominant, but most species are now resistant).

Gram-positive and Gram-negative organisms are denoted as such because of their ability to take a Gram stain, one way of identifying them. Of much more importance are the differences in their cellular structure.

What's a Gram Stain?

Hans Gram (1853–1938) found he could see bacteria more clearly under a microscope if he applied a stain made from crystal violet to them. Different types of bacteria absorb the stain differently, enabling researchers to more easily identify them.

Just as we have skin, bacteria have an external membrane surrounding their bodies, a.k.a. the cell wall. Their interior is called the *cytoplasm*; then there is the *cytoplasmic membrane*, which covers the cytoplasm, then the *cell wall*. The cell wall consists primarily of a polymer called peptidoglycan. If the bacteria happen to be Gram-negative, they will have a second wall called the *outer membrane*. Between the two membranes in Gram-negative bacteria is a compartment, the *periplasmic space*. Gram-positive bacteria, because they lack that other membrane, have much thicker cell walls to protect them from outside events.

Because Gram-positive bacteria have only a single cell wall, even though it's thicker, they are, in general, much easier to treat. With Gram-negative bacteria, two cell walls have to be penetrated, not just one. In essence, the bacteria have two chances to identify and deactivate an antibacterial that is hostile to them. Even if an antibiotic gets into the periplasmic space, it usually will not kill the bacteria. It still has to penetrate the second wall.

More than 70 percent of all pathogenic bacteria in hospitals are at least minimally resistant.

Gram-negative bacteria have a series of highly synergistic reactions to antibiotics, in essence using three primary mechanisms, all highly coordinated, to resist antibiotics. The first is the double cell wall. The second is a special group of enzymes, beta-lactamases, that are especially effective in deactivating beta-lactam antibiotics (the antibiotics most often used against them). The third is a variety of multidrug efflux pumps. These efflux pumps essentially act like sump pumps; they pump out the antibiotic substances just as fast as they come in so that the bacteria are unaffected by them.

Gram-positive bacteria rely on their thicker cell wall and very, very fast efflux pumps since they don't have a periplasmic space in which to hold the antibiotics while they deal with them. Some Gram-positive bacteria, such as the staphylococci, have incorporated the use of beta-lactamases, which they learned about from Gram-negative organisms.

Resistant Diseases and How to Treat Them

Here are some general thoughts to keep in mind when you are approaching treatment of a resistant pathogen. Always remember that you are dealing with virulent, highly pathogenic microbial infections—your treatment must be focused and continual and unremitting until the outcome is decided, one way or the other.

As a general rule of thumb, follow these recommendations when dealing with a resistant infection.

Disease	Herbal Remedy
Systemic infection	Cryptolepis, alchornea, or sida will *almost* always work. (Bidens is very good, but you will need higher doses.)
Severe diarrhea, dysentery	A berberine plant will *almost* always work.
Urinary tract infection	Juniper berry combined with bidens will *almost* always work.
Infected surface or surgical wound	Honey has *always* worked.
Meningitis	Add piperine, isatis, and either Japanese knotweed or stephania to the herbal mix—they are exceptionally good for this.
Bacteremia	Use *Echinacea angustifolia* in large doses.
Sepsis	Use Salvia miltiorrhiza/Angelica sinensis tincture in large, frequent doses.

Note: Gram-positive bacteria are often highly susceptible to hyaluronidase inhibitors. Echinacea is a potent one—if your treatment is going poorly, consider adding it.

RECOGNIZING ENDOTOXINS

Endotoxins generally come from the outer wall of Gram-negative bacteria and are released into the body when the bacteria die. In a number of diseases, bubonic plague for example, it is not the bacteria that kill you but the endotoxins. If you are treating a systemic infection by a Gram-negative bacteria, the use of an endotoxin scavenger and protectant is often important. Isatis is perhaps the best herb for this (ginger is also good).

USING SYNERGISTS

If you are treating a difficult infection, especially if it is Gram-negative, use a synergist to enhance the treatment. There are two forms of synergists: the first is active against the efflux pumps in the bacteria, the second helps move the herbs across the intestinal membrane and strongly into the blood. Licorice is the best synergist for Gram-negative bacteria. Piperine will potently move herbal compounds across the intestinal membrane, significantly increasing their presence in the blood. See chapter 6 for more specifics.

INCREASING NATURAL IMMUNITY

Always work to increase the body's natural immune function through the use of immune herbs or an immune formulation. These should be taken daily. The formulations suggested in this section were generated by looking at immune herbs that were also active against the specific organisms—kind of a two-for-one thing. Nevertheless, don't get obsessed by these, as other immune herbs that don't have any specific antibacterial activity will work, often better than these, in increasing immune function. These are only guidelines.

A note about the suggested formulations: The formulations that I have included to treat the various bacteria and the types of infections they cause *are only suggestions*. They can be varied considerably. Don't get stuck in thinking that any of these formulations are the only way to go. *Read the book* and the monographs on the herbs themselves. Tremendous sophistication is possible. These are just guidelines.

Finally, don't forget that human love and caring are an essential part of the healing process—they are medicines that you must also dispense to those you are working to heal. There is perhaps nothing

Piperine Warning

Under no circumstances should you use piperine for severe intestinal infections such as *E. coli* O157:H7 or cholera. Piperine increases intestinal permeability, which can allow the resistant organisms access to the interior of your body in significantly greater numbers. It can make you much sicker.

that the ill need more than to know that they are supported in their suffering. It is very difficult to live without love, and nearly impossible to truly heal without it.

Using This Book

The rest of this chapter is concerned with the individual resistant bacteria, what herbs are effective in treating them, and then some actual specific suggestions for treatment. These are the main ones you need to know about to be able to take care of yourself and your family.

Subsequent chapters explore viral strains and how they infect the body, as well as the properties of individual herbs; what other organisms they are active against; what else they can do medicinally; and then show how to grow, harvest, and prepare them as medicines so that you can take complete charge of your own health care if you wish to do so.

Chapter 7 contains in-depth explorations on the immune-enhancing herbs that you can use to keep your immune system strong—a number of which are also potently effective against resistant pathogens. And chapters 8 and 9 will tell you more than you ever wanted to know about making just about any kind of herbal medicine you might ever need.

Dealing with Gram-Positive Bacteria

The major resistant Gram-positive organisms are:

- *Clostridium difficile*
- *Enterococcus* spp. (*E. faecalis*, *E. faecium*)
- *Mycobacterium tuberculosis*
- *Staphylococcus aureus*
- *Streptococcus* spp. (*S. pyogenes*, *S. pneumoniae*)

Note: *All* the formulations given for treating each type of bacteria are meant to be taken simultaneously. Some offer immune support, some are directly antibacterial, and some are for a specific symptom picture.

Clostridium difficile

The *Clostridium* genus comprises about 100 different species of bacteria; four of them are human pathogens. They often form spores that, once they enter a cut or the GI tract, lead to a number of potentially dangerous diseases.

C. botulinum is the source of botulism poisoning in food (and of the drug Botox) and sometimes also causes infections in wounds; *C. perfringens* can cause anything from food poisoning to gas gangrene; and *C. tetani* is the cause of tetanus. *C. difficile* is the main resistant pathogen. The organism flourishes in people who have been on long antibiotic therapies, especially in hospitals, and because it is exposed to so many antibiotics, it is highly resistant to treatment. At the present most *C. difficile* infections are confined to hospitals, but their numbers are increasing exponentially. The disease causes severe diarrhea and inflammation of the colon and sometimes death.

The primary herbs to use to treat the condition, listed in order of strength against the organism, are the berberine plants, cryptolepis, isatis, usnea, lomatium, licorice, and echinacea. Because juniper berry is active against *C. perfringens*, I would suggest its use for *C. difficile* as well.

TREATING CLOSTRIDIUM DIFFICILE

Formulation 1 (antibacterial) Cryptolepis or any berberine plant tincture: 1 tsp–1 tbl, 3–6x daily, depending on severity of symptoms

Formulation 2 (immune support) Echinacea, ginger, and licorice (equal parts) tincture: 1 tsp, 6x daily

Formulation 3 (antidiarrheal/colon soothing) Blackberry root and marsh mallow root (equal parts) standard infusion: up to 6 cups daily (Note: Elm bark porridge will also help ease colon inflammation tremendously.)

Enterococcus spp.

This genus was considered to be part of the streptococcus genus until it was reclassified in the 1980s. Although both *E. casseliflavus*

General Protocol: Take all of the basic (numbered) formulations for the condition unless otherwise noted.

and *E. raffinosus* may sometimes cause human infections, the major problematical species are *E. faecalis* and *E. faecium*. These enterococcal organisms are often highly resistant to antibiotics, especially in hospitals. They don't respond very well to beta-lactam antibiotics (penicillins and cephalosporins), aminoglycosides, and, increasingly, vancomycin.

Enterococcal organisms cause urinary tract infections, bacteremia, bacterial endocarditis, diverticulitis, and meningitis. The primary herbs to treat them are sida, alchornea, cryptolepis, bidens, ginger, echinacea, juniper berry, usnea, *Artemisia annua*, honey (I know, it's not *exactly* an herb), licorice, oregano oil, and *Acacia aroma*. If you are treating a really tough vancomycin-resistant enterococcal infection, add ginger juice to your formulation; it strongly inhibits resistance mechanisms in these bacteria.

TREATING ENTEROCOCCUS INFECTIONS

Formulation 1 (antibacterial) Sida, alchornea, or cryptolepis tincture: 1 tsp–1 tbl, 3–6x daily, depending on severity of symptoms (Note: Bidens tincture will work but requires higher doses and must be prepared properly; see monograph, page 229.)

Formulation 2 (immune support) Licorice, astragalus, and rhodiola (equal parts) tincture: 1 tsp, 3x daily (Note: Echinacea tincture will also be of benefit for immune support.)

For systemic enterococcal infections, diverticulitis, and endocarditis: Formulations 1 and 2

For enterococcal UTI: Formulation 1 plus juniper berry–bidens tincture (1 part juniper, 2 parts bidens), 30 drops, 3–6x daily, depending on severity

For enterococcal bacteremia: Formulation 1 plus *Echinacea angustifolia* tincture, 1/2 tsp–1 tbl in minimal water, every half hour to hour

For enterococcal meningitis: Formulations 1 and 2, plus formulations 3 and 4 on the next page

Formulation 3 Piperine: 20 mg, 2x daily, with the first dose in the morning 30 minutes before taking the other formulations, and the second dose at 4 P.M.

Formulation 4 Isatis leaf (or root) and either Japanese knotweed or stephania (equal parts) tincture: 1 tsp, 3–6x daily

Mycobacterium tuberculosis

This is the primary cause of tuberculosis (TB), which has become increasingly resistant and difficult to treat. There are, however, some 130 species of mycobacteria, a number of which can cause human disease. The members of this genus are a bit different than other Gram-positive bacteria. They don't stain well, but they also don't possess the double membrane structure of the Gram-negative bacteria. Their membrane is waxy and thicker than that of other Gram-positive bacteria, making them tougher overall. Of the 130 or so species, there are eight that can cause TB. *M. leprae* causes leprosy, and the *M. avium* complex often causes pulmonary infections in AIDS patients and has been implicated in Crohn's disease.

Mycobacterium tuberculosis has been developing increasing resistance for decades. MDR-TB (multidrug-resistant TB) is resistant to the two main first-line drugs used to treat it, isoniazid and rifampicin. Some 450,000 people contract this disease each year. XDR-TB (extensively drug-resistant TB) is resistant to all of the most effective anti-TB drugs. About 45,000 people a year contract this form of the disease; the death rate is about 90 percent.

The herbs effective for treating resistant and nonresistant TB are cryptolepis, sida, bidens, piperine, *Artemisia annua*, berberine plants, juniper, usnea, lomatium, licorice, echinacea, and rhodiola.

TREATING TUBERCULOSIS

Formulation 1 (systemic antibiotic) Cryptolepis and sida (equal parts) tincture: 1 tsp–1 tbl, 3–6x daily, depending on symptoms

Formulation 2 Piperine: 20 mg, 2x daily, with the first dose in the morning 30 minutes before taking the other formulations, and the second dose at 4 P.M.

Formulation 3 (immune support) Lomatium, licorice, and rhodiola (equal parts) tincture: 1 tsp, 3x daily

Staphylococcus aureus

Methicillin-resistant *Staphylococcus aureus* (MRSA) has become an increasingly common infectious disease. It is now present in both hospitals and the general community and is passing between people, wherever they congregate, with great abandon. Individuals with compromised immune function, even if they appear healthy, are at greater risk of serious infections. There are numerous strains of the bacteria, some more resistant than others. In many respects MRSA should mean "multidrug-resistant," not merely "methicillin resistant."

Most MRSA infections in the general community initially present as small red bumps that are similar to pimples or perhaps spider bites or small boils. There may be fever or even a rash. As the disease progresses, the bumps become larger and very painful, eventually breaking open into deep, pus-filled boils. In those in whom antibiotic treatment fails, the boils continue to spread and the infection goes deeper, sometimes necessitating amputation of affected limbs.

In hospitals MRSA can infect open wounds, intravenous catheters, the urinary tract, and the lungs; the infection can be quite dangerous, spreading throughout the whole system. Unchecked, it can infect the valves of the heart, the bones and joints, the organs, and the blood (bacteremia) and cause toxic shock syndrome (sepsis) and necrotizing (flesh-eating) pneumonia. Many people worldwide die from it each year.

The main herbs to treat MRSA are cryptolepis, sida, alchornea, bidens, black pepper, the berberines, usnea, juniper berry, isatis, licorice, ginger, ashwagandha, echinacea, red root, reishi, honey, and *Artemisia annua*.

TREATING MRSA INFECTIONS

Formulation 1 (internal systemic antibacterial) Cryptolepis tincture: 1 tsp–1 tbl, 3–6x daily, depending on severity

Formulation 2 (immune support) Ginger, reishi, and licorice (2 parts ginger, 2 parts reishi, 1 part licorice) tincture: 1 tsp, 3x daily

For MRSA UTIs: Formulations 1 and 2 plus juniper berry–bidens tincture (1 part juniper, 2 parts bidens), 30 drops, 3–6x daily

Streptococcus spp.

The main species of streptococcal bacteria that cause disease in human beings are *S. pyogenes*, which causes strep throat, acute bacterial glomerulonephritis, and necrotizing (flesh-eating) fasciitis; *S. pneumoniae*, which causes bacterial pneumonia, otitis media, sinusitis, meningitis, and peritonitis; and *S. agalactiae*, which causes pneumonia, meningitis, bacteremia, intestinal infections, and infections of the female reproductive tract. Of these, the first two are the most common causes of infections in people.

The primary herbs used to treat streptococcal bacteria are cryptolepis, sida, alchornea, bidens (though you'll need to use larger doses, for longer), the berberine plants, juniper, usnea, lomatium, honey, echinacea, licorice, ginger, and red root.

TREATING ACUTE, LIFE-THREATENING STREP INFECTIONS

Formulation 1 (antibacterial) *Echinacea angustifolia* tincture: 1 tbl in minimal water, every hour

Formulation 2 Cryptolepis, sida, or alchornea tincture: 1 tbl, every hour

Formulation 3 Lomatium, rhodiola, and eleuthero (equal parts) tincture: 1 tsp, 4x daily

For streptococcal glomerulonephritis: Formulations 1, 2, and 3, plus juniper berry tincture, 10 drops, up to 6x daily

For streptococcal bacteremia, necrotizing fasciitis, pneumonia,

peritonitis, and infections of the female reproductive tract: Formulations 1, 2, and 3

For strep throat: ½ tsp *Echinacea angustifolia* tincture, undiluted, held in the mouth until saliva is well stimulated, then allowed to dribble slowly down throat, over the affected areas; repeat *every* hour

For streptococcal necrotizing fasciitis (topical): Honey is best (see monograph, page 289). If it's not available, combine equal parts *Echinacea angustifolia* root powder, berberine plant powder, juniper berry powder, and lomatium root powder; mix well, apply as poultice, replace every 2 hours.

For streptococcal intestinal infection: Tincture of equal parts berberine plant, cryptolepis, and lomatium, 1 tsp–1 tbl, 3–6x daily, depending on severity of infection

For streptococcal meningitis: Treat as you would enterococcal meningitis (see page 51).

Dealing with Gram-Negative Bacteria

One of the most important things to remember in treating Gram-negative infections is that the use of a synergist will significantly increase the impact of the herbs on the bacteria. For instance, when treating diseases caused by *Shigella* spp., *Serratia marcescens, Salmonella* spp., *Klebsiella* spp., *Enterobacter* spp., or *E. coli,* add licorice to the mix. It strongly inhibits several of the main efflux pumps in this family of bacteria (AcrAB-TolC). You can use piperine when dealing with a *non–gastrointestinal tract infection,* but this is important: Don't use it with a GI tract infection such as *E. coli* or cholera. Piperine allows more of the herbs to pass through the GI tract, increasing the presence of their antibacterial compounds in the body.

The Gram-negative organisms are:

- *Acinetobacter baumannii*
- *Campylobacter jejuni*

- *Enterohemorrhagic E. coli* (*E. coli* O157, *E. coli* O157:HM, *E. coli* O157:H7)
- *Haemophilus influenzae*
- *Klebsiella pneumoniae*
- *Neisseria gonorrhoeae*
- *Proteus* spp. (*P. vulgaris, P. mirabilis*)
- *Pseudomonas aeruginosa*
- *Salmonella* spp. (*S. typhi, S. enteritidis, S. typhimurium*)
- *Serratia marcescens*
- *Shigella* spp. (*S. dysentariae, S. flexneri, S. sonnei*)
- *Stenotrophomonas maltophilia*
- *Vibrio cholerae*

Acinetobacter baumannii

Of the many species in this genus that can infect humans, *Acinetobacter baumanii,* the most common, is multidrug resistant; its name is often abbreviated as MDRAB. As of this writing it has become resistant to nearly all the antibiotics that can affect it. The only drugs still useful for fully resistant MDRAB are the older polymyxins that have not been in use for decades due to their toxicity—tigecycline has been the most recent drug of choice, but *Acinetobacter*'s resistance to it is increasing rapidly. In some hospitals it won't work at all. It is inevitable that as they are used more regularly to treat the bacteria, the polymyxins will also become ineffective.

Acinetobacter spp. are highly responsive to the exchange of DNA strands with other bacteria that contain both resistance and virulence factors. Many of the soldiers wounded in combat overseas tend to return with active MDRAB infections that then spread across hospitals. The bacteria enter the body through wounds, breathing tubes, catheters, injection sites—anything that breaks the surface and allows foreign pathogens in. They are generally spread by health-care workers and are especially troublesome because they can live on hospital surfaces (and the hospital staff's hands) for up to 5 months.

General Protocol: Take all of the basic (numbered) formulations for the condition unless otherwise noted.

Most hospital infections from these bacteria, aside from those due to combat, come from the insertion of contaminated breathing tubes during hospital procedures; 82 percent of these patients develop severe pneumonia and die as a result. Catheter insertion can cause severe infections of the urinary tract. Injections, blood draws, intravenous lines, surgical drains, and open wounds invite infection of the bloodstream, a.k.a. bacteremia.

These bacteria like to live in aquatic conditions and are often found in the irrigating and intravenous solutions used by the physicians; they love the lungs. They may enter the peritoneal fluid during peritoneal dialysis and can also find their way into the cerebral spinal fluid under some circumstances.

The herbs active against *Acinetobacter* are alchornea, cryptolepis, sida, juniper, isatis, ginger, lomatium, honey, oregano essential oil, epigallocatechin, *Acacia aroma*, *Zuccagnia punctata*, and *Sechium edule* fluid extract.

Note: Ginger juice taken internally is especially effective in reducing the resistance of *Acinetobacter* organisms. It is crucial to use if the infection is serious and has not responded to antibiotics.

TREATING ACINETOBACTER INFECTIONS

Formulation 1 (antibacterial) Cryptolepis, alchornea, or sida tincture: 1 tsp–1 tbl, 3–6x daily, depending on severity of symptoms

Formulation 2 Lomatium, astragalus, and rhodiola (equal parts) tincture: 1 tsp, 6x daily

Formulation 3 (important) Fresh ginger juice, stabilized with 20 percent alcohol (see page 437): 1 tbl in hot water, 6x daily

Formulation 4 Oregano or juniper essential oil inhalation as aromatherapy: 3x daily

For *Acinetobacter* pneumonia: Formulations 1, 2, 3, and 4

For *Acinetobacter* surgical wound infections: Formulations 1 and 2, plus daily topical honey dressings (see monograph, page 290)

For *Acinetobacter* UTIs: Formulations 2 and 3, plus juniper berry–bidens tincture (1 part juniper, 2 parts bidens), 30 drops, 6x daily (or oregano essential oil, 3 drops in water, 3x daily)

For *Acinetobacter* septicemia: Formulations 1, 2, and 3, plus *Echinacea angustifolia* tincture, 1/2 tsp–1 tbl, every half hour to hour

Campylobacter jejuni

Campylobacter infections generally cause enteritis accompanied by abdominal pain, diarrhea, fever, and malaise. They are not usually fatal but can be debilitating. The organism is increasingly resistant to antibiotics.

The herbs for campylobacter are cryptolepis (strongly), sida, ginger, and the berberines.

TREATING CAMPYLOBACTER INFECTIONS

Formulation 1 (antibacterial) Cryptolepis or sida tincture: 1 tsp, 3x daily

Formulation 2 Any strong tannin-containing plant (oak, geranium, krameria, pine needles) as a decoction: 6 ounces, up to 6x daily

E. coli

There are, roughly, three kinds of *E. coli* to be aware of. The first is the enterohemorrhagic *E. coli* strains (*E. coli* O157, *E. coli* O157:HM, and so on). The second is the kind that cause urinary tract infections, especially ST131. And finally, there are the *E. coli* B2 strains that cause what are called extraintestinal infections.

Of the current strains of enterohemorrhagic *E. coli*, O157 is the best known. All of them create similar conditions after infection; that is, hemorrhagic diarrhea and occasionally kidney failure. The infection is generally foodborne, most frequently arising from contaminated ground beef. It can also be contracted by drinking contaminated water or juices, eating contaminated vegetables, or swimming in contaminated pools.

The early signs are abdominal cramps, then acute diarrhea,

General Protocol: Take all of the basic (numbered) formulations for the condition unless otherwise noted.

often hemorrhagic. In some cases the red blood cells in the body are destroyed and the kidneys fail. Death is most common in the very young and the elderly.

A number of *E. coli* strains, both O157 and non-O157 strains, produce a shiga toxin (very similar to those made by *Shigella* species—all named after Kiyoshi Shiga, who discovered the shigella bacteria in the late nineteenth century). The toxins cause hemolytic-uremic syndrome; hemolytic anemia, acute renal failure, and low platelet counts all occur. Sida is essential to use if there is anemia/red blood cell damage.

The *E. coli* strains that cause UTIs have been fairly easy to treat, but a new strain of *E. coli*, ST131, emerged in 2008 and has begun to spread widely. It is strongly resistant and extremely virulent. The strain is, at this writing, only one resistance gene short of being untreatable. Unlike O157, ST131 causes urinary tract infections, generally in hospital settings, that sometimes lead to death.

The B2 group causes extraintestinal infections in the body, things like septicemia, meningitis, bacteremic pneumonia, peritonitis, and ascending cholangitis.

The first two strains are relatively easy to treat, but severe extraintestinal infections call for much more focus and care.

The herbs that are effective for *E. coli* are the berberines, cryptolepis, sida, alchornea, bidens, nearly all artemisias, juniper, honey, usnea, lomatium, isatis, licorice, ginger, ashwagandha, and reishi. All oak species (*Quercus*) and pomegranate (*Punica granatum*) fruit rind or tree bark are also highly effective against the *E. coli* O157:H7 strains. They are highly bacteriostatic and bactericidal and are very effective in killing the organisms *and* correcting the diarrhea. If you can't find any of the other plants I've listed, use oak bark; oak species grow nearly everywhere.

TREATING ENTEROHEMORRHAGIC E. COLI INFECTIONS

Formulation 1 (antibacterial) Berberine plant tincture: 1 tsp–1 tbl, 3–6x daily, depending on severity

Formulation 2 Blackberry root or oak bark decoction: 3 tbl–½ cup, 2–4x daily (Note: If the intestines are highly inflamed and sore, add powdered elm bark gruel.)

For enterohemorrhagic *E. coli* with red blood cell damage: Formulations 1 and 2 plus sida tincture, 1 tsp, 6x daily, along with ginger, licorice, and reishi (equal parts) tincture, 1 tsp, 3x daily

TREATING E. COLI ST131 INFECTIONS

Formulation 1 (antibacterial) Juniper berry–bidens tincture (1 part juniper, 2 parts bidens): 30 drops, 3–6x daily

Formulation 2 Cryptolepis and either sida or (if you can't get sida) berberine plant (equal parts) tincture: 1 tsp, 6x daily

Formulation 3 Ginger, licorice, and reishi (equal parts) tincture: 1 tsp, 3x daily

TREATING E. COLI B2 INFECTIONS

Formulation 1 (antibacterial) Cryptolepis and sida (equal parts; sida is important here) tincture: 1 tbl, 2–4x daily

Formulation 2 *Echinacea angustifolia* tincture: ½ tsp–1 tbl, every half hour to hour

Formulation 3 Ginger, licorice, and reishi (equal parts) tincture: 1 tsp, 3x daily

For *E. coli* B2 with septicemia: Formulations 1, 2, and 3

For *E. coli* B2 with meningitis: Treat as you would enterococcal meningitis (see page 51).

For *E. coli* B2 with bacteremic pneumonia: Formulations 1, 2, and 3, plus eucalyptus or juniper berry essential oil inhalation as aromatherapy, 4–6x daily

For *E. coli* B2 with peritonitis: Formulations 1, 2, and 3

For *E. coli* B2 with ascending cholangitis: Formulations 1, 2, and 3

General Protocol: Take all of the basic (numbered) formulations for the condition unless otherwise noted.

Haemophilus influenzae

Four species in this genus are the main sources of *Haemophilus* infection in people, the primary one being *Haemophilus influenzae,* specifically *H. influenzae* type B. Widespread vaccination in the United States and Europe began in 1988 and rates of infection from this particular organism have since fallen, though it is still common in the rest of the world.

The four species that cause infections in people are *H. influenzae, H. parainfluenzae, H. aphrophilus,* and *H. ducreyi. H. influenzae* has a number of types that cause disease: the encapsulated types, identified as A through F (B being the most problematical), and the unencapsulated, non-typeable strains.

The encapsulated strains, especially type B, cause invasive infections: pneumonia, meningitis, epiglottitis, septic arthritis, osteomyelitis, facial cellulitis, and bacteremia, generally in children, generally under 5 years of age. Pneumonia and meningitis are the most common. These forms of infection are generally spread by inhalation of infectious respiratory droplets—in other words, someone coughs, someone else breathes in.

The unencapsulated strains generally cause otitis media (ear infections) in children and lower respiratory tract infections in both children and immunocompromised adults—often those with existing lung diseases such as cystic fibrosis. They can also cause acute sinusitis and acute exacerbations of chronic bronchitis. A unique form, *H. influenzae* biogroup *aegyptius,* causes purulent conjunctivitis and sepsis in children, usually 1 to 4 years of age, following conjunctivitis infection.

H. parainfluenzae typically has low virulence but does occasionally cause endocarditis and bacteremia. However, it carries resistance genes that help increase resistance in other members of this genus. *H. aphrophilus,* uncommonly, causes endocarditis and brain abscesses. *H. ducreyi* causes chancroid, a sexually transmitted disease accompanied by shallow and painful genital ulcers and inguinal lymphadenitis (buboes).

Haemophilus organisms are common in most people. They usually become a problem only when a person becomes immunocompromised. However, the genus is growing increasingly resistant to antibiotics; it appears that while type B is becoming less of a problem due to vaccination programs, the other types are growing more problematical. Resistant respiratory infections are more common every year, and the organisms, once more invasive of children, have now shifted to infecting adults in nearly equal numbers.

An additional concern is that influenza viruses are highly synergistic with *Haemophilus*. Dual infection is considerably more dangerous than with either alone. There is some evidence that the 1918 influenza epidemic involved a highly activated synergy with *Haemophilus*; even immunocompetent individuals become highly susceptible to the bacteria when the two activate together. This synergistic capacity seems inherent in *Haemophilus;* other studies have found the same kind of synergy between it and other respiratory pathogens such as *Moraxella catarrhalis*, respiratory syncytial virus, human parainfluenza virus 3, and rhinovirus.

Importantly, *Haemophilus* are what are called fastidious bacteria, meaning they need an iron source to grow, and unlike most other bacteria, they usually get it from the hemoglobin in our blood to which iron is bonded (giving blood its red color). Protecting the blood cells through the use of something like sida is crucial in treating this kind of infection.

The herbs that have been found active against *Haemophilus* are ginger, licorice, isatis, lomatium, honey, eucalyptus essential oil, eucalyptus leaf, and basil essential oil. Unfortunately, cryptolepis, sida, and alchornea have not been tested against this organism. However, I believe that, due to their activity against similar Gram-negative bacteria, they are usable for *Haemophilus* infections, especially sida, given its strong protective effects on red blood cells. I would use them myself without hesitation.

General Protocol: Take all of the basic (numbered) formulations for the condition unless otherwise noted.

TREATING HAEMOPHILUS INFECTIONS

Formulation 1 (antibacterial) Sida tincture: 1 tsp, 3–6x daily

Formulation 2 Isatis, ginger, licorice, and red root (equal parts) tincture: 1 tsp, 6x daily

Formulation 3 Fresh ginger juice tea (see page 438): 4–6x daily

For *Haemophilus* pneumonia: Formulations 1, 2, and 3

For *Haemophilus* epiglottitis and facial cellulitis: Formulations 1, 2, and 3

For *Haemophilus* chancroid: Formulations 1, 2, and 3. Add a topical wash of an infusion of eucalyptus and lomatium and honey 4x daily. If ulcers are severe, apply honey dressings after using the topical wash.

For *Haemophilus* meningitis: Formulations 1 and 2, along with piperine, 20 mg, 2x daily, with the first dose in the morning 30 minutes before taking the other formulations, and the second dose at 4 P.M. Also add isatis leaf (or root) and either Japanese knotweed or stephania (equal parts) tincture, 1 tsp, 3–6x daily. Echinacea will also be of benefit, as for bacteremia.

For *Haemophilus* bacteremia and osteomyelitis: Formulations 1, 2, and 3, along with *Echinacea angustifolia* tincture, ½ tsp–1 tbl, every half hour to hour

For *Haemophilus* septic arthritis: Formulations 1, 2, and 3, along with *E. angustifolia* and teasel root (equal parts) tincture, ½ tsp, 3x daily

For *Haemophilus* otitis media: Use Formulations 2 and 3 plus oil ear drops as follows: Make an oil infusion with lomatium. When done as per recipe, add 10 drops eucalyptus essential oil and 10 drops basil essential oil. Place 2–3 drops in ear 2x daily.

For *Haemophilus* purulent conjunctivitis: Use isatis or isatis-honey eyedrops.

Klebsiella

The main species that causes human infection is *K. pneumoniae*, but *K. oxytoca* and *K. rhinoscleromatis* occasionally do, too. Most infections occur in the lungs, but they also can occur in the urinary tract, the biliary tract, the lower respiratory tract, and surgical wounds. The organism can cause pneumonia, bacteremia, urinary tract infections, diarrhea, cholecystitis, osteomyelitis, meningitis, thrombophlebitis, and respiratory infections. Generally, infections are caused by hospital staff from bacteria on their hands or bacterial colonization of invasive apparatus, and sometimes patients' GI tracts are contaminated.

When *Klebsiella* infect the lung tissue, necrosis, inflammation, and hemorrhage often occur, giving rise to a thick, bloody mucus; it looks something like currant jelly (so they say).

Klebsiella organisms are often multidrug resistant, producing extended-spectrum beta-lactamases (ESBL). These strains are highly virulent and spread promiscuously. The mortality rate is around 50 percent, irrespective of antibiotic use. They are one of the fastest-growing resistant infections in U.S. hospitals and are common throughout the world. The newest resistant form is referred to as CRKP (carbapenem-resistant *Klebsiella pneumoniae*). Very dangerous.

The herbs useful for *Klebsiella* are cryptolepis, alchornea, bidens, black pepper, juniper, the berberine plants, *Acacia*, *Artemisia annua*, reishi, licorice, and honey.

TREATING KLEBSIELLA INFECTIONS

Formulation 1 (antibacterial) Cryptolepis and alchornea (equal parts) tincture: 1 tsp–1 tbl, 6x daily

Formulation 2 (to thin mucus) Ginger juice tea (page 438): 4–6x daily

Formulation 3 (immune support) Reishi, red root, licorice, and *Echinacea angustifolia* (equal parts) tincture: 1 tsp, 6x daily

Formulation 4 Juniper essential oil inhalation as aromatherapy: 4–6x daily

For *Klebsiella* pneumonia and respiratory infections: Formulations 1, 2, 3, and 4

For *Klebsiella* osteomyelitis: Formulations 1, 2, and 4, plus *Echinacea angustifolia* tincture, ½ tsp–1 tbl, every half hour to hour

For *Klebsiella* meningitis: Treat as you would enterococcal meningitis (see page 51).

For *Klebsiella* surgical wound infections: Formulations 1, 2, and 4, plus daily topical honey dressings (see monograph, page 290)

For *Klebsiella* bacteremia: Instead of the formulations above, use *Echinacea angustifolia tincture,* ½ tsp–1 tbl, every half hour to hour; cryptolepis tincture, 1 tbl, 6x daily; and piperine, 20 mg, 2x daily (the first dose in the morning 30 minutes before taking the other formulations and the second dose at 4 P.M.).

For *Klebsiella* UTIs: Instead of the formulations above, use juniper berry–bidens tincture (1 part juniper, 2 parts bidens), 30 drops, 3–6x daily; and cryptolepis–berberine plant tincture (equal parts), 1 tsp, 3x daily.

For *Klebsiella* diarrhea: Instead of the formulations above, use a berberine plant tincture, 1 tsp, 3–6x daily.

Neisseria gonorrhoeae

This organism causes gonorrhea, which is sexually transmitted. The main herbs effective for it are cryptolepis and sida.

TREATING NEISSERIA GONORRHOEAE

Formulation Cryptolepis and sida (equal parts) tincture: 1 tsp, 3x daily for 14 days

Proteus spp.

The two most troublesome *Proteus* species are *P. vulgaris* and *P. mirabilis.* Both are resistant. *P. mirabilis* generates 90 percent of *Proteus* infections in people. *Proteus* infections can cause alkaline kidney stones, but more seriously, when contracted in hospitals, they can cause wound infections, urinary tract infections, septicemia, and pneumonia.

The herbs that are effective for proteus are cryptolepis, sida, alchornea, *Artemisia annua*, juniper, usnea, *Acacia aroma*, lomatium, ginger, and honey.

TREATING PROTEUS UTIs

Formulation 1 (antibacterial) Juniper berry and bidens tincture (1 part juniper, 2 parts bidens): 30 drops, 3–6x daily

Formulation 2 Cryptolepis, sida, or alchornea tincture: 1 tsp, 3–6x daily

Formulation 3 Ginger, rhodiola, and red root (equal parts) tincture: 1 tsp, 3x daily

Formulation 4 Piperine: 20 mg, 2x daily (the first dose in the morning 30 minutes before taking the other formulations and the second dose at 4 P.M.)

TREATING PROTEUS SEPTICEMIA

Formulation 1 (antibacterial) Cryptolepis, sida, or alchornea tincture: 1 tsp, 6x daily

Formulation 2 (to prevent septic shock) Isatis tincture: 1 tbl, 3–6x daily

Formulation 3 *Echinacea angustifolia* tincture: ½ tsp–1 tbl, every half hour to hour

Formulation 4 Lomatium, rhodiola, and red root (equal parts) tincture: 1 tsp, 3x daily

TREATING PROTEUS WOUND INFECTIONS

Formulation 1 (antibacterial) Cryptolepis, alchornea, and sida (equal parts) tincture: 1 tsp, 6x daily

Formulation 2 Lomatium, rhodiola, and red root (equal parts) tincture: 1 tsp, 3–6x daily

Formulation 3 Daily topical honey dressings (see monograph, page 290)

General Protocol: Take all of the basic (numbered) formulations for the condition unless otherwise noted.

TREATING PROTEUS PNEUMONIA

Formulation 1 (antibacterial) Cryptolepis, alchornea, and sida (equal parts) tincture: 1 tsp, 6x daily

Formulation 2 Ginger juice tea (page 438)

Formulation 3 (immune support) Lomatium, licorice, red root, and *Echinacea angustifolia* (equal parts) tincture: 1 tsp, 6x daily

Formulation 4 Juniper essential oil inhalation as aromatherapy: 3x daily

Pseudomonas aeruginosa

This species is another opportunistic pathogen that takes advantage of hospital settings. It can live, even thrive, on most surfaces and is common on most medical equipment, including catheters, on which it often enters the human body. It can grow in diesel and jet fuel and survive temperatures up to 108°F, so fevers don't affect it much. It can live in oxygen, partial oxygen, or no oxygen. It can even live in distilled water in which virtually no nutrients exist. It's tough and very, very resistant to antibiotics.

Pseudomonas can infect nearly any part of the body; all it needs is an opening (which hospitals often give it). It causes pneumonia, septic shock, urinary tract infections, otitis media, gastrointestinal infections, and skin and soft tissue infections. The most common infections are from burns, surgical wounds, urinary tract infections, and otitis media. Low phosphate levels in the human body are highly stimulatory of its growth.

The primary herbs useful for treating *Pseudomonas aeruginosa* are isatis, alchornea, bidens, cryptolepis, sida, black pepper, *Artemisia annua,* the berberines, juniper, ginger, *Acacia aroma,* honey, lomatium, ashwagandha, echinacea, and reishi.

TREATING PSEUDOMONAS PNEUMONIA

Formulation 1 (antibacterial) Cryptolepis and alchornea (equal parts) tincture: 1 tsp–1 tbl, up to 6x daily

Formulation 2 Ginger juice tea (page 438)

Formulation 3 (immune support) Ginger, isatis, red root, and *Echinacea angustifolia* (equal parts) tincture: 1 tsp, 6x daily

Formulation 4 Juniper essential oil inhalation as aromatherapy: 3x daily

TREATING PSEUDOMONAS SEPSIS

Formulation 1 (antibacterial) Cryptolepis and alchornea (equal parts) tincture: 1 tbl, 6x daily

Formulation 2 (immune support) Ginger, isatis, and red root (equal parts) tincture: 1 tsp, 6x daily

Formulation 3 *Echinacea angustifolia* tincture: ½ tsp–1 tbl, every half hour to hour

Formulation 4 Tincture combination of *Salvia miltiorrhiza* and *Angelica sinensis*, ½–1 tbl, every hour in water

TREATING PSEUDOMONAS GI TRACT INFECTIONS

Formulation 1 (antibacterial) Cryptolepis and a berberine plant (equal parts) tincture: 1 tsp–1 tbl, 3–6x daily depending on severity

Formulation 2 Ginger, red root, and *Echinacea angustifolia* (equal parts) tincture: 1 tsp, 6x daily

TREATING PSEUDOMONAS UTIs

Formulation 1 (antibacterial) Juniper berry and bidens (1 part juniper, 2 parts bidens) tincture: 30 drops, 3x daily

Formulation 2 Berberine plant tincture: 1 tsp, 3x daily

Formulation 3 Ginger, licorice, and red root (equal parts) tincture: 1 tsp, 3x daily

TREATING PSEUDOMONAS INFECTIONS OF SURGICAL WOUNDS AND BURNS

Formulation 1 (antibacterial) Piperine: 20 mg, 2x daily, with the first dose in the morning 30 minutes before taking the other formulations, and the second dose at 4 P.M.

Formulation 2 Cryptolepis and alchornea (equal parts) tincture: 1 tsp, 6x daily

Formulation 3 (immune support) Ginger, licorice, and red root (equal parts) tincture: 1 tsp, 6x daily

Formulation 4 Daily topical honey dressings (see monograph, page 290)

TREATING PSEUDOMONAS OTITIS MEDIA

Formulation Ear formulation with lomatium, honey, berberine plant, or cryptolepis or use ear infection glycerite (page 564) with the addition of lomatium: 1–3 drops topically, up to 6x daily

Salmonella spp.

Closely related to both shigella and *E. coli,* salmonella organisms cause typhoid fever (*S. typhi*), paratyphoid fever (*S. paratyphi*), and salmonellosis, a.k.a. food poisoning. Most infections come from contaminated foods.

Salmonella can survive outside a host for years—active organisms have been identified in dried two-and-a-half-year-old feces. They are not destroyed by freezing and have to be heated to at least 130°F for 1 hour to kill them (or 10 minutes at 170°F). Poultry, pork, cattle, and many fruits and vegetables are now commonly infected with the bacteria. About 150,000 people in the United States sicken from eating infected chicken eggs each year.

The bacteria inhibit the innate immune system as they penetrate the body to better enable their survival. General symptoms are diarrhea, vomiting, fever, and severe abdominal cramps. Sepsis and infection of other organs can occur in severe cases.

The organisms, due to heavy antibiotic use in both plant and animal agriculture, have developed multidrug resistance and are becoming much more difficult to treat.

The primary herbs effective for salmonella are cryptolepis, sida, alchornea, bidens, the berberines, juniper, honey, licorice, lomatium, and ginger.

TREATING SALMONELLA INFECTIONS

Formulation 1 (antibacterial) Cryptolepis, sida, or alchornea tincture: 1 tsp–1 tbl, 3–6x daily depending on the severity of the infection

Formulation 2 Berberine plant tincture: 1 tsp–1 tbl, 3–6x daily, depending on symptom picture

Formulation 3 (immune support) Licorice tincture, rhodiola tincture, and ginger juice (equal parts) combined: 1 tsp, 3x daily

Note: Juniper-evergreen and sida teas are especially useful for treating salmonella.

For salmonella with sepsis: Formulations 1, 2, and 3, and add tincture combination of *Salvia miltiorrhiza* and *Angelica sinensis*, ½–1 tbl, every hour in water.

Serratia marcescens

This is primarily a hospital-acquired infection. The bacteria can colonize the urinary tract (causing UTIs, from catheters), surgical wounds, the blood (bacteremia), the eye (conjunctivitis), the respiratory tract (pneumonia), the CNS (meningitis), the bones (osteomyelitis), and the heart (endocarditis). It is becoming highly resistant.

The primary herbs active against the organism are juniper, bidens, licorice, lomatium, *Coptis chinensis*, honey, oregano oil, *Tribulus terrestris*, and *Emblica officinalis*. The following plants are also active: *Trichosanthes cucumerina, Cassia didymobotrya, Blumea lacera, Moringa oleifera, Isodon* spp., *Dendrophthoe falcata, Zuccagnia punctata,* and *Phrygilanthus acutifolius.*

Note: For all *Serratia* infections, use piperine, 20 mg, 2x daily, with the first dose in the morning 30 minutes before taking the other formulations, and the second dose at 4 P.M.

TREATING SERRATIA UTIs

Formulation 1 (antibacterial) Juniper berry and bidens (1 part juniper, 2 parts bidens) tincture: 30 drops, 6x daily for 10 days

General Protocol: Take all of the basic (numbered) formulations for the condition unless otherwise noted.

Formulation 2 Bidens fresh plant juice or tincture; or *Coptis chinensis* tincture; or *Tribulus terrestris* tincture; or a combination of the three (equal parts): ½ tsp, 3x daily

Formulation 3 (immune support) Ginger, licorice, and rhodiola (equal parts) tincture: ½ tsp, 3x daily

TREATING SERRATIA SURGICAL WOUND INFECTIONS

Formulations 2 and 3 for *Serratia* UTI infections (above), plus topical honey dressings daily (see monograph, page 290)

TREATING SERRATIA EYE INFECTIONS

Formulation 1 (antibacterial) Bidens fresh juice: 1–3 drops applied to the eye, up to 6x daily

Formulation 2 (immune support) Lomatium, licorice, and ginger (equal parts) tincture: ½ tsp, 3x daily

TREATING SERRATIA BACTEREMIA AND OSTEOMYELITIS

Formulation 1 (antibacterial) *Echinacea angustifolia* tincture: ½ tsp–1 tbl, every half hour

Formulation 2 (immune support) Lomatium, licorice, and ginger (equal parts) tincture: 1 tsp, 3x daily

Formulation 3 Bidens fresh juice or plant tincture: 1 tbl, 6x daily

TREATING SERRATIA PNEUMONIA

Formulation 1 (antibacterial) Bidens fresh plant juice or tincture: 1 tsp, 6x daily

Formulation 2 (immune support) Lomatium, ginger, licorice, and red root (equal parts) tincture: 1 tsp, 6x daily

Formulation 3 Juniper or oregano essential oil inhalation as aromatherapy: 3x daily

TREATING SERRATIA WOUND INFECTIONS

Formulations 1 and 2 for *Serratia* pneumonia (above), plus topical honey dressings daily (see monograph, page 290)

TREATING SERRATIA MENINGITIS

Formulations 1 and 2 for *Serratia* pneumonia (above), plus formulation 3 below:

Formulation 3 Isatis leaf (or root) and either Japanese knotweed or stephania (equal parts) tincture: 1 tsp, 3–6x daily

Note: Echinacea will also be of benefit, as for *Serratia* bacteremia.

Shigella spp.

The main *Shigella* species are *Shigella dysentariae*, *S. flexneri*, *S. boydii*, and *S. sonnei*. Shigella, *E. coli*, and salmonella are all closely related; all usually cause some form of severe diarrhea. *S. flexneri* causes about 60 percent of the shigella infections in the nonindustrialized nations, and *S. sonnei* about 80 percent of those in the industrialized. *S. dysentariae* is the cause of most epidemics of dysentery.

Shigella organisms destroy the cellular lining of the intestinal mucosa and invade the body; the disease is generally accompanied by mild to severe diarrhea and/or dysentery. There are some 165 million shigella infections a year and about a million deaths. The main route of transmission is fecal/oral. There is frequent loose-stool diarrhea consisting mostly of blood and mucus accompanied by fever, pain, and bowel cramping. Sepsis, intestinal perforation, toxic megacolon, dehydration, hyponatremia, encephalopathy, hemolytic-uremic syndrome, and pneumonia are common acute complications from the infection. If untreated, persistent dysentery, severe protein loss, and malnutrition commonly occur, even in uncomplicated cases. Fever, malaise, and body aches are common no matter the severity of the infection. Some strains produce shiga toxins, which exacerbate the symptoms considerably.

S. dysentariae is very prone to antimicrobial resistance and soon passes the information on to the other species in the genus (as well as to *E. coli* and *Salmonella* spp.). Most strains are now resistant to nearly all low-cost antibacterials. The bacteria developed resistance in much of the world to the last low-cost antibacterial, quinolone NA, within 6 months after it was used to treat an epidemic outbreak.

General Protocol: Take all of the basic (numbered) formulations for the condition unless otherwise noted.

The herbs that are effective for shigella are cryptolepis, sida, alchornea, bidens, the berberines, juniper, honey, licorice, lomatium, and ginger.

TREATING SHIGELLA INFECTIONS

Formulation 1 (antibacterial) Cryptolepis, sida, or alchornea tincture: 1 tsp–1 tbl, 3–6x daily depending on the severity of the infection

Formulation 2 Berberine plant tincture: 1 tsp–1 tbl, 3–6x daily, depending on symptom picture

Formulation 3 (immune support) Lomatium tincture, licorice tincture, and ginger juice (mixed in equal parts): 1 tsp, 3x daily

Note: Juniper/evergreen needle and sida teas are especially useful for GI tract shigella infections.

For shigella with sepsis: To the above formulations, add tincture combination of *Salvia miltiorrhiza* and *Angelica sinensis*, ½–1 tbl, every hour in water.

Stenotrophomonas maltophilia

Once considered to be *Pseudomonas maltophilia*, then identified as *Xanthomonas maltophilia*, now this newly emerging resistant bacteria is called *Stenotrophomonas maltophilia.* It usually occurs in hospitals, where it can cause infections in surgical wounds, pneumonia, bacteremia, endocarditis, and meningitis. Few herbs have been tested for activity against it as of 2011. Here is what is known to be active so far: *Berberis* spp., alchornea, boneset, honey, epigallocatechin (green tea constituent), *Scorzonera sandrasica* (aerial parts), eucalyptus essential oil, eucalyptus leaf tincture, thyme essential oil, oregano essential oil, *Acacia aroma, Zuccagnia punctata, Sechium edule* fluid extract, *Salvia* spp., *Menyanthes trifoliata, Artemisia dracunculus, Mammea americana, Oedogonium capillare, Centaurea cariensis, Artemisia arborescens, Artemisia afra*, rosemary, garlic, and devil's claw (*Harpagophytum procumbens*).

TREATING STENOTROPHOMONAS MALTOPHILIA INFECTIONS

Formulation 1 (antibacterial) Alchornea tincture: 1 tsp, 3–6x daily, depending on severity of symptoms

Formulation 2 Fresh garlic juice: 1/4–1 tsp, up to 4x daily

Formulation 3 Thyme, rosemary, eucalyptus, and oregano essential oils (blended in equal parts), inhalation as aromatherapy: 3–6x daily

Formulation 4 Eucalyptus leaf infusion: 8 ounces, up to 6x daily

Formulation 5 (immune support) Boneset, licorice, and red root (equal parts) tincture: 1 tsp, 6x daily

Formulation 6 Piperine: 20 mg, 2x daily, with the first dose in the morning 30 minutes before taking the other formulations, and the second dose at 4 P.M.

For *S. maltophilia* pneumonia: Formulations 1 through 6

For *S. maltophilia* bacteremia: Formulations 1, 2, 4, 5, and 6 (omitting formulation 3). Add *Echinacea angustifolia* tincture, 1/2 tsp–1 tbl, every half hour to hour.

For *S. maltophilia* wound infections: Formulations 1, 2, 4, 5, and 6 (omitting formulation 3). Add daily honey dressings (see monograph, page 290).

For *S. maltophilia* meningitis: Formulations 1, 2, and 6. Add tincture of isatis leaf (or root) and either Japanese knotweed or stephania (equal parts), 1 tsp, 3–6x daily. Echinacea will also be of benefit, as for bacteremia.

Vibrio cholerae

Cholera organisms infect the small intestine and cause extensive watery diarrhea (10 to 20 quarts a day—usually without cramping), generalized muscle cramps, and sometimes vomiting (clear fluid), which in turn lead to dehydration and electrolyte imbalances. (One of the most important interventions in cholera treatment is fluid replacement.) About five million people a year suffer from cholera, but before

> **General Protocol:** Take all of the basic (numbered) formulations for the condition unless otherwise noted.

antibiotics, cholera epidemics were much worse. Generally, contaminated water or food is the culprit.

Prior to 1977, there were no reports of resistance in cholera organisms, but now they are common. Most cholera strains, including O1 Inaba, O139, O138, and El Tor, are now resistant to many antibiotics, including tetracycline, ampicillin, kanamycin, streptomycin, sulphonamides, trimethoprim, and gentamicin.

The herbs useful against cholera are the berberines, cryptolepis, licorice, ginger, *Geranium mexicanum* (or any of the geranium species' roots), *Psidium guajava* (guava) leaf and bark tea or ethanol extract, and *Punica granatum* (pomegranate) fruit peel or bark as tea or ethanol extract. Basil (*Ocimum basilicum*), nopal cactus (*Opuntia ficus-indica*), *Acacia famesiana*, and *Artemisia ludoviciana* are also very active against cholera organisms. Extracts of those four plants (and the geraniums as well) disrupt the cell membranes of the cholera organisms, increase membrane permeability, decrease cytoplasm pH and cell membrane hyperpolarization, and decrease cellular ATP concentration in all strains tested. In fact, nearly any of the acacias will do for this use.

TREATING CHOLERA

Formulation 1 (antibacterial) Cryptolepis and berberine plant (equal parts) tincture: 1 tsp, 6x daily

Formulation 2 Geranium root strong decoction: 3 tbl, every hour

Formulation 3 Guava leaf or bark and pomegranate peel or bark (equal parts) tea: as much as possible

Alternative Effective Decoction Acacia bark decoction: 3 tbl, every hour; basil and artemisia infusion: 8 ounces, every hour

Nonbacterial Variants

The three resistant nonbacterial variants are the candidas, malaria, and the aspergillus mold.

Candida spp.

Candida species are a type of yeast that form a normal part of the human intestinal and urinary tracts and skin flora. The main species is usually *Candida albicans.* Antibiotic overuse has stimulated tremendous problems with this organism. Overgrowth in the intestinal and urinary tracts is common. Candida has traditionally been treated with antifungals and azoles, but the last 20 years have seen significant resistance emerge across the entire genus.

Resistant candida infections cause urinary tract infections, vaginal infections, mouth infections (thrush)—they love mucous membrane systems. Itching, burning, soreness, irritation, and whitish patches or discharge are common symptoms. In some instances candida can become systemic and affect multiple organs. Infections are much more serious in people whose immune systems are compromised.

The herbs to treat candida are sida, alchornea, bidens, cryptolepis (minimally), *Artemisia annua*, the berberines, juniper, honey, usnea, black pepper, lomatium, isatis, licorice, red root flowers, reishi, echinacea, chaparro amargosa (*Castela emoryi*), and desert willow (*Chilopsis linearis*).

TREATING CANDIDA UTIs

Formulation Berberine plant, alchornea, or sida tincture: 1 tsp, 3x daily; or juniper berry–bidens tincture (1 part juniper, 2 parts bidens): 30 drops, 3x daily; or lomatium, isatis, and echinacea (equal parts) tincture: 1 tsp, 3x daily

TREATING CANDIDA VAGINAL INFECTIONS

Formulation 1 (antibacterial) Alchornea or sida tincture: 1 tsp, 3x daily

Formulation 2 Lomatium, isatis, and echinacea (equal parts) tincture: 1 tsp, 3x daily

Formulation 3 Berberine tincture diluted in water, used as a douche (see page 263): 2x daily, in the morning and again in the evening

General Protocol: Take all of the basic (numbered) formulations for the condition unless otherwise noted.

TREATING CANDIDA MOUTH INFECTIONS

Formulation 1 (antibacterial) Lomatium, isatis, and echinacea (equal parts) tincture: 1 tsp, 3x daily

Formulation 2 One ounce berberine tincture diluted in 6 ounces water, take 1 tablespoon to wash mouth and gums thoroughly: 3x daily

TREATING SYSTEMIC CANDIDA INFECTIONS

Formulation 1 (antibacterial) Alchornea or sida tincture: 1 tsp, 3x daily

Formulation 2 Licorice, reishi, and echinacea (equal parts) tincture: 1 tsp, 3x daily

Formulation 3 Desert willow and chaparro amargosa (equal parts) tincture: 1 tsp, 3x daily

Plasmodium spp.

There are some 200 or more species of plasmodia, parasitic protists that infect red blood cells. Eleven of the species infect people. The disease is transmitted by mosquito bites. The organisms grow in the liver, then infect the red blood cells. Fever, shivering, shaking, muscle pain, headache, anemia, enlarged spleen and liver, and malaise are typical symptoms. Vomiting is sometimes present. In severe infections brain damage, convulsions, and death can occur. Given their life cycle, latent parasites can emerge later. This is why treatment for *Plasmodium* is often repeated after 14 days.

Worldwide, there are some 250 million cases of malaria each year, resulting in nearly a million deaths, and 80 percent of them come from *Plasmodium falciparum*. The malarial organisms are often resistant to antibiotics, hence the development of artemisinin from *Artemisia annua*. However, the use of that isolated constituent is now provoking resistance worldwide, so the constituent is often combined with antibiotics to retard resistance development. In the treatment of malaria, the whole herb or mixtures of herbs are preferable for just that reason.

The herbs effective for malaria are cryptolepis, sida, alchornea, bidens, *Artemisia annua*, juniper, isatis, and licorice.

General Protocol: Take all of the basic (numbered) formulations for the condition unless otherwise noted.

TREATING MALARIA

Formulation Cryptolepis, sida, or alchornea tincture: 1 tbl, 3x daily for 7 days, repeat in 14 days; or artemisinin: 1,000 mg the first day, 500 mg daily for 4 more days, repeat in 14 days

Aspergillus spp.

Aspergillus, especially *A. fumigatus*, is an increasing source of resistant infections. This rather common mold can cause bronchopulmonary infections and chronic sinusitis. In hospital settings or among the immunocompromised, it usually causes pulmonary disease and to a lesser extent surgical wound infections. It is resistant to most available drugs—polyenes, azoles, and echinocandins. Mortality rates in hospitals run 50 percent to 60 percent on average and as high as 90 percent in some populations (such as leukemia patients).

The herbs effective for aspergillus are sida, alchornea, cryptolepis, juniper, lomatium, isatis, ginger, honey, *Artemisia giraldii*, and *Sechium edule* fluid extract.

TREATING ASPERGILLUS INFECTIONS

Formulation 1 (antibacterial) Cryptolepis, sida, or alchornea tincture, or a combination of the three: 1 tsp, 3x daily

Formulation 2 (immune support) Ginger, licorice, and rhodiola (equal parts) tincture: 1 tsp, 3x daily

Formulation 3 Nasal spray formula for sinus infections (see page 566) prepared with *just* juniper essential oil; or juniper essential oil inhalation as aromatherapy: 3–6x daily

For sinusitis and bronchopulmonary conditions: Formulations 1, 2, and 3

For systemic treatment in the immunocompromised, pulmonary infection, or pneumonia: Formulations 1, 2, and 3; increase the dosage for formulations 1 and 2 to 1 tsp–1 tbl, up to 6x daily

For surgical wound infections: Formulations 1 and 2, plus topical honey dressing daily (see monograph, page 290)

3

EMERGING VIRUSES: WHAT WE ARE FACING

Viral diseases, caused by pathogenic virus infections which have high morbidity and mortality rates, are still the leading cause of death in humans worldwide. . . . Moreover, the emergence of viral resistance to drugs, as well as the serious adverse effects induced by antiviral drugs, has caused serious medical problems, particularly when [the drugs are] administered in combination over prolonged treatment periods. . . . And these drugs are quite costly, thus limiting their use in developing countries, where infection is most prevalent.

—Kaio Kitazato et al., "Viral Infectious Disease and Natural Products with Antiviral Activity"

For much of the twentieth century, infectious diseases in human populations of Western countries have been in retreat, as we learnt to sanitize our cities, cleanse our water supplies, improve domestic hygiene, use antibiotics, control vector organisms and vaccinate. As a result the developed world became rather complacent, naively welcoming the false dawn of a life mostly free of infectious disease. Since the 1980s things have looked much less secure, however, with the emergence of many previously unrecognized infectious diseases, and the re-emergence of known infectious diseases that were thought to be under control. This trend has continued until the present time and many infectious pathogens, predominantly viruses, have been newly identified.

—Thijs Kuiken et al., "Emerging Viral Infections in a Rapidly Changing World"

During the summer of 2006 a hitherto little-known viral disease swept across a large and diverse range of islands in the Indian Ocean. On the island of Réunion 265,000 people became critically ill—out of a population of 770,000. Very few of those infected were asymptomatic; the illness was, in nearly every case, severe. Health-care workers and the island's hospital system were overwhelmed. Even if they had not been, there was little they could do. So, they offered "supportive" care. In other words, they watched. They waited. Either the person's immune and bodily systems would fight it off, or they wouldn't. For many, they didn't.

The virus soon jumped to India, where an estimated 1.3 million people became ill. The culprit? A relatively little-known viral disease, chikungunya fever.[1] The virus is known to medical science but not well; it's not a common disease. But it had mutated. Later analysis showed that the mutation had occurred sometime between the spring and fall of 2005. Within 6 months it had become pandemic in the region. By the end of 2006 more than two million people had become infected.

The disease is attended by severe joint pain. The ankles and wrists are the most impacted; conjunctivitis and a rash often occur. The pain in the joints can last for weeks . . . or months, and it is debilitating. There is no treatment and there is no cure. The physicians recommended the use of acetominophen for the pain. The cause of death for many of those who died? Liver damage . . . from the acetaminophen.

People visiting the region who traveled back to their homes in the United States and Europe brought the disease with them. More than 1,000 in the United States were diagnosed with it; person-to-person transmission occurred in a number of instances, infecting new hosts. Then, luckily for most of us, the epidemic just . . . faded away.

The disease is primarily spread by mosquitoes (similarly to most of the viruses discussed in this book), specifically *Aedes albopictus*. This is a mosquito that was once limited in its geographical range but has, in the past 50 years, spread to every continent on Earth.

This is an example of just how fast a new viral pathogen can spread in the global village. It began with an African virus entering an Asian mosquito that traveled with people by plane and boat to the Indian Ocean and India. And from there, it went everywhere. This same dynamic is now playing out everyplace on Earth. The chikungunya outbreak is not an uncommon event. West Nile encephalitis virus emerged in the United States in a large outbreak in 1999. It soon spread throughout the world and is now endemic in Europe and Asia. In the fall of 2002, SARS emerged in China and quickly spread throughout the pan-Asian region. The epidemiologists who studied the SARS outbreak discovered that it had initially emerged in a small region in China. The physician who attended the ill then visited Hong Kong, where he infected 16 people. Some of them traveled and in doing so spread the disease worldwide in a matter of weeks.

Then came swine flu and headlines like these:

460 Flu Victims Fighting for Life as Experts Admit 24 Deaths from Swine Strain May Be Only a Fraction of the True Number

—Sophie Borland, *Mail Online*, December 24, 2010

Flu Crisis Hits Cancer Surgery: Hospitals Struggle to Cope as Deaths Rise and Britain Teeters on the Brink of an Epidemic

—Sophie Borland, *Mail Online*, December 27, 2010

Fears Over Outbreak After 12 Infected with New Swine Flu Strain (H3N2v) in U.S.

—Nina Golgowski, *Mail Online,* January 12, 2012

"Swine Flu" Strain Returns: Dramatic Rise in Deaths of Young Adults, Children

—Ariana Eunjung Cha, *Washington Post,* February 19, 2014

And only a year later, in the fall of 2011, a worldwide epidemic of dengue fever began in northern Africa. It soon spread to the Philippines and Puerto Rico, crossing the ocean in both directions. Finally it hit Brazil. By April of 2012 more than 50,000 people had been admitted to hospitals in Brazil. Five hundred newly infected people were being admitted each week.

Viral diseases such as these are emerging in new and potent forms everyplace on Earth. There are few medical treatments for them if a reliable vaccine does not exist. And for most of them it does not.

Welcome to the twenty-first century.

But We Won . . . Didn't We?

As you read in Chapter 1, when the first antibiotic, penicillin, came into common use in 1946, it was heralded as the beginning of the end for infectious diseases. And as each new antibiotic was discovered, and ever more diseases conquered, the voices proclaiming the end of infectious diseases grew louder. The success of antibiotics stimulated concerted medical assaults on epidemic viral diseases, primarily through the development and use of vaccines. The first widespread success was the polio vaccine.

Though it is not widely known, nearly everyone in a given region, when the polio virus spread to that area, became infected. It was, in fact, a very common virus with very few symptoms for most people. For more than 90 percent there were no symptoms at all. Only about 8 percent or so had mild to moderate symptoms, generally a self-limited flu-like condition (which nearly every virus causes). But for about 1 percent of the population, the virus entered the nervous system and those people developed what most people think of as polio. It caused shrunken limbs or paralysis or even, for some, the loss of the capacity to breathe on their own. For those, the rest of life was lived encased in a shell that raised and lowered the chest mechanically.

Oddly enough, given the memories that some people still have of the disease—and the fear it engendered prior to the late twentieth century—it was relatively uncommon. Polio epidemics, as such, were unknown throughout most of human history. But by 1910 major epidemics of the disease began to sweep the world. It became the scourge of the industrialized nations.

The success of antibiotics after World War II combined with the deep public fear of the disease drove a powerful medical movement in the search for a cure. And as with most viral diseases, the focus was on a vaccine. It didn't take long. The Salk vaccine was discovered in 1955, and, after trials, in 1962 it was licensed for widespread use. Worldwide epidemics soon faded from memory, and infections declined from the millions to the hundreds of thousands, and by 2007 to a mere 1,652, almost all in Asia and Africa. It was a powerful success story, and the belief that medical science could defeat all infectious diseases spread. For a while, it seemed that this belief might be well founded, for the next viral disease they attacked was smallpox.

Though they rarely get credit for it, it was Russian physicians in 1958 who began to press for a worldwide program to permanently eradicate smallpox. By 1967 the program was in full swing with some 250 million vaccinations occurring throughout the world each year. Within a decade, mostly due to the efforts of an American physician and epidemiologist, Donald Henderson, the last regions still endemic for the disease were cleared. And the world celebrated. For the first time a major human disease pathogen had been eradicated from the planet. (Though to be fair to the virus, both the Russians and the Americans kept just a little around, in case they needed it later—you know, for the kids.)

The triumph over smallpox was the apex of the success of the medical assault on microbial disease pathogens—though few knew it at the time. It was thought to be the beginning of the end for every disease pathogen on Earth. The hubris level, already immense by 1963, grew larger. If humans could defeat smallpox, they could defeat every virus on Earth. The word spread; the newspapers were filled with optimistic scenarios of a future without disease. Researchers were quoted extensively (as they still are) as saying that, soon, in just a few years, none of us would die from infectious diseases. Most people in the industrialized world accepted this at face value . . . as they still do. It is, regrettably, part of the utopian future-myth of science (especially medical science) that many people take for granted. But it never has, and never has had, much to do with reality. As physician and researcher Frank Ryan comments, "Perhaps it reflected, in part, a regrettable separation of clinicians from basic scientists."

> In fact those people whose living depended upon a study of microbes, of their potential and durability, were never deluded. A prescient few, such as René Dubos, warned us openly that the optimism was unjustified. But on the whole people were not inclined to listen. Most doctors, never mind members of the public, were infected with the prevailing overconfidence, hardly perceiving

> the growing threat of social changes to the "global village." They seemed unable to grasp the new potential afforded to a very ancient peril arising from world travel. . . . Today, as one after another of the dismissed plagues returns to haunt us, as new plagues every bit as deadly as anything seen in previous history threaten our species, it is obvious that the postwar years were an age of delusion. It was comforting, a very understandable delusion, but a delusion nonetheless.[2]

As it happens, the scientific and medical beliefs about the Earth and its interrelated life-forms, including bacteria and viruses, that have been widely spread are not very accurate. Lynn Margulis and Dorion Sagan, in their book *What Is Life?*, note that once "the germ theory of contagion finally caught on, it did so with a vengeance. Different types of bacteria were implicated in anthrax, gonorrhea, typhoid, and leprosy. Microbes, once amusing little anomalies, became demonized. . . . [They] became a virulent 'other' to be destroyed."[3] But there are many problems with this belief about microbes. Two stand out for me. The first comes from the particular medical paradigm in use in the West and the second from a very inaccurate, outmoded nineteenth-/early-twentieth-century view of nature.

The medical paradigm problem is simple enough, though it's rarely recognized for the problem it is. Specifically: Most physicians and medical researchers commonly speak of the "cause of death" when speaking of mortality. The assumption, deeply embedded within that communication, is that the bacteria or virus (or heart disease or stroke) caused the death. Even deeper is the communication that if all "causes" of death were defeated, then there would be no more death. As Harvard researcher and zoologist Richard Lewontin puts it, "The claims made by medicine imply this possibility without explicitly stating it. Medical scientists speak of 'preventing' deaths by curing disease, but the evidence is that death cannot be prevented, only postponed at best. Moreover, the postponement has not been as effective as is sometimes claimed during the last 50 years of great progress in physiology, cell biology, and medicine. . . . [The truth is] that although the proximate causes of death can be dealt with, death itself cannot.

So, there must be a cause of death as a *phenomenon*, as distinct from the individual cases."[4] In other words, if *every* "cause" of death were removed, in spite of what physicians (and news reports) say, there would still be death. Death is inherent in this place. The unstated and deeply buried assertion that microbes "cause" death is not only false, it stimulates people to view microbes as enemies, as participants in a war against us—and this is very far from the truth.

Bacteria and viruses are not a "virulent other." They are, instead, intimately interwoven into the underpinnings of life on this planet. They cannot be killed off without killing off every form of life on Earth. This is the great error of the nineteenth-/early-twentieth-century view of nature that continues to plague us. We are, counterintuitively and most upsettingly, only a form of bacteria ourselves—in extremely elegant, symbiogenic, innovative shapes. Bacteria are the foundation of every life-form on this planet. Had bacteria not developed resistance to antibiotics, all life on this planet would have already become extinct simply from the millions of tons of antibiotics now present in the environment.

With bacteria the paradigm problem is bad enough, but when viruses enter the picture, the complexity rises by orders of magnitude. Viruses are not and never have been parasites, though they may act as or seem to be parasites when we fall sick with one. They, in fact, perform highly elegant ecosystem functions—as everything on this planet does. Viruses, as Frank Ryan comments, "weave in and out of the genomes of every form of life on earth. As a result, terrestrial life [has] become a dense web of genetic interactions."[5]

DNA is not, and never has been, a computer program (and neither is RNA). It is, as Nobel Prize winner Barbara McClintock once noted, a living organ of the cell. DNA and RNA are both similar structures, and they are deeply interactive with the world around them. DNA is a double-stranded molecule, RNA is single-stranded, but both of them are intimately involved in the structural formation of life-forms. DNA contains information about the genetic development of living organisms. RNA is a messenger molecule used to carry genetic information that directs, in part, the synthesis of proteins, proteins that are needed for the structural formation of organisms. But again, these nucleic acids are not fixed in form. They change. We live in the midst of constant genetic rearrangements. And these gene rearrangements occur not only in response to impulses within the organism but also, as Barbara McClintock observed, to communications from the environment around it.

There is, in fact, no discrete inside and outside, no "us" and "them," even though it seems (within our nineteenth-century paradigm) that there is. The life-forms on this planet are living organisms, and that means they possess soft boundaries, *very* soft boundaries. There is a constant exchange (of energy, for example) between the inside and outside in all living systems. But to be more direct, there is a constant inflow and outflow of life through those soft boundaries. The nature of the ecological reality of this world demands it.

As Richard Lewontin observes,

> Even virus particles, which do not metabolize energy, can reproduce only when they become integrated into the metabolic apparatus of the cells they infect. At the time of viral replication, there is a complete abolition of the previously existing boundary between the virus and its cellular environment. . . . Organisms do not find already existent ecological niches to which they adapt, but are in the constant process of defining and remaking their environments. At every moment natural selection is operating to change the genetic composition of populations in response to the momentary environment, but as that composition changes it forces a concomitant change in the environment itself. Thus organism and environment are both causes and effects in a coevolutionary process. . . . Small changes in environment lead to small changes in the organism which, in turn, lead to small changes in the environment. . . . In general the organism and the environment must track each other continuously or life would long ago have become extinct.[6]

Specifically, viruses have the capacity to enter cells, snip off sections of DNA (or RNA), and weave them into their own genetic structure. They can then weave those sections, as well as sections of their own genome, into other living organisms. One of their main functions in fact is the genetic intermingling of all life-forms on Earth. Or as Frank Ryan puts it, "Viruses are vehicles for genetic exchange between the disparate species that make up the matrix of life on earth."[7] Our genome, as that of all life on this planet, contains snippets of the genetic codes of multiple other life-forms. It also contains snippets of viral genes. Our forms, our shapes, are an expression of a communication that has been ongoing since life has been. We *are* the enemy we have been fighting.

In short, the perspectives of most scientists at the beginning of the antibiotic era were limited, more limited than even the most prescient knew. And the view of the world that they disseminated was deeply flawed. Viruses are deeply interwoven into the ecological matrix of this planet, and they serve functions that are essential. Further, they are extremely adaptable. They can alter their structure very rapidly and take on new forms seemingly at will—all based on their analysis of the environment that surrounds them. They are highly intelligent. They are not in fact stupid. But we certainly were (and are) when we thought them so.

The paradigm of medicine that emerged in the twentieth century was wrong, and we are now paying the price for applying it so comprehensively. We now face the emergence of epidemics more devastating than any known before. If *we* are to adapt, we have to see with different eyes, understand through a different paradigm. We have to realize that viruses are not what we thought them to be. We have to learn to see them as they are.

Viruses

To begin with, if you have ever read much about viruses, or if you have looked closely at some of the words I have used while writing this, you might have noted that many people refer to viruses as "particles." There is a widely held belief among scientists that viruses are not alive. Many insist that they are merely organic structures that interact with living organisms. Some say they are "organisms at the edge of life" but really aren't organisms in any meaningful sense. This is, they say, because they lack a cellular structure, don't have their own metabolism, and can only reproduce *inside* cellular structures—and besides they don't use cellular division to do it either. If asked where the definition of life comes from, a definition that precludes viruses, biologists will admit, under duress, that people invented the definition but nevertheless, it's true anyway. (This explains why manufacturers put a warning label on those sun shields people occasionally place in the front windows of their cars to protect the interior from the sun: "Warning: Do not drive with shield in place.")

Oddly enough some bacteria such as rickettsia and chlamydia are considered bacteria and thus living despite having similar limitations. (And the Earth is not alive, though it may "act" like a living system. Why? Because it consumes its own waste, which, as everyone knows, living organisms *never* do . . . apparently they have not met my neighbor's dog.)

There are a lot of viruses on this planet. Estimates are that the Earth contains 10^{31} viruses, that is, a 10 with 31 zeros after it. Technically (for wonks) that is somewhere between a nonillion and a decillion (though if you just say bajillion you are close enough). Essentially—a whole lot. And there are multitudes of different kinds. In every 200 liters of water (about 50 gallons or the contents of a typical hot water tank) some 5,000 different viral genotypes are present. There are viruses in the coldest, most inhospitable parts of this planet and viruses inside boiling hot springs. There are viruses high in the atmosphere and in the deepest wells on Earth. They live on top of mountains and in the farthest depths of the ocean. And, sometimes, they even travel into space. They are a part of life on this planet; there is no avoiding them.

Viruses, unlike bacteria, have no nucleus and no cell wall. They are the minimum of life honed to a structural simplicity. Though there are many kinds, in general, a virus is a strand of DNA or RNA surrounded by a mathematically elegant polyhedron, called a capsid, whose shape is virus specific. For what are called "enveloped" viruses, the capsid is surrounded by one or more protein envelopes. This simplified structure makes them different than bacteria, for example, but no less alive. They *are* a unique life-form (but that is no reason to discriminate against them). They are very much like seeds (or spores): They only grow when they find the right soil in which to do so. And like seeds, even though in a suspended state, they constantly monitor the exterior world around them.

The surface of the viral protein envelope is studded with receptors, specific kinds of sensory organs that tell viruses about their surroundings. Viruses use these elegant sensory organs to analyze the environment in which they find themselves and to help them find the cells they are most suited for. As physician and researcher Frank Ryan comments,

> Viruses have a kind of sensation that could be classed as intermediate between a rudimentary smell or touch. . . . They have a way of detecting the chemical composition of cell surfaces. . . . This gives a virus the most exquisite ability to sense the right cell surfaces [allowing it to find its unique host cell]. It recognizes them through a perception in three-dimensional surface chemistry.[8]

Viruses have a highly sophisticated capacity to sense the environment around them, to determine its nature, to find the cellular organisms within which they can most easily reproduce, and to then stimulate the organisms in which those cells reside in order to spread the viruses to new hosts. And they are very good at surviving. They can analyze the nature of the immune response that occurs against them and they can alter themselves—or alter the host immune defense itself—in order to avoid it. They can *reason* by any useful definition of the term, that is: analyze inputs and create new behaviors based on what they have determined the meaning of those inputs to be.

Viruses are typed in a number of ways: by size or shape, presence or absence of an enclosing capsule (not all have one), whether DNA or RNA based (and from that whether single or double stranded, positive or negative sense), their type of protein structure, and their manner of replication. DNA viruses are fairly reliable as viruses go because they have a kind of "copy-check" mechanism that RNA viruses lack. This means that when a DNA virus is making more of itself within a host cell, it uses a biofeedback loop to make sure the copies of itself are reasonably accurate. In contrast an RNA virus can't. It tends to make a whole lot of copies that vary, sometimes a great deal, from the original. Some of these copy differences are initiated intentionally by RNA viruses to increase their genetic variation and, hence, survivability in the host. Because of this, while it is often possible to come up with a lasting vaccine for a DNA virus, it is very hard, if not impossible, to make one for an RNA virus. This also makes RNA viruses very hard to treat with pharmaceuticals; they, like bacteria, begin creating solutions to synthetic drugs the moment they encounter one. Evidence indicates that the mutation rate of the hepatitis C virus, for example, accelerates in response to interferon and ribavirin therapy in much the same way that bacterial alteration occurs in the presence of antibiotics. Infection with an RNA virus like West Nile or Japanese encephalitis is actually quite different than infection with a DNA virus.

> We live in an era of rapidly changing global landscapes and local environments. Viruses with RNA as their genetic material can quickly adapt to and exploit these varying conditions. . . . It comes as no surprise, then, that several prominent recent examples of emerging or re-emerging viruses are caused by RNA viruses.
>
> —*Stuart Nichol et al.*, "Emerging Viral Diseases"

While DNA viruses make billions more of themselves, RNA viruses make billions of similar but not identical viruses. It is something like a swarm of honeybees—all similar but all different. In fact it is much more accurate to think of an RNA infection as infection by a viral swarm. The ones most similar to each other are the ones that die off when the human immune system is first activated or a pharmaceutical drug that can recognize them is used. This leaves the others free to multiply unchecked, and they multiply very fast indeed (some viruses producing a new generation every *minute*) while still making subtle changes in each new virus produced.

There is also evidence that both DNA and RNA viruses, like bacteria, share information among themselves in order to remain unaffected by medical treatments or immune systems. Similar viruses will actively share genetic structure to create very difficult-to-treat infections. Influenza viruses (for instance) specifically (and intentionally) both rearrange their genetic structures and insert entirely new genes within themselves on a regular basis in order to remain invisible to the human immune system. And they gather these new gene sequences from pigs and birds in Asia. This is why a new vaccine is needed every year for the flu.

Viruses, when not in a living cell, go into a state of hibernation much like plant seeds. In this state of dormancy they move with air currents, in water, or simply rest dormant on the ground until they come into contact with a life-form that contains the cells they need to awaken from their long sleep. At that moment a virus's first task is to get inside the new host organism, bypass its protective mechanisms, and find the proper host cell. Viruses use highly elegant analysis to address these challenges; they actually begin experimenting with new combinations of genes to adapt to the environment they face. Most of them have also generated a genetic structure that facilitates their entry into other host organisms after an initial infection begins. The rabies virus, for instance, affects a part of the brain that then causes uncontrolled biting. At the same time, the virus swarms in its billions into the saliva of infected animals. Then, every time the animal bites something, the virus is transmitted to a new host. Influenza, and other respiratory viruses, enter respiratory droplets and then stimulate coughing or sneezing. Those droplets are then breathed in by new hosts. And still other viruses, spread by mosquitoes, flood into the blood and there stimulate the release of chemicals through the host skin surface that calls mosquitoes to the infected host so that the virus can be picked up and spread to others. Viruses are very good at getting from *here* to *there*.

Viruses spread by ticks or mosquitoes take advantage of the compounds in the arthropod saliva to facilitate their entry into the new host. The salival compounds reduce certain immune responses in the host to allow the arthropod to feed and often anesthetize the bite location as well. The lowered immune responses at that location allow the viruses to enter the new host in a place where there will be little resistance. Once inside the viruses will make their way to the draining lymph node nearest the bite location and be carried to the spleen via the lymph. There they will begin altering the host's immune function, reducing the capacity of immune cells to recognize and kill invading microbes. Once that occurs, the viruses will catch a ride on immune cells, macrophages or monocytes usually, and begin spreading throughout the body. This is common for encephalitis viruses, for example. They will then travel in the lymph to the barrier between the brain and the rest of the body, release compounds that make the barrier more porous, enter the brain, and find the cells they really prefer: brain neurons.

Other viruses enter through being inhaled (influenza) or through sex (HIV) or through being eaten on food (enteroviruses). Once in the body, they hitch rides on whatever cells they have developed a taste for (usually immune cells, for those cells travel *everywhere*) and actively seek out their preferred location. Such is the case with HIV, which views T4 lymphocytes as the perfect host cells, or the Epstein-Barr virus, which has an affinity for human B cells, or the Japanese encephalitis virus, which loves monocytes.

To hitch rides, a virus uses chemotactic compounds that allow it to stick to its preferred "taxi" cell. The receptors on the surface of the virus fool the cell into thinking it is a compatible protein that has attached, and through a series of chemical communications, the virus gets the cell to let it inside. Basically, it gets the cell's confidence, then abuses it. From there the virus is carried everyplace it might need to go in the body. Once near its preferred location, it leaves its ride, attaches to the cell that is most specific for it, and once again fools the cell into taking it inside. Now it begins to replicate in its millions.

Once inside the primary habitat cell, the virus sheds its protein coat and begins taking over the cell. First it stops the cell from dying, which infected cells are programmed to do, and there it remains, protected from the rest of the immune system. It then breaks off pieces of itself and sends them into the nucleus of the cell, which is then tricked into making copies of the virus, using the viral proteins as a template. These new viral particles exit the nucleus, travel to the interior of the cell wall, and bubble out (viral budding, they call it). The cell dies during this process and bursts apart, and the viruses take up parts of the cell membrane and make themselves new viral protein coats with receptors for new host cells. And it all happens very quickly.

> The present period of unprecedented ecological change and the growing economic and social crises that are driving vast movements of hosts are together contributing to the resurgence of old pests and the appearance of new ones. Important components in this rapid evolution are the vulnerabilities of ecosystems and instabilities in climate.
>
> —*Paul Epstein,* "Emerging Diseases and Ecosystem Instability: New Threats to Public Health"

Thus the ancient struggle begins: finding out which is in better shape—the organism's immune system or the replicating virus. If the virus is particularly strong or if the immune system is compromised in any way, the virus can really take hold and illness, sometimes severe illness, is inevitable.

Emerging Pathogenic Viruses

Similarly to antibiotic-resistant bacteria, many of the viruses long thought conquered are making comebacks. They are doing this through genetic rearrangements, through learned resistance to antivirals, and, most of all, because of changes in the world in which all of us live. And those changes are profound.

Here are some of the major alterations affecting the planet that researchers have identified as being behind the emergence of so many new (and old) pathogenic viruses. There is no place on the planet that has escaped them.

- **Demographic changes:** human population and refugee increases, accelerated mobility, worldwide urbanization, increasing population density in confined spaces such as inner cities and prisons
- **Medical care and technology:** medical-related infections in hospitals, concentrated microbial intermingling in hospitals and nursing homes, blood transfusions, organ transplantation, reuse of medical equipment, pharmaceutical contaminants, viral and antibiotic resistance
- **Economic and commercial trends:** overly extensive industrial agriculture with the resultant damage of ecosystem homeodynamis; worldwide disbursement of commercial food animals, food plants, and agricultural pharmaceuticals
- **Ecosystem disturbance:** deforestation, waterway disturbances, reduction in predator populations, destruction of wild plant populations
- **Climatic changes:** disruptions in climate homeodynamis by anthropogenic factors such as global warming, CO_2 increases, and pollutant gases

Viruses have lived for millions of years in balance with their host species (such as wild bee or buffalo populations). The disruption of healthy ecosystems by human incursions and the resultant loss of host species and their habitats stimulates viruses to jump species. And one of the species into which they jump is us (or the animals that survive well with us: pigeons, mice, pigs, and chickens—from whom they then easily move into us). After all, there are a lot more of *us* now (and our food animals) than any other large life-form; we aren't that hard to find. As a matter of fact, many of us live in the same places the viruses' former hosts did. And a home is a home. Our bodies are not all that different from the other animals on this planet. It is a simple adjustment for the viruses to make *us* their new hosts.

Some of the most common emerging, resistant, or newly virulent viruses are dengue virus (which infects millions worldwide every year), hepatitis C, enterovirus 71, HIV, and the eight members of the herpes family that affect humans, including cytomegalovirus and Epstein-Barr virus. But by far the ones that are causing the most worldwide concern (outside HIV) are the influenza and encephalitis viruses.

Influenza, which often seems a somewhat mild disease in many people's minds, just another "case of the flu," is actually a very potent viral pathogen. Epidemiologists have been warning, with increasing insistence, that a worldwide pandemic similar to the one that covered the globe in 1918, a pandemic that infected more than 500 million people and caused some 100 million deaths, is due soon. Our factory farms (in whose pigs and chickens the viruses increase their virulence), our growing populations, the hubris and outdated nature of our medical system, and the intelligence of viruses make it certain that a pandemic strain will emerge again. It is only a matter of time. As Robert Heinlein once said, "Population problems have a horrible way of solving themselves."

The viruses are learning. We should, too.

4

COMMON VIRAL ILLNESSES AND HOW TO TREAT THEM

Persistent host-specific viral agents are the origin of emerging acute epidemic disease following adaptation of that virus to new host species. . . . These acute viruses have a high dependence on host population structure as described by the apparently accurate mathematical models that resemble predator-prey dynamics in which the viruses act as predators on their host prey. . . . Acute human influenza A represents a host species jump of a persisting viral agent of aquatic birds.

—Luis Villarreal et al., "Acute and Persistent Viral Life Strategies and Their Relationship to Emerging Diseases"

The major animal reservoirs of Influenza A are migratory birds and the majority of all the possible combinations of HA-NA subtypes have been isolated from them.

—Andrew Pekosz and Gregory Glass, "Emerging Viral Diseases"

Most of us think of the flu as a fairly minor disease, and for most of us, it is. At worst we lie in bed for a week or so, feeling miserable. But for the old and the very young, the flu can be deadly; it kills those with the weakest or least developed immune systems, some 30,000 people a year in the United States. But sometimes a real pandemic happens and the death rate rises. It has never risen more than it did in 1918.

The 1918 world influenza pandemic is the most deadly plague that human beings have *ever* experienced. It began in 1918, just as war was drawing to a close, and lasted until December of 1920. World War I (which ended in 1918) killed some 17 million people. In contrast, the influenza pandemic, spread around the world by returning soldiers, killed six times as many in half the time—perhaps as many as 130 million people. The first wave of the pandemic began in January of 1918, and it was fairly routine. People became ill, but only the very old and very young died; it was, so far, a pretty typical flu. But the virus soon mutated. And the second wave? It was deadly. It killed those with the strongest immune systems. Half of those who died were between the ages of 20 and 40; nearly all were under age 65. And it killed them by the millions.

Instead of the usual respiratory infection, with death occurring as the lungs filled with fluid, massive hemorrhages took place. The infected lung cells, and those nearby, damaged by the virus-stimulated cytokine storm (see page 103 for more on cytokines), literally burst open from the inflammation. And unlike most viral influenzas, this one did not stay confined to the respiratory system. It spread to the GI tract, the brain, and every mucous membrane system in the body. First it destroyed the infected mucosal epithelial cells, then the blood vessels that fed them inflamed and burst open. Bleeding was extensive from the nose, stomach, and intestines; hemorrhages from the skin and ears were common. The infected literally bled out. And nothing physicians tried would stop it.[1]

To understand the impact, consider the fact that, in a world reeling from war, *one-third* of the entire world's population contracted the disease—more than 500 million people. In some places half the population was bedridden. As troops demobilized, the ships returning them home from war stopped at hundreds of ports along the way, and the infection spread across the globe. On the islands of Western Samoa 90 percent of the population fell ill—*simultaneously*. Thirty percent of the men, 22 percent of the women, and 10 percent of the children died.

In an attempt to stop the infection, port quarantines were put into effect around the world. Most were too late to do any good. One out of every three persons on Earth fell ill. One out of every five of those died. Five percent of the total world population—one out of every 20 people—did not survive the pandemic. Within the first 6 months 25 million people died, more than were killed in 5 years of war. Entire towns and cities were shut down.

There were few professionals to help the sick. Doctors and nurses were the first responders, and they succumbed immediately. (The morticians followed soon after.) The infected filled the hospitals, school gymnasiums, auditoriums—every large building that could hold masses of people was pressed into service. The beds and the floors were awash in blood as the people died . . . and hemorrhaged by the hundreds and the thousands while doing it. And the bodies piled up. Steam shovels were brought in and mass graves dug—row after row after row of identically sized holes stretching across empty fields in a terrible mockery of industrial expediency. Then the trucks came, the bodies piled high on the wooden beds, and the masked workers dropped them in, hour by hour, day by day, month after month. And behind them, the steam shovels covered them over . . . one by one, day by day, for the 2 terrible years of the pandemic. There were few coffins and often no headstones. The system was completely overwhelmed. Not even a full century of the Black Plague had killed like this. In the history of human habitation of Earth, never had a disease spread so quickly around the world nor killed so many in so short a time. Only one place on Earth reported *no* infections: the tiny island of Marajó near Brazil in South America. And then, as inexplicably as it had begun, in a 1-month period of time, between November and December of 1920, the pandemic ended, simultaneously, around the globe.

Much effort has been expended in recent years in an attempt to understand what made that particular influenza strain so much more deadly than all the others people have known. It turns out that there were two interrelated events that came together in just the right way at just the right time in a terrible serendipity of the universe. From that intermingling came the worst pandemic the human species has ever experienced.

The first event was the emergence of a new strain of influenza at just the right time in human history. An analysis of the viral genome from 1918 has revealed that a new influenza strain had jumped species (from birds) just prior to 1913. By 1915 the virus had split into two types: one infecting pigs, the other humans. The second event was the war itself, which began with perfect timing in 1914.

Normally, when people fall ill with the flu, they go home and rest. The soldiers could not, and the new influenza strain rapidly spread throughout the troops on both sides of the conflict. Constrained in cramped, unhealthy conditions, in hospital tents and in trenches, the soldiers were a perfect breeding ground for the virus. And sometime between 1915 and late 1917 the virus mutated again, this time into a form that could powerfully infect just that kind of population: the young. Then, the war over, the soldiers, millions of whom were infected, were crowded together in ships (there was no air travel then) that sailed from port to port to port, infecting as they went. Once home port was reached, the soldiers took trains, buses, and cars to their individual towns and cities. And the virus went with them, infecting everyone.

Re-created forms of the strain, patiently assembled in laboratories, when given to primates, have been found to generate the same symptoms as those described, in depth, by the physicians who treated the 1918 pandemic. An analysis of the physiological damage that occurs found that the reason the disease is so severe is that the virus creates a tremendously potent cytokine cascade in the body—a cytokine storm. A perfect storm. These cytokines are immunoregulatory proteins stimulated by the body's innate immune system in response to infection. The cytokine cascade is how the body attempts to kill off the invading pathogen. But this was much more than the usual immune response. The immune reaction was extreme, somewhere between 100 and 1,000 times what would be normal in those who were infected. And that overreaction, much more pronounced in those with strong immune systems, is what killed so many so quickly.

It is just this kind of influenza pandemic that epidemiologists and viral researchers fear will emerge once more. Given the current population density (and the crowding in prisons, nursing homes, hospitals, day care centers, and inner cities), the ecological disruptions that are occurring worldwide, the number of viruses that are jumping species, the rate of mutation, *and* the vast and very rapid movement of people via air travel, they say it is only a matter of time. And in spite of the many advances in medical technology, there is very little that modern medicine can do to treat a widespread pandemic of deadly influenza. Pharmaceutical antivirals are only partially effective for this kind of infection, and the stocks of those antivirals are insufficient to deal with a true pandemic. And vaccines? Vaccines take time.

Flu vaccines have to be made for the specific virus that emerges *in that year*. This means that the disease will already be moving throughout the world before production even begins. And if it is a true pandemic of a deadly strain, by the time the vaccine is produced and shipped (normally a 3- to 6-month process), the infrastructure of the world will already be failing. The health-care workers, hospitals, and transportation workers will be the first to fall. Then the morticians and cemetery workers. The system will begin to shut down. Quarantines, forcing people to stay in their homes, will be put into effect to try to stop the spread. And people will survive as best they can, just as they always have.

The Influenza Virus

The influenza virus is a member of the Orthomyxoviridae family. It is an RNA virus, and that means it alters its genetic structure very quickly. That is why a new flu shot is needed every year (for those in the Western world who have such things available). The old vaccine can only help prevent infection by the strain that has emerged in that particular year. The next year, it is not the same virus, merely a similar one. Influenza viruses spread around the world every year in seasonal epidemics; 250,000 to 500,000 people die from them each time.

About one-third of people who are infected remain asymptomatic; the rest get some degree of the "flu." The first symptoms are usually a feeling of being cold or achy and perhaps the beginnings of a fever. High fever alternating with severe chills sets in as the infection spreads. As the virus enters the lungs and sinus tissues, mucous congestion begins. Coughing, body aches, fatigue, headache, and irritated eyes, nose, and throat are common. Some people will have diarrhea and abdominal pain. Vomiting. Sometimes. Yes.

The symptoms of the infection usually begin the third day after infection. But the virus is already well established by then. It starts replicating the second day, then begins "shedding" viral particles that are released in increasing numbers for the next 5 to 7 days. The higher the fever, the more viral organisms that are being released. Children are *extremely* infectious compared to adults, with very high viral loads. They also tend to have very high fevers.

As the virus invades the lungs, it stimulates inflammation in the tissues. The lung cells, filled with viruses, soon bulge outward and explode—the essence of viral shedding. Then the virus stimulates coughing, spreading the virus to new hosts via respiratory droplets. Pneumonia, a severe inflammation of the lungs accompanied by massive fluid retention and an inability to breathe, is the main cause of death. People, in essence, drown.

There are three different groups of influenza viruses, denoted A, B, and C. Influenza A is the most virulent. Influenza B is a relatively stable virus and mutates much more slowly than A. Most people develop, in childhood, at least some immunity to it; it is much less dangerous. Influenza C is fairly rare. It does infect people, sometimes severely, but it usually causes only a mild illness, generally in children. When people talk about an influenza pandemic, what they are talking about is influenza A in one of its many genetically altered forms. The 1918 pandemic was caused by an influenza A strain.

There have been numerous pandemics of influenza over the years, each caused by a different strain of the virus. The one in 1918 was the beginning of the modern influenza pandemic era; such pandemics were much less common before then. There was a long rest after 1918. Since 1957, however, they have been occurring with greater frequency.

The most dangerous strains, currently, are H1N1, which caused the flu pandemic of 1918; H2N2, which caused the Asian flu pandemic in 1957; H3N2, which caused the Hong Kong flu pandemic in 1968; and a relatively new one, H5N1, known as avian or bird flu, which caused a pandemic in 2004. Then H1N1 came again. It was the source of the swine flu pandemic in 2009 and is a modified descendant of the 1918 H1N1 strain.

The influenza virus alters its genetic structure rather significantly every year by passing through both pigs and birds. And on that trip it exchanges genetic material with other viruses and reworks its own. Then it spreads around the world again by plane and boat, rail and car, infecting millions, causing what we call the yearly flu season. But every so often it develops a much more virulent strain, sometimes through unique genetic rearrangements, sometimes through species jumps, sometimes through both. The Asian flu pandemic in 2004 was a species jump. The swine flu epidemic of 2009 was a unique genetic rearrangement. It occurred when the virus took advantage of giant agribusiness animal crowding.

Viral geneticists have traced the lineage of the 2009 swine flu epidemic, a virulent H1N1 strain, to an H3N2 strain that emerged in 1998 in U.S. factory farms, specifically huge hog farms in which the animals are so tightly packed together that they literally cannot move. This H3N2 strain combined with another swine strain, a European H1N2 variant, rearranged genetic material into a new and very potent H1N1 form, and then emerged into the human population. The earliest infections occurred in La Gloria, Veracruz, Mexico, just adjacent to a huge hog farm. The workers became infected with the new strain, went home, infected others, many of whom traveled to other cities and towns, and the pandemic began. And it was particularly deadly for those who were infected. Among those hospitalized, depending on location, up to 31 percent were in intensive care units, and as many as 46 percent of those receiving intensive care died.

One of the main fears that epidemiologists and viral geneticists have is the possibility of a combined swine and avian flu strain. The crowding of human food animals, similar to the crowding of soldiers in trenches in World War I, continually allows for the emergence of potently virulent strains. Chicken farms, in which unique avian flu strains can emerge, and hog farms, in which unique swine strains can emerge, are perfectly positioned to allow the combination of the two into one potent, and very deadly, influenza strain. This kind of combined strain can then pass easily into farm workers and thence into the population at large.

Researchers have found that, indeed, the H3N2 swine flu virus easily combines with H5N1 strains of avian flu. When that occurs, a tremendously pathogenic form of the virus emerges. It is, they insist, only a matter of time until it occurs on its own. In fact, studies of pigs on large farms adjacent to poultry farms have found such viral combinations already infecting pigs. That combined viral strain has not infected people . . . yet.

Infection Dynamics and the Cytokine Cascade

Cytokines are physiological signaling molecules produced by the body for a variety of reasons. They are produced in the largest numbers during infections. Cytokines (and their cousins, chemokines) are generally part of the innate (rather than the adapted) immune system. They are intended to respond to incursions into our bodies by viruses and bacteria. Another way to think of them is as inflammatory molecules. They cause various sorts of inflammation in the body—they are why, when you cut yourself, the wound gets red and tender and swells. The cytokines rushing to the area create conditions in which many bacteria and viruses find it difficult to survive. Unfortunately for us, bacteria and viruses have also learned how to use our own immune responses for their purposes. They subvert them, quite often, to facilitate their infection of the body *and* their destruction of certain areas of the body. This facilitates their reproduction and allows them to gather nutrients. Influenza viruses love the lungs, and it is where they cause the greatest damage.

Unlike encephalitis viruses, which love brain neurons but have to find their way to the brain after being injected into people by mosquitoes, influenza viruses don't have to work nearly so hard. They are taken to the location they like best simply because we need to breathe.

Once inhaled, the viruses begin attaching to lung epithelial cells. They use a kind of agglutinin (a substance that glues things to itself—its name shares a root with the English word "glue"), a hemagglutinin, to bind to what are called sialic acid linkages on the surface of airway epithelial cells. (This is one mechanism by which plants such as Chinese skullcap and ginger stop influenza infections; they are hemagglutinin inhibitors.) All viruses do this in their own way; they have an affinity for a unique receptor on the surface of specific cells, and in one way or another they get to that location and those particular cells. Once there, they attach to that part of the cells. In a sense they use that part of the host cells' membrane as a docking port.

As soon as it is attached to a cell, the virus begins to alter the permeability of the cell wall, inducing alterations in the cell's cytoskeleton and initiating endocytosis. In other words, it makes the cell surface more soft, causes the skeletal structure of the cell to bend apart, and tricks the cell into taking the virus inside it where it can't be found by the immune system. It does this by using a particular kind of enzyme, neuraminidase—which is sometimes also called a sialidase because such enzymes catalyze, or break apart, the sialic acid linkages on the host cell surface. This is why neuraminidase inhibitors (such as Tamiflu, i.e., oseltamivir) are effective in the treatment of influenza; they inhibit the ability of the virus to enter host cells. This stops the infection. (Chinese skullcap, elder, licorice, rhodiola, ginger, isatis, *Lespedeza bicolor*, *Angelica keiskei*, *Amorpha fruticosa*, quercetin, *Alpinia zerumbet*, *Erythrina addisoniae*, and *Cleistocalyx operculatus* are all neuraminidase inhibitors.) Neuraminidase inhibitors are effective against both influenza A and B strains.

During the process of endocytosis, the virus stimulates the cell to create what is called a vacuole, essentially a sealed bubble that will be held inside the cell. Cells do this to sequester substances that can damage them. Microbes have learned to use such vacuoles for their own purposes, usually to protect the virus or bacteria from intracellular antimicrobial actions.

The virus uses its hemagglutinin to bind itself to the inside of the vacuole membrane, where it opens a pore to the cell's cytoplasm, i.e., its interior spaces. To do this, the virus uses what is called the M2 ion channel—ion channels are tiny pores in cells that allow charged molecules to enter and exit cells, bringing food in and allowing waste out. Using an M2 inhibitor blocks this process and literally stops the virus from replicating. (Lomatium is one of the most potent M2 inhibitors known, stronger than the pharmaceutical amantadine.) Use of the M2 channel is specific to the influenza A virus, which is why the development of blockers for it was considered crucial. Unfortunately, the extensive use of chemical M2 inhibitors such as amantadine in poultry farms has now created nearly complete resistance to them in all influenza A strains.

Once the pore is open, the virus disassembles itself and releases viral RNA and core proteins into the cytoplasm. (Chinese skullcap inhibits this kind of viral RNA release.) The core proteins and viral RNA form a complex that is taken into the nucleus of the cell, where the cell is stimulated to begin making copies of the viral RNA (each slightly different). The new viral RNA is combined with other newly manufactured virus components such as neuraminidase and hemagglutinin and assembled into new viruses. These attach to the inside of the host cell membrane, a bulge forms in the membrane, and the new viruses are expressed (viral budding or shedding) into the extracellular matrix surrounding the cell.

The cell is taken over by the virus in this process, its own components depleted during the creation of new viruses. Once its resources are gone, the cell dies and the newly created viruses move on to new host cells, beginning the process all over again.

The alveolar epithelial cells are specific sites for this process to occur. The alveoli are tiny sacs that are the terminal end of the respiratory tree. The air we breathe travels throughout the bronchial tree, eventually emerging into the alveoli, where the oxygen transfuses across very thin membranes into the blood. This is how our bodies remain oxygenated. In the cells lining those tiny sacs the viruses breed. They cause extreme inflammation, or swelling, of the cells in that location with resulting edema (fluid accumulation). All the infected cells burst open and die as new viruses are made. So, fewer alveoli are functional. Breathing is more difficult, and the infected person has much less energy because oxygen is not making it into the blood in sufficient quantities. (This is why hospitals sometimes give the infected oxygen.) Pneumonia is when this process becomes severe, the sacs filling with increasing amounts of fluid while there are fewer and fewer functional alveoli.

Throughout the cellular infection and replication process, the virus is also stimulating the release of cytokines by the cell. These cytokines make the tight junctions between cells (and the cellular membranes) more porous and allow easier movement of viral particles through the extracellular matrix (and into the cells themselves). The cytokines are also stimulated in just such a way as to keep the parts of the immune system that can kill the viruses suppressed for as long as possible.

Toll-like receptors (TLRs) are pattern recognition receptors that can identify different types of microbes. The virus particles stimulate TLR3, which begins inducing the release of nuclear factor kappa-B (NF-κB) cytokines. NF-κB is an upstream cytokine, meaning that it is a powerful initiator of other inflammatory cytokines. NF-κB *begins* very specific types of cytokine cascades. Other types of initiators such as RIG-1, NOD2, and MDA5 are also released as part of the body's reaction to a viral infection. Normally, these would strongly stimulate type 1 interferon (IFN) production (IFN-α and IFN-ß). And influenza viruses are generally very susceptible to these interferons. However, the influenza virus uses a protein, the NS1 protein, which blocks the induction of type 1 IFNs long enough to get established in the body.

(Upregulating the production of type I interferons with herbs such as licorice will help reduce the severity of the infection.) The virus also inhibits dendritic cell maturation and activation, lowering the response levels of T and B cells. (Increasing T cell counts is particularly effective in reducing influenza severity. Licorice, elder, red root, and zinc are specific for this.) These cells are part of the adaptive immune response; suppressing them protects the virus from attack. The body response also stimulates the release of type III interferons, to which the virus is less susceptible and which it does nothing to suppress. These interferons have general, rather than specific, antiviral qualities and are upregulated within 3 to 6 hours of infection. This is what begins causing the general flu-like feelings that presage a full-blown flu episode. The virus itself does not make you feel "fluey."

During this same time period, the infected airway cells (tracheobronchial and alveolar epithelial cells) begin generating specific cytokines and chemokines: interleukin-1 beta (IL-1ß), IL-6, IL-18 (which causes spikes in IFN-γ production), C-C chemokine ligand 5 (CCL5, also known as RANTES, "regulated and normal T cell expressed and secreted"), C-X-C chemokine ligand 10 (CXCL10). Then, some 12 to 16 hours later, other cytokines are produced: tumor necrosis factor alpha (TNF-α), IL-8, and CCL2 (also known as monocyte chemoattractant protein-1 or MCP-1). The expressed cytokines make the epithelial structures more porous. This assists faster viral penetration of the cells. It also stimulates the migration of immune cells to the sites of infection.

Interferon-gamma (IFN-γ) is a type 2 interferon, sometimes called macrophage-activating factor. It is this IFN that is crucial in the cytokine overinflammation that occurs during severe influenza. By stimulating it, the virus initiates a positive feedback loop in the cytokine process that leads, in severe infections, to cytokine storms.

CCL2 causes the migration of blood-derived monocytes into the alveolar airspaces. TNF-α and IL-1ß upregulate adhesion molecules (which include intercellular adhesion molecule 1, a.k.a. ICAM-1, and E-selectin) on the surface of the endothelial cells that line blood vessels. This helps the endothelial lining become more porous and stimulates the transendothelial migration of neutrophils to those locations. TNF-α induces monocyte and neutrophil movement across the epithelium through ICAM-1 and VCAM-1 (vascular cell adhesion molecule-1) upregulation. The consequence of this is increasing amounts of white-blood-cell-filled mucus in the lungs. (This is what we cough up during a flu infection.)

The size of the drainage lymph nodes in the lungs begins to increase. This helps, during a healthy resolution of infection, to drain more of the fluids from the lungs, preventing suffocation. Within those lymph nodes, areas called the germinal centers increase their size and development. The germinal centers are the sites where B lymphocytes are produced and are differentiated in order to attack the specific infection that is occurring. This is part of the adaptive humoral immune response. These lymph node locations (as well as those in peripheral tissues) can become overfull during severe infections, slowing drainage and healthy adaptive immune responses. They can also, during severe influenza infections, be specifically attacked and damaged so that they do not function at all. This is a contributor to the mortality that sometimes occurs during cytokine storms. (This is why herbs such as red root, inmortal, and pleurisy root are useful; they all support the lymph structures in the lungs and periphery. Red root—*Ceanothus* spp.—is particularly useful in the periphery for spleen and lymph enlargement and lymph drainage; inmortal—*Asclepias asperula*—is specific for optimizing lymph drainage from the lungs; pleurisy root—*Asclepias tuberosa*—is specific for reducing inflammation in the pleurae and lungs. They can be used interchangeably to some extent.) The lymph centers in the lungs are heavily affected during influenza, much more so than the periphery.

Similarly to many viruses, while influenza viruses reproduce most efficiently in the alveolar epithelial cells, they can also infect other cells, specifically dendritic cells, monocytes, macrophages, neutrophils, T cells, B cells, and natural killer (NK) cells. In response to being infected those cells also begin releasing cytokines and chemokines:

IFNs, IL-1α and IL-1ß, IL-6, TNF-α, CXCL8, CCL2 (MCP-1), CCL3 (a.k.a. macrophage inflammatory protein-1 alpha, or MIP-1α), CCL4, CXCL9, and CXCL10 through the ERK-1, ERK-2 (extracelluar-signal-regulated kinase 1 and 2), p38 MAPK (p38 mitogen-activated protein kinase), and JNK (c-Jun N-terminal kinase) pathways.

TNF-α, IL-1ß, IL-6, and IFN-γ are responsible for most of the negative effects of the cytokine cascade. Mice that are unable to produce TNF-α consistently show decreased mortality, a reduced symptom picture, and less severe course of the disease. This holds true even if they are infected with the reconstituted, and very virulent, 1918 virus. Inhibition of TNF-α (especially) and IL-1ß has been found to significantly reduce the cytokine-based inflammation that occurs during influenza, alleviating symptoms and inhibiting viral spread. (Herbs specific for inhibiting TNF-α are kudzu, Chinese senega root, Chinese skullcap, elder, ginger, houttuynia, licorice, boneset, and cordyceps. Herbs specific for inhibiting IL-1ß are Japanese knotweed, Chinese senega root, Chinese skullcap, cordyceps, kudzu, and boneset.)

The virus can also inhibit the production of macrophages over time. This occurs because, over time, macrophages will begin producing anti-inflammatory cytokines such as IL-4 and IL-10. Once the bodily system is macrophage-depleted, a prolonged inflammatory process occurs, keeping the infection going. Lung levels of IL-1ß, IL-6, and TNF-α all increase considerably at that point. Stimulating monocyte and dendritic cell maturation (cordyceps) and inducing IL-4 and IL-10 (Chinese skullcap, elder, houttuynia, licorice, cordyceps) will help counteract this.

The virus is exceptionally sophisticated in its impacts. There are three stages of chemokine stimulation. The first, 2 to 4 hours postinfection, is attended by the production of CXCL16, CXCL1, CXCL2, and CXCL3. These chemokines are specific for attracting neutrophils, cytotoxic T cells, and NK cells. At 8 to 12 hours postinfection CXCL8, CCL3, CCL4, CCL5, CXCL9, CXCL10, and CXCL11 are being produced, which attract effector memory T cells. At 24 to 48 hours postinfection, when dendritic cells are most present in the lymphoid tissues, the chemokine profile changes again in such a manner as to attract naive T and B cells. The effect of all this is the virus playing the immune system as a virtuoso plays a violin. Eventually the immune system catches up (usually) and the infection is stopped as influenza-specific antibodies are created.

Plants that reduce the other main cytokines that the virus stimulates will also help lessen disease severity and prevent lung damage. I think the most important are inhibitors of NF-κB (Chinese senega root, Chinese skullcap, ginger, houttuynia, kudzu, licorice, boneset, astragalus), IL-6 (kudzu, Chinese skullcap, isatis), IL-8 (cordyceps, isatis, Japanese knotweed), RANTES (licorice, isatis), MCP-1 (houttuynia), CXCL10 (boneset), CCL2 (boneset), the ERK pathway (kudzu, Chinese skullcap, cordyceps), the p38 pathway (Chinese skullcap, houttuynia, cordyceps), and the JNK pathway (Chinese skullcap, cordyceps, lion's mane). The reduction of these cytokines and pathways will reduce IFN-γ.

Each type of influenza has a slightly different cytokine profile with slightly different cytokines more strongly represented. However, the protocols herein, directed to this form of cytokine profile, will be specific enough for every strain, including the low pathogenic avian strain H9N2, which strongly upregulates transforming growth factor beta 2 (TGF-ß2), a different dynamic entirely. Medicinal plants already in use in the developed protocol are, however, specific for TGF-ß2, i.e., astragalus (the strongest) and Chinese skullcap. *Magnolia officinalis, Ginkgo biloba, Folium syringae, Nigella sativa, Paeonia lactiflora,* and *Lonicera japonica* are other plants specific for inhibiting TGF-ß2. (This is why lonicera, or Japanese honeysuckle, is commonly used in the treatment of respiratory infections in China—it alleviates wind heat and expels wind heat invasion. In other words, it reduces inflammation in the lungs and expels the virus or bacteria responsible.)

Normally, influenza viruses stay in the upper respiratory tract. However, during more severe infections they will infect the lower respiratory tract as well. Pneumonia is one serious complication from that. So are cytokine storms, should the disease really take hold.

Cytokine Storms

The more serious pandemic viruses (1918 H1N1, 2009 H1N1, and 2004 H5N1) cause severe pulmonary injury and inflammation. In these cases, the cytokine cascades become storms and the death rate correspondingly climbs. H5N1, for example, has around a 60 percent death rate in those who are infected, usually from acute respiratory distress and organ failure. The 1918 rate had a much lower mortality rate, around 20 percent, but the strain is much more infective, reaching about one-third of the population. (The emergence of a highly infective avian H5N1 strain is one of the things that keeps viral researchers up at night.)

While there is (usually) not a corresponding increase in viral replication during a viral storm, the cytokine increases in severe pandemic influenzas are significant, and this is where the mortal damage comes from. Interferon-gamma (IFN-γ) production is usually increased, as is the expression of TNF-α, IL-1ß, CXCL10, RANTES, MIP-1α, MCP-1, MCP-3, and IL-6. The IFN-γ levels and the virus synergistically interact to significantly increase CXCL10 in airway epithelial cells. This causes a tremendous infiltration of immune cells into the airways. Blocking IFN-γ through the use of inhibitors has been found to significantly reduce airway infiltrates (houttuynia, cordyceps, Chinese skullcap, and licorice; note that licorice is an IFN-γ *modulator*—it inhibits its production when levels are high and stimulates its production, especially in T cells, when levels are low).

In particular, the inhibition of TNF-α, IFN-γ, IL-1ß, and IL-6 is crucial during infection with severe influenza pandemic strains. Those cytokines are found in exceptionally high levels in such instances, and damage to the lungs is specific to them. If their levels rise high enough, the inflammation does not stay confined to the respiratory system but goes systemic. This kind of condition is called sepsis, essentially a whole-body inflammatory state. If severe enough, it can lead to organ failure and cardiac arrest.

A particular cytokine-like protein has been implicated in sepsis-induced cytokine storms: high-mobility group box 1 protein (HMGB1).

This cytokine-like protein is highly elevated in all patients who die from sepsis, including sepsis generated by influenza. HMGB1 is also unique in that once stimulated, its secretion continues for a very long time. TNF-α, in comparison, lasts at peak levels for about 90 minutes once stimulated. HMGB1 peak levels last 18 hours before they begin to decline. Once HMGB1 is released, it stimulates further cytokine releases *and* has the additional property of being synergistic with the other cytokines already present in the body, amplifying their effects. HMGB1 release is stimulated by macrophages and monocytes when a particularly potent cytokine cascade begins, specifically with high levels of NF-κB, TNF-α, RANTES, IL-6, and IFN-γ, in pretty much that order. The amount released is directly dose-dependent. In other words, the higher the cytokine levels, the more HMGB1 is released. And the more that is released, the higher the cytokine levels go. As examples, levels of IL-6 are nearly four times higher, IL-8 nearly three times higher, and IFN-γ more than two times higher during severe infections than in milder cases. Higher IL-6 concentrations are positively correlated with prolonged illness and hospitalization. As the storm progresses, levels of IL-8, MCP-1, and H_2O_2-myeloperoxidase also significantly increase. Endothelial cells are strongly stimulated and begin to amplify the storm's cytokines. Hyperactivation of p38 MAPK with an accompanying inhibition of the adaptive immune system is a marker for these kinds of cytokine storms.

HMGB1 is also released when the nuclei of cells are damaged, as they are during influenza infections. HMG proteins are held in the nucleus to help in forming DNA complexes and regulating gene expression. When HMGB1 is expressed in lung tissue, as it is during severe influenza episodes, it causes massive neutrophil infiltration into the lungs and acute lung injury. As the storm progresses, respiratory failure (requiring mechanical ventilation), acute renal failure, and systemic shock all occur. In severe cases such as these, antivirals (oseltamivir), antibiotics, and corticosteroids have all been found to be ineffective.

Common steroidal drugs (e.g., dexamethasone and cortisone) have consistently been found to have no effect on HMGB1 levels, and the same can be said for NSAIDs such as aspirin, ibuprofen, and indomethacin—even at superpharmacological concentrations. However, a number of herbs and herbal constituents do have direct suppressive actions against the protein.

Direct inhibition of HMGB1 with herbs such as *Angelica sinensis* and *Salvia miltiorrhiza* protects mice both before and 24 hours after infection with normally lethal influenza viruses. The licorice constituent glycyrrhizin directly binds HMGB1, inactivating its actions in the body. The green tea component epigallocatechin gallate (EGCG) also inhibits HMGB1, as does quercetin. Counterintuitively, nicotine also significantly lowers HMGB1 in the lungs. The pharmaceutical minocycline has also shown the ability to reduce HMGB1 levels; its use should be explored in hospital and pharmaceutical settings.

During severe influenza infections reducing HMGB1 is essential.

Lung and Tissue Pathology During Severe Influenza Infections

Influenza viruses specifically invade lung tissues and cause both direct and inflammatory-mediated damage. There are four primary pathological changes that occur: 1) diffuse alveolar damage; 2) necrotizing bronchiolitis; 3) intense alveolar hemorrhage; and 4) severe fluid accumulation.

The viruses infect specific cellular structures, in fact any that possess linked sialic acids (alpha-2,6 and alpha-2,3) on their surface membranes. But cells in the respiratory system express those acids differently, and different influenzal strains create different infection profiles. The nonciliated cells of the lungs contain a higher proportion of alpha-2,6-linked sialic acids, while ciliated cells contain both alpha-2,6- and alpha-2,3-linked sialic acid. H3N2 viruses prefer the nonciliated-cell sialic acids, while the avian flu types (H5N1) exclusively infect ciliated cells. This is part of the reason that the avian strains tend to be more deadly. The cilia, when infected, are often killed and their ability to move mucus up and out of the lungs destroyed. This substantially increases mucous buildup in the lungs. The H5N1 strains prefer the alpha-2,3-linked sialic acids that are most strongly present on the ciliated cells, but those acids exist on ciliated cells in higher quantities in the lower respiratory tract. So, the H5N1 strains infect not only the cilia but also the lower respiratory tract, causing a much deeper infection.

In severe cases, irrespective of strain, alveolar hemorrhage is often present, as is intra-alveolar edema and interstitial inflammation. The tissues surrounding blood vessels and lymph nodes and channels all inflame (perivasculitis). Microthrombi or tiny blood clots occur throughout the blood vessels in the lungs. IFN-γ levels are high in macrophages, alveolar epithelial cells, and vessels. TNF-α levels are high in alveolar macrophages and bronchial and vascular smooth muscle. There are massive infiltrates surrounding airways and in the alveolar walls. The spleen typically atrophies and presents with nonreactive white pulp. In the lymph nodes nonreactive follicles and sinusoidal erythrophagocytosis are common.

Protecting spleen and lymph structures and their function, cilial structures, and mucous membrane structures is essential.

Medical Interventions

If influenza is pharmaceutically treated, neuraminidase inhibitors such as oseltamivir (Tamiflu) or zanamivir (Relenza) are usually used. Sometimes adamantanes (amantadine and rimantadine) are as well; they inhibit the M2 ion channels. These pharmaceuticals are commonly referred to as antivirals, but they are not, at least not in the same way that an antibiotic is an antibiotic, that is, something that specifically kills bacteria. They, more accurately, inhibit viral penetration of host cells (thus stopping or slowing the infection) or prevent the vacuole-enveloped virus from releasing viral proteins into the host cell interior (thus stopping or slowing the infection). They don't directly kill the virus. Ribavirin, a drug that interferes with RNA metabolism, is sometimes used, but its effects are mixed and it has many serious side effects.

If there is significant inflammation, corticosteriods may be used to try to reduce it—but if HMGB1 levels are in play, corticosteroids will do nothing to reduce them. Hospitalization is common in severe cases, but other than passive care and the use of oxygen, little can be done. Intravenous liquids may be given, but they may have serious side effects, since the main approach has been the use of a combination nutrient solution/glucose IV in an attempt to keep the patient's nutrient/energy levels high. Unfortunately, it turns out that the use of glucose during influenza infections significantly increases viral load and illness parameters. Insulin, on the other hand, reduces them considerably and also has the added benefit of lowering HMGB1 levels.

There is the bare beginnings within hospital settings of the use of cytokine inhibitors such as minocycline and HMGB1 inhibitors (e.g., anti-IFN-γ antibodies, intravenous immunoglobulin), but their use is not widespread. If microthrombi proliferate in the lungs, then anti-coagulants may be used. Interestingly, both antithrombin III and thrombomodulin decrease HMGB1 in vitro. Very few of these HMGB1 interventions are commonly used, or known of, by practicing physicians.

To make matters worse, many influenza strains are developing resistance to the primary neuraminidase inhibitor used to treat them, oseltamivir, as well as to the primary adamantane M2 ion channel inhibitor, amantadine. Influenza virus samples from the 2007–2008 season showed 0.06 percent resistance, from the 2008–2009 season 1.5 percent resistance, and from the 2009–2010 season 28 percent resistance—a normal exponential learning curve for resistance. Research in late 2009 began finding strains resistant to the other major neuraminidase inhibitor, zanamivir. Resistance has become common as well to the other primary M2 ion channel inhibitor, rimantadine. Some areas report 100 percent resistance to amantadine and more than 90 percent resistance to oseltamivir. Besides their overuse in agribusiness, there is another reason for resistance: human excretion.

Oseltamivir is immediately metabolized in the body to oseltamivir carboxylate. It is only active in this form. Unfortunately this form *is* the metabolized form and it is excreted out of the human body without any further alterations. It flows unaffected through wastewater treatment plants and ends up in waterways in low doses, where it comes into contact with waterfowl and thus is exposed to avian influenza strains. The avian strains develop resistance, and as the avian, human, and swine strains commingle, the resistance is passed on into strains that can infect humans.

These drugs are also often used in large quantities during epidemic outbreaks. And the viruses quickly develop resistance to them. About 30 percent of those treated will develop resistant strains and will shed them for days afterward. The newly infected are then resistant to the drugs.

Less severe cases of the flu, if one sees a physician, are rarely treated (though, irresponsibly, some physicians will prescribe antibiotics, which are not active against viruses, for the flu). The usual medical advice is to "rest in bed, drink plenty of fluids, and take over-the-counter medications as needed." In other words, it is left up to the individual's immune system and some very limited self-care options to treat the infection. The Chinese don't have this kind of technological bias in place. Unlike those of us in the West, they have been developing both herb-alone and herb/pharmaceutical combination approaches in their treatment protocols. And their outcomes are very good when compared to Western approaches.

There are a great many interventions that are possible with plant medicines, and unlike pharmaceuticals, viruses don't develop resistance to them.

Natural Treatment Protocols for Influenza

Again, just to emphasize this: *There are thousands of combinations of plant medicines that can be created to treat respiratory infections.* These are just the ones I have found useful. Please feel free to experiment, combine, innovate, and find your own unique combinations. There is no one right way to the truth.

An influenza infection can run the range from extremely mild to extremely severe. I break the disease down into four types, each needing a different approach: 1) early onset; 2) mild infection; 3) moderate infection; and 4) severe infection. I will go into some of the unique aspects of treating severe infections on page 120.

Early-Onset Treatment

I have found two approaches that can short-circuit a developing episode before it gets a good hold in the body: oscillococcinum and an herbal tincture combination.

OSCILLOCOCCINUM

I have found this homeopathic remedy to be extremely good for stopping the development of the flu *if you take it at the first signs of the flu*, that is, the *moment* you feel that first tingling sensation in your body that tells you that you are about to get sick.

Oscillococcinum comes as little sugar granules in tiny tubes. Take one tube every 6 hours, three per day, for 2 or 3 days in a row. This is often enough to stop the infection.

HERBAL TINCTURE COMBINATION

For many years I used a particular tincture combination: *Echinacea angustifolia* (now I use ginger juice—see page 118; and note: *E. purpurea* is useless for this; it won't work), red root, and licorice, in equal parts. The dosage is a full dropperful of the tincture (30 drops) *every hour*, every day, until the symptoms resolve themselves.

I have found this useful for stopping the development of a flu infection *if you take it at the first signs of tingling or soreness in your throat.* The tincture mix should be held in your mouth, liberally mixed with saliva, then swallowed, *slowly*, letting it dribble down the back of the throat.

For *Echinacea angustifolia* to work for a cold or flu, *the herbal tincture must touch the affected membranes.* Echinacea *is* antiviral; it's been found active against HIV and influenza H5N1, H7N7, and H1N1 (swine origin). However, in order to inactivate the influenza strains, it needs *direct contact* with the affected cells just prior to or right at the moment of infection. Echinacea inhibits the receptor cell binding activity of the virus, interfering with its entry into the cells while at the same time strengthening the protective power of the mucous membranes through hyaluronidase inhibition. In essence, it strengthens the cellular bonds in the mucous membranes and makes it harder for a virus to penetrate. If the virus does penetrate deeper into the body, the herb just won't work because direct contact is not possible.

Goldenseal has some similar actions on mucous membranes, which is why the deplorable echinacea/goldenseal combinations are so common. They are only effective at the first signs of infection. (I reiterate: They are *only* effective at the first signs of infection. If the infection is full-blown, you are just wasting your money.) Again, *E. purpurea* (in the form in use in most of the West) will not work. The Germans use *only* the fresh, stabilized juice of the stalks, not the root, and it is the root that nearly every American herbalist and company use in their products. (Capsules, of any species, are completely useless for viral and bacterial infections.)

Mild Infection

If you do get sick but have a relatively mild case developing, then the following protocol, composed of two parts, will usually get rid of it.

FRESH GINGER JUICE TEA

Ginger is useful for the flu *only* if the juice of the fresh root is used. Dried ginger is useless.

At the first signs of an infection that is not going to stop, juice 1–2 pounds of ginger. (Squeeze the remaining pulp to get all the juice out of it, and keep any leftover juice refrigerated.) Pour 3–4 ounces of the juice into a mug, and add one-quarter of a lime (squeezed), a large tablespoon of honey, 1/8 teaspoon of cayenne, and 6 ounces of hot water. Stir well. Drink 2–6 cups daily.

This will usually end the infection within a few days. *If it does not,* it is still tremendously useful as it will thin the mucus, slow the spread of the virus in the body, and help protect mucous membranes from damage.

Comment: Some people find that an elderberry syrup will provide the same effects.

Other Anti-Influenza Herbs and Supplements

A number of other plants have been found effective for influenza during in vitro, in vivo, or human studies:

Achillea millefolium (yarrow)
Aegle marmelos (bael)
Agathosma betulina
Agrimonia pilosa
Allium oreoprasum
Allium sativum (garlic)
Alpinia officinarum
Andrographis paniculata
Androsace strigilosa
Angelica keiskei
Aronia melanocarpa
Asparagus filicinus
Azadirachta indica (neem)
Bergenia ligulata
Camellia sinensis (green tea, EGCG)
Cephalotaxus harringtonia
Chaenomeles sinensis
Cistus incanus
Clinacanthus siamensis
Cocos nucifera (coconut oil, monolaurin)
Commelina communis
Eleutherococcus senticosus
Elsholtzia rugulosa
Geranium sanguineum
Ginkgo biloba
Holoptelea integrifolia
Hypericum japonicum
Justicia pectoralis
Myrica rubra
Narcissus tazetta
Nerium indicum
Ocimum sanctum (holy basil)
Olea europaea (olive)
Panax spp. (ginseng)
Pandanus amaryllifolius
Phyllanthus emblica
Propolis
Prunus mume
Punica granatum (pomegranate)
Rhinacanthus nasutus
Sanicula europaea
Saponaria officinalis
Schefflera heptaphylla
Terminalia chebula
Thalictrum simplex
Tinospora cordifolia
Toddalia asiatica
Trachyspermum ammi
Tussilago farfara (coltsfoot)
Uncaria rhynchophylla
Verbascum thapsus (mullein)

HERBAL TINCTURE COMBINATION

Tincture combination of 2 parts lomatium, 2 parts red root, 2 parts licorice, and 1 part isatis (e.g., 2 ounces of each of the first three, 1 ounce of the latter). Dosage: 30–60 drops each hour until the condition improves.

Moderate and Severe Infections

I treat moderate and severe influenza infections similarly, though with severe infections there needs to be a great deal of focus and persistence. The doses often need to be higher as well and additional formulations used as symptoms develop.

The primary interventions are:

- Direct antivirals that will inhibit viral penetration of host cells and replication. (The primary antiviral herbs for this are Chinese skullcap, isatis, licorice, houttuynia, lomatium, cordyceps, astragalus, rhodiola, boneset, elder, *Strobilanthes cusia, Forsythia suspensa*, and *Sophora flavescens*.)
- Reducing cytokine levels, thus inhibiting damage in tissues.
- Thinning the mucus and promoting fluid drainage from the lungs.
- Repair of damaged tissues.
- Normalization of immune responses.
- If sepsis is a potential problem, large quantities of HMGB1 inhibitors should be used.

Treatment of moderate to severe influenza is composed of three main formulations, to which others can be added if necessary. These are an antiviral tincture formulation, an antiviral ginger juice tea, and an immune complex tincture formulation.

ANTIVIRAL TINCTURE FORMULATION

Equal parts of Chinese skullcap, isatis, licorice, houttuynia, lomatium, red root, yerba santa (*Eriodictyon* spp.), elephant tree (*Bursera microphylla*), osha (*Ligusticum porteri*), and either inmortal (*Asclepias asperula*) or pleurisy root (*Asclepias tuberosa*).

This formulation contains potent antivirals, specifically Chinese skullcap, isatis, licorice, houttuynia, and lomatium. These are designed to kill the virus and inhibit its entry into the body. And of course many of them have alternate actions as well. Licorice, for example, is muco-protective, strongly anti-inflammatory, and expectorant. Chinese skullcap is potently anti-inflammatory for the cytokine cascades that influenza creates, provides splenic protection and activation, will help lower fevers, and is an expectorant. All of these antiviral herbs have multiple functions in respiratory diseases.

The four herbs added to this protocol that are not discussed in depth in this book (yerba santa, osha, elephant tree, and inmortal or pleurisy root) do not have to be included in this formulation, though they do help considerably, primarily through helping with the tastiness of the formulation, thinning the mucus, stimulating expectoration, and promoting lymph drainage from the lungs.

Both yerba santa and osha are added for taste as well as their medicinal actions (isatis really does taste foul to me). Osha is a relative of lomatium and has its own antiviral and expectorant actions. It has

Complex Formulations

For nearly 30 years I tended to use formulations that contained only three herbs, occasionally five. With the emergence of more intense forms of influenza, and my increasing age, I have found that a more complex formulation works better. I do think a major factor in that is aging. There are, in myself and in many of the people I help, considerable age-related alterations in our physiology. There are preexisting inflammations in many parts of our bodies, from age-related memory dysfunction to arthritis. Our bodies are wearing out, biodegrading, and that deterioration makes them more susceptible to infections such as influenza, and in more severe forms. Further, our immune systems are not as vital as they once were and have a great deal more trouble counteracting the infection.

strong impacts on inflammation in the lungs and increases the degree of oxygen intake during respiration. It also has the added benefit of anesthesizing the throat tissues, helping reduce throat soreness. Yerba santa is a very good expectorant, bronchial dilator, and decongestant. Elephant tree is anti-inflammatory, thins and softens bronchial mucus, and stimulates expectoration. It is a major source of copal and a close relative of myrrh. (Myrrh can be substituted for elephant tree in this formulation if the tincture is stabilized with 20 percent glycerin.) I consider all three of these herbs to be specific for maintaining the mucous membranes of the lungs, thinning the mucus, and increasing expectoration. Inmortal (or, as an alternative, pleurisy root) improves cilia function and is a bronchial dilator, an expectorant, a febrifuge (lowering fevers), and most especially a potent medicinal for stimulating lymph drainage from the lungs.

Dosage needs to be high for two reasons. The first is that there are so many herbs in the formulation that each herb has a reduced presence in the formulation. The second is the nature of moderate to severe influenza infections. As the disease progresses up the scale of severity, the cytokine cascade increases in intensity. The body needs to be *bathed* in the plant compounds in high enough quantities that the cytokine cascade is potently inhibited. In addition, the body needs to be suffused with enough of the antiviral compounds that the viral entry into host cells and its presence in the body are severely curtailed.

For moderate influenza: 60 drops or 3 ml (a little more than 1/2 tsp) every hour

For severe influenza: 1–2 tsp every hour

Dividing the formulation: You can if you wish divide the formulation in two. The first would contain Chinese skullcap, isatis, licorice, houttuynia, and lomatium and would be primarily an antiviral formulation (and would taste from okay to bad). The second would contain red root, yerba santa (*Eriodictyon* spp.), elephant tree (*Bursera microphylla*), and either inmortal (*Asclepias asperula*) or pleurisy root (*Asclepias tuberosa*) and would taste very good. (I would skip the osha if the formulation is split in two.) This second formulation would primarily be for lymph and spleen optimization and protection, expectorant and decongestant actions, mucus thinning, cilia protection, and lymph drainage from the lungs. The dosage for each would be half the dosage as when combined.

GINGER JUICE TEA

This is the same as discussed earlier, in essence: ginger juice tea, hot. Again, ginger is useful for the flu *only* if the juice of the fresh root is used. Dried ginger is useless.

Juice 1–2 pounds of ginger. (Squeeze the pulp to get all the juice out of it.) Keep it refrigerated. Pour 3–4 ounces of the juice into a mug, and add one-quarter of a lime (squeezed), a large tablespoon of honey, 1/8 teaspoon of cayenne, and 6 ounces of hot water. Stir well. Drink 4–6 cups daily.

Ginger in this form is potently antiviral for influenza. The fresh juice tea will also thin the mucus, help protect mucous membranes from damage, *and* act as a potent diaphoretic, lowering fever during the infection.

IMMUNE COMPLEX TINCTURE FORMULATION

Equal parts of the tinctures of astragalus, cordyceps, and rhodiola. All of these herbs are active against influenza viruses. They are also potently adaptogenic, that is, they increase the resistance of organisms to stressors, whether microbial or external. Additionally, astragalus and cordyceps are highly specific for the cytokine cascades that are initiated by influenza. These herbs will help through their antiviral actions, modulate the overactive immune response, lower cytokine levels, and enhance a healthy immune response to the infection.

Again, dosage levels should be highish, for the same reasons as outlined above.

For moderate influenza: 1/2 tsp of the tincture 3x daily

For severe influenza: 1–2 tsp of the tincture 6x daily

Supportive Additions

There are a few additional things that can be very helpful during acute influenza episodes. These are treatments for high fever, severe headache, cough, high HMGB1 levels during cytokine storms, and protecting cilial structures and mucous membranes in the lungs. Two supplements have also been found to be helpful (in a number of studies). And essential oil inhalants can help with the infection in the lungs, coughing, and mucous flow and secretion.

For Fever

There are a number of interventions that can help. The ginger juice tea previously described (page 123) can often lower the high fevers that occur during influenza, but if you want more:

- **Boneset tea:** Boneset is specific for influenza and a number of the cytokines it stimulates. It is also highly specific for diseases that alternate fevers and chill episodes. If I am going to use boneset, and I am already ill, it is easier to make up a lot at one time. Getting out of bed over and over again is too difficult. So . . . add 3 ounces of dried boneset herb to 1 gallon of hot water, let steep 30 minutes, then drink 8 ounces every few hours. *The tea must be consumed hot for it to be effective for fever.* The herb will stimulate sweating, thus lowering the fever. It will help interrupt the chill/fever, chill/fever cycles. It's bitter, so add honey.
- **Pasque flower (*Pulsatilla patens*) tincture:** 10 drops each hour as needed.
- **Any diaphoretic (causes sweating) tea:** Peppermint is a good choice, children like it, and it will also help calm the stomach. Yarrow is more bitter but is also good for this. Both of them do have some antiviral activity against influenza.
- **Wet cloth:** A wet washcloth, applied regularly over the entire body, will mimic the action of sweat in helping lower a fever. The higher the fever, the more often you have to do it.

For Headache

- **Indian pipe (*Monotropa uniflora*) tincture:** The best I have found for the kinds of recalcitrant headaches that can sometimes occur during the flu. Dosage is from 30 drops to 1 tsp every few hours.
- **Coral root (*Corallorhiza* spp.) tincture:** Up to 1 tsp every few hours. It does help and for some people it is specific.
- **Tinctures of motherwort (*Leonurus cardiaca*) and American wood betony (*Pedicularis* spp.):** Combined, equal parts. Dosage is up to 1 ounce (yes, that's right) of the combination at a time, in water. I usually use 1/4 ounce, but the high dosage can help occasionally when nothing else does. Go slow and work up, every 4 hours or so.

For Cough

I make a cough syrup every fall just before the flu season. It comes in handy. The recipe varies all the time, depending on what I have on hand and what I have wild-harvested in any particular year. But the recipe below gives you a good idea of what kinds of herbs are in it. I do keep it refrigerated, though it will last awhile if it is not.

Cough Syrup Recipe

INGREDIENTS

- 3 ounces horehound
- 2 ounces cherry bark
- 2 ounces elderberries
- 2 ounces elecampane
- 2 ounces licorice
- 2 ounces mallow (or marshmallow)
- 1 ounce Russian or slippery elm bark
- 1 ounce vervain
- 1 ounce lomatium (or osha)
- 7 pints water
- 3 ounces glycerin
- Wildflower honey
- 2 ounces mullein tincture
- 1 ounce yerba santa tincture

Combine the horehound, cherry bark, elderberries, elecampane, licorice, mallow, elm bark, vervain, and half of the lomatium (or osha) in 7 pints of water in a large pot. Bring to a boil. Stir frequently as it heats to prevent sticking. Once it boils, reduce the heat and let simmer, stirring constantly. Cook until the liquid is reduced by half. Remove from the heat and let cool. (You can put the pot in a bath of cold water to cool it faster. Don't let it tip over.) Strain the liquid, pressing the marc (the spent plant matter) through a cloth to get as much liquid as you can.

(With mucilaginous herbs—the licorice, mallow, and elm bark—as part of the mix, it can be hard for the liquid to pass through the weave of the cloth you are using. So, alternatively, you can keep the mucilaginous herbs out of the mix and once the marc is pressed, heat all the liquid again, adding the licorice, mallow, and elm to the pot in a muslin bag to keep them out of the liquid. Bring to a boil and simmer, stirring constantly, for 30 minutes. Remove the bag, let it cool, then squeeze out the liquid as best you can.)

Gently warm the liquid again and add the glycerin, then the honey to taste. Heat just enough to dissolve the glycerin and honey. Grind the remaining lomatium (or osha) to a fine powder—a nut or coffee grinder or mortar and pestle is good for this—then add it to the liquid. Let the mix cool, then add the mullein and yerba santa tinctures. (Keep in mind that you can substitute similar herbs for any used in this recipe.)

The honey, glycerin, and two tinctures help stabilize the syrup, keeping it from going bad. I do keep the whole thing in the refrigerator though. It will last a year very easily. Generally, it is best to make this kind of a syrup in the fall, after the berries are ripe and ready for harvest, and just before flu season. It is very effective.

To use:

I keep this by the bed and take as desired. Really, none of that 1-tablespoon-at-a-time stuff, that won't help at all. Just drink it as needed, right out of the bottle. It will help soothe the mucous membranes, reduce coughing, and ease the aches and pains that come with the flu.

To Reduce HMGB1 Levels during Cytokine Storms

The herbs that are already being used will help this considerably. However, if the condition significantly worsens, then the following specific intervention is warranted. Take both formulations.

Formulation 1: Tincture combination of *Angelica sinensis* and *Salvia miltiorrhiza*, in equal parts. Dosage: 1 tbl every hour. Or . . .

Formulation 2: Strong infusion of the two herbs, 4 ounces of each in 1 gallon of just-boiled water. Remove from the heat, let sit 4 hours, and strain. Dosage: Drink 12 ounces every hour.

To Protect Cilial Structures and Lung Mucosa

There are a number of herbs that are specific for protecting the cilia: cordyceps, olive oil and leaf, the berberine plants, and, my favorite, *Bidens pilosa*. Bidens is a very strong systemic antibiotic that is used in Asia and Africa for systemic bacterial infections (including respiratory) *and* influenza (though it has not been tested against that virus). If the mucous membranes have been infected by a microbe and you start to get well, relapse, start to get well, relapse, this is the herb to use. The herb is specific for healing and protecting mucous membrane structures, including the cilia. Tincture of the fresh herb should be used. The dry herb is not as antimicrobial, though it will still help the mucous membranes' tone. Dosage: 1/4–1/2 tsp up to 6x daily.

Some Comments on Treating Severe Influenza

When people become severely ill with influenza, they often present with high fever, extreme lethargy, and significantly reduced vital energy. They are usually bedridden and very, very afraid.

The interventions in such cases need to be highly focused and attentive. It takes a lot of work. They need to be nurtured continuously, fed if they will eat (chicken broth is very good), helped to the bathroom (if they can even get out of bed), and ministered to. The fever will often need to be brought down, and you will have to monitor the plant medicine intake. It needs to be constant (every hour at minimum), and in fairly high dosages in order to lower the cytokine cascade, reduce the viral load, and get the immune system back online. It will often take a week to begin to turn the situation around, and several more weeks before the person really begins to get well. It can be done. Of all the herbs useful for this, lomatium, licorice, Chinese skullcap, and cordyceps are the most essential.

Supplements

Zinc and selenium are very helpful during influenza infections. Both have been found to protect mice from severe influenzal strains. Dosage: 200 mcg daily of selenium; 25–40 mg daily of zinc.

Essential Oil Inhalants

Essential oils of thyme, eucalyptus, rosemary, and sage can all help. They are all antiviral for influenza (to varying extents), will help reduce the coughing reflex, thin and help expectorate mucus, and improve airflow in the bronchial tract. To use: Bring a gallon of water to a boil in a pot on the stove. Turn off the heat, add 20 drops of each of the essential oils to the pot, and bring the pot to a comfortable location where you can sit with your head over it. Hold your head over the pot and breathe in the steam for as long as you can take it, every few hours.

A Few Other Respiratory Viral Infections

The main ones that people encounter are the adenoviruses, parainfluenza viruses, respiratory syncytial virus, and rhinoviruses.

Adenoviruses

Adenovirus infections tend to be mild and are generally easy to treat. However, acute conditions such as pharyngoconjunctival fever, acute respiratory disease, pneumonia, and meningitis can also occur.

Adenovirus 14 is an emerging serotype that can cause serious infection, essentially acute respiratory disease, which can sometimes lead to death. Conjunctivitis, high fever, pneumonia, and gastrointestinal involvement can all occur. The virus sheds in both respiratory droplets and feces and can remain highly infective in feces for long periods.

The herbs specific for adenovirus infections are astragalus, Chinese skullcap, elder, isatis, and licorice. Other herbs that are active are *Ardisia squamulosa*, *Artemisia princeps*, *Boussingaultia gracilis*, *Caesalpinia pulcherrima*, *Ocimum basilicum*, and *Serissa japonica*.

Treatment: The same as for mild influenza. If it becomes serious, the same as for moderate to severe influenza.

Parainfluenza Viruses

Parainfluenza viruses generally cause what is called croup. It is an acute infection of the upper respiratory tract accompanied by barking cough (the croup part) and hoarseness. The throat is often swollen, which can interfere with breathing. The herbs specific for parainfluenza are Chinese skullcap, elder, and licorice. *Allium sativum* and *Cicer arietinum* have also been found active.

Treatment: Tincture combination of elderberry, Chinese skullcap, and licorice tinctures, in equal parts. Dosage: 30 drops every hour.

Respiratory Syncytial Virus

Respiratory syncytial virus is also a single-strand, enveloped RNA virus with high variation in its genome. It is a very common infection, especially in young children, throughout the world. It causes bronchiolitis and other types of respiratory infections, especially in the lower respiratory tract. It generally presents as a common cold but can sometimes become serious, turning into pneumonia if left untreated.

The herbs specific for respiratory syncytial virus infections are Chinese skullcap, *Eleutherococcus senticosus*, elder, isatis, licorice, and *Sophora flavescens*. Other herbs found active are *Barleria prionitis*, *Blumea laciniata*, *Elephantopus scaber*, *Laggera pterodonta*, *Markhamia lutea*, *Mussaenda pubescens*, *Narcissus tazetta*, *Selaginella sinensis*, *Scutellaria indica*, and *Schefflera octophylla* (in vitro).

Treatment: The same as for mild influenza. If it becomes serious, the same as for moderate to severe influenza.

Rhinoviruses

These viruses cause the common cold. The herbs/supplements specific for rhinovirus infections are ginger, *Echinacea angustifolia*, elder, *Eleutherococcus senticosus*, quercetin, *Papaver pseudocanescens*, and

Raoulia australis. A Japanese traditional formulation, hochu-ekki-to, has been found highly effective, as has *Prunus mume*.

Treatment: I have found the use of an *E. angustifolia*, licorice, and red root tincture combination, as outlined earlier (see page 117), *and* the prolific use of the ginger juice tea, also discussed earlier (see page 118), to be very effective.

The Encephalitis Viruses

There are some viruses that specifically infect the brain and cause encephalitis (West Nile), and there are others that sometimes get into the brain and cause encephalitis (herpes simplex). Many of them are spread by insect vectors (mosquitoes and ticks). For some of them, there are vaccines (tick-borne encephalitis—TBE). Others will sometimes respond fairly well to pharmaceuticals (acyclovir for instance for nonresistant herpes encephalitis). Most of the viruses that cause encephalitis show similar initial symptoms; all of them can be treated with plant medicines. (And yes, pharmaceuticals can be used along with plant-based protocols. The plant protocol tends to *increase* the effectiveness of the pharmaceutical protocol while at the same time significantly relieving the symptom picture.)

Here is a look at the most common encephalitis viruses and their geographical distribution:

- **Togaviruses, the alphavirus complex:** eastern equine encephalitis (eastern and Gulf coasts of the United States, Caribbean, South America), western equine encephalitis (western United States and Canada), Venezuelan equine encephalitis (South and Central America, Florida, southwest United States). All are spread by mosquitoes.
- **Flaviviruses, the West Nile complex:** St. Louis encephalitis (United States), Japanese encephalitis (Japan, China, southeast Asia, India, southeast Russia, northern Australia, New Guinea), Murray Valley encephalitis (Australia and New Guinea), West Nile (United States, Africa, Europe, Middle East, Asia), Ilhéus

(South and Central America), Rocio (Brazil). All are spread by mosquitoes.

- **Flaviviruses, the tick-borne complex:** Far Eastern tick-borne encephalitis (eastern Russia), central European encephalitis (central Europe), Kyasanur forest disease (India), louping ill (England, Scotland, northern Ireland), Powassan (Canada and northern United States), Negishi (Japan). All spread by ticks. In general, this group is usually just referred to as TBE or tick-borne encephalitis virus and treated accordingly.
- **Bunyaviruses, the bunyavirus complex:** California encephalitis (western United States), La Crosse encephalitis (mid- and eastern United States), Jamestown Canyon (United States, including Alaska), snowshoe hare (Canada, Alaska, northern United States), Tahyna (Czech Republic, Slovakia, former Yugoslavian states, Italy, southern France), Inkoo (Finland). All spread by mosquitoes.
- **Phlebovirus:** Rift Valley fever (eastern Africa). Spread by mosquitoes.
- **Reovirus, orbivirus:** Colorado tick fever (Rocky Mountains, western United States and Canada). Spread by ticks.

The most common, in the United States, are West Nile, St. Louis encephalitis, La Crosse encephalitis, and California encephalitis. Japanese encephalitis virus (JEV) is the most common in Asia (estimates are that in some areas the infection rate is 100 percent). From all reports, it is the main member of the common viral encephalitides that causes the most damage. The most common viral encephalitis in Europe and Russia is West Nile and TBE; West Nile is, in fact, becoming a worldwide phenomenon and is present in most of the world. Most of the other encephalitis viruses are somewhat uncommon in people. Vaccines have been created for both Japanese viral encephalitis and TBE, but they can't be used on those younger than 15 to 17 years of age.

In spite of the existence of vaccines, there are large outbreaks of both Japanese viral encephalitis and TBE every year, especially in the young. The vaccine needs to be repeated every year (Japanese) or every 3 years (TBE). For many cultures, the cost is often prohibitive and many people simply never get the vaccines. There are also certain groups of people for whom it is considered risky to give the vaccine, primarily the old and the young. Specifically: 1) those over 60 years of age; 2) those allergic to formaldehyde, neomycin, gentamycin, protamine sulfate, latex, eggs, or chickens; 3) those with a brain or central nervous system problem; 4) those with high temperatures; 5) those with weakened immune systems; 6) those with autoimmune conditions; 7) women who are pregnant; 8) those under 15 years of age (17 for the Japanese viral encephalitis vaccine). There remain a large number of people who can't be vaccinated, many of whom succumb to the infections each year.

Symptoms

Nearly all, 90 percent, of people infected by an encephalitis virus have flu-like symptoms: fever, sore throat, cough, general ill feeling, aches and pains, weakness, and malaise. About 10 percent have no symptoms at all. And for most people the infection passes, just like the flu; they really have no idea that they were infected with viral encephalitis.

If the infection is severe, the symptom picture alters accordingly: Headache, confusion, disorientation, photophobia, agitation, optic neuritis, myelitis, personality alterations, seizures, coma, and death can all occur, depending on the severity of the infection. Depending on which part of the brain is affected, language skills may be impaired and voluntary movement affected, and severe muscle weakness, uncontrollable tremors, partial paralysis, involuntary movements, and loss of ability to regulate body temperature may occur.

Medical Treatment

Most neural encephalitis infections have no established pharmaceutical treatment approaches—though there are a few treatments that are showing promise.

Immunoglobulin therapy has helped with a number of different viral encephalitides including West Nile. Interferon-alpha and ribavirin have also been used, though with mixed to moderate success for West Nile. Minocycline has been found effective in West Nile encephalitis, and I think it a good treatment approach if the disease becomes serious. Erythromycin can significantly reduce the endothelial hyperplasia that sometimes occurs during West Nile encephalitis.

Anticonvulsant medications are sometimes used to treat seizures. Steroid medications given by IV are used for inflammation in severe cases.

Some of the nonspecific viruses that can sometimes infect the brain, such as herpes, do respond to pharmaceuticals. The usual treatment for them is antivirals: acyclovir (for herpes simplex, Epstein-Barr, and varicella zoster encephalitis) and ganciclovir (for cytomegalovirus and herpes simplex 1 encephalitis).

Mechanisms of Viral Infection

West Nile virus (WNV), tick-borne encephalitis virus (TBE), and St. Louis encephalitis virus are all flaviviruses, they are closely related, and they have very similar impacts in the body. In other words, with slight differences, what they do once they are in the body, how they affect brain structures, and the kinds of cytokines they stimulate are all very similar. (The treatment protocol for each, in consequence, is also very similar.) I will look in the most depth at WNV, then just a bit at TBE (which, being tick spread, has some unique features) and a bit at La Crosse, the most common nonflavivirus encephalitis virus. I will also take a brief look at dengue and its encephalitis aspects.

West Nile Encephalitis

Although discovered in 1937, the first large outbreak of West Nile did not occur until the 1990s; research did not begin in earnest until the latter part of that decade—after outbreaks occurred in the United States. Thirty-two hundred of the 3,600 studies on the virus have occurred since then; the Chinese database CNKI has a mere 74 journal articles on the virus.

Four in five of those infected have few or no symptoms at all. One in five experiences a flu-like febrile illness of limited duration. One in 150 develops encephalitis or meningitis or both. The older a person is, the worse the outcome and the greater likelihood they will be seriously ill. The virus seems to specialize in attacking the aging brain. The younger the person, the younger the neural structures, the less likely the disease is to be severe, or even to be symptomatic. Children and young adults tend to be asymptomatic. The median age of those who present with just fever and flu-like symptoms is 43; the median age of those who develop severe symptoms is 59. The old are also especially at risk because the aging immune system is less strong (immune senescence) and, at the same time, they tend to have preexisting conditions that affect brain function (such as higher reactive oxygen species and other cytokines already active in the brain from Alzheimer's and similar conditions). The incubation period is 3 to 11 days, with the average at 5 days.

Most of the people who experience severe infection have similar symptoms: muscle weakness, gastrointestinal symptoms, fever, headache, alterations in mental status, and movement disorders such as tremors, myoclonus, and Parkinsonism. A smaller proportion have an erythematous macular rash of one sort or another that can appear in various places on the body. Meningoencephalitis is common. A polio-like paralysis appears in a small subset of those infected. If meningitis occurs, neck stiffness, headache, hypothermia, photophobia, and/or phonophobia are common. With encephalitis, especially severe, depressed or altered consciousness, lethargy, personality alterations, fever, and hypothermia are common.

Ribavirin and interferon-a2b are the most common pharmaceuticals used, but they show a very mixed success rate. The main intervention is hospitalization ("supportive" treatment, as most journal articles refer to it) and observation; there is little medical intervention. Mostly the people just get well on their own . . . or don't.

INFECTION PROGRESSION

After infection (by mosquito bite) nothing appears amiss for about 5 days or so, but on day 6 or 7 lethargy sets in, food intake slows, and weakness begins to develop. By days 7 to 10 (in severe cases) tremors and difficulty walking, thinking, and communicating start to occur.

The virus travels first to the spleen and then to the CNS. The blood-brain barrier is made more permeable, and once into the brain, the virus begins to seek out its preferred areas. Those are the cerebral cortex, cerebellar cortex, subcortical gray matter, hippocampus, and basal ganglia. As the infection progresses, the cerebral cortex and the hippocampus are more heavily affected; severe degeneration begins in the neurons in those areas, then escalates as the virus reproduces. The virus then spreads to the brain stem and spinal cord (which is when a general paralysis can occur).

There is direct infection of neurons and an inflammatory stimulation of the host immune system, which the virus uses during the disease process. In essence, it stimulates an autoimmune response to break down cellular structures in the CNS. The microglia are infected, and microglial nodules form, filled with lymphocytic infiltrate, the nodules surrounded by degenerated (exploded) neurons. As the disease progresses, the brain stem is more deeply affected and begins showing tremendous neuronal degeneration and the inflammation in the spinal cord is much more developed. The lumbar region of the spinal cord can become severely affected, with inflammatory infiltrates along the entire length of the cord. The brain stem, temporal lobes, and basal ganglia are, generally, the most severely affected regions of the brain.

In those who survive the illness, persistent neurological problems can remain. The virus can, in some, develop into a long-term, chronic infection that does not heal. Long-term chronic infection with West Nile is almost totally dependent on the failure of CD8+ T cells to become active or highly present in the body. As with Japanese viral encephalitis, the higher the CD8+ T cell activity prior to infection, the less chance there is for infection, especially serious infection, to occur.

THE CYTOKINE/CHEMOKINE CASCADE

The cytokines TNF-α, IL-1ß, IL-5, IL-6, IL-8, IL-13, interferon-inducible protein-10 (IP-10), matrix metalloproteinase-1 (MMP-1), MMP-3, MMP-9, NF-κB, COX-2, and the chemokine MCP-1 are all increased. Interferon-gamma levels are strongly increased, as are the levels of IDO (indoleamine 2,3-dioxygenase), ICAM-1 (intercellular adhesion molecule-1), VCAM-1 (vascular cell adhesion molecule-1), E-selectin, p38 MAPK, RANTES, and PGE2 (prostaglandin E2).

Researchers have looked intensively at the presence of a number of chemokines in West Nile encephalitis; CCR1, CCR2, CCR5, CCL2, CCL3, and CCL4 all showed increases. IL-10 levels are initially upregulated by the virus upon infection in order to keep the innate immune response as low as possible. Once the virus is established in the body and cytokine levels begin to rise, the levels of IL-4 and IL-10 are inhibited in order to stop their cytokine regulatory actions. The longer the infection, the lower the levels become. Perforin levels are reduced as well. Perforin is a protein in cytotoxic T cells that creates pores in target cells that allows the T cells to enter the infected cells and kill them.

The virus stimulates the production of MMPs (MMP-1, MMP-3, and MMP-9) once it enters the spleen. The MMPs are a kind of enzyme that especially degrade extracellular matrix proteins. These proteins make up much of the connective tissue in animals, including crucial elements of the blood-brain barrier. In essence, once MMPs are activated in a location, the connective tissue in that location begins to degrade. West Nile uses these to degrade the blood-brain barrier enough that it can gain entry to the brain and spinal cord. The tight junction protein bonds are weakened, making the barrier more permeable. Once inside the brain, the virus attaches strongly to astrocytes and stimulates them to continue releasing MMPs. Astrocytes are, in fact, the main source of these compounds in the brain. (The endothelial cells of the brain's microvascular system are also activated to produce MMPs.) This makes the blood-brain barrier significantly more porous and keeps it that way. This creates an enhanced infiltration of immune cells into the brain, and they cluster around the sites of viral infection and contribute to the inflammation in those locations. The cellular structures are weakened, helping the virus gain entry to their host's cells. In other words, the virus makes the blood-brain barrier porous and actively damages neural structures, which stimulates the production of cytokines and chemokines, which then call to themselves a variety of immune cells at the specific neural locations the virus wants them. The use of MMP inhibitors (such as Japanese knotweed root, Chinese skullcap, and cordyceps) has been found to stop the process by inhibiting astrocyte production of MMPs and restoring blood-brain barrier integrity.

WNV also manipulates cholesterol content in cellular membranes. It upregulates host cell cholesterol biosynthesis and redistributes the produced cholesterol into viral replication membranes.

The cytokines stimulated by the virus (specifically TNF-α and IL-1ß) in turn stimulate the production of ICAM-1, VCAM-1, and E-selectin by both astrocytes and endothelial cells in the brain. These are chemotactic for immune infiltrates that form the microglial nodules. Basically, they act like magnets, calling the immune cells to them. The leukocytes that are called to those locations bind to cells and then transmigrate into tissues, in this instance making the cells more accessible to the viral particles. PGE2, which is stimulated by COX-2, is strongly involved in the inflammation process and the aggregation of platelets; it has a number of potent impacts on spinal neurons and is a stimulant of IDO in the body. TNF-α inhibitors (kudzu, Chinese senega root, Chinese skullcap, elder, ginger, houttuynia, licorice, boneset, cordyceps) and IL-1ß inhibitors (Japanese knotweed, Chinese senega root, Chinese skullcap, cordyceps, kudzu, boneset) have all been found to stop this process. Inhibitors of ICAM-1 (Japanese knotweed, elder, cordyceps), VCAM-1 (Japanese knotweed, kudzu, elder, licorice), and E-selectin (Japanese knotweed, kudzu, licorice) can significantly reduce leukocyte infiltration and congregation.

The stimulation of the endothelial cells in the brain's microvascular network also causes a hypertrophy of those cells, interfering with blood flow to the brain. A central nervous system vasculitis can occur that can, sometimes, lead to stroke or other complications. Plants such as Japanese knotweed (or compounds such as EGCG and resveratrol), which are specific inhibitors of endothelial hypertrophy, can not only reduce MMP production but also inhibit this process. (Erythromycin is also specifically indicated for this.) Cerebral vasculitis from West Nile infection is somewhat more common than understood. In severe cases endothelial cell normalizers (Japanese knotweed root, EGCG, hawthorn berry, *Salvia miltiorrhiza,* licorice) really should be used. COX-2 (and PGE2) inhibitors are also helpful, especially because they help reduce IDO levels (Japanese knotweed, kudzu, Chinese skullcap, Chinese senega root, elder, ginger, houttuynia, isatis, cordyceps). COX-2 inhibitors also specifically block the production of WNV-induced cytokines in astrocytes (essentially the same herbs).

One of the first things that the virus does is to, in a specific process, increase levels of interferon-gamma (and TNF-α) in order to stimulate the production of indoleamine 2,3-dioxygenase (IDO). During WNV infection, high levels of IFN-γ, TNF-α, IL-1ß, and IL-2 are present in the brain. (TNF-α is synergistic with IFN-γ in stimulating IDO production.) Additionally, once the virus enters the spleen and infects dendritic cells, it begins stimulating them to produce IDO (which reduces T cell proliferation, thus protecting the virus from the most effective immune response). IDO is an enzyme that breaks apart (catalyzes) the amino acid L-tryptophan. There are a number of wide-ranging effects from this, all of which have deleterious effects in the body.

Normally, when infection occurs, the body creates IFN-γ to catalyze tryptophan because tryptophan degradation limits protein biosynthesis by depriving cells of an essential amino acid. But West Nile doesn't need tryptophan. It, instead, uses this natural immune response to limit T cell proliferation and to create specific, and very potent, inflammations in the brain. IDO is a potent inhibitor of T cells (it also induces apoptosis of competent T cells) and through its degradation of tryptophan creates powerful inflammatory molecules in the brain. The degree of tryptophan degradation is a specific indicator of the progression, and seriousness, of the infection.

L-tryptophan is normally degraded into L-kynurenine and then into three intermediary compounds that are highly neuroactive in the brain: 3-hydroxykynurenine (3-HK), quinolinic acid (QUIN), and kynurenic acid (KYNA).

High QUIN levels in the brain will cause an overstimulation of neurons, excitotoxic lesions, degradation of brain tissue, high levels of reactive oxygen species in the brain, and convulsions. The precursor to QUIN, 3-HK, is highly neurodestructive, causing cellular disintegration, primarily through the generation of free radicals. Neurons are particularly vulnerable to its actions. KYNA, on the other hand, is neuroprotective, and ameliorates the impacts of QUIN and 3-HK. Unfortunately, the amount of KYNA depends on healthy neuron function, which in WNV infection is inhibited severely. Compromised cellular energy metabolism (i.e., mitochondrial function) will also significantly reduce KYNA levels. In WNV infection 3-HK and QUIN levels are very high, and KYNA levels are very low. Upon microglial and astrocyte activation 3-HK and QUIN levels can increase 100 to 1,000 times; this is especially true if there is the kind of macrophage infiltration that occurs during West Nile encephalitis. The number and seriousness of seizures, convulsions, and paralysis that people with West Nile experience are directly proportional to the level of IDO generated in the brain (and its subsequent generation of QUIN and 3-HK).

IDO stimulation also has the regrettable ability to significantly inhibit serotonin and melatonin production in the brain. Melatonin, besides its potent sleep regulatory actions, is also an incredibly strong antioxidant, more powerful than most. It very specifically deactivates the oxidants that 3-HK and QUIN create. During WNV infection, however, melatonin levels fall very low in the brain. (Keeping melatonin levels high will reduce, or eliminate, the ability of West Nile—and other encephalitis viruses—to cause infections. Increasing melatonin levels, by using plants such as Chinese skullcap that are very high in melatonin, will reduce vulnerability to infection, symptom picture, and mortality. It specifically reduces paralysis and convulsions and is highly protective of the brain's neural structures.)

IDO inhibitors (and exogenous melatonin) can stop this process (*and* reduce IFN-γ and TNF-α levels), thus protecting brain tissues and reducing symptom severity, postinfection complications, and mortality. The most potent inhibitors of IDO are Chinese skullcap, Japanese knotweed, isatis, and, most especially, *Crinum latifolium*.

The high levels of IDO also create tryptophan depletion in the body. Tryptophan is an essential amino acid that cannot be synthesized by the body; it has to come from outside sources. During severe West Nile encephalitis, tryptophan supplementation should occur. (This will *not* feed the viruses, making the disease worse, but will, in fact, help repair CNS damage.) Studies have found that exogenous tryptophan can help restore healthy T cell function and responses.

There are several other interventions that have been found to reduce WNV impacts in the body. The inhibition of p38 MAPK (Chinese skullcap, houttuynia, cordyceps) significantly decreases chemokine production in response to WNV. CD8+ T cells require perforin to clear West Nile virus from infected neurons. Low perforin levels correlate to a much higher viral load, worse symptom picture, and increased mortality. Increasing perforin levels (by using plants such as astragalus) stimulates clearance of the virus and reduces symptoms.

Tick-Borne Encephalitis

TBE is very similar to the other members of this group. It has a higher affinity for the lymph system, with subsequent involvement of the nodes. And this is where it first replicates before traveling to the brain (via the spleen and lymph system). The spleen is particularly infected (making the use of spleen herbs essential), and the virus can remain in the body, including the spleen, for months, perhaps years. Acute symptoms (beyond the initial flu symptoms) are hyperemia, petechial hemorrhages, inflammatory infiltration, necrosis of microglial cells, and hyperplastic and hypertrophic glial nodules. Lesions are most common in the periventricular regions of the brain stem, including the cerebellum and reticular formation. The cerebellar cortex and basilar portions of the pons, thalamus, and olivary nuclei can also be affected. Perivascular inflammation around the blood vessels and cerebral interstitial edema are common. Laminar necrosis can occur. The cranial nerve and cervical anterior horn motor neuron cells are commonly affected during deeper progressions of the disease. Meningitis is common.

The cytokine/chemokine profiles are similar to those of other encephalitides: IL-6, TNF-α, IL-1ß, and IL-1α are all high; IL-10 is initially high, then decreases substantially—as usual with these kinds of viruses. One difference is that if the pH of the blood moves from its normal alkaline state (around 7.3) to an acidic state, it strongly facilitates the ability of TBE virus to infect the body. Using a combination of sodium bicarbonate, calcium citrate, and magnesium citrate (and isatis) supplementation will reliably increase pH and reduce the ability of the virus to fuse with host cells.

Presenting symptoms in serious cases are high fever, headache, vomiting, and vertigo. Then tremors, profuse sweating, paresis, delirium, psychosis, coma, and death. There is no pharmaceutical treatment for TBE, though tetracycline hydrochloride has been found to significantly reduce the inflammatory cytokines during infection. Corticosteroids have as well been found to inhibit inflammation, decreasing the severity of symptoms.

There are two specific physiological differences during TBE (when compared to West Nile encephalitis): Edema is often pronounced in TBE, and the microglia are often necrotic.

La Crosse Encephalitis

La Crosse encephalitis virus (LCEV) infections decrease with the age of the host; the younger the person, the more susceptible they are to infection, and the more likely the disease is to be severe. Those under age 8 are the most affected.

There are about 300,000 new LCEV infections each year in the

United States. As with most encephalitis infections, many cases are asymptomatic or present as a mild to moderate flu that passes without serious effects. In severe cases, the same kinds of inflammatory lesions that are seen in TBE are found, either diffuse or as microglial nodules. The cerebral cortex is most adversely affected, including the frontal, parietal, and temporal lobes. Inflammatory foci are also present in the pons and basal ganglia. Unlike in TBE the spinal cord is rarely affected, but if the infection travels down the spinal cord from the brain, it will cause perivascular cuffs of lymphocytes and nerve degeneration.

There has been, oddly, little study of the cytokine profile of the disease, though what has been done shows that it is similar to most viral encephalitis infections. LCEV stimulates the production of IL-1ß, TNF-α, and IL-6. Bcl-2 is downregulated as well.

Symptoms during severe infection are meningoencephalitis, high fever, seizures, vomiting, photophobia, stiff neck, confusion, paresis, aphasia, chorea, dysarthria, ataxia, and coma. Fever, headache, behavioral changes, and vomiting are the most common symptoms. Those who recover often show lower IQ scores, and a high proportion show ADHD behaviors. Some continue to experience seizures.

The virus is spread by mosquitoes. Once in the body the virus begins replicating in the muscle tissue and spreads to the blood, lymph, and spleen and thence to the brain, where it begins to infect neurons, its preferred replication site. It, like the other encephalitides, is present in high quantities in both the spleen and lymph. There are sometimes areas of necrosis in the spleen. Unlike other such viruses, it also infects the respiratory passages.

Although there is no accepted pharmaceutical treatment, ribavirin and recombinant glycoproteins have been found to help. Corticosteroids are sometimes used to reduce the inflammation.

The infection is considered to most closely resemble herpes simplex encephalitis, with which it is often confused. However, I think the infection dynamics are very similar to those of Japanese encephalitis, and natural treatment should follow that protocol with one addition: Endothelial swelling can commonly occur with La Crosse viral encephalitis; Japanese knotweed (or an equivalent) should be added to the protocol to help alleviate it.

Natural Treatment for Encephalitis

This treatment protocol is specific for all viral encephalitis infections. Some adjustment is needed for West Nile, TBE, and dengue, and those adjustments are detailed at the end of the protocol.

If seizures occur, Chinese skullcap and lion's mane should be used, in large doses. If cerebral edema, ischemia, or hypoxia are present, *Ligusticum wallichii* (or the extract ligustrazine) is specific. Rhodiola is also specific for hypoxia.

Note: Chondroitin sulfate has been found to enhance the infection of brain cells by JEV and the damage it causes in the brain. This supplement should be avoided during active infection.

The treatment protocol is followed by a brief look at some of the more important herbs that are neuroprotective and neuroregenerative: Chinese senega root, Japanese knotweed root, kudzu root, lion's mane, and *Crinum latifolium.*

The Protocol Overview

Treatment approaches that can reduce the impacts of the encephalitis infections consist of the following steps:

1. Antiviral systemics
2. Stimulation of the spleen and lymph system to actively attack the infection, thus reducing movement into the brain by the virus and promoting the induction of splenic T cell activation
3. Reduction of cytokine/chemokine cascades through the use of specific inhibitors
4. Protection of neural cells and neural mitochondria
5. Inhibition of viral infection of neural cells
6. Regeneration of damaged neural structures

7. Enhancement of healthy immune system responses through the use of adaptogenic agents
8. Inhibition of HMGB1 if sepsis appears likely

Protocol Specifics

The protocol contains elements to address all these aspects of the infection.

1. ANTIVIRAL SYSTEMICS

Specific antivirals for encephalitis viruses are licorice, Chinese skullcap, isatis, and houttuynia. I personally also use lomatium for West Nile and consider it specific.

Formulation: Equal parts of the tinctures of each herb, combined.

Dosage: Depending on the severity of condition, from 1/4 tsp to 1 tbl of the combination tincture up to 6x daily. My normal use for mild to moderate West Nile, for example, is 1 tsp 4–6x daily for 2 to 4 weeks. Note: The dosage needs to be moderated for children, depending on their weight.

2. STIMULATION OF THE SPLEEN AND LYMPH SYSTEM

Red root (or poke if you can't find red root) will stimulate spleen function, reduce inflammation in the spleen, and enhance T cell counts.

Formulation: Red root tincture.

Dosage: 1/4–1 tsp up to 6x daily depending on the severity of the condition.

3. REDUCTION OF CYTOKINE CASCADES

The herbs specific for this are Chinese skullcap, licorice, isatis, houttuynia, cordyceps, rhodiola, and astragalus. They're all included in antiviral and immune formulations (steps 1 and 7, respectively).

4. PROTECTION OF NEURAL CELLS AND NEURAL MITOCHONDRIA

The main herbs for this are Chinese skullcap, cordyceps, Japanese knotweed, rhodiola, kudzu, and olive oil (oleorupin). They're all included in the antiviral and immune formulations (steps 1 and 7, respectively).

5. INHIBITION OF VIRAL INFECTION OF NEURAL CELLS

The main herbs for this are cordyceps, licorice, and Chinese skullcap. They're included in the antiviral and immune formulations (steps 1 and 7, respectively).

6. REGENERATION OF DAMAGED NEURAL STRUCTURES

The best herbs are Chinese senega root (*Polygala tenuifolia*) and lion's mane (*Hericium erinaceus*). Both contain substantial amounts of nerve growth factor.

Formulation and dosage:

- **Chinese senega root:** 30 drops of the tincture 3x daily for 30 days, and . . .
- **Lion's mane:** 3–8 grams per day or 1 tsp of the tincture 2x daily.

7. IMMUNE HERBS/ADAPTOGENS

The best for this are astragalus, cordyceps, and rhodiola.

Formulation: Tincture combination of all three herbs, with 1 part astragalus, 1 part rhodiola, and 2 parts cordyceps.

Dosage: 1 tsp of the combination tincture 6x daily during active infections.

Note: Cordyceps is very specific for the kinds of neuroinflammation that occur in the brain during encephalitis infections. In severe cases the dosage of cordyceps can be substantially increased. There is no toxic upper range to the herb.

8. INHIBITION OF HMGB1

The best herbs for this are licorice, *Angelica sinensis*, and *Salvia miltiorrhiza.*

Formulation: Equal parts of the tinctures of *Angelica sinensis* and *Salvia miltiorrhiza*, combined.

Dosage: 1 tsp to 1 tbl of the combination tincture up to 10x daily (or more), depending on the degree of inflammation occurring.

Strong infusions of these herbs will also work just fine.

Formulation: 8 ounces of herb per gallon of water; pour boiling water over the herb, cover, and let stand for 4 hours. Strain and use.

Dosage: An entire gallon should be consumed daily as the primary liquid source.

Note: There is no upper dosage range for these herbs. The inhibition is dose dependent.

For West Nile Encephalitis

Add the following to the basic protocol described above:

- **Astragalus:** Increase the dosage of astragalus by taking 3,000 mg daily or 1/2 tsp of the tincture 3–6x daily.
- **Japanese knotweed (*Polygonum cuspidatum*):** Tincture, 1/2 tsp 3–6x daily (or resveratrol, from knotweed root, 4,000 mg daily).
- ***Crinum latifolium* leaf:** Tea, 4–6 cups daily, or, if you wish, capsules, 8,000 mg daily. (Aqueous extracts are best.)

For Tick-Borne Encephalitis

Add the following to the basic protocol described above:

- **Greater celandine (*Chelidonium majus*) tincture:** 1/4 tsp 3x daily (not to exceed 30 days).
- **Motherwort (*Leonurus cardiaca*) tincture:** 1/4–1/2 tsp up to 6x daily.
- ***Ligusticum wallichii* tincture (for edema):** 1/4–1/2 tsp up to 6x daily, or a strong infusion 6x daily. (This herb will also reduce many of the cytokines TBE induces; the related herbs *Ligusticum porteri* and *Lomatium dissectum* may possibly be legitimate substitutes.)
- **Reduce blood acidity:** Reduce purine intake in the diet, explore acid/alkaline diet modification, and supplement with beta-alanine (750–2,250 mg daily).

For Dengue Encephalitis

To the basic protocol described above, add velvet leaf (*Cissampelos pareira*), which is active against all four serotypes of the virus (see the discussion of dengue on page 155 for more). Sea buckthorn leaf

(*Hippophae rhamnoides*), boneset, and cat's claw (*Uncaria tomentosa*) are all antivirals specific for dengue as well. Cat's claw is also a decent immune-enhancing herb. The specifics:

- **Velvet leaf tea:** A strong decoction of velvet leaf. Take 2 ounces 4x daily.
- **Tea from sea buckthorn and boneset leaves:** Add 1 ounce each of sea buckthorn leaf and boneset leaf to a quart jar (that can take heat), add boiling water, cover, and let steep 1 hour. Drink throughout the day, every day, for 2 weeks.
- **Sea buckthorn oil:** ½–1 tsp 3x daily.
- **Cat's claw:** Tincture, 1 tsp 3–6x daily, or capsules, 1,200 mg 3–6x daily, for 2 weeks.

A Brief Look at Some Neural Herbs for Encephalitis Treatment

There are a few herbs that are very specific for protecting or stimulating the regrowth of the neural structures of the brain. They are Chinese senega root, Japanese knotweed, kudzu root, lion's mane, and pink-striped trumpet lily.

Chinese Senega Root (*Polygala tenuifolia*)

This is one of the 50 fundamental herbs of Chinese medicine and is known there as *yuan zhi*. It is used in China primarily as an expectorant and to help lung inflammations. But it also has strong impacts on cognitive function, enhancing memory, alleviating neurotoxicity, and producing positive impacts in the treatment of Alzheimer's, dementia, depression, and degenerative diseases. It is a very good anti-inflammatory and inhibits NF-κB, nitric oxide, iNOS, COX-2, PGE2, TNF-α, and IL-1ß in microglial cells. One of the more important activities of the herb is that it enhances the secretion of nerve growth factor (NGF) in the brain, spinal cord, and peripheral nervous systems. NGF is a small protein that is crucial for the growth, maintenance, and survival of neurons. When neuronal damage occurs, higher levels of

NGF are essential in stimulating axonal regeneration. This is perhaps the best plant for stimulation of NGF.

PREPARATION AND USE

Take 30 drops of the tincture 3x daily for 30 days. It is contraindicated in those with ulcers or gastritis.

Japanese Knotweed (*Polygonum cuspidatum*)

Japanese knotweed is a world-class invasive originally native to Japan, north China, Taiwan, and Korea. It is another significant invasive that is specific for emerging infections. The root is the part of the plant used for medicine.

The herb has a wide range of actions; among other things, it is an antiviral, antimicrobial (widely), antifungal, immunomodulant, anti-inflammatory, angiogenesis modulator, central nervous system relaxant, central nervous system (brain and spinal cord) protectant and anti-inflammatory, antioxidant, inhibitor of platelet aggregation, inhibitor of eicosanoid synthesis, antithrombotic, tyrosine kinase inhibitor, antipyretic, cardioprotective, analgesic, hemostatic, and astringent.

A broadly systemic plant, Japanese knotweed modulates immune function, reducing and balancing cytokine cascades; is anti-inflammatory for arthritic, viral, and bacterial inflammations; protects the body against endotoxin damage; and is a potently strong angiogenesis modulator, highly protective of the endothelia of the body. It is specifically inhibitive of endothelial hyperplasia. It crosses the blood-brain barrier and is potently anti-inflammatory in the brain and CNS. It is highly specific for all CNS infections.

Knotweed is a very strong inhibitor of cytokine cascades initiated by pathogens, especially MMP-1, MMP-3, and MMP-9. These can be stimulated through various pathways, but knotweed is highly specific for reducing MMPs *and* mitogen-activated protein kinases (MAPKs), specifically c-Jun N-terminal kinase (JNK), p38 mitogen-activated protein kinase (p38 MAPK), and extracellular-signal-regulated kinase

1 and 2 (ERK-1 and ERK-2). Resveratrol (one of the plant's constituents) is also directly active in reducing MMP-9 levels through both the JNK and protein kinase C-delta pathways; it has been found to specifically inhibit MMP-9 gene transcription. The plant root is so high in resveratrols that it is the main source of the supplement throughout the world. Another component of the plant, rhein, inhibits the JNK pathway for MMP-1, MMP-3, and MMP-9 expression. The plant is also high in emodin, a constituent that has been found specifically active against a range of encephalitis viruses. Knotweed is also a formidable inhibitor of NF-κB, TNF-α, ICAM-1, VCAM-1, IL-1ß, IL-6, COX-2, IL-8, PI3K (phosphoinositide 3-kinase), E-selectin, IDO, and VEGF (vascular endothelial growth factor).

Polygonum cuspidatum's constituents cross the blood-brain barrier, where they act on the central nervous system as antimicrobials, anti-inflammatories, protectants against oxidative and microbial damage, and calming agents. The herb specifically protects the brain from inflammatory damage, microbial endotoxins, and bacterial infections. The compounds easily move across the gastrointestinal mucosa and circulate in the bloodstream.

The whole herb and its constituent, resveratrol, are both strong antioxidants. People who consume the herb (or constituent) have been found to have significantly increased antioxidant activity in their blood. This potent antioxidant action has been detected throughout the body. Interestingly, resveratrol seems to be an antioxidant modulator in that it will increase antioxidant action when needed (most of the time) but will lower it in instances where necessary, e.g., in leukemia cells.

Another component of knotweed, emodin, is highly protective of brain neurons and reduces pain by inhibiting the activation of the P2X7 receptors in the brain. It reduces impacts on the P2X2/3 receptors as well.

The herb, in fact, is a potent immunomodulator. It normalizes immune response, especially in diseases where autoimmune reactions are stimulated (such as Lyme disease and lupus). It seems able to bring up immune function when necessary and reduce its local manifestations when overstimulated, e.g., in rheumatoid arthritis. This is a very strong aspect of the plant's actions.

The herb and its constituents have also been found to enhance and potentiate the action of other drugs and herbs when taken with them.

Japanese knotweed and its constituents also possess strong actions in the central nervous system and brain, and this range of activity is where a great deal of interest in the plant is being generated.

Knotweed and the constituents trans-resveratrol and resveratrol have been found to be strongly neuroprotective through a variety of actions in numerous studies. One of the herb's mechanisms of action in this regard is as an antioxidant. Resveratrol and trans-resveratrol have been found to protect rat embryonic mesencephalic cells from a powerful pro-oxidant, tert-butyl hydroperoxide. Another study found that regular use of trans-resveratrol prevented streptozotocin-induced cognitive impairment and oxidative stress in rats (an Alzheimer's-like condition). And yet another found that trans-resveratrol protected against and reversed many of the impacts of induced stroke in rats.

While the herb's antioxidant actions are important, trans-resveratrol, for example, has been found in a number of studies to strongly protect neuronal structures from damage through mechanisms other than antioxidant activity alone. Resveratrol has been found specific for protecting the brain from neurotoxic substances such as the beta-amyloid peptides, which are associated with Alzheimer's disease.

Resveratrol and trans-resveratrol are specific for reducing inflammation in the brain and central nervous system. In spinal cord injuries resveratrol "remarkably" reduced secondary spinal cord edema, significantly suppressed the activity of lactate dehydrogenase, reduced malondialdehyde content in the injured spinal cord tissue, and markedly improved NA+/K+-ATPase activities. It immediately stimulated microcirculation to the injured tissues.

Low-level, chronic inflammation in the brain and central nervous system plays a major role in many neurodegenerative conditions. Both the herb and its constituents are specific for such inflammations. They have been found active for such things as amyotrophic lateral sclerosis and other motor neuron diseases, Parkinson's disease, Alzheimer's disease, bulbar atrophy, dementia, Huntington's disease, myasthenia gravis, stroke, multiple sclerosis, frontotemporal dementia, encephalomyelitis, traumatic brain injury, cerebral ischemia, and so on. The resveratrols specifically protect brain cells from assault, whether chemical or microbial in origin. The herb and its constituents, as well, stimulate microcirculation in the brain.

PREPARATION AND USE

Capsules or tincture can be used. Capsules of pure knotweed root can be had from Green Dragon Botanicals (see Sources of Supply on page 599) or you can buy resveratrol, which is in fact only a standardized knotweed root formulation. That is, it is knotweed root standardized for the presence of a certain percentage of resveratrols. Most of the brands on the market are usable. Just make sure they are made from knotweed root (it will say on the package someplace in tiny print) and not grapes. As for dosage:

- **Capsules:** 3 or 4 capsules 3 or 4x daily (or 1 tbl of the powdered root in juice 3 or 4x daily).
- **Tincture:** 1/4–1/2 tsp 3–6x daily.

The major side effect, in about 0.5 percent of those who use it, is loss of taste. This corrects upon discontinuance of the herb (in a week or so). Metallic or odd taste is moderately common. GI tract disturbances are rare but do occur. Note: Some people have reported rather strong negative physical responses to the Source Naturals resveratrol. I am not sure why this is; however, those who do, having switched to another product by Paradise Herbs, report a better outcome. Just an FYI on that one.

Japanese knotweed should not be used with blood-thinning agents. Discontinue use of the herb 10 days prior to any surgery. The plant is a synergist and may potentiate the effects of pharmaceuticals and other herbs.

Kudzu Root (*Pueraria lobata*)

Kudzu root and its major constituents (puerarin and kakkalide and irisolidone—a metabolite of kakkalide produced by intestinal microflora that is more potent than kakkalide) inhibit TNF-α, IL-1ß, NF-κB, ERK, iNOS, PGE2, COX-2, AP-1 (activator protein-1), ICAM-1, VCAM-1, E-selectin, C-reactive protein (CRP), and the phosphorylation of the 1κB-α protein. It has targeted and potent effects on cytokine-activated microglial cells and will reduce damage by cytokines in the CNS.

Kudzu (and puerarin) are strongly protective of the brain and CNS, especially in ischemia/reperfusion injury. They have a strong protective effect against beta-amyloid-induced neurotoxicity in hippocampal neurons, protect mitochondria from reactive oxygen species (ROS), and stimulate peripheral nerve regeneration. Neuron pain receptors P2X3 and P2X2/3, similar to P2X7, in the brain are inhibited by puerarin, making this a very good companion herb to use with greater celandine. The root is, in fact, strongly anti-inflammatory in the brain and CNS. It significantly inhibits neutrophil respiratory bursts, reducing autoimmune dynamics in the brain. It modulates Bax/Bcl-2 actions in the mitochondria in the brain and inhibits caspase-3 and iNOS expressions. It is strongly neuroprotective during inflammation disturbances in the brain and CNS.

It is a good herb for viral encephalitis types of cytokine cascades, especially so since it is invasive and there is no dearth of supply. *Anywhere* encephalitis occurs and kudzu grows, use kudzu.

PREPARATION AND USE

In traditional Chinese medicine the usual dose is 6–12 grams per day of the powdered root. Normally dosing in the West is 1 gram per day. The tincture dosage in encephalitis infection is $^1/_2$ tsp 3 or 4x daily.

Lion's Mane (*Hericium erinaceus*)

Lion's mane is a highly edible mushroom, a member of the tooth fungus group of mushrooms. (It should look sort of like a waterfall of beautiful white threads. If it does not, be suspicious.) The mushroom has a long history of use in Asia. Like most mushrooms, it is high in polysaccharides and possesses strong immunomodulating and immune-activating properties. It strongly activates T cells and strongly downregulates iNOS, nitric oxide, ROS, PGE2, COX-2, NF-κB, and JNK during inflammatory overreactions.

However, its strongest actions are in its effects on nerve cells and brain function. The herb stimulates peripheral and CNS nerve regeneration after damage (specifically by inducing nerve growth factor in the body), increases remyelination of nerve sheaths, improves cognitive impairment after neural damage (including amyloid peptide-induced), and significantly alleviates depression and anxiety.

PREPARATION AND USE

The herb can be used as either an aqueous or alcohol preparation; I tend to prefer the alcohol tincture made from the fresh mushroom. Dosage for encephalitis is 1/4–1/2 tsp 3–6x daily, depending on the severity of the condition. I think the herb is highly indicated to alleviate or in the treatment of postencephalitis conditions.

Pink-Striped Trumpet Lily (*Crinum latifolium*)

Pink-striped trumpet lily is a typical-looking lily, a perennial that grows from a bulb. The herb is commonly used in Asia as a medicinal for inflammatory problems of various sorts, especially rheumatoid complaints. It is most commonly used in the West now to reduce prostate enlargement, either benign prostatic hyperplasia or prostatitis.

The herb is a potent inhibitor, perhaps the best currently known, of indoleamine 2,3-dioxygenase (IDO). In consequence it is a potent stimulant of T cell activation in cases where IDO has been overexpressed by pathogens. It is strongly inhibitive of IFN-γ, stopping the particular cytokine cascade that it starts during infections. It also inhibits NF-κB. The plant is a pretty good free radical scavenger, reducing ROS in the body and CNS. The herb is anti-angiogenic, protecting the endothelial cells from inflammation, hyperplasia, and overstimulation by cytokines. It has been found to possess antiviral activity against some vaccinia viruses. And it is active, in vitro and in vivo, against a variety of cancers, including prostate.

PREPARATION AND USE

The leaf, prepared as a tea (aqueous extracts are best), 4–6 cups daily, or, if you wish, in capsules, 8,000 mg daily. The bulbs are easy to find and the herb grows easily. You can find the tea most easily on the online site eBay.

Cytomegalovirus

Cytomegalovirus (CMV) is a member of the Herpesviridae family of viruses, a very large group of DNA viruses that also includes the herpes simplex viruses, Epstein-Barr virus, and varicella zoster virus (chicken pox/shingles). It is sometimes referred to as human herpesvirus 5 (HHV-5). It usually causes minor problems in people with healthy immune systems, but if immune function drops (especially in those with AIDS, those taking immunosuppressive drugs, or those whose immune function is simply becoming weak from either age or illness) or if the immune system has not yet developed fully (babies, in and out of utero), it can cause severe problems up to and including death.

Infection rates are high. In the United States somewhere between 50 percent and 80 percent of the adult population are asymptomatically infected. When people first become infected, the usual signs are fever, fatigue, muscle tenderness, and tender and enlarged lymph nodes. Just like the flu. Then it passes, you feel fine, and you are an asymptomatic carrier.

As the years go by, the virus periodically blooms, sending viruses to body fluids: saliva, tears, urine, blood, semen, vaginal secretions, and breast milk. From there it spreads to new hosts. It is a pretty good parasitic virus, and it usually doesn't cause much trouble. However, in people whose immune function is impaired, the virus can cause a wide range of symptoms: encephalitis, myelitis, seizures, coma, psychosis, dysphagia, weakness, numbness in the legs, retinitis, visual impairments including blurred vision or blindness, pneumonia, gastritis, enteritis, colitis, diarrhea, ulcers in the GI tract, and hepatitis.

In babies, CMV is the most common congenital infection in the United States. For most it will not be a problem, but for some it can cause severe and long-term difficulties: neurological problems, hearing impairment or loss, visual problems, seizures, or mental and physical disabilities. The worst problems occur in infants whose mothers become infected while the infants are in utero.

CMV is normally treated with the intravenous antibiotic ganciclovir (or valganciclovir), usually along with CMV-specific immune globulin. Treatment usually lasts 2 to 4 weeks, followed by a transition to oral valganciclovir. Unfortunately the virus is becoming fairly resistant to ganciclovir. Generally, this drug will not cure the infection but only lessen its effects. Again, the search is for a vaccine; however, early trials show that the vaccines in development only tend to lessen the effects of the disease, not eliminate it, for the majority of people using them.

Dengue Fever

Dengue viruses (DENVs) are single-stranded RNA viruses in the Flaviviridae family, specifically in the *Flavivirus* genus. This genus includes many of the encephalitis viruses such as West Nile, tick-borne encephalitis, Japanese encephalitis, Murray Valley encephalitis, St. Louis encephalitis, and so on. Yellow fever virus is also in this group. There are various serotypes of dengue (1, 2, 3, and 4). Each one produces a slightly different spectrum of symptoms. DENV-3 produces more musculoskeletal and gastrointestinal symptoms; DENV-4 has more respiratory and cutaneous symptoms.

Dengue fever, a.k.a. breakbone fever, is a mosquito-transmitted disease and is not infectious except through that route. There are about

100 million people infected with dengue each year; several hundred thousand develop dengue hemorrhagic fever, which is very serious, and about 22,000 die.

The disease is endemic pretty much everywhere, including the southern United States. Outbreaks have occurred in recent years throughout the Caribbean including Puerto Rico, the U.S. Virgin Islands, and Cuba. The disease is common in Tahiti, Singapore, the South Pacific, Southeast Asia, the West Indies, India, and the Middle East as well as throughout South America. The incidence of the disease is growing each year.

Once a mosquito bites a person, the virus enters the body and begins seeking out monocytes and macrophages, the primary parts of the body it infects. The symptoms develop in 3 to 15 days (normally 5 to 8). The symptoms are sudden-onset fever, headache, pain on eye movement, and low backache. Muscle and joint pain (which is often very severe—it's called "breakbone" fever for a reason) occurs soon after a fever, often as high as 104 degrees Fahrenheit, develops; heart rate and blood pressure drop. The eyes redden, a rash may occur on the face, and lymph nodes often swell.

The fever tends to last several days, then a sudden drop in body temperature occurs accompanied by extreme sweating. This passes, you feel fine, then it starts all over again. This time the rash covers the whole body except for the face.

Dengue hemorrhagic fever (DHF) usually affects children under 10 years of age. It causes severe abdominal pain, hemorrhage, and shock. Sore throat, cough, nausea, and vomiting all occur. Somewhere from 2 to 6 days after symptoms begin there is sudden collapse, with cool, clammy extremities, weak pulse, and cyanosis around the mouth. The skin bruises easily; there is bleeding, spitting up of blood, blood in the stool, bleeding gums, nosebleeds. Pneumonia is common; inflammation of the heart may occur. The disease is associated with high levels of circulating von Willebrand factor. Normal treatment for DHF is transfusions, oxygen, and fluid replacement.

There are no pharmaceutical treatments for either form of dengue fever. There is no vaccine. However, recent research has shown that the antibiotic Geneticin is active against the virus. Its effectiveness in practice is unknown.

Enterovirus 71

Enterovirus 71 (sometimes called hand, foot, and mouth disease) is a single-stranded, nonenveloped RNA virus in the Picornaviridae family. Rhinoviruses (common cold), hepatitis A, and the polio virus are some of the better-known members of the family.

Enterovirus 71 was first identified in 1965; the first known outbreak was in 1969 in the United States. There are severe outbreaks every 3 to 4 years throughout the world with smaller annual episodes here and there. A huge outbreak in Taiwan in 1998 infected more than 130,000 people, mostly children. The virus is usually spread by respiratory droplets or contact with an infected person's body fluids. It is excreted in feces for weeks or months after infection.

The virus initially colonizes the GI tract, and from there, if the disease does increase in severity, it invades the spinal cord and ascends to the brain. In the CNS and brain it produces high levels of cytokines: IL-1ß, IL-6, IL-8, and TNF-α. Enterovirus 71 is considered to be an emerging pathogen, with the number of cases increasing each year.

The most common symptoms of infection are fever, headache, fatigue, malaise, ear pain, sore throat, body rash, blisters on the palms of the hands or soles of the feet (they may also occur in the nostrils and buttocks), oral ulcers, loss of appetite, diarrhea, and vomiting. Fever and sore throat are usually the first signs.

Unfortunately, there are some more serious complications that can occur during infection: high fever, meningitis, encephalitis, paralysis, cardiopulmonary edema, and sometimes coma and death.

There is no pharmaceutical treatment or vaccine.

Epstein-Barr

Epstein-Barr is a member of the Herpesviridae or herpesvirus family; it's sometimes referred to as human herpesvirus 4 (HHV-4). It is the cause of mononucleosis and a very common cause of chronic fatigue syndrome. It is considered an oncovirus, meaning it can, under some circumstances, over long periods of time, cause certain forms of cancer. Most children become infected with it at a young age, in which case the symptoms are usually mild—it looks like a mild case of the flu. The older the person at infection, the more severe the symptoms. In teenagers it causes infectious mononucleosis. This is usually accompanied by a severe sore throat, fever, and extreme fatigue and malaise. The infected may also experience swollen throat, loss of appetite, enlarged lymph nodes, swollen spleen and liver, jaundice, and petechiae. Some of the very serious complications are splenic rupture or hemorrhage, meningitis, peripheral neuritis, and pneumonitis. An autoimmune hemolytic anemia can occur as well, though it is much rarer.

There are no reliable pharmaceutical treatments for the disease. Acyclovir can help reduce viral shedding. Valacyclovir has been found to, sometimes, significantly reduce the viral load and thus the symptoms of the disease.

Herpes Simplex 1 and 2

Herpes is probably the most famous (or infamous) member of the Herpesviridae family of viruses. There are two types, herpes simplex virus 1 (HSV-1) and herpes simplex virus 2 (HSV-2). The most common sites of infection are around the lips (cold sores, fever blisters) and on the genitals (herpes). Cold sores are usually caused by herpes simplex 1, genital herpes by herpes simplex 2. A less common form is infection of the fingers, called herpetic whitlow. It is caused by either type. There are some more serious forms of infection: ocular herpes (which infects the eyes, causing a form of keratitis), herpes gladiatorum (which broadly infects the skin), herpes encephalitis (which infects the brain), Mollaret's meningitis (which infects the protective membranes covering the brain and spinal cord), and neonatal herpes (where the baby is infected as it is born or in utero).

Herpes, either oral or genital, is usually cyclic with long (or short) periods of remission between episodes. With genital herpes, once the virus enters a new host, it travels along the nerve paths, where it takes up residence. For many people, after an initial outbreak, the virus may become dormant indefinitely. For others, every so often, the virus becomes active. It then travels back along the nerve paths to the surface of the skin, where it creates blisters that shed viruses, spreading the disease.

Just prior to a new episode, there may be a feeling of pain in the nerves in the genitals. Soon small blisters may appear; they eventually break open and produce very painful sores that scab over and heal after several weeks. Sometimes people with an active infection feel as if they have the flu, and the lymph nodes may be swollen.

Oral herpes and herpetic whitlow symptoms are similar but occur around the lips and fingers respectively.

There are generally three types of ocular, or eye, herpes. Herpes keratitis is the most common form; it's a viral infection of the cornea or surface of the eye. This usually heals without damage to the eye. Stromal keratitis is a deeper form, where the virus penetrates deeper into the layers of the cornea. It can cause scarring of the cornea and, sometimes, blindness. The final type is iridocyclitis. Here the iris and surrounding tissues of the eye are infected and become inflamed. There is often severe light sensitivity and blurred vision, and the infected eye is red. Sometimes this kind of infection can occur in the retina or inside lining of the back of the eye; it's then called herpes retinitis.

Signs and symptoms of herpetic eye infections are swelling, tearing, irritation, foreign body sensation, redness, eye sores, discharge, and light sensitivity.

The normal treatment for eye herpes is ganciclovir as an ophthalmic gel, 5 drops daily. Sometimes steroid eyedrops are used to decrease the inflammation. The infected cornea is sometimes scraped away. There is no effective cure; these interventions reduce the impact of the episode and, hopefully, prevent permanent damage.

Herpes gladiatorum is tremendously infective and is transmitted by skin-to-skin contact. It is essentially a cutaneous form of herpes, usually herpes simplex 1 (the same form of the virus that causes cold sores). It is somewhat common in sports clubs (which is where it got its name). In this condition, the sores, instead of being confined to the genitals or lips, are found in clusters over the body: neck, chest, face, stomach, legs. The lymph nodes are often enlarged, with fever, sore throat, and headache. The blisters are very painful and take weeks to heal.

Herpes encephalitis and meningitis are uncommon but severe complications of herpes infection. Herpes meningitis is usually caused by the HSV-2 serotype and is an inflammation of the meninges, the tissue surrounding the brain and spinal cord. The normal symptoms are stiff neck, headache, fever, light sensitivity, fatigue, nausea, appetite loss, and vomiting (sometimes). It is usually a self-limiting disease and clears on its own. For some people it recurs at periodic intervals just as genital and oral herpes do. In rare instances it may cause minor mental dysfunctions, slight confusion, and difficulty in problem solving that fail to resolve.

Herpes simplex encephalitis is usually caused by HSV-1. During herpes simplex encephalitis, the temporal and frontal lobes are usually infected when the virus travels along the nerve lines into the brain. The usual encephalitic processes occur: inflammation of the brain, confusion, psychological alterations, fever, and—in anywhere from 30 percent to 70 percent of those infected—seizures, coma, and death. The infection is usually treated with IV acyclovir, but there is still a 30 percent mortality rate. There is often long-lasting brain damage.

The usual treatment for herpes infections is valacyclovir, acyclovir (a.k.a. aciclovir), or famciclovir. All are forms of guanosine analogue antiviral drugs that, when taken, are metabolized by the body into an active form. These drugs are widely used to help control outbreaks of herpes simplex viruses, chicken pox, shingles, Epstein-Barr, and cytomegalovirus, all of which are closely related herpesviruses. They are strongest against the simplex types and have no effect on the viruses in their latent form in the nerve sheaths; they are effective only when the viruses become active. The drugs can shorten the course of the disease to some extent and help prevent spread. They do not cure it.

Herpesviruses are becoming resistant fairly rapidly to acyclovir, especially in those with compromised immune systems.

Varicella Zoster Virus (Chicken Pox/Shingles)

Varicella zoster virus is also a member of the Herpesviridae family; it's sometimes referred to as human herpesvirus 3 (HHV-3). HHV-3 usually occurs first as chicken pox (i.e., varicella), later as shingles (herpes zoster).

During the initial infection, normally during childhood, spread via respiratory droplets in the air, the virus enters the bloodstream and travels everywhere, making spots all over the surface of the body. It takes about 2 weeks for the spots to appear, and the infection period lasts for up to 3 weeks after that, until the spots crust over. At that point, still spotted, the child is no longer infected. ("Yes, you still have to go to school.")

Though the disease was usually self-limiting and fairly benign, vaccines are now commonly used in the West for chicken pox. However . . .

Regrettably, the virus, once the initial infection has passed, settles in the dorsal ganglion, part of the nerve structure of the central nervous system. There it lives quite happily for decades, until in later age, usually as a result of lowering immune function, it sometimes reappears as shingles.

The virus leaves its happy home, travels along the nerves, and emerges at the surface of the skin, often on the face, and makes life intolerable. There is often hemorrhage, edema, and lymphocytic infiltration of the affected nerves. Usually, the person can feel the event beginning—as the virus travels along the nerves, it creates odd feelings, tingling, burning, numbness, and a very definite feeling that something is wrong. Then, quite quickly, the virus emerges out of the body onto the surface of the skin, creating tiny blisters filled with virus particles. The pain is often excruciating, and little in the pharmaceutical armamentarium can help. Occasionally there can be fever, enlarged lymph nodes, chills, malaise, loss of appetite, and stomach upset. The lesions can last up to a week or so once they emerge. There can also, rarely, be more difficult complications such as encephalitis, peripheral nerve palsies, hemiparesis, and myelitis.

The most problematic aspect of shingles is postherpetic neuropathy, i.e., pain, at the site of the eruption. It can be an unrelenting sharp, burning, or stabbing pain that can become highly debilitating. About half the people who get shingles also develop postherpetic neuropathy. The neuropathy is usually caused by the infection itself as it blooms at its emergence location. The local nerves are damaged by the inflammation, and it takes them time, sometimes a very long time (7 to 10 months), to recover. The older the person, the longer they take to heal. As long as the damage lasts, postherpetic neuropathy will remain.

The usual medical treatment is the use of antivirals such as acyclovir, valacyclovir, or famciclovir. Corticosteroids may also be used to lessen the inflammation, especially if the complications are serious. Over-the-counter analgesics are often used, with varying success. The pain is sometimes so severe that opiates are necessary. Pharmaceuticals don't heal the disease, but they can help reduce the length of an episode and help with pain.

One of the better natural approaches for shingles is the use of herbs to increase immune function to reduce outbreak frequency and herbs that protect and restore the nerves. Specific herbs for nerve pain will also help tremendously, especially those that affect the P2X receptors in the brain.

Gastrointestinal Viruses (Rotaviruses and Noroviruses)

There are a number of common (and a few uncommon) viruses that cause gastrointestinal infections in people. The two primary ones are rotavirus and the Norwalk (norovirus) virus. Some countries now use vaccines against rotaviruses; there is none for the Norwalk virus, which is thought to cause 90 percent of all nonbacterial epidemic gastroenteritis worldwide and as much as half of all U.S. gastroenteritis infections. There is also an emerging group of viruses, discovered in the 1970s, the astroviruses, that are GI tract infectives. And the orthoreoviruses that are thought to only rarely cause human disease.

These groups of viruses are specialists in infecting human food plants and bind quite strongly to lettuce leaves, for example. They are the main cause of diarrheal outbreaks from agricultural food products. The symptoms are much the same for all: nausea, vomiting, diarrhea, abdominal pain, lethargy, weakness, muscle aches, headache, low-grade fever, and dehydration. The diseases are usually self-limiting, but they can be quite debilitating and a few people in the United States always die from them every year. Rotaviruses are still a major cause of child mortality throughout the world.

In essence this is what is usually called the stomach flu in the United States. It is a food-borne illness from virus-contaminated food, usually vegetables, and is commonly spread via salad bars or prepackaged spinach, bean sprouts, and so on.

The Treatment Protocols

Again, the protocols suggested in this section are *only* suggestions. There are many ways to approach treating these viruses; this is just a starting point. Comment: If encephalitis occurs from any of these viruses, the encephalitis protocol, with slight alterations for each virus, which would mean adding specific herbs to the protocol, should be used.

Cytomegalovirus (CMV)

Herbs (and supplements) that have been found active for this virus in vitro, in vivo, and in human clinical use are (in alphabetical order) *Artemisia annua* (or artemisinin), *Astragalus membranaceus* (astragalus), the berberine plants, *Bidens pilosa* (bidens), *Bupleurum kaoi*, *Forsythia suspensa*, *Geum japonicum*, *Glycyrrhiza glabra* (licorice), houttuynia, *Hypericum perforatum*, isatis, *Lomatium dissectum*, *Nigella sativa*, quercetin, *Scaevola spinescens*, *Syzygium aromaticum* (cloves), *Terminalia chebula*, *Urtica dioica* (nettles), and *Zingiber officinale* (ginger).

Geum japonicum, licorice, isatis, and the berberines have been found as effective as ganciclovir in the treatment of CMV in vivo.

TREATMENT

To begin: Bidens is a potent systemic antimicrobial herb (it must be prepared from fresh leaves; for more information, see page 229), and I would include it in any protocol for treating CMV. A systemic formulation that would be good is *Bidens pilosa*, houttuynia, isatis, licorice, and lomatium, equal parts of each of the tinctures, combined. Dosage: 1/4–1/2 tsp of the tincture combination from 3–6x daily depending on severity of the infection.

Then, based on specific symptoms, add to this systemic formulation any of the following:

For GI tract symptoms: Berberine-containing plants are specific in this instance: goldenseal, phyllanthus, barberry, Oregon grape root, coptis, and so on will all work fine. My preference is for phyllanthus, barberry, or goldenseal. Dosage: 1/4–1/2 tsp of the tincture 3–6x daily depending on severity of symptoms. The systemic tincture should also be used, with the same dosage range described above. The licorice will help any ulceration that has occurred.

For neurological symptoms: The encephalitis protocol (see page 143) plus bidens.

For pneumonia: Moderate to severe influenza protocol (see page 120) plus bidens.

Dengue Fever Virus

Some herbs and supplements effective for dengue are (in alphabetical order) *Alternanthera philoxeroides*, *Andrographis paniculata*, *Artemisia douglasiana*, *Azadirachta indica* (neem), the berberine (and palmatine) plants, *Cissampelos pareira, Cladogynos orientalis, Cryptocarya chartacea, Daucus maritimus, Distictella elongata, Ellipeiopsis cherrevensis, Eupatorium patens, Eupatorium perfoliatum* (boneset), *Flagellaria indica, Garcinia multiflora, Gastrodia elata, Glycyrrhiza glabra* (licorice), grape seed proanthocyanidins, *Hippophae rhamnoides* (sea buckthorn leaf), houttuynia, *Kaempferia parviflora, Lantana grisebachii, Momordica charantia, Ocimum sanctum* (mildly active), *Punica granatum* (pomegranate juice), *Quercus lusitanica* (gall oak seed), *Rhizophora apiculata, Salvia miltiorrhiza* (Chinese or red sage), *Stemona tuberosa, Tephrosia* spp., and *Uncaria tomentosa.* Oligomeric procyanidins (OPCs) are also specifically antiviral for dengue. They are common in cranberry juice, pomegranate juice, grape seeds, and unripe apple peels (for example). Any source can help, but that is the reason that pomegranate is included here. In addition pomegranate is a fairly potent synergist with a wide range of antimicrobial activity.

Many of the studies did not mention the serotype of dengue tested. Most of the herbs and supplements that did specify serotype have only been tested against type 2 (out of the four serotypes). The exceptions (that I can find) are andrographis, *Momordica charantia* (type 1), *Ocimum sanctum* (type 1), and *Cissampelos pareira* (all four serotypes). It is possible that many of these herbs are active against other serotypes, but no testing has yet been done.

TREATMENT

I would suggest beginning treatment with the following: *Cissampelos pareira,* sea buckthorn leaf, boneset, houttuynia, licorice, pomegranate juice, and cat's claw. *Salvia miltiorrhiza* is for hemorrhagic dengue as an adjunct.

Cissampelos pareira (in English, velvet leaf) is a widely used herb in Chinese medicine, Ayurveda, and South and Central America (where it is called *arbuta*). It is moderately findable, if you look for it. It is somewhat invasive in Florida and should be harvested for use in that region.

The herb is antipyretic, anti-inflammatory, immunomodulatory, antiplasmodial, antinociceptive, antiarthritic, antioxidant protective, antileukemic, cardioprotective, constipative, and abortifacient. It should not be used if you are pregnant or wanting to become pregnant. You can use it either as a strong decoction or as a 50 percent alcohol/ water tincture. It is the only herb that is considered to have strong action against all four serotypes of dengue.

Sea buckthorn leaf and boneset are both antivirals specific for dengue. The boneset, additionally, will help lower fever, reduce pains in the body, and stimulate the immune response. Houttuynia and licorice are good supportive antivirals, and both are active against dengue. (Unfortunately, all have only been tested against serotype 2.) Licorice will also act as a synergist and anti-inflammatory. Pomegranate juice constituents are antiviral for dengue, and it is a good synergist and anti-inflammatory, so it is perfect for keeping up fluids. Cat's claw will protect the macrophages and monocytes from dengue infection (it is very specific for this). Chinese sage should be used in cases of hemorrhagic dengue; it will lower circulating levels of von Willebrand factor in the blood. Here is a suggested protocol:

- **Strong decoction of velvet leaf:** Take 2 ounces 4x daily.
- **Tea from sea buckthorn and boneset leaves:** Add 1 ounce each of sea buckthorn leaf and boneset leaf to a quart jar (that can take heat), add boiling water, cover, and let steep 1 hour. Drink throughout the day, every day, for 2 weeks.
- **Sea buckthorn oil:** ½–1 tsp 3x daily.
- **Cat's claw:** Tincture, 1 tsp 3–6x daily, or capsules, 1,200 mg 3–6x daily, for 2 weeks.
- **Tincture combination** of houttuynia, licorice and Chinese skullcap, equal parts of each, 1 tsp 3–6x daily for 2 weeks.
- **Pomegranate juice:** Drink throughout the day.
- **Vitamin C effervescent salts:** As needed if the velvet leaf causes constipation.

For dengue encephalitis use the dengue protocol outlined on page 146.

Enterovirus 71

Some herbs and supplements effective for enterovirus 71 are, in alphabetical order, *Amomum villosum, Ampelopsis brevipedunculata* (porcelain berry, invasive), *Azadirachta indica* (neem), *Elaeagnus oldhamii, Euchresta formosana* (shan dou gen), *Ficus pumila, Forsythia suspensa* (lian qiao), *Glycine tomentella, Glycyrrhiza glabra* (licorice), houttuynia, *Kalanchoe gracilis, Laminaria japonica* (kombu), *Ledebouriella divaricata* (fang feng), *Lemmaphyllum microphyllum, Lonicera japonica* (Japanese honeysuckle, invasive), *Melastoma candidum* (invasive), *Melissa officinalis* (lemon balm), *Ocimum basilicum* (basil), *Origanum vulgare* (oregano), *Phragmites communis* (a.k.a. *P. australis*; invasive), *Polygonum chinense* (Chinese knotweed), *Polygonum multiflorum* (fo-ti), *Psidium guajava* (guava), *Pueraria lobata* (kudzu, invasive), *Rheum officinale* (rhubarb), *Rosmarinus officinalis* (rosemary), *Schisandra chinensis* (schisandra), *Spatholobi caulis, Thymus vulgaris* (thyme), *Toona sinensis*, and *Zingiber officinale* (ginger).

TREATMENT

Enterovirus 71 is an emerging pathogen that has no reliable pharmaceutical treatment. Numerous invasives are specific for this disease. I would begin with these herbs as systemic antivirals (then add others specific to the symptom picture): porcelain berry, neem leaf, licorice, houttuynia, fo-ti, ginger.

Japanese knotweed (*Polygonum cuspidatum*), a.k.a. hu zhang (huchang), has not been tested for activity against enterovirus 71 to my knowledge, but its constituents and actions are very similar to the two polygonums that have been tested. This is of interest to me because Japanese knotweed is an invasive and thus presents a large, easily available source of medicine.

Interestingly, a Chinese combination used for measles for several millennia has been found effective in the treatment of enterovirus 71. It is composed of black cohosh rhizome, kudzu root, red peony root, and licorice. It's a nice combination, though I don't know where you can easily find it already prepared in the West. The kudzu and the licorice are antiviral. The licorice is synergistic and immune potentiating, the kudzu and peony neuroprotective, and to some extent so is the licorice. The black cohosh is pain relieving. You can, however, buy the herbs, most of them, from 1stChineseHerbs.com. Just because of my own preferences, I would approach my own formulation slightly differently.

In addition to the systemic antibacterials, lemon balm, especially a prepared oil infusion, is specific for the blistering that enterovirus 71 can cause on the palms and soles of the feet. If neurological complications occur, you need to add specific anti-inflammatories for the brain and neural protectors. Kudzu is a good one, and a decent choice since it is active against the virus. My general preferences for anti-inflammatories in the brain these days are Japanese knotweed, Chinese skullcap, greater celandine, and lion's mane.

For simple, uncomplicated enterovirus 71, here is a suggested protocol:

- **Tincture combination** composed of equal parts of licorice, houttuynia, and porcelain berry. Dosage: From 1–5 ml, 3–6x daily, depending on the severity of the symptoms and age of child.
- **Tea** of ginger juice, neem leaf, honey, squeeze of lime, pinch of cayenne. Dosage: 3–6x daily.

For specific symptoms or complications, incorporate these additional formulations into the protocol:

For blisters: Lemon balm infused oil or cordial, applied topically to blisters, as many times daily as seems appropriate.

For diarrhea: Blackberry root infusion, consumed throughout the day as tea, with honey added as desired. Pomegranate juice is highly suggested as it is antiviral, will reduce the cytokine cascade in the body, replaces fluids, helps reduce diarrhea, and is a good synergist. A combination of pomegranate and cranberry juice is just about perfect for this.

For fever: Boneset tea, 4–6x daily. Pasque flower tincture, 5–10 drops every hour or so, can also help. It will also help reduce anxiety levels.

For encephalitis and meningitis: I would essentially use the protocol outlined earlier in this chapter. However, add a tincture combination of fo-ti, cordyceps, and Chinese skullcap, in equal parts, 1/4–1/2 tsp (or more, depending on the severity of symptoms) up to 6x daily. This will reduce the cytokine cascade in the brain and CNS, protect neural structures, and reduce the symptom picture. Lion's mane tincture, at the same dosage, will help restore neural function. If neurological symptoms are very severe, add greater celandine tincture, 30–60 drops, 3–6x daily for a max of 30 days.

Note: When treating a child, all dosages need to be adjusted for the child's weight and age; see page 577 for specifics.

Epstein-Barr Virus

Some of the herbs and supplements effective for Epstein-Barr are *Ailanthus altissima, Alpinia galanga, Andrographis paniculata, Artemisia annua* (or artemisinin), *Azadirachta indica* (neem), *Calendula officinalis, Chrysanthemum indicum, Cochlospermum tinctorium, Coix lacryma-jobi, Curcuma longa* (turmeric), *Eucalyptus* spp., *Ganoderma lucidum* (reishi), *Glycosmis arborea, Glycyrrhiza glabra* (licorice), isatis, *Morinda citrifolia* (noni), *Opuntia streptacantha* (prickly pear cactus), *Passiflora incarnata* (passionflower), *Polygonum cuspidatum* (Japanese knotweed), *Prunus persica* (peach tree leaves), *Scutellaria baicalensis* (Chinese skullcap), *Thelypteris torresiana, Thuja* spp., *Usnea* spp., *Wolfiporia extensa* (a.k.a. *Poria cocos,* a.k.a. fu ling), and *Zingiber officinale* (ginger).

Epstein-Barr acute episodes can often lead to severe chronic fatigue. Part of the fatigue comes from its impacts on mitochondrial function. It scavenges and damages mitochondria, so protecting mitochondria is important. The best herbs and supplements for this are cordyceps, *Leonurus cardiaca* (motherwort), *Passiflora* spp. (passionflower), rhodiola, schisandra, *Pueraria lobata* (kudzu), *Scutellaria baicalensis,* and N-acetylcysteine. Some of these are also very good immune herbs that will help raise immune function. Motherwort and passionflower will also help reduce anxiety and sleeplessness.

Epstein-Barr, during acute attacks, usually presents with a very severe, very painful sore throat, usually confined mainly to one pinpoint location just at the back of the throat from the mouth. I haven't found *anything* that will truly relieve it. *Echinacea angustifolia* (**not** *E. purpurea*) tincture will help a bit, if you use the tincture full strength. Keep it on the tongue a bit, let the saliva be stimulated, then let the whole mix flow *slowly* over the affected area. (But it won't do anything for the disease itself.) The root of *Artemisia absinthium* can also help if you chew a fresh root, just a bit when needed. It will really cool (almost creating a freeze sensation) the back of the throat.

TREATMENT

- **Tincture combination** of Chinese skullcap, isatis, and licorice, in equal parts, 1/2–1 tsp 3–6x daily depending on the severity of the infection.
- **Ginger juice tea** (see page 118), 3–6x daily.
- **Andrographis capsules or tablets,** 1,200 mg 3x daily for 30 days. (Caution: About 1 percent of people who use andrographis get a bad case of hives; if you do, discontinue the herb, and it will clear up in a week or so.)
- **Tincture combination** of motherwort and passionflower, in equal parts, 1/4–1/2 tsp 6x daily.
- **Tincture combination** of cordyceps and rhodiola, in equal parts, 1/4–1/2 tsp 3x daily.

If spleen enlargement occurs, use red root (*Ceanothus* spp.). With enlarged liver, milk thistle. With meningitis, use the protocols mentioned earlier in this chapter for encephalitic swelling.

Herpes Simplex Virus 1 and 2

There are many herbs (and supplements) useful against herpes simplex viruses; here are some of them: *Actinidia chinensis* (kiwi tree root), *Agrimonia pilosa* (hairy agrimony), *Andrographis paniculata* (andrographis), *Aristolochia debilis*, *Artemisia annua* (artemisinin), *Artemisia anomala*, *Astragalus membranaceus* (astragalus), *Azadirachta indica* (neem), the berberine plants, *Bidens pilosa* (bidens), *Boussingaultia gracilis*, *Byrsonima verbascifolia*, *Caesalpinia pulcherrima* (a strong decoction of the flower is strongest, followed by stem/leaf preparations), *Carissa edulis* (root bark), *Centella asiatica* (gotu kola), *Cordyceps sinensis* (cordyceps), *Crossostephium chinense*, *Cryptolepis sanguinolenta* (cryptolepis), *Cynanchum paniculatum*, *Distictella elongata*, *Ganoderma lucidum* (reishi), *Geum japonicum*, *Glycyrrhiza glabra* (licorice), honey, houttuynia, isatis, *Juniper* spp., *Limonium brasiliense*, *Lindera strychnifolia*, *Melia azedarach* (chinaberry leaves, invasive in the United States), *Melissa officinalis* (lemon balm), *Ocimum americanum* (hairy basil), *Ocimum basilicum* (basil), *Ocimum sanctum* (holy basil, strongest of the three), *Patrinia villosa*, *Phyllanthus niruri*, *Pinus massoniana*, *Pithecellobium clypearia* (a.k.a. *Archidendron clypearia*), *Pongamia pinnata* (seeds), *Prunella vulgaris* (self-heal), *Psidium guajava*, *Punica granatum* (pomegranate juice), *Pyrrosia lingua*, *Rheum officinale* (rhubarb root), *Rhus aromatica* (fragrant sumac), *Rhus chinensis* (Chinese sumac), *Rhus javanica*, *Rosmarinus officinalis* (rosemary), *Salvia officinalis* (sage), *Sargassum fusiforme*, *Scutellaria baicalensis* (Chinese skullcap), *Serissa japonica* (a.k.a. *S. foetida*), *Sida acuta* (sida), *Stephania cepharantha* (stephania), *Syzygium aromaticum*, *Taraxacum mongolicum*, *Terminalia chebula*, *Thymus vulgaris* (thyme), *Usnea* spp., zinc, zinc sulfate cream.

Byrsonima verbascifolia is a South American herb; it is particularly antiviral for these two viruses but is hard to get in the United States. Bidens, reishi, licorice, and houttuynia are also especially strong. A combination Chinese formula, yin chen hao tang, composed of *Artemisia capillaris*, *Rheum officinale*, and *Gardenia jasminoides*, has shown good effect against HSV-1 and HSV-2.

Terminalia chebula, *Syzygium aromaticum*, *Rhus javanica*, and *Geum japonicum* have all been found potent against HSV serotypes. They have particularly strong actions in the brain and are synergistic with acyclovir, enhancing its actions and impacts. The use of these herbs, singly, or in combination, has been found to prevent recurrence of HSV blooms in vivo (mice). All are traditional herbs, long used in community medicine. They all have activity against a variety of viruses.

TREATMENT

- **Systemic antiviral formulation:** A combination tincture with equal parts of licorice, isatis, houttuynia, and sida, 1/2 tsp 3x daily. Houttuynia is particularly effective in reducing the cytokine cascade the virus starts, thus strongly inhibiting it. (In severe systemic infections, double the dose to 6x daily.)
- **Immune formulation:** A combination tincture with equal parts of astragalus, cordyceps, and reishi. (Reishi is particularly strong against these viruses.) Tonic dose: 20–60 drops 3x daily. In acute episodes: 1/2 tsp up to 6x daily.
- **Zinc,** internally, 25 mg daily. Double that for a few days if you feel an attack coming on.

To prevent outbreaks, try L-lysine, in a tonic dose of 1,000 mg 3x daily. (Note: If you do have an outbreak anyway, increase the dosage, up to 3,000 mg 3x daily. However, if taken regularly, the tonic dose can help prevent outbreaks from occurring.) Another helpful supplement is vitamin B_{12}, 500 mcg daily (a good B-complex is very helpful as well). Avoid L-arginine supplements and foods containing L-arginine such as nuts and chocolate. These can stimulate outbreaks.

To treat active sores, you can use zinc sulfate cream, applied 6–10x daily. This can reduce and eliminate sores within 3 to 5 days. The sore-relief concentrated herbal cream on page 174 can do the same even more quickly, within 3 days.

To reduce nerve pain, some of the things that can help are:

- **Geranium oil,** topical, applied as needed. If the pure essential oil is too strong, you can dilute it with olive oil if necessary.
- **Greater celandine (*Chelidonium majus*) tincture.** Typical American dosage is 10–30 drops 3x daily for 30 days. English dosage is higher,

generally 40–80 drops 3x daily, again for 30 days. In rare instances use for longer than 30 days can cause severe inflammation of the bile ducts, so only use it for 30 days in a row.

- **Pasque flower tincture,** 10 drops every hour or so.
- **Kudzu root (*Pueraria lobata*) tincture,** 1/2 tsp 3 or 4x daily. This alters certain neural receptors in the brain and peripheral nervous system.
- **Theramine** can also help, sometimes a lot. It is a prescription nutriceutical that is very good for certain kinds of recalcitrant pain.

For some specific expressions of HSV, incorporate these additional formulations into the protocol:

For vaginal herpes: Prepare a douche by combining 1 ounce of a berberine plant (e.g., goldenseal, barberry) tincture and 1 ounce of lemon balm tincture in a pint of water and use it to douche 3x daily.

For herpes eye infection: Prepare eyedrops by combining 1 ounce each of dried licorice, houttuynia, and isatis in a heat-proof quart jar. Bring water to a boil, then pour it over the herbs, stir well, cover, and let sit overnight. Strain well the next day. Pour some of the infusion into a 1-ounce brown bottle with dropper. Store the rest in the refrigerator. Use the eyedrops throughout the day, a minimum of 6x daily. Just 1–3 drops in each eye every hour or two until the condition clears.

For herpetic encephalitis/meningitis: Use the protocols for viral encephalitis delineated in depth earlier in this chapter. An ethanol extract of *Cynanchum paniculatum* has been found to be very effective in protecting the brain and neural structures in some studies and may prove useful here.

Caution: The use of L-arginine during an *active* herpes outbreak can sometimes exacerbate the condition excruciatingly.

Varicella Zoster Virus (Chicken Pox/Shingles)

Although chicken pox (varicella zoster virus) tends to be a self-limiting disease, a vaccine has been developed in the West; a variety of it has also been crafted for herpes zoster (shingles). Shingles tends to be the most problematic element of this virus; it is often extremely painful and somewhat difficult to treat well.

I won't explore the use of herbs for chicken pox itself since, with the vaccine, episodes in the West are becoming rare. However, modifications of the protocols outlined for shingles will help with chicken pox, especially the systemic and topical formulations. Treatment protocols in this section are specific only for shingles.

Some of the herbs and supplements effective for herpes zoster (shingles) are *Ampelopsis brevipedunculata, Astragalus membranaceus* (astragalus), *Clinacanthus nutans, Ficus binjamina* (leaves), *Garcinia multiflora, Glycyrrhiza glabra* (licorice), isatis, *Lonicera japonica* (Japanese honeysuckle), *Melissa officinalis* (lemon balm), *Polygonum cuspidatum* (Japanese knotweed), *Quillaja saponaria* (Chilean soapbark tree, inner bark infusion/decoction, low dosing), *Rhus succedanea*, and *Ribes nigrum* (black currant).

Concentrated Sore-Relief Herbal Cream

INGREDIENTS

- 3 ounces licorice root
- 2 ounces birch bark
- 2 ounces lemon balm leaf
- 2 ounces rosemary leaf

To make:

Combine the herbs in a slow cooker with 32 ounces of water. Bring to a boil. Reduce the heat to barely under a simmer. Cook for 3 days. Turn off the heat, let cool, and strain out the herbs. Return the liquid to the cleaned slow cooker, bring to a boil again, then reduce heat to just under a simmer. Let cook until the liquid is reduced to 2 ounces. (Caution: It can easily burn once it gets close, so watch it.) When reduced sufficiently, turn off the heat, let cool, and place the cream in a jar.

To use:

Apply 6–10x daily. This combination will eliminate sores, reduce pain, and promote healing very quickly, usually within 3 days or so.

TREATMENT

The basic treatment for shingles comprises 1) systemic antivirals, 2) immune formulations, 3) topical creams for skin outbreaks, and 4) treatments to reduce nerve pain and regenerate nerve cells.

1. **Systemic antivirals.** I would suggest both of the following:
   - **Tincture combination** of licorice, isatis, and Chinese skullcap, in equal parts, 1/4–1/2 tsp 3–6x daily, depending on the severity of the outbreak. This will actually help heal the nerves of the infection and prevent recurrences, if you use it over time.
   - **Lemon balm tincture** (I suggest the Herb Pharm brand), 1/4 tsp 3–6x daily. This is *very* helpful over time. It is also very calming to the nerves and helps prevent recurrences.
2. **Immune formulation.** Tincture combination of astragalus, rhodiola, and cordyceps, in equal parts, 1/2 tsp 3x daily. This will increase immune function and help reduce the incidence of future outbreaks. (Lowered immune function due to age is the main cause of shingles outbreaks after age 50.)
3. **Topical healing.** A couple of formulations can help here:
   - **Lemon balm infused oil or cordial,** applied topically daily. This really does help.
   - **Pine pollen cream,** applied topically daily. This really does help if you can find the cream.
4. **Nerve pain.** The herbs and supplements recommended for reducing the nerve pain of herpes simplex virus outbreaks (see page 172) will also help reduce the nerve pain that accompanies a shingles outbreak.

Herbs can also help prevent or cure the postherpetic nerve pain that comes from nerve damage after outbreaks by regenerating the damaged nerves. Two of the best regenerators (both very high in nerve growth factor) are Chinese senega root and lion's mane; vitamin B_{12} is also very helpful:

- **Chinese senega root:** 30 drops of the tincture 3x daily for 30 days, and . . .

- **Lion's mane (*Hericium erinaceus*):** 1 tsp of the tincture 2x daily. Note: The fresh mushroom tincture, not the dried, is preferable if you can find it. Long-term use of this herb is fine. And . . .
- **Vitamin B_{12}:** 500–2,000 mcg daily.

  Supplements for both deep healing and nerve pain:
- **L-lysine:** as a tonic dose, 1,000 mg 3x daily; during a shingles outbreak, up to 3,000 mg 3x daily.
- **L-carnitine:** 500–700 mg 3x daily.
- **Alpha lipoic acid:** 200 mg 3x daily.
- **Inositol:** 500–1,000 mg 3x daily.

Regular fruit intake can also be important. Low fruit intake (less than one serving per week) can lead to more frequent outbreaks.

Note: L-arginine intake can sometimes *cause* a shingles outbreak. If you have a history of shingles, I would recommend avoiding L-arginine supplementation. (Nuts and dark chocolate are fairly high in L-arginine; caution is warranted.)

Rotavirus and Norovirus

Rotaviruses are the best studied of the viral gastroenteritis diseases, in terms of herbal treatments, but for all of them, tannin-containing plants are indicated for one big reason: They inactivate the viruses. In the case of the Norwalk virus, for example, tannic acid inhibits the binding of the viral proteins to HBGA (histo-blood group antigen) receptors, thus preventing infection. There have been a number of double-blind studies using tannic-acid-containing plants in the treatment of viral gastroenteritis, and all have shown good success. Researchers have tested plants traditionally used for this kind of condition and found many of them active. The most common and strongest: *Musa* spp. (the green, unripe banana fruit, usually cooked), *Potentilla erecta* (leaves), *Potentilla tormentilla* (root), and *Psidium guajava* (guava).

The plants found effective for rotaviruses are *Aegle marmelos* (unripe fruit), *Artocarpus integrifolia* (bark), *Byrsonima verbascifolia*, *Eugenia dysenterica* (a.k.a. *Stenocalyx dysentericus*), *Glycyrrhiza glabra* (licorice), *Haemanthus albiflos* (bulb), *Hymenaea courbaril, Lomatium dissectum, Myracrodruon urundeuva, Myristica fragrans* (seeds), *Panax ginseng, Potentilla erecta* (leaves), *Potentilla tormentilla* (root), *Wolfiporia* (a.k.a. *Poria*) and *Polyporus* in combination (as a decoction), *Psidium guajava* (leaves), *Punica granatum* (pomegranate leaves and juice), *Quillaja saponaria, Sophora flavescens, Spondias lutea* (a.k.a. *S. mombin*; leaves and bark), *Stevia rebaudiana,* and *Vaccinium macrocarpon* (cranberry juice).

Plants have not been tested to any extent against astroviruses, though *Detarium senegalense* and *Dichrostachys glomerata* are both active against the viruses. For orthoreoviruses, the barks of both *Castanea* (chestnut) and *Schinopsis* (quebracho) are active antivirals as well as tannin sources in general.

In essence, any plant that is strongly drying on the tongue is going to work: oak leaves or bark, *Krameria* (rhatany) root, pine needles (mature), acacia, agrimony, pinedrops (*Pterospora*), rose, raspberry, blackberry, and so on. Roots, leaves, and bark tend to be the most astringent parts of such plants. In my experience rhatany root, blackberry root, and pinedrops are some of the strongest, followed by quebracho, oak, and pine needles, but really, any astringent plants will do. It is just that the stronger they are, the faster they work.

Other useful plants are:

- **Berberine-containing plants.** These plants do have some antiviral properties, but they also have strong actions on the GI tract membrane and help it resist any microbial infection.
- ***Bidens* spp.** These plants are strong, systemic antimicrobials and prostaglandin inhibitors and are very specific for diarrheal diseases and healing damaged mucous membrane systems.
- ***Alchornea cordifolia.*** This plant is a potent systemic antibacterial and antimicrobial that is used in traditional African medicine for a variety of conditions, including diarrhea. It has been found to reduce water and electrolyte loss during diarrheal diseases.
- ***Baccharis teindalensis, Carica papaya, Croton lechleri, Euphorbia hirta, Jatropha curcas, Jussiaea suffruticosa, Mangifera indica,***

Terminalia avicennoides, and Zingiber officinale. All have been found in a number of studies to help reduce diarrhea, limit water and electrolyte loss, and help with cramping.

TREATMENT

The treatment of these viral gastroenteritis diseases is straightforward, and while you can get fancy with this, it primarily entails the use of any plants strong in tannins, in large quantities. My preference is for their use as decoctions but even that is not necessary; unripe banana is especially useful in the regions in which it grows, for example, and is usually used as a mashed, cooked ingestible. Plants high in tannins bind the viruses while, at the same time, reducing fluid loss through firming up the stool.

Some suggestions:

- **Combination tincture** of *Alchornea cordifolia* (or any berberine-containing plant), licorice, and lomatium, in equal parts, 30 drops to 1 tsp 3–6x daily depending on the severity of the condition and age of the person.
- **Strong infusion of blackberry root:** Add 4 ounces powdered or roughly ground blackberry root to a large heat-proof jar. Add 1 quart of very hot water, cover, and let steep overnight. Drink the whole thing over the next day. Repeat daily. Increase the dosage if diarrhea is not substantially helped within 24 hours. Or . . .
- **Strong decoction of blackberry root:** 4 ounces blackberry root to 1 quart of water; boil until the water is reduced by half. Let cool and consume in equal parts throughout the day. Repeat daily.

5

ABOUT HERBAL MEDICINES

Facts are subversive of lies, half-truths, myths; of all those easy speeches that comfort cruel men.

—Timothy Garton Ash

In 1998, when I wrote my first book on herbal medicine, the Internet was very new; the world was a different place. A lot has changed.

For one thing, the Internet has become the greatest reference library human beings have ever known. A tiny part of that library, though enormously huge compared to what was available in the past, has to do with medicinal plants and the vast amount of research now being conducted on them. This facilitated the writing of this book enormously. During my research for the first book, despite the size of my personal library (huge) and my access to a great university library at the University of Colorado in Boulder, I had access to only a tiny portion of the research and other material on medicinal plants that existed in the world. Now I have access to a great deal more; it's as close as my office computer.

But that is only a small part of the changes that have taken place over the past 15 years; something a great deal more interesting has been happening. As I spent weeks on the Web, following the scent of medicinal plants through the Internet forest, what struck home the most was a deep and visceral impact of just how much the human world itself has changed.

It is a new world out there. And it is a world with which the United States has an increasingly tenuous connection. The rest of the

Western nations are nearly as lost. During the past 15 years nations on the African continent, in Asia and South America, within the Russian sphere, and in most of the old Eastern bloc have realized that the medical model used by the West is unworkable, and to a great extent, they have begun abandoning it as the dominant approach to their people's health care.

Nations in those regions, especially in Africa, Asia, and South America, have realized they can't afford a pharmaceutical/technological medical model as their primary approach to health care. They know that the problems of antibiotic resistance, petroleum depletion (most pharmaceuticals and all medical technology are made from or highly dependent on petroleum products), population expansion, top-down care models, and most especially cost and cost inflation cannot be solved and are only going to worsen over time. With that realization, they have begun abandoning industrialized medicine as a legitimate model for providing health care to their populations. (Industrialized medicine will still play a part, but a much smaller, more affordable, and considerably less dangerous one.)

Unlike in the United States, researchers in those nations aren't exploring *whether* plant medicines work (nor are they spending their time and money trying to discredit what they feel is "primitive" medicine or unscientific quackery); they are exploring which herbal medicines work best and in what form and at what dosage. Their research and their journal papers are looking for the herbs that can treat malaria most successfully (for example) and how those plants, once identified, can be grown by the people who need them so they can be used when, and where, and by whom they are needed.

Many non-Western researchers are actively addressing the health problems of their populations with little if any profit motive. They have simply realized that corporate profit making and human health are not compatible. Shorthand: They are tired of seeing their cultures get screwed by international corporations that make billions out of the misery of others. They want to solve the problems facing them, simply, repeatedly, cheaply, ecologically, and with a great deal of personal empowerment for the people who are most directly affected. Reading the journal articles of U.S. researchers and comparing them with those of other nations and cultures is an illuminating and sobering experience.

The African and Asian journal articles tend to have titles like this: "Antibacterial activity of guava (*Psidium guajava* L.) and neem (*Azadirachta indica* A. Juss.) extracts against foodborne pathogens and spoilage bacteria" or "Evaluation of antimicrobial activities of extracts of five plants used in traditional medicine in Nigeria" or "Antimicrobial activity of ethanolic and aqueous extracts of *Sida acuta* on microorganisms from skin infections."

The U.S. journal articles are more along these lines: "Severe hypernatremia and hyperosmolality exacerbated by an herbal preparation in a patient with diabetic ketoacidosis" or "Metal content of ephedra-containing dietary supplements and select botanicals" or "Hypereosinophilia associated with echinacea use."

The abstract for that last study contains the kind of commentary common to many Western researchers, especially in the United States:

> Echinacea, believed by herbal practitioners to enhance the immune system, is one of the most widely used herbal supplements in the United States. Like most herbal products, it lacks strict FDA regulation and more information is needed about its potential adverse reactions. Here, we report the case of a patient with eosinophilia of unclear etiology whose condition resolved after cessation of this supplement. We feel this likely represents an IgE-mediated allergic process to echinacea.[1]

The article ignores the in-depth research on echinacea done in Germany over decades and the fact that it is a part of primary care medicine in that country. It uses words and phrases such as "believed by" and "we feel" and "likely." Its writers *assume* that the echinacea is the cause of the eosinophilia even though they have conducted no research to make sure of it. It's not science, not research, but rather guesswork and opinion that reflect the orientation, and bias, of the technologically focused, pharmaceutically dominated medical world, especially in the United States.

Now compare that with this abstract from an article by Nigerian researchers, "Antimicrobial activity of ethanolic and aqueous extracts of *Sida acuta* of microorganisms from skin infections."

> The antimicrobial effect of the ethanolic and aqueous extracts of *Sida acuta* was investigated. Phytochemical analysis revealed the presence of saponins, tannins, cardiac glycosides, alkaloids and anthraquinones. The test isolates from human skin infections were *Staphylococcus aureus, Bacillus subtilis, Pseudomonas aeruginosa, Escherichia coli, Scopulariopsis candida, Aspergillus niger* and *Aspergillus fumigatus.* The zone of inhibition for the ethanolic extract varied from 10 mm for *P. aeruginosa* to 43 mm for *S. aureus* and from 4 mm for *P. aeruginosa* to 29 mm for *S. aureus* in the aqueous extract. Though the zone of inhibition increased with increase in the concentration of the extract, the highest concentration of the ethanolic extract revealed a higher significant (P. 0.05) inhibition against *S. aureus* and *B. subtilis* compared to the inhibition effect on these organisms by gentamicin used as control. The aqueous extract had no significant effect on the test organisms. The extracts had no inhibitory effect on the fungi isolates. This study has shown that the extract of *S. acuta* if properly harnessed medically will enhance our health care delivery system.[2]

This herb "will enhance our health care delivery system." I have never seen that sentiment in a research article in the United States, and I've read thousands of them. (Gentamicin, by the way, is what is called an aminoglycoside antibiotic, often used to treat Gram-negative bacteria. *Sida acuta* at higher doses was more active against the test organisms than the antibiotic was.)

The authors of this study tested both aqueous (water) and ethanolic (alcohol) extracts of the plant—infusions and tinctures—to see which were most effective. Most plants are used by indigenous cultures as water infusions (strong teas) or in whole form of one sort or another, either eaten or placed directly on the affected area of the body. Some cultures do use simple alcohol extractions. Of the active ingredients in plants, some are soluble in water, some in alcohol, and the researchers clearly wanted to find out which form of preparation was the most effective for this plant. It's *usable* information they were after. And they found it. They came to *Sida acuta* by looking at what traditional healers and herbalists in Nigeria were using in their practice, and they decided to test it for activity. If it was effective, they wanted to find out how it was *most* effective. And they planned then on supporting the use of that plant widely throughout Nigeria to enhance their country's health care system. Nothing could be more alien to the medical establishment in the United States.

To be fair, there are some good studies occurring in the United States, but to be clear, virtually *none* of them support the use of herbal medicines by the general populace or even by educated herbal practitioners. Their focus, rather, is on the identification of an "active" constituent that can then be modified chemically, patented, and subsequently produced by a pharmaceutical company for profit. U.S. researchers, in spite of often being affiliated with universities, generally work for or in concert with pharmaceutical companies. They are not looking for something the general populace can use without a prescription; they are not working to empower self-care. In most instances they don't trust the general populace to be intelligent enough to provide their own health care, nor do they want to interrupt their own financial income stream.

We in the Western world, especially in the United States, are being left behind in an outmoded model that has no effective place in the real world. By the time we realize it, the rest of the world will be generations ahead. The rest of the world has abandoned our approach; they understand the problems they face and what lies ahead. In the meantime, we spend our time making better and better buggy whips, not realizing the automobile really is here to stay.

Some Comments on the Herbs Discussed in This Book

To find the top herbs that can be effectively used for treating antibiotic-resistant organisms and emerging viral strains, I have relied on decades of my own experience, the cumulative experience of a great many other practitioners, many thousands of journal papers of very good research by committed researchers from many countries around the world, and the history of use of these plants by local peoples over centuries.

I have put the herbs in this book into four categories: systemic antibacterials, localized antibacterials, antivirals, and facilitative or synergistic herbs.

Systemic antibacterials are herbal medicines that are broadly systemic, that are spread by the bloodstream throughout the body, thus affecting every cell and organ within the body, and that are active against a range of bacteria. These herbs are good for treating infections such as MRSA that have spread throughout the body and are not responding to multiple antibiotic protocols.

Localized antibacterials are those that do not spread easily throughout the body but are limited in their movement. Because they don't easily cross membranes, they are effective in the GI and urinary tracts and for external infections. These kinds of herbs are useful for infections such as *E. coli* O157:H7 or cholera or for infected skin wounds that refuse to heal.

Antivirals are active against a wide range of viruses, and most potent antivirals are also synergistic (see below). These herbs inhibit viral activity, either by interfering with the mechanisms of the virus itself or by stimulating the body's immune response to fight the invading organism. Elder, for example, inhibits the replication of influenza viruses and blocks the production of proteins needed to invade a host cell.

Facilitative or synergistic herbs are just that: plants that facilitate the action of other plants or pharmaceuticals. They either enhance the action of the antibacterial being used or affect the bacteria so that the antibacterial is more effective. Most plants contain both antibiotic substances *and* a potent synergist, quite often one or more efflux inhibitors. Goldenseal, which contains berberine, is an example.

Berberine, a strong antibacterial, is very active against a number of resistant organisms. It is considerably more active, however, in the presence of another constituent in goldenseal,

5′-methoxyhydnocarpin (5′-MHC), which is a multidrug efflux pump inhibitor. It reduces or eliminates MRSA's ability to eject antibiotic substances that might harm it from inside its cellular membrane. 5′-MHC has no known function other than to do exactly this, and it is one of the reasons goldenseal is so effective in the treatment of resistant infections of the GI tract.

Compounds such as 5′-MHC are why plants are often more effective than single constituents in treating disease conditions. Other compounds in plants do still other things; some have no known function in the plant other than to reduce the side effects of the more pharmacologically active constituents. This is one reason plants tend to be strange medicines in the minds of medical reductionists—they can't understand that kind of complexity or see the reason for its existence. Nevertheless, newer generations of researchers have grasped that the old paradigm is unworkable and they are looking toward plants with new eyes. They are understanding that plant medicines are much more sophisticated than pharmaceuticals (something those in older cultures innately understand).

As some specific examples: The anticonvulsant actions of yangonin and desmethoxyyangonin, kavalactones found in *Piper methysticum*, are much greater when the lactones are used in combination with other kava constituents. Concentrations of yangonin and another lactone, kavain, are much higher in the brain when the whole plant extract is used rather than the purified lactones themselves. In other words, some of the other constituents in kava help move the bioactive lactones across the blood-brain barrier into the brain. Blood plasma concentration of kavain is 50 percent less if the purified compound is used rather than an extract of the plant itself. Plant compounds in *Isatis tinctoria*, a potent antiviral and anti-inflammatory herb, are highly synergistic. Tryptanthrin, a strong anti-inflammatory in the plant, possesses very poor skin penetration capacity. However, when the whole plant extract is applied to the skin, penetration of tryptanthrin is very good. In other words, applying a salve of pure tryptanthrin to the skin, despite how anti-inflammatory that compound is, won't do you much good. But if you make the plant itself into a salve, the tryptanthrin moves rapidly into the skin and helps reduce skin inflammation.

Artemisinin is much more active against malarial parasites if administered with artemetin and casticin, flavonoids normally contained in the artemisia plant. Additional flavones in the plant, chrysophlenetin and chrysospenol-D, also act as potent synergists in this way. They are also permeability glycoprotein (P-gp) inhibitors (see monograph on piperine, page 447), thus facilitating the movement of artemisinin and the plant's other constituents through the intestinal membrane and into the blood.

As a final example, side effects such as tinnitus and stomach ulcers that can occur from the use of acetylsalicylic acid don't occur if whole extracts of willow bark are given rather than that purified constituent; other compounds in the plant specifically ameliorate its side effects.

Combining Plants for Greater Effect

When it comes to plant combinations, things get even more complex. For example, constituents from licorice (glycyrrhizin and its related compounds) significantly enhance the solubility of other plant compounds, such as the saikosaponins from Asian ginseng, in water. Thus, marrying plants *during the medicine-making process*—a field almost completely unexamined in Western herbal approaches—can produce much stronger tinctures than when they are produced singly.

Quercetin (an anti-inflammatory and moderate anticancer flavonol found in many plants and vegetables) is poorly soluble in water, but that solubility is strongly enhanced by complex mixtures of saponins if plants containing them are added to the mix when the medicine is being made.

So . . . while some plants such as goldenseal are synergistic within themselves from the presence of efflux inhibitors and potent antibacterial constituents, other plants, such as *Dalea spinosa*, are relatively mild as antibacterials but contain compounds that are multidrug resistance (MDR) inhibitors, making them synergists for other plants.

Adding synergists to a systemic antibacterial when creating an herbal compound increases the potency of the primary herb being used, sometimes considerably. (This has long been recognized in the actions of such plants as licorice and western red cedar, though the reasons *why* were not known.)

Synergists, while known throughout herbal history, have been only mildly recognized for their actions, usually in the Chinese and Ayurvedic systems, but they have not been accepted as a legitimate and unique category of herbal medicines that should be studied in their own right. Given the seriousness of emerging resistant pathogens, it is time to begin developing this category of herbal medicines in more depth, to begin to understand how to use them in practice, and to find the most potent ones that can be used for healing. The material in this book is, I hope, the beginning of that development.

The Importance of Preparation Methods

I remember, growing up, how often the physicians in my family made fun of the old plant doctors and herbalists insisting that some plants must be harvested only at such and such a time or they would be too weak to work or their insistence that certain plants must be used together to work. Turns out there is a great deal of truth to those old assertions. So . . . considerable attention is paid within this book to *how* and *when* the plants should be harvested, prepared, and made into medicine.

There are other complexities that come into play when it comes time to actually make your plants into medicine. There is a synergy between the plant and the medium in which it is extracted. Regrettably, there has been an unfortunate lack of attention paid to this in much of the world, especially among us American herbalists. For example: The word *alkaloid* means *alkaline-like*, a clue that has been overlooked in every herbal preparation manual I have read over the past 30 years. In practical terms: Plant alkaloids won't extract easily in alkaline waters; they need more acidic waters to do so. Extracts of plants with highly bioactive alkaloids increase in strength if the plants are extracted in liquid mixtures that are at least minimally acidic. The water being used to make extracts (tinctures and infusions) needs to be "soft," or else an acid such as vinegar needs to be added in minimal amounts to make it so (see box, page 194).

Understanding these kinds of complexities in plants and the medicines they become comes from long exposure to them, from the same kind of intuitive sensing (holistic nonlinear perception) that all artisans use (in things from writing to house building to making music), and, most importantly, from a lack of intellectual hubris. If you understand up front that plants are highly complex living beings that are a great deal older than the human species, it is much more difficult to place an intellectually reductionistic paradigm on them. *You can't see what you assume is not there.*

Herbalism is an art; it is, and always will remain, much too complex to be approached from a reductionist and linear orientation with any expectation of success. "Phytorationalism" is an oxymoron. A practitioner with such an orientation will never grasp the essential nonlinearity of the world, of healing, of plant medicines.

The synergy within and among plant medicines, a prime example of the nonlinear complexity in this field, *means* that the combined effect of different substances will be greater than that which can be expected from the individual components alone. Combination produces outcomes beyond rational expectation. To face the challenges before us, we ourselves have no choice but to synergize within ourselves: to develop our abilities to feel and think *simultaneously*, neither in competition with the other, and blend those capacities together into a unique perceptual tool of tremendous elegance. I am talking about developing forebrain elegance here, not just tentative understandings of the hindbrain. As Erich Fromm once commented: "Reason flows from the blending of rational thought and feeling. If the two functions are torn apart, thinking deteriorates into schizoid intellectual activity and feeling deteriorates into neurotic life-damaging passions."[3]

6

THE MATERIA MEDICA

Included in this chapter is the collective knowledge about the most effective antibacterial and antiviral herbs—the herbal equivalent of the pharmacology notes you receive with your medications when you pick them up at the drug store. The herbs are divided into systemic antibacterials, localized antibacterials, antivirals, and synergistic herbs. Note that despite the categorical divisions, these herbs serve multiple roles. Many antiviral herbs are naturally synergistic, and in the listings for antibiotic herbs, there are also notes about their antiviral properties, and vice versa. For example, *cryptolepis* is excellent against Gram-negative bacterial infections but also serves as a mild antiviral treatment. And elder flowers work against two strains of influenza virus as well as *Staphylococcus areus* bacteria.

Under the listings for each herb, you can find the recommended species; which parts of the plant are used for medicine; preparation and dosage instructions for tinctures, capsules, teas, and other forms; side effects and contraindications; any known interactions with pharmaceuticals; where to find the herbs and how to cultivate them; and a summary of the research supporting the herb's effectiveness.

Systemic Antibacterials

Our epitaph [as a species] may well read: "They died of a peculiar strain of reductionism, complicated by a sudden attack of elitism, even though there were ready natural cures close at hand."

—**Gary Paul Nabhan, *Cultures of Habitat***

Most herbalists, irrespective of culture or country, do know of the antibacterial activity of plants and they do use them to heal bacterial disease on a regular basis, but, in general, our understanding of herbal antibiotics has been thin. By *thin* I mean we've been stuck in a paradigm of "take this for that" or "what's that plant good for" or even (among the reductionist herbal schools that have adopted the medical model; that is, the phytorationalists) "the active constituent of *Hypericum perfoliatum* should be standardized in order for the plant to be effective in the treatment of mild depression." Given the seriousness of the emerging bacterial diseases, we need to have a more comprehensive paradigm in place, one that takes into account the potential sophistication of herbal medicine as a very ancient art form of healing, one that uses both perceptual and intellectual awareness, as well as a focus on outcomes, in its expression.

The importance of systemic herbal antibacterials cannot be overstated.

Many resistant diseases, such as staph, are widely spread throughout the body. They can affect internal organs, invade difficult-to-reach parts of the body, or, very commonly, infect the skin (from the inside rather than outside), appearing as skin ulcerations in various locations. To treat a systemic infection like staph, an herbal antibiotic that is systemically spread throughout the body is necessary.

I remember the first time someone told me she had a community-acquired systemic staph infection; it was a woman who'd come to hear me teach. She said that she had undergone numerous courses of antibiotics, and that after the last one failed the physicians had told her, "Well, let's just observe it and see what happens." Her furious response was, "I know what's going to happen, I'm going to lose my foot."

I began to understand then just how important systemic antibacterials are in herbal practice. With resistant bacterial infections spreading at the rate they are, we *need* systemics—we need to know them as a category and we need to *really* know how to use them. We need to move from herbalism as a kind of "let's-eat-organic-today" choice (unless we're really sick; then we'll go to the emergency room) to a "we-can-depend-on-this-for-our-life" form of healing.

When herbs are taken into the body, some just stay pretty much in the GI tract, whereas others cross the intestinal membranes and circulate in the body, often concentrating in particular locations; the liver or kidneys, for instance. But one class of herbs is always broadly systemic. Once ingested they concentrate in the bloodstream (and sometimes the liver) and are widely circulated, reaching every cell that needs a constant blood supply, which is pretty much every cell in the body. These are the herbs that have traditionally been used to treat malaria. Many, if not most of them, also tend to possess rather strong antibacterial actions, sometimes broadly so. It is important, however, to make a distinction between the two common types of malarial herbs, for not all malarial herbs are true antimalarials.

Some malarial herbs are widely systemic and actually do kill the parasites responsible for malaria, but others only treat some of the symptoms of the disease such as fever or chills. Many researchers have not understood the distinction, and so they may list an herb as being used for malaria when in fact it is *only* being used as an adjunct herb to treat one of the symptoms of malaria; for instance, when yarrow is used to treat malarial fevers.

Yarrow isn't a systemic antimalarial (even though it does have some mild actions against the parasite) but, rather, is a diaphoretic adjunct. It helps reduce fevers because it induces sweating, which cools the body. When researching the ethnobotanical literature, it is crucial to understand this distinction between the different kinds of malarial herbs. Once you do, their study begins to open up the wider world of systemic antibacterials. Systemic antibacterial herbs have often been used for centuries in the treatment of malaria simply because one of their antimicrobial actions is against malarial organisms. But they are often widely active against other organisms and can be very powerful. (Systemic antibacterials may also be found in a particular category of Chinese medicine—plants for toxic blood.)

The first systemic herbal antibiotic I began to understand was

Cryptolepis sanguinolenta, a traditional herbal medicine from Ghana. I was introduced to it by a healer from Ghana, Nana Nkatiah, and it was this herb that I recommended to the woman who approached me at the workshop. Her family had become infected through exposure to her, and at this point they were all ill. They used cryptolepis and it worked very well. Since then I have used cryptolepis on numerous occasions to treat systemic staph infections that have not responded to multiple antibiotic regimens. It has, so far, never failed. I consider this plant, along with alchornea, sida, and bidens, to be *the* primary systemic herbal antibiotics for use in treating resistant organisms at this time.

While cryptolepis is sometimes hard to find, many of the other herbs in this section are not—at least in the wild. They are often widely distributed throughout the world; a number of them are considered invasive plants, which is a plus.

Invasive plants—Earth's way of insisting we notice her medicines.

Cryptolepis

Family: In flux, given the propensity of botanical PhD students to write dissertations on minutiae; probably Apocynaceae (subfamily Periplocoideae) or perhaps Asclepiadaceae

Common Names: *Cryptolepis (in the West) • delboi • gangamau (among the Hausa) • Ghanian quinine • kadze (among the Ewe) • koli mekari (among the Mpiemo peoples in the Central African Republic and the eastern part of Cameroon) • nibima (among the Twi-speaking people of Ghana) • ouidoukoi • yellow dye root*

Species Used: There are about 20 or maybe 30 (taxonomists are so irritating) species of cryptolepis, 10 or more in Africa, two in Madagascar, four in Asia, three in Papua New Guinea, and one in Australia, and probably others elsewhere if that larger number is accurate. The primary systemic antibacterial among the genus is *Cryptolepis sanguinolenta.*

The potency of *C. sanguinolenta* has generated a lot of interest in this genus of plants. *C. triangularis,* native to Angola, Lagos, Belgian Congo, and Gambia, has, like *C. sanguinolenta,* been found to contain cryptolepine, one of the more potent antimalarial alkaloids known. (Some sources consider these two to be the same plant; others list them as distinct species.) Some sources say that *all* the members of this genus contain the antibacterial alkaloids cryptolepine, quindoline, and neocryptolepine. I have been unable to verify this by finding any in-depth chemical analysis of the other species. A number of sources do list cryptolepine and similar alkaloids as present in *C. buchanani,* a traditional Ayurvedic plant, commonly used as a medicinal in Thailand, Nepal, and India. It may be true; the traditional uses of *C. buchanani* show the same range of action as that of *C. sanguinolenta,* so I tend to give the reports credence. *C. hypoglauca* is reported in one study to contain cryptolepine, but I can't find anything definitive on that either.

The Top 5 Systemic Herbal Antibiotics

- Cryptolepis
- Sida
- Alchornea
- Bidens
- Artemisia

Of all the plants in the genus, *C. buchanani* and *C. obtusa* have stimulated the most interest outside *C. sanguinolenta.* Given the importance of *C. sanguinolenta,* in-depth chemical research needs to be done on the entire genus to determine whether the other species within it can be used as effectively.

Parts Used

The root is usually the part used medicinally (or in dyeing). The leaves *can* be used medicinally (see the description of the plant's chemistry on page 199) but rarely are. The root of the plant is generally about the thickness of a pencil, appears to be fairly consistent in thickness over long lengths, and has a light tannish color on the thin exterior bark and a brilliant yellow on the interior. It's pretty. The root is exceptionally bitter due to the many alkaloids present.

Preparation and Dosage

Cryptolepis can be prepared as powder, capsules, tea, or tincture.

POWDER

For bacterial infections of the skin and wound sepsis, liberally sprinkle cryptolepis powder on the site of infection as frequently as needed.

TINCTURE

1:5, 60 percent alcohol, 20–40 drops, up to 4x daily

For resistant staph: In the treatment of severe systemic staph infection, the usual dose is ½–1 tsp, 3x daily. In very severe cases increase the dose to 1 tbl, 3x daily. (I prefer to not use dosages this high for longer than 60 days. That is usually sufficient.)

For malaria: 1 tsp–1 tbl, 3x daily for 5 days, repeat in 14 days

TEA

Use 1 teaspoon cryptolepis in 6 ounces water to make a strong infusion.

As a preventive: Drink 1 or 2 cups daily.

In acute conditions: Drink up to 6 cups daily.

Check the pH of Your Water

The alkaloids in cryptolepis are water soluble, but if the pH of the water is alkaline, the alkaloids will not dissolve well. The pH scale ranges from 1 to 14, where 1 is the most acidic, 14 the most alkaline, and 7 is neutral. The word alkaloid means "alkaline-like." The more alkaline water is, the less well alkaloids will dissolve in it. You have to have a pH of at least 6 for the alkaloids to dissolve in water. "Hard" water is alkaline. (A water softener makes hard water soft; that is, acidic rather than alkaline.) If you have hard water (you can call your city's water department to find out the average pH) or if you don't know, add a teaspoon of vinegar or lemon juice to the boiling water you are using to make your cryptolepis tea.

Note: While the herb will work if infused in cold water, studies have found that the hot-water extraction is more effective. It is nearly as strong as the alcohol tincture.

CAPSULES

As a preventive: Take 3 "00" capsules 2x daily.
In acute conditions: Take up to 20 capsules daily.

Side Effects and Contraindications

None noted. Considerable research has taken place to determine the potential adverse reactions from using the plant, and none have been found, either in human clinical use or with in vivo testing on mice, rats, and rabbits. The herb is taken as a regular tonic for years at a time in some parts of Africa and India. One or 2 cups of the tea or 2 or 3 droppers of the tincture (60–90 drops) a day are fine for extended, long-term use.

Researchers in some instances have noted that people taking cryptolepis have elevated levels of ALP (alkaline phosphatase) and uric acid, which return to normal after the herb is discontinued. There have been no reported side effects from this. And though there is one report in the literature of adverse effects of cryptolepis in mouse pregnancy, I can find nothing in traditional use that substantiates an extrapolation to humans nor any studies in the literature that show negative effects in pregnancy in people.

Cryptolepine has been found to be cytotoxic, which raises concerns in some people. A few points:

- Cryptolepine is an isolated constituent, and like most isolated constituents that are made into pharmaceuticals, it produces side effects that don't appear when the whole herb is used. *Cryptolepis itself has not been found to be cytotoxic to people.*
- The word *cytotoxic,* when used in reports, generally means it kills cancer cells, and indeed, cryptolepine does.
- Cryptolepine is cytotoxic because it intercalates DNA. DNA is a double helix, two joined twisted ladders. Cryptolepine inserts itself

(continued on page 198)

Properties of Cryptolepis

Actions

Antibacterial	Antimuscarinic	Antiviral (mild)
Anticomplementary activity	Antiparasitic	Hypoglycemic
Anti-inflammatory	Antiprotozoal	Hypothermic
Antimalarial	Antipyretic	Noradrenergic
Antimicrobial	Antithrombotic	Renal vasodilator

Active Against

Aspergillus spp.	*Escherichia coli*	*Proteus vulgaris*
Babesia spp.	*Herpes simplex*	*Salmonella* spp.
Bacillus subtilis	*Klebsiella* spp.	*Shigella dysentariae*
Campylobacter spp.	*Mycobacterium* spp.	*Staphylococcus aureus*
Candida spp.	*Neisseria gonorrhoeae*	*Streptococcus pyogenes*
Entamoeba histolytica	*Plasmodium* spp.	
Enterobacter cloacae	*Proteus mirabilis*	

Tests have found the plant to be a stronger antibacterial than the pharmaceutical antibiotic chloramphenicol. Generally, it is more broadly active against Gram-positive bacteria (which are usually easier to treat due to their cellular structure), but it does have potent activity against a number of Gram-negative bacteria.

A number of studies have found cryptolepis active against *Pseudomonas aeruginosa*; other studies have found it ineffective. A balanced review of the journal papers, in my opinion, indicates that it is active against *Pseudomonas.* Examination of the studies does not give an easy clue as to the discrepancy in findings, but preparation differences seem to be involved.

Cryptolepis possesses little antifungal activity, though again, some studies have found it effective against candida while others have not. Again, a review of the studies, in my opinion, indicates that it is effective against candida and that preparation problems are the source of the discrepancy.

Use to Treat

Systemic infections, especially malaria, MRSA, streptococcus, babesia, campylobacter, urinary tract infections, tuberculosis, wound sepsis. It is very good for several Gram-negative bacterial infections: klebsiella, salmonella, shigella, *E. coli*, enterobacter, gonorrhea, and most likely pseudomonas.

Other Uses

The root has long been used as a brilliant yellow dye in the regions in which it grows; hence its common name, yellow dye root. The dye is usually used for dying leather, generally goat skins. The roots are gathered, dried, then ground in a wooden mortar. The powdered root is blended with hot water in a large vessel. The goat skin is coated with groundnut oil and then dipped in the dye bath. The extract is hand-rubbed into the leather during soaking. Then a tamarind fruit paste is added and rubbed in. The skin is exposed to air for a few minutes, then reimmersed in the bath and rubbed once more. The fruit paste purifies the color.

Though the roots are the primary part of the plant used (both for dye and medicine), the leaves are used as a vegetable in Burkina Faso.

Finding Cryptolepis

The herb is somewhat difficult to obtain in the United States. The only tincture I currently know of is available from Woodland Essence. *Cryptolepis buchanani* may (I repeat, *may*) be a decent substitute for *C. sanguinolenta*, and it is somewhat easier to find. Raksa Thai Herbs is a good source.

between the two ladders—that is, intercalates—and as a result interferes with cellular division, which is why it is useful in cancer treatment. Cryptolepine is a potent inhibitor of topoisomerase II, which it inhibits once it intercalates. The function of topoisomerase II is to allow DNA replication by unwinding the DNA helix, using it as a template, then winding it again after replication. If topoisomerase is inhibited, DNA replication, and cellular division, can't occur.

Herb/Drug Interactions

None noted. However . . . cryptolepis has been used in traditional medicine to help rectify insomnia. One mouse study has supported that effect of the plant. There is some potential for the plant to synergize with hypnosedatives or central nervous system depressants. Caution should be exercised, although there have been no reported adverse effects in these situations to date.

Habitat and Appearance

Cryptolepis sanguinolenta is a slender, thin-stemmed climbing shrub whose stem produces a blood-red to deep orange juice when cut (*sanguinolenta* means "tinged or mixed with blood; bloody"). Essentially it's a tropical plant that likes it hottish and a bit humid. It is common from sea level to 2,500 feet in altitude in savanna, dry forest, and gallery forest—that is, the riparian forests that develop along rivers and wetlands.

Cultivation and Collection

From reports, though it is usually wildcrafted, cryptolepis seems fairly easy to cultivate from seed and root cuttings. The seeds can be broadcast if desired. Due to its climbing nature, the plant needs a trellis to do well. Because of the growing international interest in the plant, commercial planting in Africa is on the increase.

The seeds are collected when semi-ripe and red/black in color. Normally they are then planted in raised mounds to facilitate harvesting of the roots. The seeds lose viability fairly quickly; they have a 90 percent to 100 percent germination rate for 4 weeks after harvesting and then begin to decline.

Roots can be collected after the plant is 1 year old, at any time of year. The side of the mounds are dug into and the root harvested. Up to one-third of the root from an individual plant can be taken without damaging the plant or its growth.

Cryptolepis would probably grow well in the American South, the northwest Olympic Peninsula, and parts of the West, or in any climate similar to its natural home. Given its importance, it should be cultivated wherever and whenever it can grow.

Plant Chemistry

There is some confusion in the naming of some of the more potent alkaloids in *C. sanguinolenta*, as researchers in different parts of the world named them with different names at about the same time. It still isn't sorted out. However, the primary ones are cryptolepine, neocryptolepine (a.k.a. cryptotackieniene, quinindoline), several other forms of neocryptolepine, hydroxycryptolepine, cryptolepine hydrochloride, isocryptoline (a.k.a. cryptosanguinolentine), quindoline, cryptoheptine, biscryptolepine, cryptoquindoline, cryptospirolepine, and cryptomisrine.

Most cryptolepis species contain phenolic compounds, but *C. sanguinolenta* does not. Screening has found alkaloids (numerous), polyuronoides, and reducing sugars but little else. Polyphenols, saponins, flavonoids, and cyanogenic glycosides have been reported in at least one study. Cryptolepine is considered to be the strongest constituent (see the sida monograph, page 202, especially the "Scientific Research" section), though many of the others are nearly as potent.

An analysis of the leaves has found many of the same alkaloids that are present in the root, including cryptolepine. Aqueous and ethanolic extracts of the leaves are highly active against malaria (and presumably other microorganisms), giving a 90 percent inhibition of multidrug-resistant malarial strains in vitro. The leaves contain at least two novel alkaloids not present in the roots: cryptolepinoic acid and methyl cryptolepinoate, as well as the usual cryptolepine, hydroxycryptolepine, and quindoline.

C. buchanani, *C. hypoglauca*, and *C. triangularis* have all been listed as containing similar alkaloids as *C. sanguinolenta*. The research is thinner than I would like, and *triangularis* may be a synonym of *sanguinolenta*. *Buchanani* has been studied in the most depth. It's a traditional herb in Ayurvedic practice (see that description, opposite page). Several sources list it as containing cryptolepine and quindoline as well as sarmentogenin, sarmentocymarin, nicotinoyl glucoside, glucopyranose, buchananine, buchanin, n-triacontanol, n-triacontanoic acid, alpha-amyrin, beta-sitosterol glucoside, cryptosin, cryptanoside A-D, germinocol, cryptolepain, sarverogenin, and isosaverogenin. These latter two compounds appear to have potent antibacterial and antiparasitic properties. Given its traditional uses in India, it appears that *C. buchanani* may in fact be a good substitute for *sanguinolenta*.

C. obtusa contains some novel steroidal alkaloids, but not much work has been done on this plant—and on the rest of the family even less.

Traditional Uses of Cryptolepis

Cryptolepis has been successfully used for centuries by traditional African healers in the treatment of malaria, fevers, and diarrhea, as shown in the chart below.

Country/Region	Use Cryptolepis For
Congo	Amoebic infection, including dysentery
DR Congo	Colic, stomach complaints
Ghana	Malaria, fever
Guinea-Bissau	Fever, hepatitis, jaundice
Nigeria	Urinary tract infections, upper respiratory tract infections, colic, stomach complaints, venereal disease, rheumatism, as a general tonic
Senegal	Colic and stomach complaints, venereal disease, rheumatism, as a general tonic
Uganda	Colic and stomach complaints, wounds, snakebite, hernia
Zaire	Stomach and intestinal diseases

AYURVEDA

Cryptolepis buchanani has been used in traditional Ayurvedic practice for millennia. It is widely distributed throughout Pakistan, India, Nepal, Bhutan, Myanmar, China, Thailand, and Sri Lanka. It is considered an invasive weed in many areas (a useful sign of medicinal importance). There are a multitude of local names for the plant in those regions, 60 that I have identified so far. *Maranta* is a common one. It's been used as an antidiarrheal, antibacterial, anti-inflammatory, antiulcerative, blood purifier, demulcent, diaphoretic, and diuretic, and for treating paralysis and rickets and as a general tonic for overall health. It is commonly used for urinary tract infections, for coughs as an expectorant, as a febrifuge (antipyretic), and for abdominal disorders such as dysentery.

A Clinical Trial

Parameters: 44 outpatients with uncomplicated malaria were given a strong tea (steeped for 5 to 10 minutes) three times daily for 5 days, with posttreatment follow-up for 28 days.

Results: More than half cleared the malarial parasite from their blood within 72 hours (mean clearance time was 82.3 hours). Fever clearance time was 25.2 hours compared with chloroquine's clearance time of 48 hours. Chills, vomiting, and nausea were cleared in all patients in 72 hours. There were two instances of late recrudescence (return of the disease), but the researchers are unsure whether this resulted from reinfection or relapse; no genetic testing was done on the initial infection. Overall the cure rate was 93.5 percent. Nii-Ayi Ankrah, of the Department of Clinical Pathology at the University of Ghana, remarked (in a separate article), "The present result is indeed welcome news since it advances the vision to incorporate plant medicine into the health care delivery system in Ghana."[1] How different than in the United States.

Other studies, in mice, have found that the intake of a cryptolepis tea prior to inoculation with the malarial parasite does confer some degree of protection against infection. Taking it daily as a preventive as so many in Africa do seems to work well.

In Thailand alcohol extracts of the plant have been used as a primary anti-inflammatory in the treatment of arthritis, muscle and joint pain, and rheumatism.

Scientific studies of *C. buchanani* conducted in India and based on traditional use have found it is strongly antibacterial, effective against *Staphylococcus aureus, E. coli, Salmonella typhimurium, Klebsiella pneumoniae, Proteus vulgaris,* and *Bacillus subtilis.* Research has found it to possess immunopotentiating properties (useful in immunodeficiency), to act as a cardiotonic and cardio-protector, to be hepatoprotective, and to be strongly anti-inflammatory. It has shown some hypotensive actions and is considered to be, in one study, antiamphetaminic (a truly strange category—I gave him the amphetamines but they didn't work because . . .).

TRADITIONAL CHINESE MEDICINE

Given the plant's presence in China and nearby countries, it is certain that it is used in TCM, but none of my sources, though rather extensive in places, give a listing for the plant.

WESTERN BOTANIC PRACTICE

Until recently, this plant was not known to Western practice.

Scientific Research

Cryptolepis was discovered by the West because of the resurgence of pharmaceutically resistant plasmodial parasites. In an attempt to find new treatments for malaria, researchers began looking at traditional treatments. Initial studies revealed both *Cryptolepis sanguinolenta* and *Artemisia annua* (see monograph, page 242) to be powerfully active against resistant strains. Artemisia was the first to be developed into a drug (with the same predictable problems ensuing). Cryptolepis lagged behind, but in the past 15 years a tremendous amount of research has been conducted on the plant. Initially, most of it was concerned with malaria.

Cryptolepis is potently active against the malarial parasite, *Plasmodium falciparum.* (It is also active against other members of the genus: *P. berghei berghei, P. berghei yoelii,* and *P. vinckei petteri.*) Scores of studies have found it to be effective against the malarial parasite *no matter the degree of its resistance to pharmaceuticals.* Five of the plant's constituents — cryptolepine, cryptolepine hydrochloride, hydroxycryptolepine, cryptoheptine, and neocryptolepine—have been found to be exceptionally active against the parasite, and one other, quindoline, is also active, though not as strong. Studies looking solely at inhibition of beta-haematin formation, which is one of the primary ways that antimalarials deal with malarial infection of blood cells, have found that seven compounds in cryptolepis are active in that respect.

The herb has been remarkably potent against malaria in human clinical trials. One such trial compared the effectiveness of cryptolepis (a hot water infusion of the powdered root) with chloroquine, the usual synthetic drug for malaria treatment, in comparative patient populations at the outpatient clinic of the Centre for Scientific Research into Plant Medicine at Mampong-Akuapem in Ghana, West Africa. Clinical symptoms were relieved in 36 hours with cryptolepis, and 48 hours with chloroquine. Parasitic clearance time was 3.3 days in the cryptolepis group, and 2.3 days in the chloroquine group—a remarkably comparable time period. Forty percent of the patients using chloroquine reported unpleasant side effects necessitating other medications, whereas those using cryptolepis reported *no* side effects.

Because many of the antimalarial compounds in cryptolepis are water soluble, and water-soluble extracts have worked well in clinical trials, a local company in Ghana hopes that a premade tea of cryptolepis will work well against malaria. Using 2.5 grams of powdered root per tea bag, the preparation is called Phyto-Laria and can be purchased over the counter in Ghana. (Similar products, Malaherb and Herbaquine, are also available in Ghana, and one called Malarial is sold in Mali.)

Pharmaceutical companies have created a number of cryptolepine analogues in an attempt to generate a patented drug they can control. Side effects from these analogues are unknown (isolated cryptolepine, unlike the plant it comes from, has shown a number of serious side effects during in vitro and in vivo studies), and like artemisinin and artesenuate (constituents isolated from *Artemisia annua*; see monograph, page 242), these analogues are likely to prove futile in the long run since the malarial parasite does develop immunity to single chemical compounds with regularity. Even though the analogues are molecularly close to cryptolepine, studies have found their mode of action to be different from cryptolepine's—the researchers really don't know what they do in the body or the likely long-term impacts. Because the herb itself is so tremendously safe and effective, I would not recommend the use of analogues if they do in fact ever come on the market.

ANTIBACTERIAL AND OTHER PROPERTIES

Cryptolepis is also broadly antibacterial. It has been tested against more than 100 strains of campylobacter bacteria and found strongly effective against all of them. The tincture is more effective than co-trimoxazole and sulfamethoxazole, and equal to ampicillin. Cryptolepis is active against cholera but is not as strong in its effects as tetracycline. It has been found to be broadly active against a number of enteropathogenic microorganisms including *Shigella dysentariae*, *Entamoeba histolytica*, and *E. coli*. It is especially potent in the treatment of resistant staph, *Streptococcus pyogenes*, numerous strains of tuberculosis (*Mycobacterium* spp.), and urinary tract infections caused by enterobacter and klebsiella bacteria. The activity against such a wide range of organisms bears out its traditional use for many of the diseases that these organisms cause.

Cryptolepis also possesses antihyperglycemic properties, making it a potential antidiabetic herb. The isolated constituent cryptolepine lowered glucose levels in mouse models of type 2 diabetes, caused a decline in insulin levels, and enhanced glucose uptake. Several patents have been granted in this area.

The herb is strongly hypothermic, which means it lowers body temperature, a main reason why it has been found so effective in the treatment of fevers. It is also hypotensive due to its vasodilating effects, and it has been found to be active against a number of cancer lines and is stimulating interest as a potential anticancer agent.

Sida

Family: Malvaceae

Common Names: *Most of the species in this genus are commonly called something to do with "fanpetals," and in fact the sidas are sometimes referred to as the fanpetals.* S. cordata, *for example, is heartleaf fanpetals,* S. neomexicana *is New Mexico fanpetals,* S. spinosa *is prickly fanpetals, and so on. If it has fanpetals as part of its common name, it is probably a sida.*

Oddly, the most medicinally inclined tend to be called something else: S. cordifolia *is country mallow,* S. rhombifolia *is Cuban jute,* S. acuta *is common wireweed or teaweed or ironweed—all of which give an indication as to its nature, as does the Australian common name: spinyhead sida. Sometimes it is called hornbeam-leaved sida, morning mallow, or broomweed (the immensely durable branches are used everywhere the plant grows to make brooms), but most prefer a nastier name.*

The sidas are so widely distributed around the world and used in so many medicinal traditions that their non-English common names are legion. *(See the Traditional Uses section on page 215 for some examples.)*

Species Used: There are 125 or 150 or 200 species of the genus *Sida* (taxonomy is an *exact* science). They are distributed throughout the world, mostly in the tropics and subtropics, but some species extend into temperate regions.

The main medicinal species that has been studied is *Sida acuta*. However, as research has deepened on this species, other sidas are coming to light as similarly potent, particularly *S. rhombifolia* and *S. cordifolia*. Two other species, *S. tiagii* and *S. spinosa*, have not been studied as extensively, but their traditional uses, and some research, indicate they may possess the same medicinal actions.

Given the potency of some of this genus, it makes sense for more research to occur. As far as I can determine, little has been done along this line, but it may well be that many sidas contain similar constituents. If so, given their wide range, they would be one of the world's most accessible systemic herbal antibacterials.

This section will primarily concentrate on where the most research has been done: *Sida acuta*, with some depth on *S. rhombifolia*, *S. cordifolia*, *S. spinosa*, and *S. tiagii*.

Note: *Sida carpinifolia* is considered to be a synonym of *S. acuta*.

Parts Used

The whole plant—roots, leaves, stems, seeds. Most people tend to just use the aerial parts for the simplicity of harvest and ecological soundness. More practically, harvesting the root of a mature plant in this genus is as difficult as conveying to a politician the meaning of the word *integrity*. It is a tough, tough root to dig up. Nevertheless, *S. acuta* is considered an invasive botanical in many countries, and most people are happy if you just take the whole damn thing.

Preparation and Dosage

The tincture and the hot-water extract are the strongest medicinal forms of sida for internal use. The plant can be prepared as powder, capsules, hot tea, or alcohol tincture. Most people use the leaves.

POWDER

For bacterial infections of the skin, wound sepsis, and eczema, liberally sprinkle the powder on the site of infection as frequently as needed.

CAPSULES

As a preventive: Take 3 "00" capsules 3x daily.

In acute conditions: Take up to 30 capsules daily. Or you can just use 1–3 tbl powder in water or juice.

TINCTURE

1:5, 60 percent alcohol, 20–40 drops, up to 4x daily

For resistant staph: In the treatment of severe systemic staph infection the usual dose is ½ tsp–1 tbl, 3–6x daily. (I prefer to not use dosages this high for longer than 60 days. That is usually sufficient.)

TEA

Use 1–2 tsp of the powdered leaves in 6 ounces water; let steep 15 minutes.

As a preventive: Drink 1 or 2 cups daily.

In acute conditions: Drink up to 10 cups daily.

For eye infections: Use the cool tea as eyedrops, 1–3 drops as needed, 3–6x a day.

Not Good for Goats

The plant is a good forage plant for all animals except goats. Goats react negatively to swainsonine and will develop ataxia, hypermetria, hyperesthesia, and muscle tremors of the neck and head. Essentially the plant induces alpha-mannosidosis in goats, something other animals get if they eat too much "locoweed"—usually that is swainsonine-containing plants of the *Oxytropis* or *Astragalus* genera. This constituent does not affect people. Oddly enough, many foraging animals tolerate sida very well; the only report of adverse effects has been in goats.

Note: While the herb will work if infused in cold water, studies have found that the hot-water extraction is more effective. It is nearly as strong as the alcohol tincture. Also, because the plant's primary active constituents are alkaloids, the water used for the infusion must be acidic; see the box on page 194.

Side Effects and Contraindications

None noted, known, or reported; however . . .

- The herb is traditionally used to prevent pregnancy. It does interfere with egg implantation in mice. The herb should not be used in patients who are trying to get pregnant or are newly pregnant.
- Even though the herb is traditionally used in later pregnancy, caution should be exercised with pregnant patients. I would be uncomfortable using it if I were pregnant, but then I would be uncomfortable anyway if I were pregnant.
- Since the herb contains cryptolepine, it is a DNA intercalator and interferes with DNA replication. (See page 195 in the cryptolepis monograph, for more.)
- The herb contains ephedrine, although not in large quantities (see the box on page 214, for an explanation of just how minute those amounts are). There has been a lot of inaccurate, hysterical reporting on ephedra, even among researchers who should know better. Weight loss and "natural energy" companies marketed supplements containing the herb (usually along with caffeine and other stimulants). People wanting to lose weight or increase their energy took the supplements—often in huge doses, far beyond sanity. Herbalists did not support this use of the herb. Ephedra is very safe when used properly; it really didn't need to be banned. The companies using it improperly just needed to be prohibited from doing so. Nevertheless, be aware that sida contains minute amounts of ephedra and that a mild raciness or wakefulness may occur from using the herb—but it probably won't.

(continues on page 210)

Properties of Sida

Actions

Adaptogenic
Analgesic
Anthelmintic (fresh leaf juice)
Antiamoebic
Antibacterial
Anticancer (antineoplastic, antiproliferative)
Antifertility activity (inhibits egg implantation in mice)
Anti-inflammatory
Antimalarial
Antimicrobial
Antioxidant (mild)
Antiprotozoal
Antipyretic
Antiulcerative
Antivenin activity
Hematoprotectant
Hematoregenerator
Hematotonic
Hepatoprotective
Hypoglycemic
Insecticidal

Active Against

Sida acuta is active against:

Babesia spp.
Bacillus spp.
Escherichia coli
Herpes simplex
Listeria innocua
Mycobacterium phlei
Pasteurella multicocida
Plasmodium spp.
Salmonella typhimurium
Shigella boydii
Shigella dysentariae
Shigella flexneri
Staphylococcus aureus
Streptococcus pyogenes

The plant is apparently less active against *Pseudomonas aeruginosa*, *Candida* spp., *Aspergillus niger*, and *A. fumigatus* (however, see the Scientific Research section on page 218).

Sida rhombifolia is active against:

Aspergillus niger
Bacillus spp. (various)
Candida albicans
Entamoeba histolytica
Escherichia coli
Klebsiella pneumoniae
Micrococcus luteus
Morganella morganii
Proteus vulgaris
Pseudomonas aeruginosa
Salmonella enteritidis (mildly)
Salmonella paratyphi
Salmonella sonnei
Salmonella typhi
Shigella boydii
Shigella dysentariae
Staphylococcus aureus
Vibrio mimicus
Vibrio parahaemolyticus

Use to Treat

- Anemia
- Cancer of the blood
- Diarrhea
- Dysentery
- Eye infections (as eyedrops)
- Fevers
- Infected wounds
- Malaria
- Skin rashes such as eczema and impetigo
- Systemic staph infections
- Tuberculosis

Early indications are that sida is moderately virucidal against herpes viruses and can help prevent outbreaks. It is also useful as an adaptogenic in long-term debilitating infections such as Lyme, malaria, and dysentery.

Other Uses

Sida is very high in protein, being 16 percent to 25 percent protein depending on how it is grown. Some cultures use it as a pot herb; it is possible to use it as a primary protein source, especially if you are an "invasivore." Yes, they do exist. Invasivores eat only invasive species—though none have yet (publicly) admitted to consuming *Homo sapiens*.

I have not eaten sida, but the tincture is delicious, one of the few that delights the tongue. If you do try the herb as a vegetable, let me know what you think.

Many cultures use the plant's twigs in making brooms. From all reports they are exceptionally long lasting and useful given the hardiness of the wood. The bark from the stems of most species has been used for making cords, ropes, and twine; the bark from *S. acuta* can be used for making canvas and fishnets as well, hence the "jute" designation for some of the species.

Finding Sida

From what I can tell, based on traditional use and what research there is, *Sida acuta*, *S. cordifolia*, and *S. rhombifolia* can all be used similarly, and most likely *S. spinosa* and probably a number of others can as well. My preference is for *S. acuta* if you can get it, as the most research has been done on that species, then *S. rhombifolia*, then *S. cordifolia.*

Sources for the seeds in-the-year-of-our-plant-2014 are rare, but hopefully the material in this book will stimulate enough interest to make them more easily available. They are certainly available in quantity wherever the plant grows. Seeds of *Sida acuta* can be ordered from e*species Tropical Seeds. Horizon Herbs has *Sida cordifolia* seeds.

Because a number of weight loss companies are adding it to some of their "lose-weight-while-eating-all-you-want" formulations and bodybuilder supplement companies are also going gangbusters with it, some of the sidas may be banned. At this writing the only one that I have heard *may* be illegal in the United States is *rhombifolia,* but I have been unable to confirm that. If you search for *S. cordifolia,* you will find a number of capsule forms of it for sale. Use only the pure herb—many of those weight loss formulas have adulterants or other herbs mixed in. Again, I think the tincture and hot-water extracts are the most potent forms to use for healing, especially with resistant bacteria.

Unfortunately, due to the ephedra content in some of the sida species, at least one, *Sida rhombifolia*, has been reported to be illegal to harvest. Entheogenic adherents have also, sigh, been using the plant to get high by smoking it. (It is reputed to be an aphrodisiac stimulant in a number of cultures.)

Herb/Drug Interactions

None known or reported; however . . .

- Since the herb is hypoglycemic, it *may* affect medications for diabetes. Just watch blood sugar levels of diabetic patients.
- Since the herb contains ephedrine, it probably should not be used with pharmaceuticals that possess similar effects.

Habitat and Appearance

Many of the sidas are typical-looking mallow-like plants with the usual five-lobed pale yellow to orange flowers. They get their name from the spreading or fanning of their flower petals. Some of the species are ground covers, while others grow into sturdy bushes as much as 6 feet tall. They can be perennials, annuals, or biennials—and I am talking about the same plant here; they alter their behavior depending on where they are growing and the climate. They are often considered wasteland weeds irrespective of the species.

Sida acuta grows from 3 to 6 feet tall and may appear as either an annual or a perennial. It is a *potently* invasive medicinal wherever it gets established. In general, when the sidas get loose, they just keep on going, and they don't like to be controlled once they're established.

S. acuta has a very deep and strong taproot that endures droughts, mowing, and tillage with impunity. The plant easily survives extensive foraging by animals. With age the stem gets tough and woody, which helps the plant resist the phytopolice who wish to send it back to Mexico. Once established, the plant is highly competitive, loves and spreads easily into disturbed ecosystems, and doesn't share or play well with others. It can be found as high as 5,000 feet and is often found in pastures, wastelands, cultivated farmland, roadsides, lawns, forests, and any human-planted or disturbed environment. It grows well in clay soils and desert as well as your typical black humus and survives heavy rainfall as well as drought. The seeds (spinyhead) adhere well to clothing and animals, are picked up in mud on tires and shoes, hide in hay and grass bales, and germinate easily wherever they end up. They are very sharp and puncture the skin, and feet, with abandon.

Truly one of the great invasives.

NORTH AMERICAN RANGE

Sida acuta can be grown in much of the United States and should be cultivated wherever it can be. It has been reported in Alabama, Florida,

Georgia, Hawaii, Louisiana, Mississippi, New Jersey, Pennsylvania, South Carolina, Texas, Puerto Rico, and the U.S. Virgin Islands. Although it is said to grow most easily in zones 8 to 11, given that it grows in New Jersey and Pennsylvania, there is no reason it cannot grow throughout that region as well as in Northern California, Oregon, and the Olympic Peninsula and most likely other regions as well.

Sida cordifolia grows in Alabama, Florida, Hawaii, Texas, Puerto Rico, and the U.S. Virgin Islands.

Sida rhombifolia is widely distributed: Alabama, Arizona, Arkansas, California, Florida, Georgia, Hawaii, Kansas, Kentucky, Louisiana, Maryland, Mississippi, New Jersey, North Carolina, Oklahoma, Pennsylvania, South Carolina, Tennessee, Texas, Virginia, Puerto Rico, and the U.S. Virgin Islands.

Sida spinosa grows throughout those states and also in Connecticut, D.C., Delaware, Illinois, Indiana, Iowa, Maine, Massachusetts, Missouri, Nebraska, New York, Ohio, West Virginia, and Ontario, Canada.

WORLDWIDE RANGE

Sida acuta is considered to be native to Mexico and Central America, but it has spread around the world with great abandon (the seeds are great hitchhikers—the Spanish colonizers in South America and Mexico took some with them everywhere they traveled). In Australia's northern territories biological control has been instituted to try to stop its spread, with only mixed success.

This species is common in China, Japan, Taiwan, the Philippines, Malaysia, Singapore, Indonesia, Papua New Guinea, Fiji, Tonga, Tahiti—it's common throughout the entire Pacific Rim and Pacific Islands, in fact—India, Sri Lanka, Thailand, Cambodia, Vietnam, Burkina Faso, Togo, Nigeria, Kenya, Peru, western Colombia, Panama, Honduras, El Salvador, Guatemala, Mexico, and other similar places and regions around the world. In most places where it has been introduced it is considered invasive and noxious and is often deeply disliked (the seeds, rather nasty, contribute to its poor reputation). It is considered a plant threat to Pacific ecosystems. However, in some regions (Florida) people grow it as an ornamental. Go figure.

Sida rhombifolia is even more widespread than *S. acuta*. It is invasive throughout the Pacific Rim and Islands, Australia, and New Zealand. It is widely found in China, Japan, Taiwan, Thailand, Cambodia, Vietnam, Malaysia, Indonesia, the Indian Ocean chain, Peru, Ecuador, Colombia, Costa Rica, Nicaragua, Honduras, El Salvador, Guatemala, and Mexico.

Sida cordifolia also grows widely throughout the Pacific Rim and Islands (invasive status) as well as in Japan, Taiwan, Australia, El Salvador, and Honduras.

Sida spinosa is invasive throughout the Pacific Rim and Islands and grows widely in Japan, Australia, Chile, Peru, and Mexico.

Cultivation and Collection

Sida acuta grows well from seed. In fact, its seeds are very hardy, with at least a 30 percent survival rate over several seasons of drought. Each plant produces several hundred seeds every year. They attach to any passing animal and drop off later to spread the plant even further. The seeds need a period of high temperature to break their seed coat and do best if there is a period of alternating high and low temperatures.

The seeds are collected in the fall and can be top-seeded where you want them to grow, with average watering.

Note: *Sida acuta* is as good at healing damaged land as it is ill people; it is exceptionally good at detoxifying polluted soils. It removes cadmium, lead, nickel, iron, zinc, cobalt, mercury, molybdenum, copper, manganese, arsenic, and chromium from industrially polluted or dump sites. It is particularly good at scavenging lead, zinc, iron, nickel, cadmium, chromium, molybdenum, and arsenic. The plant should *not* be harvested for medicine from such sites as it will contain high levels of heavy metals.

Plant Chemistry

Sida acuta (and several others in the genus) is one of the few medicinals known besides *Cryptolepis sanguinolenta* to contain cryptolepine. This is one of the more potent constituents in the plant. The plant, like *C. sanguinolenta*, also generates a number of cryptolepine derivatives: quindoline, quindolinone, cryptolepinone, and 11-methoxy-quindoline.

Other constituents include ecdysterone, beta-sitosterol, stigmasterol, ampesterol, evofolin A and B, scopoletin, loliolide, 4-ketopinoresinol, ephedrine, beta-phenethylamine, quinazoline, carboxylated tryptamine alkaloids, alpha-amyrin, hentriacontane, hypolaetin-8-glucoside, campesterol, heraclenol, acanthoside B, daucoglycoside, choline, betaine, trans-feruloyltyramine, vomifoliol, ferulic acid, sinapic acid, syringic acid, syringaresinol, vanillic acid, swainsonine, vasicine, vasicinol, vasicinone, and peganine.

The seeds of both *Sida acuta* and *Sida rhombifolia* contain numerous ecdysteroids including ecdysone and 20-hydroxyecdysone. *Sida filicaulis* seeds contain lesser amounts. There is some indication that the plants, as opposed to the seeds, contain these compounds as well. This is the presumed source of the adaptogenic actions of the sidas when used as medicine. *Sida acuta* plants also contain alkaloids,

Not a Good Source of Ephedrine

The ephedrine content of *Sida acuta* and the other sidas is tiny when compared to that of the true ephedra species. *S. acuta* has 0.006 percent in the roots and 0.041 percent in the leaves and stems. *S. cordata* has 0.005 percent and 0.036 percent; *S. cordifolia* has 0.007 percent and 0.112 percent; *S. rhombifolia* has 0.031 percent and 0.017 percent. In contrast *Ephedra distachya* contains about 3 percent in the plant; *E. sinica* has about 2.2 percent. *Sida cordifolia* root at 0.112 percent is the closest in strength to the ephedras' percent. Essentially, *S. cordifolia* has about 1/20th the ephedrine content of *E. sinica*. Nevertheless, companies are once again selling the sidas for weight loss and energy, and for weight lifters—a practice I consider to be unscrupulous.

flavonoids, steroids, tannins, cardenolides, polyphenols, terpenoids, and cardiac glycosides.

Sida acuta and *Sida rhombifolia* contain a number of cyclopropenoid fatty acids. The same alkaloids present in *Sida acuta* have been found in *Sida humilis*, *S. rhombifolia*, and *S. spinosa*.

Traditional Uses of Sida

Sida acuta is widely used in traditional medicinal practice around the world to treat malaria, fevers, headache, skin diseases, infected wounds, diarrhea, dysentery, snake bites, asthma, GI tract problems, and systemic infections. James Duke's database lists 12 species of sida that have been used in traditional medicine, all for a similar range of complaints. The heaviest hits occurred with *acuta, cordifolia, rhombifolia*, and *veronicaefolia*. *S. acuta* and *rhombifolia* are sometimes smoked in Mexico for their euphoric effects.

Country/Region	Use *Sida* For
Australia	Aborigines use to treat diarrhea and indigestion
Burkina Faso	Fever, diarrhea, pulmonary infection, snake and insect bites
Colombia	Snakebite
Guatemala, Nicaragua	Asthma, renal inflammation, colds, fever, headache, ulcers, intestinal worms
Hawaii	Used by native islanders for vaginal infections, the flowers chewed as a laxative, the whole plant pounded and the juice taken for asthma or for general debility
Kenya	Tonic and common plant food
Malacca	Influenza, wounds, toothaches, ulcers, chest pains, scabies, abscesses, impotence, gonorrhea, and rheumatism
Nigeria	Malaria, typhoid fever, toothache, sore gums, teeth cleaning, ulcer, fever, gonorrhea, abortion (but also to stop diarrhea during pregnancy), hysteria, bruises, eye infections (as eyedrops), nosebleeds (fresh leaf juice), breast cancer, poisoning, inflammation, and sores and wounds, to stop bleeding, and as an antipyretic and emollient
Sri Lanka	Hemorrhoids, fevers, impotency, gonorrhea, and rheumatism; *S. acuta* is used in the treatment of neuralgia, *S. cordifolia* for hysteria, *S. rhombifolia* for fever
Togo	Eczema, kidney stones, headache
Trinidad and Tobago	Eczema

AYURVEDA

Various sida species have been used in India for more than 5,000 years; some species are native, others were introduced from the Americas. The primary species used is *Sida cordifolia,* but all are common medicinals. *Sida acuta* is considered an invasive menace by some and listed as such in some government writings. Practitioners in India commonly use the various species interchangeably, which has led to calls for stricter identification of which sidas are being used and for what. Species commonly used are *S. acuta, S. carpinifolia, S. cordifolia, S. humilis, S. indica, S. rhombifolia*, and *S. spinosa.*

Bala is the primary term in Sanskrit for the main medicinal species—*acuta* and *cordifolia*—while lesser species are distinguished by a linguistic modification of that term: *S. carpinifolia* is *bala phanijivika, S. rhombifolia* is *atibala* (or *mahabala*), *S. spinosa* is *nagabala, S. humilis* is *bhumibala*. However, every local ethnic group that uses the genus for medicine has its own local name for the plants. There are scores of them. The plants, again, are considered to be interchangeable for the most part in practice; the roots, leaves, seeds, and stems are all used.

Sida cordifolia is considered to be cooling, astringent, stomachic, tonic, aromatic, bitter, febrifuge, demulcent, diuretic. The seeds are used as an aphrodisiac and to treat gonorrhea, cystitis, hemorrhoids, colic, and tenesmus. The leaves are used for strangury, hematuria, gonorrhea, cystitis, leukorrhea, chronic dysentery, nervous diseases, facial paralysis, and asthma, and as a cardiac tonic. They are cooked with rice and used for bloody diarrhea and bleeding hemorrhoids. An infusion of the roots is effective for nervous and urinary diseases and disorders of the blood and liver, while a decoction of the root (with ginger) is used for fever accompanied by cold shivering fits (essentially malarial fevers). The root juice is good for wounds, and an infusion of the dried root for bloody diarrhea, dandruff, and scalp problems. The juice of the plant is used for spermatorrhoea, rheumatism, and gonorrhea. All parts of the plant are used as a stomachic and cardiac tonic.

Sida acuta is used as a diaphoretic and antipyretic and to treat fevers, dyspepsia, and lingering debility from previous illnesses. The juice of the root is used for intestinal worms, an infusion of the root for intermittent fever and chronic bowel complaints and for asthma, and the powdered root is made into a paste and applied to boils and abscesses. The leaves are used as a demulcent and diuretic and to treat chronic diarrhea and dysentery, rheumatic conditions, and gonorrhea. It is a common food plant in some districts.

Sida rhombifolia is used as a diuretic and aphrodisiac and to treat hemorrhoids, gonorrhea, rheumatism, kidney stones, fever, and scorpion sting. An infusion of the root is used for asthma.

Sida spinosa is used for cooling fevers (as a decoction, 2x daily) and to treat gonorrhea, gleet, scalding urine, debility. It was used as a primary trauma medicine in Chhattisgarh, India, during the wars of the twentieth century. The leaf juice was used to stop bleeding, decrease pain, prevent infection, and hasten healing time.

Other Ayurvedic uses of sida include the treatment of eye problems (infections), sinusitis, cramps, joint pain, fracture, swelling, Parkinson's disease, colic, whooping cough, uterine problems, vaginal infection, bronchitis, TB, emaciation, and cystitis. All the sidas are used as veterinary medicine for treating diarrhea in farm animals throughout India.

TRADITIONAL CHINESE MEDICINE

Sida acuta—*huanghuaren* or *huang hu aren*—is used in Chinese medicine, as is *Sida rhombifolia*—*huan hua mu*—and presumably other sidas as well. I can find little on the plants even though they seem to have a longish history of use there. The plants are usually used as decoctions, with a dosage range of up to 30 grams, or about 1 ounce. The Chinese consider sida to clear heat and benefit dampness. They have found it to be antibiotic, anti-inflammatory, analgesic, diuretic, and tonic.

Sidas are commonly used for depression, bronchitis with cough and wheezing, and urinary tract inflammations. Less common uses are for dermatosis, itching, eczema of the scrotum, sores and boils, stomach pain, dysentery, gastritis, enteritis, tonsillitis, liver problems, jaundice, cervical tuberculous lymphadenitis, malaria, colds and flu, and kidney stones.

WESTERN BOTANIC PRACTICE

Sida (*S. rhombifolia* primarily) was apparently introduced into the United States in the nineteenth century as a fiber plant, but it wasn't much used as a medicinal. The Eclectics listed it in a tiny reference under *Althea*, a.k.a. marsh mallow, as being highly mucilaginous, useful as a poultice, and effective for respiratory complaints.

Scientific Research

The recent focus on cryptolepine-containing plants as well as traditional malarial plants has stimulated a lot of interest in *Sida acuta* and some of the more commonly used Asian sidas. Most of the scientific studies have focused on phytochemical analysis and in vitro studies of the plants' antimicrobial actions, with a smattering of in vivo studies. The scientific exploration of these plants is still in its infancy and no clinical trials have been conducted that I am aware of.

There have been a number of studies of the antimicrobial activity of *Sida acuta*, and while they do give a good indication of its potency, nearly all the studies are flawed. Inexplicably, very few of the researchers appeared aware of the importance of proper preparation of the plant extracts.

Looking only at the ethanol and water extract preparations in the studies, the problems are twofold. First, they tended to use 90 percent to 95 percent pure alcohol to make the ethanol extracts. This means that *only* the alcohol-soluble constituents would be present in the extract. (There would be a tiny amount of water-soluble constituents from the 5 percent to 10 percent water that was present in the alcohol.) Many of the most potent constituents in the plant, such as cryptolepine, are only water soluble, so the preparation method will affect the impact of the extract on microorganisms.

Second, when making the water-based extracts, many of the researchers used a neutral-pH distilled water. Additionally, some made it as a cold maceration. This is problematical for these reasons: The alkaloids in the plant, most important cryptolepine and its derivatives, are primarily soluble in water that is somewhat acidic and the plant constituents are less soluble in cold water than in hot.

For the studies to be truly relevant, the water extracts should have used water with a pH of from 1 to 6 to make sure they were acidic enough to extract the alkaloids and the water should have been hot. With the ethanol extracts, preparation should have been made using half water and half pure grain alcohol; the water should have been hot, the herb inserted, the mixture allowed to cool, and then the alcohol added. The differences in preparation techniques are the most likely reason that the antimicrobial actions of the plant vary as much as they do from study to study.

Nevertheless, in all studies *Sida acuta* has been shown to be potently active against malarial parasites, staph bacteria, and TB, though beyond that there is a lot of variance. The best study took these factors into account but was exploring *only* alkaloid activity.[2] That study found more activity from the alkaloids against Gram-negative bacteria than previous research, which makes sense, as cryptolepis has been found to be active against Gram-negative bacteria simply due to the presence of cryptolepine and its derivatives. In fact the alkaloidal extract of *Sida acuta* was nearly as effective against Gram-negative as Gram-positive bacteria.

A close examination does indicate, however, that both cryptolepis and sida more easily kill Gram-positive organisms than Gram-negative. This does not mean they are not active, it simply means that the dose needs to be higher if you are dealing with Gram-negative organisms, an observation confirmed by studies on both plants. The plant should also be taken for a longer duration—the Gram-negative bacteria did need a longer exposure to the herb than the Gram-positive. The use of a synergist that enhances

Neutralizing Hemotoxins

Importantly, sida has been found in vivo to neutralize venom from the snake *Bothrops atrox*, a common and very poisonous pit viper in South America. The snake's venom is a hemotoxin that destroys red blood cells (rather than the neurotoxin more common to cobras and rattlesnakes). The constituents in sida are particularly protective of red blood cells, which is one reason they are effective for treating malaria and babesia. With the snake venom, compounds in the plant neutralize a hemotoxic compound, rather than the plant's antimicrobial actions killing an infective organism. In this sense sida represents a unique category of herbal medicines: hematotonic, hematoregenerator, and hematoprotectant. It is especially useful for treating anemia, and I believe there are strong indications that the herb will be significantly useful for the treatment of certain forms of myeloma—cancer of the red blood cells. It is the only herb I know of that is specific in this way for red blood cells.

Given that the actions of cryptolepis are similar to sida's and that it contains some similar constituents, it makes sense to explore cryptolepis for similar protectant actions; e.g., from hemotoxins.

antibacterial activity against Gram-negative bacteria would be helpful. (See piperine monograph, page 447.)

In spite of the problems in the in vitro studies, tests for antimicrobial activity have borne out the traditional uses of the plants against microbial diseases. They have found sida to be strongly active against *Plasmodium* spp., *Staphylococcus aureus*, and *Mycobacterium phlei*—resistant and nonresistant strains. It is highly active against *Streptococcus pyogenes, E. coli, Bacillus subtilis, Pasteurella multicocida*, and *Salmonella typhimurium*. It is also active against herpes simplex, *Shigella boydii, S. flexneri, S. dysentariae*, and *Listeria innocua* but less active against *Pseudomonas aeruginosa, Candida* spp., *Aspergillus niger*, and *A fumigatus* yet still effective, especially if the dosage is increased. In many instances the plant was more effective against the bacterial strains than pharmaceutical antibiotics.

Sida increases glutathione levels in the blood, increases red blood cell numbers (making it good for treating anemia), and increases total white blood cell count, indicating an immune potentiation effect that may tie in with its reported adaptogenic actions in traditional practice.

In vivo studies have found *Sida acuta* to have a strong and reliable antiulcerative effect; that is, it protects the stomach lining from the formation of induced ulcers. In vivo research has also found a strong analgesic action.

Another in vivo study found sida hepatoprotective against induced liver damage (the plant is used in India for liver disease among other things). Several compounds from the plant have been found to inhibit induced preneoplastic lesions in mouse mammary tissue. In vivo studies have also found sida to be hypoglycemic, lowering blood sugar concentrations in diabetic mice, and to be antihyperlipidemic, lowering blood cholesterol and triglyceride levels, again in diabetic mice.

An analysis of four sidas—*S. acuta, humilis, rhombifolia*, and *spinosa*—found them to have similar alkaloidal constituents, including cryptolepine.

An analysis of five sidas—*S. acuta, alba* (a synonym of *spinosa*), *cordifolia, rhombifolia*, and *urens*—found varying levels of polyphenols in the plants (see chart below).

The antioxidant activity of the plants followed that order as well, with

Species	Compound			
	Phenolic (mg GAE/100mg extract)*	**Flavonoid (mg QE/100mg extract)****	**Flavonol (mg QE/100mg extract)****	**Tannin (mg TAE/100 mg extract)*****
S. alba	32.53	5.17	2.33	25.83
S. acuta	15.35	4.36	1.95	9.30
S. cordifolia	10.25	1.92	0.57	7.83
S. rhombifolia	5.75	1.02	0.68	4.35
S. urens	4.21	0.43	0.31	2.28

*Gallic acid equivalents **Quercetin equivalents ***Tannic acid equivalents

Sida alba having the highest, *S. urens* the lowest. The plants were tested for anti-inflammatory activity, exploring their lipoxygenase (LOX) and xanthine oxidase (XOX) inhibition. For LOX, *alba* inhibited 80 percent, *acuta* 79 percent, *cordifolia* 21 percent, *rhombifolia* 52 percent, *urens* 47 percent; for XOX, *alba* inhibited 47 percent, *acuta* 43 percent, *cordifolia* 13 percent, *rhombifolia* 46 percent, *urens* 35 percent.

All these species of sida are successfully used to treat liver diseases including hepatitis B in Burkina Faso; the authors of the study were exploring some of the mechanisms that might explain their effectiveness.

Sida alba (i.e., *S. spinosa*) is fairly high in ecdysteroids, which are adaptogenic and explain, in part, the plant's use for debility in traditional practice.

Numerous studies have found *Sida cordifolia* to possess very potent anti-inflammatory and analgesic activities. An alkaloid with a tremendously long name, one of the quinazoles—a group of which cryptolepine is a member—was found to be the most potent source of the activity. In vivo studies: An aqueous extract of *cordifolia* stimulated liver regeneration in 67 percent partial hepatectomy in rats; birds treated with cyclophosphamide, which causes immunosuppression, experienced a reversal of that condition when given *cordifolia*. In vitro studies: The plant is strongly antimicrobial and acts as an antistressor/adaptogenic in stressed mice; use of the plant after myocardial injury showed significantly increased endogenous antioxidants in heart tissue; other studies found evidence of a protection from neurotoxicity caused by quinolinic acid.

Sida tiagii during in vivo research has been found to have antidepressant and antiseizure effects in mice.

Alchornea

Family: Euphorbiaceae

Common Name: *Christmas bush*

Species Used: The genus *Alchornea* is a pan-tropical group of plants comprising some 60 species, six of which are indigenous to Africa. *Alchornea cordifolia* is the main medicinal species, though *A. laxiflora* is a reliable substitute. Regrettably, there has been little study on the members of this genus other than *A. cordifolia*.

Parts Used

Mostly the leaves, but the stem bark, pith, root bark, roots, and fruits are all used.

Preparation and Dosage

TEA

Add 7 ounces of herb to 1 quart of water and boil for 20 minutes. Strain, then drink 6–8 ounces of the tea every 4 hours. Studies have shown that the tea, takes about 3 hours to begin getting into the blood, and it tends to hit peak presence 1 to 2 hours after that depending on the dose; dosage presence lasts about 4 hours. This means that if you are using the tea, you need to have another cup every 4 hours or so. Recommended dosage times: 8 A.M., 12 P.M., 4 P.M., 8 P.M., or beginning whenever you rise and then going to a 4-hour period.

For eye disease: Use the cool tea as eyedrops, 1–3 drops every 3 to 4 hours.

TINCTURE

1:5, 50 percent alcohol, 50 percent water; take 1/4 tsp of the tincture every 4 hours

POWDER

For wounds and infected skin, liberally sprinkle the powder on the site as frequently as needed.

Side Effects and Contraindications

None noted, and no toxicity has been found. There are no reports in the literature or by traditional practitioners of side effects, although large doses may have a sedative or depressant effect on the central nervous system.

Herb/Drug Interactions

None noted; however, large doses should not be taken along with CNS depressants or sedatives.

Note: Some people indicate that *Alchornea castaneifolia* can be used interchangeably, but I can't see this as accurate—I would never recommend using it interchangeably. See Beware of *A. castaneifolia,* opposite page.

Habitat and Appearance

Alchornea cordifolia is a common plant throughout much of the largish middle of Africa, from Senegal to Kenya and Tanzania and from just north of South Africa to Angola. It's a straggly shrub or small tree up to 25 feet in height. It is widespread in secondary forest and likes riparian habitat and marshy areas but does spread into drier ecosystems, especially in disturbed soils. It will grow in terrain up to 5,000 feet in altitude. It likes acid soils and is an active soil modulator, restoring calcium levels to depleted soils. *Alchornea laxiflora* grows in the same regions and has virtually the same appearance.

Cultivation and Collection

Propagates well from cuttings; they root solidly in a few months. The seeds are considered to be difficult germinators, needing to be scarified and tended diligently. Germination takes up to 3 months.

The plant can be harvested at any time. The leaves are taken when healthy and vital in appearance. The plant is normally wildcrafted as

Beware of *A. castaneifolia*

A few normally reliable companies list scientific studies on the activities of *Alchornea cordifolia* under an entirely different plant—*Alchornea castaneifolia*. *A. castaneifolia* has become popular because it is sometimes used in indigenous ayahuasca ceremonies. The Internet now has scores of sites selling it under the identifier *iporuru* or some version of that name.

Unfortunately most of the sites selling *A. castaneifolia* indicate that it has the same actions as *A. cordifolia* and point to studies on *A. cordifolia* to prove it. This just isn't accurate. The plants are definitely *not* interchangeable. There is very, very little research on the pharmacology of *A. castaneifolia*, and while there may be some overlap in actions—for instance, it *may* be useful for staph infections—there probably is not. Under no circumstances should you believe that *A. castaneifolia* will act as a reliable systemic antibacterial for resistant infections.

Properties of Alchornea

Actions

Amoebicidal
Anthelmintic
Antiamoebic
Antianemic
Antibacterial
Antidiarrheal
Antidrepanocytary
Antifungal
Anti-inflammatory
Antimalarial
Antimicrobial
Antioxidant
Antiprotozoal
Antiseptic
Antitumor
Antiviral
Bronchial relaxant
Smooth muscle tissue relaxant
Trypanocidal

Active Against

Aspergillus spp.
Babesia spp.
Bacillus subtilis
Candida albicans
Entamoeba histolytica
Escherichia coli
Helicobacter pylori
Klebsiella pneumoniae
Plasmodium spp.
Proteus mirabilis
Proteus vulgaris
Pseudomonas aeruginosa
Salmonella enteritidis
Salmonella typhi
Shigella flexneri
Staphylococcus aureus
Streptococcus pyogenes

Use to Treat

Malaria, systemic staph infections, pseudomonas, anemia, fevers, infections from *Streptococcus pyogenes*, and diarrhea and dysentery from such things as severe *E. coli*, *Salmonella*, *Entamoeba*, *Shigella*, or amoebic organisms. Generally, resistant Gram-positive and Gram-negative infections, systemic or of the GI tract. Infected wounds. Sickle cell anemia, sleeping sickness, resistant respiratory infections, conjunctivitis (as an eyewash), UTIs.

Other Uses

Alchornea is a potent alley-cropping plant and soil restorer: Rows of the trees are planted as windbreaks to protect other crops while returning calcium to depleted soils. The fruits produce a black dye traditionally used for fishing nets, cloth, pottery, and leather. The wood is used for construction and crafts.

it is widespread and vigorous once established. It is not yet an agricultural crop.

It coppices well and is very hard to get rid of once established.

Plant Chemistry

A. cordifolia contains the usual terpenes, sterols, flavonoids, tannins, carbohydrates, glycosides, saponins, and alkaloids. It also has alchorneine, alchornine, and alchornidine (all are imidazopyrimidine alkaloids), several guanidine alkaloids, allic acid, gentisic acid, anthranilic acid, protocatechuic acid, ellagic acid, hyperoside, various quercitrins, daucosterol, acetyl aleuritolic acid, beta-sitosterol, epoxy fatty acids (in the seeds, lots), and a lot of other stuff no one has discovered yet.

Traditional Uses of Alchornea

A. cordifolia is widely used throughout every region of Africa in which it grows. It is used as a wash for eye infections and powdered for ringworm and other skin infections. It is an anti-inflammatory, a carminative, an anodyne, a diuretic, an emmenagogue, a blood purifier, and a tonic and has antitumor actions. See chart on next page for a comprehensive list of traditional uses.

Finding Alchornea

The herb is not readily available in the West. I have found only one supplier (Woodland Essence) that carries the herb in tincture form. Part of the point of listing this wonderful plant here is to stimulate suppliers to import it or gardeners to begin planting it in the United States. It would do well here. If you can plant alchornea in your region, do so; it will be worth the effort.

Seed stock is available from the National Forestry Seeds Centre of Burkina Faso (Centre National de Semences Forestières de Burkina Faso) at $14 per kg (about 2.2 pounds). The website is cnsf.bf. The primary government language is French, but an English version of the website was under construction at the time this was being written.

Traditional Uses of Alchornea		
Amoebic dysentery	Epilepsy	Snakebite
Anemia	Fever	Sore throat
Asthma	Gastrointestinal disorders	Tachycardia
Bronchitis	Gonorrhea	Thrush
Buccal ulceration	Headache	Toothache
Chancre	Hemorrhoids	Trypanosomiasis
Chills	Jaundice	Tuberculosis
Conjunctivitis	Leprosy	Ulcers
Constipation	Malaria	Urinary disorders
Cough	Mouth ulcers	Urogenital infections
Dental caries	Myalgia	Worms
Diarrhea	Postpartum hemorrhage (topical)	Wounds
Edema	Respiratory	Yaws
Enlarged spleen	Rheumatism	

AYURVEDA

Not known as far as I can tell.

TRADITIONAL CHINESE MEDICINE

Not known as far as I can tell.

WESTERN BOTANIC PRACTICE

Not known as far as I can tell, though some species have been used for a long time in South American indigenous practice. They don't seem to be similar in action to the two African species discussed here.

Scientific Research

In vitro studies have found *Alchornea cordifolia* active against 15 MRSA isolates and to be strongly active against *Pseudomonas aeruginosa*. Low concentrations of the herb are active against *E. coli, P. aeruginosa*, and *Staphylococcus aureus*; it is as or more active than pharmaceutical antibiotics such as gentamicin and ampicillin. In vivo studies have confirmed the MRSA action in mice. A 50 percent ethanol extract (normal tincture) of alchornea was tested against 74 microbial strains: aerobic, facultative, anaerobic, and fungi. It was active at low concentrations against all except three strains, all filamentous fungi. Like most systemic antibacterial herbs, it was a bit stronger against Gram-positive strains than Gram-negative. It has been found to be active against *Helicobacter pylori, Salmonella typhi, Shigella flexneri, Salmonella enteritidis,* and enterohemorrhagic *E. coli* (EHEC), bearing out its traditional uses for treating dysentery and diarrheagenic bacterial pathogens. Ethanolic and water extracts have been found to be equally active except that only the ethanolic extract was active against EHEC. Other studies have found the ethanolic extract reliably effective in vitro for *E. coli, Pseudomonas aeruginosa, Staphylococcus aureus, Klebsiella pneumoniae,* and *Proteus mirabilis*—at the proper dosage, it is as effective as ciprofloxacin.

In vitro screening of 45 Congolese medicinal plants found alchornea to be highly antiamoebic, with strong activity against *Entamoeba histolytica.* Other studies have confirmed this, including finding a strong spasmolytic action. The plant exhibited a more than 70 percent reduction of spasms in guinea pig ilea.

A. cordifolia has been found to produce its activity in the treatment

Treating Sickle Cell Anemia

Sickle cell anemia is a genetic disease resulting from a mutation in the hemoglobin structure. The cells undergo alterations, ending up as a sickle shape rather than round. This reduces the ability of the cells to carry oxygen and starves the body of enough oxygen to function. About 25 percent of people in sub-Saharan Africa have the disease, which is passed from parent to child genetically; half of those in whom the disease becomes active die before the age of five, about 60,000 in Nigeria each year. Traditional healers have used *Alchornea cordifolia* for centuries in the treatment of the disease, and recent scientific study has found it highly effective. Essentially the plant prevents sickling of the cells (antidrepanocytary activity) and reverses cells that have already transformed. Of all the plants tested for sickle cell treatment, *A. cordifolia* was the most potent. In Lagos a relative, *A. laxiflora*, has been found to have the same activity. The use of *A. cordifolia* reduced sickling by 85 percent and reversed 69 percent of sickled cells. The pharmaceutical approaches normally used for sickle cell anemia are highly toxic, but researchers commented that with this herbal preparation "toxicity . . . is not a problem." The herb is sold as a standardized product, as a tea or capsules, in Lagos and called Cellod-S. Good outcomes have been reported in clinical practice.

of dysentery and diarrheal diseases through three mechanisms: antibacterial, antiamoebic, and antispasmodic actions that are apparently synergistic. In vivo study has found the plant to be highly antidiarrheal against castor-oil-induced diarrhea in mice.

Given the traditional use of alchornea for treating malaria across Africa, it is odd that only two in vitro studies have been conducted on its activity against *Plasmodium falciparum.* One study found it potently active, the second mildly so. *A. cordifolia* is fairly high in ellagic acid, which has been found to be strongly active, in vivo and in vitro, against the malarial parasites. The former study also found it strongly active against *Trypanosoma brucei.* (*A. cordifolia* is used in ethnoveterinary practice to treat that disease, and studies have found it active against both resistant and nonresistant forms.)

Like a number of plants in this chapter, *Alchornea* appears to be hemotonic, a hemoregenerator, and hemoprotectant, but the research has not focused that broadly. It does have a long history of use against anemia, malaria, and sickle cell anemia, as well as for trypanosomiasis (a.k.a. African sleeping sickness), which is also a parasitic disease of the bloodstream, similar in some respects to malaria and babesia.

The research on *Alchornea laxiflora* is limited, but both its traditional use and the studies that exist seem to confirm that its actions are very similar to those of *A. cordifolia.* It grows in the same eco-ranges and is considered interchangeable by the traditional practitioners. In vitro studies have found that the plant has anticonvulsant and sedative actions (in vivo studies have found this action in *A. cordifolia* as well) and is strongly antioxidant, anti-inflammatory, antimicrobial, and antibacterial against both Gram-positive and Gram-negative bacteria. The chemistry of the two plants is very similar.

One study found *A. laxiflora* strongly active against HIV-1 and HIV-2 in vitro, more so than AZT. Another found the plant to possess immune modulatory and stimulant actions. It generates a lymphoproliferative effect on naive murine splenocytes and thymocytes and modulates the effects of the phagocytic and lysomal enzyme activities of murine macrophages. It increases phagocytosis and intracellular killing capacity. Lysosomal phosphatase activity of peritoneal macrophages increased significantly.

Of 42 plants tested in one study, *Alchornea cordifolia* was found to have the most potent antioxidant effects. In vitro study found that the plant was highly protective of rat liver against hepatotoxins. In vivo study in mice found the same.

A number of in vivo studies have found the plant to be strongly anti-inflammatory and very effective in the treatment of induced edema in rats. In vitro studies have found *Alchornea cordifolia* strongly anti-inflammatory by inhibiting human neutrophil elastase and superoxide anion.

Histological changes occur in rat pancreas after use of an ethanolic extract of the plant—28 days of use resulted in regenerative alterations. Islet cells in the pancreas of rats with induced type 1 diabetes regenerated. Quiescent cells proliferated and replaced lost cells. The plant also decreased blood glucose levels and increased B-cell levels in other studies.

The plant is used as an antiasthmatic in Ghana, and an in vivo study found it to act similarly to isoprenaline, which is sometimes used in bronchial inhalers for asthma. Another study found the plant to have a marked effect on the aorta of Wistar rats, essentially inducing elastogenesis.

Bidens

Family: Asteraceae (Compositae)

Common Names: *Spanish needles, beggarticks, demon spike grass, needle grass, *$%#*%!, and a lot of other names in hundreds of languages. It appears to grow everywhere and people either hate it or loathe it or both. They certainly do name it.*

Species Used: There are 200 species in the *Bidens* genus. Maybe. Anal-retentive phytospecific maniacs are continually messing about with which species belong in the genus and, as usual, making problems for everyone. In consequence, the taxonomy of *Bidens* is considered "unsatisfactory," which is a massive understatement.

Bidens pilosa is the main species used medicinally (or at least on which most of the studies have been done), but there do seem to be a number of others in the genus that historical use and early research indicate can almost certainly be used similarly: *B. frondosa, B. tripartitus, B. ferulaefolia,* and *B. alba* are all fairly potent, *frondosa* and *tripartitus* more so than *pilosa* in their antimalarial effects. *B. maximovicziana, B. pinnata,* and *B. campylotheca* are all fairly strong as well but, in terms of impact on the malarial organism, a bit less strong than *pilosa*.

Note: *Bidens leucantha* is a synonym for *B. pilosa*.

Parts Used

Usually the aerial parts, but the entire plant is active, and in some instances the roots seem to be a bit stronger as a medicinal. Normally, however, the leaves tend to be the most potent part of the plant, followed by the roots. The fresh leaves are often used, and a number of studies show the fresh leaves and juice of the plant to be the most antimicrobial. Drying the plant reduces its antimicrobial action considerably.

Preparation and Dosage

There are some important things to know about using and preparing bidens:

- The most potent forms of this herb are alcohol tinctures and the fresh juice.
- The most potent constituents are considerably more soluble in alcohol than in water. Water infusions have a decent range of potency (as can be seen from the plant's traditional uses as a tea in Africa) but are not nearly as effective as a cold alcohol/water maceration.
- Some of the plant's most potent constituents oxidize easily and begin to degrade as soon as the plant is dried. Heat also destroys them.
- Expect about a two-thirds reduction in antimicrobial activity if the plant is not prepared fresh.
- The older the dried plant is, the less potent it will be in either water or alcohol. The fresher the dried plant material, the better.
- Water infusions lose potency fairly rapidly; they should be made and used daily. The rapidity of degradation of the plant chemicals is, in part, why so many cultures that don't normally make alcohol tinctures resort to using the juice of the leaves of this plant, internally and externally, for disease.
- Water extractions of the plant (teas, infusions, decoctions), especially if it is dried, possess about half the antibacterial activity of an alcohol tincture (depending on how old the extractions are), but they do possess most or all of the other actions described in this material (anti-inflammatory, antiallergenic, immune-modulating, and so on), especially the anti-inflammatory and antipyretic actions.

- A tincture is the strongest form of the herb as medicine. The use of piperine as a synergist will increase the potency of the plant considerably.

TINCTURE

Fresh plant, 1:2, 95 percent alcohol, 45–90 drops in water, up to 4x daily. Tincture made from the dried plant, if you must, would be 1:5, 50 percent alcohol, triple the dose.

For acute conditions (malaria, systemic staph): ¼–1 tsp and up to 1 tbl in water, up to 6x daily for up to 28 days, depending on severity. The tincture can also be used topically on infected wounds.

WATER EXTRACTION

Possible, but not really recommended.

Tea: 1 tsp herb in 8 ounces hot water; let steep 15 minutes. Drink 2–4 cups daily.

Decoction: Not recommended; heat degrades the herb. But if you must: For external use, boil 1 ounce herb in 1 quart water for 20 minutes, then strain. Cool and use on skin inflammations. For internal use, boil 2–4 ounces herb in 1 quart water for 20 minutes, then strain. Drink by the cup 2–4x daily.

Cold infusion: Steep 2–4 ounces herb in 1 quart cold water overnight. Drink by the cup 2–4x daily.

FRESH JUICE

You can run the leaves through a juicer to obtain a decent quantity of the fresh juice—the plants are pretty prolific. Be aware that they have strong fibers that will bind the juicer and you'll have to clean it often. Use the juice on infected wounds, for eye infections, or internally for systemic infections. If you want, you can stabilize the juice with the addition of 20 percent alcohol so that it will keep (see page 437). It can then be taken internally much like the tincture, though it will be more potent in its actions. Dosages are similar to those listed for the tincture.

(continues on page 234)

Properties of Bidens

Actions

Antibacterial	Blood tonic	Mucous membrane tonic
Antidiabetic	Carminative	Neuroprotectant
Antidysenteric	Diuretic	Prostaglandin synthesis inhibitor
Anti-inflammatory	Galactagogue	Styptic
Antimalarial	Hepatoprotective	Vulnerary
Antimicrobial	Hypoglycemic	
Antiseptic	Hypotensive	
Astringent	Immunomodulant	

Active Against

Bacillus cereus	*Escherichia coli*	*Plasmodium* spp.
Bacillus subtilis	Herpes simplex 1 and 2	*Pseudomonas aeruginosa*
Candida albicans	*Klebsiella pneumoniae*	*Salmonella* spp.
Human cytomegalovirus	*Leishmania amazonensis*	*Serratia marcescens*
Entamoeba histolytica	*Mycobacterium tuberculosis*	*Shigella flexneri*
Enterococcus faecalis (Streptococcus faecalis)	*Neisseria gonorrhoeae*	*Staphylococcus aureus*
		Staphylococcus epidermidis

Bidens is not very active against *Aspergillus*.

Like a lot of studies for antimicrobial activity, a number of those on *Bidens* are contradictory. For every study that finds it active against *E. coli,* another says it is not. Same for *Pseudomonas*, *Klebsiella*, *Streptococcus*, and *Candida*. Some studies show very strong activity, others mild, others none at all.

The differences come from the time of year the plant was gathered, the ecosystem in which it was found, whether wild or domesticated plants were used (wild plants have been found to be much stronger antibacterials), and differences in how the plants were prepared—the main problem being preparation. (See Preparation and Dosage, page 230.)

For this plant to act as a potent antimicrobial, it must be prepared as a tincture of the fresh plant or the fresh juice must be used.

Use to Treat

In order of potency:

1) *Any* systemic infections that are accompanied by problems in the mucous membranes anywhere in the body, especially chronic diarrhea, dysentery, UTI, vaginitis, and inflamed respiratory passages
2) Systemic staph
3) Malaria, babesia, leishmania
4) Any of the other resistant organisms bidens is active against

Other Uses

As a pot herb. The plant comes up early in the spring, is very hardy, and is used by many cultures as a food staple. However, see Side Effects and Contraindications (page 234) for a caveat on the plant as food.

Finding Bidens

Look outside in the yard. If for some reason the plant has overlooked you, ask around and you can probably find someone to send you some seeds. Soak them in some water for a day or two, then scatter them outside on the ground and cover with a bit of soil. Don't tell your neighbors.

Side Effects and Contraindications

None noted; however, be aware that *Bidens pilosa*'s leaves have numerous sharply pointed microhairs around the margins that are very high in silica. This kind of silica formation has been linked to esophageal cancer in certain domesticated animals (cows) and humans. Tribal cultures that eat large quantities of the plant as a primary food source show increased levels of that type of cancer. Cultures that use the plant only sporadically for food do not have an increased incidence of cancer. Exercise caution if using bidens as a food plant; it appears fine for occasional use but not as a steady diet.

Note: *Bidens pilosa* is a toxic-waste reclamation plant. Unless you want more heavy metals in your body, be careful where you get the plant. It should not be harvested from sites where there is heavy metal contamination. Numerous studies have found it to be a potent phytoremediation plant for cadmium, and one study showed the same for arsenic; another indicates it may have an affinity for heavy metals in general.

Herb/Drug Interactions

None noted, although one study does show it potentiating tetracycline.

Caution should be exercised when using the plant with people on diabetic medications as it will alter blood glucose and insulin levels.

Habitat and Appearance

A native of South America, *Bidens pilosa* is a world-class invasive species. Spread by the Spanish during colonization, it is now widespread seemingly everywhere. If it does not currently grow someplace, it eventually will.

Bidens grows from sea level to 10,000 feet in altitude. It tolerates moist soil, sand, clay, lime rock, infertile soil, or drylands. It thrives best in high sunlight, dry soils, and disturbed areas but has been found in nearly every type of eco-range on the planet. It can withstand long periods of drought and survives temperatures as low as 5°F (–15°C). It isn't fire tolerant but rapidly invades burned areas and is quite happy about any opportunity to do so.

It loves the southern and southwestern United States and has spread up the West and East Coasts into eastern Canada.

It is found throughout the Caribbean, Central America, South America, Europe, Russia, China, most of Africa, Southeast Asia, southern India, Japan, the Pacific Islands, and Australia. It may not grow in Ulan Bator or Nebraska, but then again, it may.

At its initial appearance in spring, bidens is quite a beautiful ground-coverish sort of plant, but as the season develops and it grows taller, it develops a rather straggly, weedy appearance. The flowers are the usual white, five-petaled things with an orange interior. The seeds are longish, thin, black needles with a sharp, extended pronged tip. There are often three or four prongs in spite of the fact that *Bidens* means "two-toothed" (*bi* means two and *dens*—as in dental—being tooth). The seeds can attach themselves to about anything, hence the name beggarticks. If you walk through a patch of bidens during seeding season, your shoelaces and pants to the knees will be covered with hundreds of the hard-to-remove seeds—a thousand seeds weigh only about 1 gram. They take hours to pick out, hence the name *$ %#*%!

The plant loves disturbed places, especially agriculturally disturbed fields, and actively tries to colonize cultivated land. It is allelopathic (toxic to other plants) and can reduce domesticated crops up to 50 percent once it invades a planted field. It is considered highly noxious in scores of countries just for that reason. The plant has very few natural predators.

I like it.

Cultivation and Collection

Bidens grows best from sea level to 10,000 feet within a temperature range of 75° to 90°F during the growing season. The edges of its growing temperature are from about 55° to 115°F.

Bidens grows easily from seed and is a tenacious grower. The seeds can still be viable after 3 years. The plant grows very fast, flowering as few as 6 weeks after its emergence from the ground. The first seeds mature just 4 weeks after flowering. Each plant produces a minimum of 3,000 seeds a year and in some climates will reproduce four times before dying back.

The seed germinates best if buried about 1½ inches in the soil; deeper than 2⅓ inches and it won't germinate at all. Soaking the seed in water prior to planting increases germination rate and numbers. The seed can be broadcast or sown in rows.

The plant is an annual and can be harvested within 4 to 6 weeks of its emergence in the spring; it is generally considered to be harvestable until it sets seed (unless of course you are interested in making medicine from the seeds). The older the leaves, the more bitter and astringent they become. If you are using it for its astringency, gather late in the year. If you are gathering it for food, get it early in the year.

If you are growing it as a medicinal, remove the flowers to retard old age and stimulate leaf growth. The leaves can be harvested throughout the year as long as you don't allow the plants to go to seed early on. If the plants are topped, you can get up to six harvests a year depending on your climate.

If you must dry bidens, do so out of the sun. And collect a lot of it, as it dries to almost nothing; a big bag of the fresh plant will give you a handful of dried powder. The plant will oxidize, so keep it in paper bags or, if well dried, in plastic, inside a plastic bin out of the sun. Replace every year or two, depending on how you store it. But ideally it should be used fresh.

A great deal of research has found that the plant leaves if used fresh or tinctured fresh possess significantly stronger antimicrobial activity than if dried. The herb's ability to inhibit malarial parasites drops from 90 percent in the fresh leaf tincture to 38 percent in the dried (in vivo studies). If you are using the plant as an antimicrobial for resistant pathogens, harvest the leaves before flowering and tincture them fresh.

If you do grow bidens intentionally, you may irritate your neighbors. Nevertheless, its ease of growth, widespread habitat, and medicinal nature make it an essential herb to know, grow, and use for the treatment of resistant pathogens.

Plant Chemistry

There has been a lot of work on the constituents of *Bidens pilosa*, and around 100 different plant chemicals have been identified so far. There are numerous aurone flavonoids, butoxy lipids, coumaric acids, and erythronic acid phenylpropanoids, a number of heptaphenyl and phenylheptatriyne benzenoids, a lot of okanin flavonoids, numerous stigmasterol steroids, a lot of quercetin flavonols, daucosterol, and a whole lot more. A very comprehensive plant in terms of flavonoids, terpenes, phenylpropanoids, lipids, and benzenoids.

The most active constituents are thought to be the polyacetylene compounds and the flavonoids. The acetylenes have shown the broadest-spectrum antimicrobial activity.

Traditional Uses of Bidens

The plant is one of the great easily available systemic antibacterial herbs. It does not appear to have as wide a range of action as *Sida* or *Cryptolepis* and is definitely not as strong. But it is reliable for the treatment of a number of resistant bacterial infections and is very simple to use. Because it grows so easily and is so prevalent in so many countries, it is a crucial herb to know about as resistant organisms extend their reach.

Wherever the plant grows it is often used by the local peoples for similar problems: to treat mouth and stomach ulcers, headaches, ear infections, hangovers, diarrhea, kidney problems, malaria, jaundice, dysentery, burns, arthritis, ulcers, abdominal problems, swollen spleen, coughs, colds and flu, rheumatism, boils, diabetes, skin rashes, and infected wounds. It is also used as an anesthetic, a coagulant, a poison antidote (especially for snakebite), and to ease childbirth.

AYURVEDA

Bidens pilosa grows primarily in the south of India, where it is known as *ottrancedi*. It is frequently used for glandular sclerosis, wounds, colds, flu, acute or chronic hepatitis, and urinary tract infections. Another species, *Bidens trifada*, is used for chronic dysentery, eczema, skin problems, ulcers, headache, earache and ear problems, toothache, cough, inflammation, and leprosy.

TRADITIONAL CHINESE MEDICINE

Called *xian feng cao* (abundant weed), *gui zhen cao* (demon needle grass), or *nian shen cao* (I don't know but probably unflattering) by the locals, all parts of the plant are used to clear heat and toxins. Dosage runs from 15–60 grams (½–2 ounces) per day, or as high as 120 grams (4 ounces) in acute conditions such as appendicitis.

It is used for treating cardiac spasm, itching, gastroenteritis, appendicitis, colitis, irritable bowel syndrome, hemorrhoids, diarrhea, dysentery, difficulty swallowing, sore throat, tonsillitis, esophageal enlargement, jaundice, acute or chronic hepatitis, malaria, boils, abscesses, infections, fever, chills, joint pain, traumatic injury, sprains, swelling, contusions, rheumatoid arthritis, gastric and esophageal cancer, epilepsy in children, infantile fever with convulsions, malnutrition in infants, colds and flu, bronchitis, chest congestion, hemoptysis, allergies, lung irritation, pneumonia, insect bites, scorpion sting, and snakebites.

WESTERN BOTANIC PRACTICE

Herbalists in the United States have consistently failed to understand this species, generally listing it as of little importance and having only minimal medicinal uses. The Eclectics knew it but used it little, primarily as an emmenagogue and expectorant, for amenorrhea, dysmenorrhea, uterine problems, severe cough, asthma, and as an infusion. An infusion of the seeds sweetened with honey was used for whooping cough. The plant was thought useful for heart conditions including palpitation, for colds, and for acute bronchial and laryngeal attacks.

The Seminole tribe used bidens similarly, as did the native Hawaiians. Numerous tribes used it as a pot herb.

Michael Moore was the first contemporary herbalist to begin to understand its actions, and he wrote about it extensively in the early 1990s. He didn't explore its antimicrobial activity but rather focused on its potency as a mucous membrane tonic. In his words, bidens "is probably the best herbal therapy we have for irritation, inflammation, pain, and bleeding of the urinary tract mucosa."[3]

The plant is a mucous membrane tonic that not only stops the inflammation and acts as a potent antibacterial in UTI infections but also heals the mucous membranes themselves. Moore felt it good for recurrent UTI infections and inflammations that didn't respond to antibiotics. The pain will usually go away in a day or two if you use bidens; he recommends using it an additional few days to completely clear up the problem.

Moore also considered bidens specific for reducing elevated levels of uric acid in the blood; i.e., for treating gout or urate-based kidney stones. It is a decent diuretic and does in fact stimulate uric acid elimination in the urine.

Because it is a mucous membrane tonic and is astringent, powerfully anti-inflammatory, and strongly antibacterial, it is specific for a number of troublesome diseases caused by resistant pathogens: UTIs, chronic diarrhea and dysentery, gastritis and ulcers (anywhere in the GI tract, from mouth to anus), inflamed mucous membranes in colds and flu and respiratory infections of any sort, sore throats from coughs or infection or even overuse of the throat, and vaginal infections.

Moore notes that bidens has the "ability to tighten, shrink, and tonify the structural cells of the mucus membranes, thereby preventing congestion and edema, while simultaneously increasing the circulation, metabolism, and healing energy of the functional cells of those tissues."[4]

It's a good plant, too often overlooked.

Scientific Research

Bidens pilosa is highly active against the malaria parasite in in vivo and in vitro studies, bearing out its traditional use for that disease. The linear polyacetylenic diol extracted from bidens was found to be highly active against the malarial parasite in vivo and in vitro, especially in the fresh plant. The constituent is unstable in the dried state.

It is generally believed that the plant's polyacetylenes are the most active constituents, the most potent antimicrobials. The research seems to bear this out. Alcohol tinctures of the fresh plant showed a 90 percent inhibition of the malarial parasite in vivo, while dried plant tinctures ran about 65 percent and water extracts about 38 percent. That activity is the same whether resistant or nonresistant strains are tested. In comparison, chloroquine-susceptible strains, when treated with chloroquine, will show a 99.2 percent inhibition of the malarial parasite. So the plant is nearly as strong as the pharmaceutical but not quite. It is definitely not as potent a plant as sida or cryptolepis, so larger doses need to be taken and for longer if you are using this plant for malaria.

An interesting in vivo study comparing the effectiveness of wild bidens versus domesticated found the wild species to be consistently stronger in its actions (the domesticated worked, just not as well).

As noted earlier, bidens possesses good antibacterial activity, as many antimalarials do. It has been found active against a wide range of microbial organisms, but some of the results are contradictory. (See Active Against, page 232, for more depth.)

Several of the plant's isolated polyacetylenes were found to be more active than ampicillin, tetracycline, norfloxacin, and amphotericin B during in vitro studies. Ciprofloxacin and ofloxacin were more potent than the plant extracts. In one study, water extracts of the plant were found to be more effective against *E. coli* and *Bacillus cereus* than gentamicin.

Bidens has been found to potentiate the activity of tetracycline if taken along with that pharmaceutical.

It is effective against herpes simplex 1 and 2 in in vitro studies, being nearly as strong as acyclovir but without the side effects.

Bidens pilosa during in vitro testing was found more active than metronidazole in the treatment of *Entamoeba histolytica*, a cause of amoebic dysentery around the world. The organisms weren't completely inhibited but were significantly reduced in number. *B. pilosa* was also found to be highly active in the treatment of the parasite *Leishmania amazonensis*. An ethanolic extract inhibited both the intracellular amastigotes and the promastigote form. The extract had very low toxicity.

Bidens pilosa is as effective as atropine, promethazine, neostigmine, and hydrocortisone in protecting mice from the venom of *Dendroaspis jamesoni*, a snake in Cameroon whose venom contains a potent neurotoxin. The plant extract also potentiated the antivenom normally used to treat those snakebites (as did atropine and promethazine). It is a very potent protector against neurotoxins. However, the plant is only weakly effective against viper venom, which causes hemorrhage and necrosis.

A number of in vivo studies reveal the herbal tincture to be highly antiulcerogenic, inhibiting gastric lesions induced by alcohol, and to be more effective than sucralfate. The herb significantly protected gastric mucosa and initiated mucosal healing through a number of mechanisms. (See Western Botanic Practice, page 238.)

A number of studies have found the plant to possess antitumor activity. It inhibits angiogenesis (the formation of abnormal blood vessels, common in cancer and certain forms of macular degeneration), is antiproliferative, and directly reduces viable tumor cells (stimulates apoptosis). It possesses a strong antileukemic activity and numerous cell regulatory actions that normalize cellular function and growth.

The plant also has a strong antipyretic effect, comparable to acetaminophen. It is specific for lowering fever during acute infections.

Bidens has been found to be a strong antioxidant and anti-inflammatory. A double-blind, randomized crossover trial with 20 participants found the herb effective in the treatment of allergic rhinitis. In vitro and in vivo studies have found it highly effective in protecting erythrocytes from oxidative damage. The water-soluble fractions are more antioxidative than the ethanol-soluble fractions. The plant inhibits COX-2 expression (similarly to ibuprofen) and prostaglandin production by inhibiting prostaglandin synthesis. It's a significant free-radical scavenger, comparable to alpha-tocopherol. It inhibits histamine release.

A number of in vivo studies note bidens to be an effective hepatoprotector. It protects the liver from chronic obstructive cholestasis and decreases the rate of necrosis and liver fibrosis. It normalizes liver enzyme levels and restores superoxide dismutase and glutathione peroxidase levels in liver-injured mice. It is strongly protective against induced liver damage.

The plant possesses oxytocic-like actions on the uterus, tones the uterine muscle, and helps in labor contractions (in vivo studies).

It possesses relaxant activity on vascular tissue, is a vasodilator, and relaxes cardiac action. It reduces the aorta resting tone and inhibits KCL- and CaCl2-induced contractions by 95 percent. The effects are relatively long lasting. It attenuates high-fructose and salt-loaded hypertension in rats and reduces insulin levels in their blood. The effects are marginal in normotensive rats, but marked in hypertensive ones.

The plant possesses antidiabetic properties: It lowers glucose levels in the blood of mice, increases insulin sensitivity, and stimulates the release of insulin from the pancreas. A single daily dose for 28 days (in mice) also was found to protect islet structure in the pancreas and potentiate its activity. It was successfully used to reverse type 2 diabetes in mice. It reduces hypoglycemia. One of the herb's constituents, cytopiloyne, a polyacetylene, has been found to prevent type 1 diabetes in nonobese mice.

Bidens pilosa is a strong and reliable immune modulator. It has been found to modulate the differentiation of helper T cells and prevent Th1-mediated autoimmune diabetes in nonobese diabetic mice. This has been attributed to a number of polyacetylenic compounds and a butanol fraction. The butanol fraction also reduces Th2-mediated airway inflammation in mice. Hot-water extracts of the plant stimulate interferon-gamma expression. The plant will increase immune action if such action is low, and decrease it if it is high.

Artemisia

Family: Asteraceae

Common Names: *Sweet Annie • sweet wormwood*

Species Used: There are approximately 400 artemisias in the genus, but *Artemisia annua* contains the most artemisinin—a potent antiparasitic—and this section will focus primarily on that species. Artemisinin is famous for its effectiveness in treating malaria. Many other artemisias contain artemisinin (contrary to earlier reports saying they did not), and I will discuss some of them in this section.

All the plants in the genus do have some antibacterial and antimicrobial actions; however, those constituents are not nearly as systemic as those in the other plants in this chapter. *Artemisia annua*, artemisinin, and its related constituents are best thought of as systemic antihematoparasiticals; that is, specific for killing blood parasites, rather than systemic antibacterials. Nevertheless, for treating diseases in their range of action, they are great.

Parts Used

The aerial parts, including the flowers, which have the highest artemisinin content.

ANTIBACTERIAL ACTIVITY

The whole herb has a much broader range of actions than the isolated constituent artemisinin.

Because the studies are few and plant preparation differs from study to study, the outcomes in the antibacterial studies of the artemisias are contradictory. They do find a range of antibacterial activity across the artemisias—bearing out traditional uses of the genus—but the studies tend to vary on which bacteria the species are active against, leading to confusion. There is a tendency to extrapolate the clinical use of the plant based on its in vitro antibacterial activity, but that is a mistake, as it is with numerous other plants.

This same problem exists with goldenseal. Goldenseal is highly active against a number of bacterial organisms, but berberine, the strongest constituent, does not make it across the GI tract membrane in any quantity, so the plant (and the constituent) is not a systemic antibacterial; it is mostly limited to the GI tract. Artemisinin, and some of the other antiparasitics in artemisia, are strongly systemic, but they have limited antibacterial activity. They are primarily antiparasitics for the blood and liver and antitumor agents.

The activities of the essential oils are more broadly antibacterial, but they are primarily confined to the GI tract when the plant is taken internally. This makes them useful for GI tract infections—or for use directly on the skin—but useless as systemic antibacterials. The traditional use of *Artemisia annua*, which gives a very good indication of its range of medicinal activity, has been primarily:

- For reducing fever—the plant stimulates sweating
- For topical use—it's useful for infected wounds and skin infections
- For GI tract problems and infections
- For female reproductive problems—primarily as an emmenagogue
- For liver problems
- As a steam inhalant for respiratory problems—which utilizes the essential oils
- For parasitic diseases of the blood and liver

Most of the antibacterial studies have been on the essential oils of various species, but again, these oils do not disseminate widely in the bloodstream, which means they will be useful only for respiratory infections when used as steam, internally in the GI tract when prepared as a cold infusion (which keeps the oils in the liquid), or topically when used as a poultice or cold infusion wash. Nevertheless, when used in these ways, the artemisias are very good medicines for resistant organisms other than blood parasites.

A study of *Artemisia nilagirica* leaf extracts found the plant active against a range of both Gram-positive and Gram-negative organisms: *Bacillus subtilis, Clavibacter michiganensis, Enterobacter aerogenes, Pseudomonas aeruginosa, Pseudomonas syringae, Salmonella typhi, Shigella flexneri,* and *Yersinia enterocolitica.* It was not active against *Enterococcus faecalis, E. coli, Klebsiella pneumoniae,* or *Staphylococcus aureus.* A number of studies have found most artemisias inactive against *E. coli, Klebsiella, Pseudomonas,* and staph, but others, such as one looking at the activity of *Artemisia anomala* against *Bacillus subtilis, E. coli, Proteus vulgaris, Salmonella typhi,* and *Staphylococcus aureus,* have found the plant to be active. In that example a methanol extract was used. Given the solubility dynamics of artemisia constituents (including artemisinin), it seems likely that the variability in the studies is coming from solubility differentials (hexane, for example, is a much better solvent for artemisia constituents than anything else and artemisinin is much more highly soluble in fat—whole milk—than water).

Preparation and Dosage

Artemisinin: The effective dosage for malaria is 500–1,000 mg on the first day and 500 mg daily thereafter for 2 to 4 more days. This will completely clear the malarial parasite from the blood. However, at 400 mg per day for 5 days, the recrudescence rate is 39 percent. Dosage at 800 mg drops the rate nearer to 3 percent. Chinese dosage runs from 500–1,600 mg for 3 days, repeated in 2 weeks (to treat newly hatching parasites). I do think there is some evidential support for 800–1,200 mg for 5 to 7 days, repeated for another 5 to 7 days in 2 weeks. The relapse rate is definitely smaller at the higher dose.

Note: Artemisinin becomes less present in the blood the longer it is taken, so that by day 7 the constituent is present at only 24 percent of its day-1 levels. *The isolated constituent is not very effective if taken for longer than 7 days at a time for parasitical infections.* If it doesn't work for babesia, for instance, within a few weeks, it is not going to. Pulsing will not help.

There are several things to keep in mind when preparing the whole herb for use:

- The fresh plant is the strongest.
- Whether fresh or dried, the plant should never be boiled.
- Fat helps extraction of the active constituents.
- The plant, while still potent for blood parasites, loses a lot of its antioxidant activities if dried.
- Dosage and length of use are crucial.

Traditional Chinese texts, thousands of years old, recommend preparation of the fresh herb, infused in room-temperature water, then pounded and wrung out to extract the plant juice as well. Examination has indeed shown that this produces the most potent infusions.

Many of the constituents in artemisia are not very water soluble, including the artemisinin. However, they are highly soluble in fats and alcohol.

FRESH HERB INFUSION FOR MALARIA

Place 100 grams (about 4 ounces) of fresh herb (leaves and flowers) cut into pieces in a container, pour ½ quart (2 cups) hot water over the herb, cover, and let stand 12 hours. Wring out; drink it all. Do this daily for 7 days. Repeat after 2 weeks.

FRESH HERB JUICE FOR MALARIA

Run the fresh plant through a juicer. Take 1 tablespoon of the fresh juice every day for 7 days—you can stabilize the juice with the addition of 20 percent alcohol (see page 437). Repeat after 2 weeks.

Note: The fresh juice is 6 to 17 times more potent than pure artemisinin; this and the tincture are the two most potent forms of the herb.

DRIED HERB INFUSION FOR MALARIA

Pour 1 quart hot water over 100 grams of dried herb (leaves and flowers), and let stand 12 hours. Strain and drink. Do this daily for 7 days. Repeat after 2 weeks.

(continues on page 248)

Properties of Artemisia

Actions

Antibacterial	Antiparasitical	Immunomodulant
Antifungal	Antitumor	Plasmodicide
Anti-inflammatory	Antiviral	Schizonticide
Antimalarial	Calcium antagonist	

Active Against

Babesia spp.	Epstein-Barr virus	*Opisthorchis viverrini*
Bovine diarrheal virus	*Fasciola hepatica*	*Plasmodium* spp.
Clonorchis sinensis	Hepatitis B and C	*Schistosoma* spp.
Eimeria acervulina	*Leishmania* spp.	*Toxoplasma gondii*
Eimeria tenella	*Neospora caninum*	*Trypanosoma* spp.

Also active against various cancer cell lines. Broadly active against dermatophytes—fungi that cause infections in hair, skin, and nails. *A. annua* is active against a number of bacteria in vitro, but the data in the various studies is contradictory, as usual. Specific for parasitic infections in the blood and liver and to some extent in the GI tract.

Decoctions of the herb are active against *Bacillus cereus, Bacillus subtilis, Bordetella bronchiseptica, E. coli, Klebsiella pneumoniae, Micrococcus flavus, Proteus vulgaris, Pseudomonas aeruginosa, Salmonella typhi, Salmonella typhimurium, Sarcina lutea, Staphylococcus aureus, Staphylococcus epidermidis*, and *Streptococcus mutans*.

A different extract (type not stated) was found to be active against *Mycobacterium avium*. Methanol extracts were found active against *Bacillus cereus, Bacillus pumilus, Bacillus subtilis, E. coli, Micrococcus luteus, Pseudomonas aeruginosa, Salmonella* spp., and *Staphylococcus aureus*.

The essential oil has been found active against *Candida albicans, Enterococcus hirae, E. coli*, and *Staphylococcus aureus* but not *Pseudomonas aeruginosa*.

Other Actions

The oil of *Artemisia tschernieviana* has been found active against *Bacillus cereus*, *Bacillus subtilis*, *Candida albicans*, *Enterobacter aerogenes*, *E. coli*, *Klebsiella pneumoniae*, and *Staphylococcus aureus*. This same antibacterial activity has been found in other artemisias: *A. absinthium*, *A. douglasiana* and *A. ludoviciana* (also *Helicobacter pylori*), *A. echegarayi* (also active against *Proteus mirabilis* and various *Listeria* species), *A. gilvescens* (also MRSA), *A. giraldii* (also *Aspergillus* spp., *Proteus* spp., *Sarcinia lutea*, *Trichoderma viride*), *A. herba-alba*, *A. iwayomogi*, *A. kulbadica*, *A. leucodes*, *A. monosperma* (also TB and staph), *A. princeps* var. *orientalis* (also *Bacteroides fragilis*, *Bifidobacterium*, *Clostridium perfringens*, and staph), and *A. vulgaris* (also *Streptococcus mutans*).

The artemisias in general are considered to be active against intestinal parasites, but again, little actual study has occurred. *A. absinthium* is often considered the most potent against intestinal parasites in historical practice. Leaf extracts are active against *Syphacia* parasites, nematodes that infect the intestinal tracts of mice; the plant is also active against multidrug-resistant malarial parasites in vivo.

Artemisia maciverae is active in vivo against *Trypanosoma brucei*, showing complete clearance after 7 days of treatment (10 mg/kg body weight). The same plant is also strongly antiplasmodial at the same dosage, clearing the parasites from mice in 3 days.

Various artemisias have been found active against plant pathogens (which is why artemisias are used to protect crops in some locations) and various fungi.

Use to Treat

Any parasitic infection in the blood and liver or for systemic cancers (artemisinin does have good activity as an antitumor drug). These are the real strengths of the plant if it is being used as a systemic. There is nothing else comparable in potency for these uses. The plant, if properly prepared, is also active against microbial and parasitic infections, especially in the GI tract (see Preparation and Dosage, page 244) and on the skin.

INFUSION IN MILK FOR MALARIA

Pour 1 quart hot, whole milk over 100 grams fresh or dried herb, cover, and let stand 4 hours.

Note: This will extract 80 percent of the artemisinin in the herb while water infusions extract much less (about 25 percent in dried herb formulations).

TINCTURE FOR MALARIA

Chop fresh herb finely, and measure its weight in ounces. Place the herb in twice that amount (now using liquid ounces) of pure grain alcohol. (For example, you'd mix 1 ounce of herb with 2 ounces of alcohol; see Fresh Plant Tinctures, page 559, for more depth on this). Let stand 2 weeks. Press out the liquid. Take 1 tbl twice daily for 7 days. Repeat after 2 weeks.

TINCTURE WITH SIDA AND CRYPTOLEPIS FOR MALARIA

Take 2 ounces each of the tinctures of sida, cryptolepis, and *Artemisia annua* and combine together. Take 2 tbl of the mix each day for 7 days. Repeat in 2 weeks.

The herb is very effective if used properly. The dose can be increased fairly high, as it is a very safe herb. Remember: The reason that this herb was discovered was that in the region of China where it

Finding Artemisia

The herb grows pretty much everywhere it is planted; seeds are widely available (try Horizon Herbs for some of the best). It is a good herb to have growing in the garden—as are any of the other artemisias that contain artemisinin, such as *Artemisia absinthium*.

Artemisinin is, currently, easily found for sale everywhere, and an online search will turn up sources for both the herb and the supplement. However, there is a movement to prohibit over-the-counter sales of the supplement due to overuse and improper use. The overuse of the supplement is already beginning to stimulate resistance in malarial organisms.

is used there were few or no incidences of malaria. The secret is in the dose, as with all medications.

Side Effects and Contraindications

About 25 percent of people using *Artemisia annua* as an antimalarial report a mild nausea, which does not progress to vomiting. It may also cause occasional dizziness, tinnitus, pruritus, and mild abdominal pain.

Artemisinin itself can cause gastrointestinal upset, loss of appetite, nausea, cramping, diarrhea, and vomiting. About 4 percent of people who take it experience these symptoms, usually in a more severe form than that experienced from ingesting the herbal infusion. Very high doses (5,000 mg per day of artemisinin for 3 days) have caused liver inflammation, which corrects upon stopping the supplement. Artemisinin has a slightly chronotropic effect on the heart. It causes mild hypotension. This has not been, apparently, a problem in any users.

Both the herb and the constituent should be used with caution in pregnancy, especially in the first trimester. In vivo studies have found a number of adverse effects in rats and mice if the herb is used in the first trimester. However, one clinical trial with 16 patients in the first trimester of pregnancy taking the herb found the miscarriage rate to be the same as that for the general population.

Herb/Drug Interactions

Artemisia annua, like many antimicrobial plants, contains synergists that make its compounds more active against microbial organisms. In this instance, chrysospenol-D and chrysophlenetin, two flavonols in the plant, have been found to potentiate the activity of berberine and norfloxacin against resistant staph. Artemisinin does induce certain liver enzymes and may interact with drugs such as omeprazole.

Habitat and Appearance

A. annua is native to China, western Asia, northern India, Japan, Korea, Vietnam, Myanmar, southern Siberia, and southeastern

Europe. An emerging invasive plant species, it is naturalized in the United States and many other countries. It loves places like roadsides, fallow fields, neglected gardens—especially in eastern North America. It can grow pretty much anyplace but is stronger and more aromatic when grown in poor, dry soil. Its artemisinin content is about 20 percent higher when it grows in mildly potassium-deficient soils.

The plant, once established, grows into a large straggly bush. The leaves look a bit like celery's leaves, though *A. annua*'s are much broader, bushier, and more extensive in their growth. The plant grows 4 to 6 feet tall with a typical attractive, weedy, bushy look. It blooms in late summer.

Cultivation and Collection

Artemisia annua is an annual (hence its species name) and cultivates easily from seed. Sow the tiny seeds outdoors in the fall or seed them indoors before the last frost. They like it best on top of well-aerated soil; they need light to germinate. Once established, the plant self-sows and will never go away.

The aerial parts should be harvested just after flowering. The flowers and leaves both contain artemisinin. The artemisinin content is higher in the fall than in spring; it takes the plant time to create the chemical. The longer you wait, the better the yield, so take even the older, dying-back leaves. The stems and root contain only very low amounts of the compound and aren't generally worth the trouble.

Once the plant is picked, let it dry in the sun for a week. The light helps the artemisinin precursors keep producing after the plant is harvested. After a week, the sun does more harm than good, so finish drying in a dry, dark spot inside.

Several hybrid plants (*Artemisia annua* var. *artemis*, var. *campinas*, var. *anamed*) have been bred for higher artemisinin content. They are available from Anamed (anamed.org) as part of an artemisia antimalarial starter kit that includes a lot of useful information on growing and using the plant. One problem with the hybrids is that they don't reseed themselves well and the artemisinin content of those that do is poor (so it is not as sustainable an alternative as it should be). If you want a continual supply of the plant, non-hybrids are the way to go.

Plant Chemistry

Artemisia annua contains a great many chemical constituents, more than 150 at last count, and that is most likely just a tiny fraction of the total. There are a minimum of 28 monoterpenes, 30 sesquiterpenes, 12 terpenoids and steroids, 36 flavonoids, 7 coumarins, 4 aromatics, and 9 aliphatic compounds.

Artemisinin is considered to be the active antiplasmodial compound, but numerous other compounds with malarial activity have been found. Others, such as arteannuin B and artemisinic acid, are antibacterial and antifungal. Arteannuin B, while found to be ineffective against malarial parasites, strongly potentiates the activity of artemisinin. Many of the flavonoid compounds have been found to be antimalarial in vitro. Some of them (artemetin, casticin, chrysophlenetin, chrysosplenol-D, and cirsilineol) have been found to also potentiate artemisinin's ability to kill plasmodial parasites. Many of these flavonoids are abundant in the plant; they induce a three- to five-fold reduction in the amount of artemisinin needed to kill malarial organisms. Some of the sesquiterpene lactones are also antiplasmodial, with

Lyme Disease Caution

I have heard from several people with Lyme disease that they have been taking artemisinin for 1 to 2 years at relatively high doses. This is highly contraindicated and should *not* be done under any circumstances. I repeat: This is a really bad idea. Artemisinin is extremely safe when used appropriately; that is, in doses around 1,200 mg daily for 7 days. If it is used long term in high doses, there is significant risk of neurotoxicity; that is, damage to the central nervous system and brain. Sida, alchornea, cryptolepis, and bidens are all much safer alternatives for long-term use, especially if you are treating babesia.

ridentin, some of the guainolides, and germacranolides being the most important.

The artemisinin content of *A. annua,* if the leaves and flowers are harvested in the fall before the plant goes to seed, can run anywhere from 0.75 percent to 1.4 percent (several high-yield varieties are in development or are just on the market).

A relatively new development is the finding of another strongly active antiplasmodial constituent, tehranolide, in a number of artemisia species. In vivo studies show it to be strongly antiplasmodial. Treatment with the tehranolide extracts of *Artemisia diffusa* resulted in complete clearance of parasites from the blood in mice at similar dosages to artemisinin.

Traditional Uses of Artemisia

Artemisia annua (and many of the other artemisias) is somewhat unusual in its actions. The *systemic* constituents of the plant primarily act in two ways: 1) as highly potent antiparasitics for blood and liver parasites; and 2) as antitumor agents. These same constituents have two other actions that are useful: 1) they stimulate sweating and thus help reduce fever; and 2) they are emmenagogues; that is, they stimulate menstruation. The emmenagogue action is why the plant is generally not recommended in the first trimester of pregnancy. Caveat: *Artemisia annua* has much less emmenagogue activity than some of the other artemisias; the stimulatory activity has been found to be only minimal.

Although other artemisias have been used to effectively treat malaria and other blood parasites, the most potent species for this, at this time, is *Artemisia annua.*

The plant has been used in Chinese medicine for more than 2,000 years, but its current status as an antimalarial emerged from its use by the North Vietnamese during the Vietnam War. Malarial infections were exceptionally high among the North Vietnamese troops. Appeals to the Chinese leader Mao for help resulted in the discovery of *Artemisia annua* for use as an antimalarial.

Chinese researchers had discovered that in one region of China the people had little incidence of malaria infection. Looking closer, they discovered that the local people took the herb at the first sign of symptoms. In 1972 Chinese researchers isolated artemisinin.

AYURVEDA

This plant is unknown in India, though a number of other artemisias are used. *Artemisia absinthium* is used for intermittent fevers, for stomach complaints (as a bitter and digestive), as a vermifuge for intestinal worms, and for nervous system complaints (from hysteria to depression). *Artemisia maritima* (wormseed) is specific for intestinal worms, especially ascarides and oxyuris. Most of the other artemisias are used similarly.

TRADITIONAL CHINESE MEDICINE

Called *qing-hao* in traditional Chinese medicine, *Artemisia annua* is used for clearing fevers from the blood, especially in conditions with

Artemisinin in Other Artemesias

A number of other artemisias do contain artemisinin (18 identified so far), none to the degree of *Artemisia annua*, though some are close. The flowers of *A. bushriences* have nearly as much artemisinin as *A. annua* (about 80 percent), then the leaves of *A. dracunculus* (about 60 percent), then flowers of a number of species (in descending order): *A. roxburghiana* (about half), *A. vestita* and *A. sieversiana* (40 percent), and *A. moorcroftiana* and *A. absinthium* (about 30 percent). Most species do have about 10 percent to 15 percent of the amount of artemisinin as is found in *A. annua*. Other species that contain artemisinin are *A. vulgaris*, *A. indica*, *A. roxburghiana* var. *gratae*, *A. japonica*, *A. tangutica*, and *A. lancea*. An exception is *A. desertorum*, which has virtually none. As usual, in the species that contain artemisinin, the flowers and leaves will have the most. Again, skip the roots and stems.

headache, dizziness, low fever, and a stifling sensation in the chest. Also for febrile diseases, for malaria, and for scabies, pruritus, and malignant ulcers.

WESTERN BOTANIC PRACTICE

For many years *A. annua* was unknown, although many other artemisias have long been used. *Artemisia absinthium* was a primary herb among the Eclectics in the late ninteenth century in the United States. The herb was used for intermittent fevers, for malaria, as a vermifuge in the treatment of intestinal worms, for dyspepsia, nervous conditions, diarrhea and liver complaints, for amenorrhea and leukorrhea, and for jaundice. Other artemisias were used similarly.

The indigenous peoples throughout the United States used the plants similarly.

Scientific Research

There have been hundreds of in vitro and in vivo studies and clinical trials on the antiparasitical actions of artemisinin (and its analogues), most on malaria and schistosomiasis. I will just touch on them here.

Every one of the several hundred clinical trials shows the effectiveness of artemisinin in the treatment of malaria. (There have been a number of clinical trials with the whole herb as well; see Whole Herb vs. Artemisinin, page 256.)

Artemisinin has become the choice for malarial treatment worldwide because it is effective against resistant strains of the organism. Ninety-eight percent of malarial parasites are generally killed within 24 hours with use of the herb or its isolated constituent. If low, short-term doses are used (less than 5 days), however, relapse rates can be as high as 39 percent. Higher dose ranges for a longer period of time (5 instead of 3 days) lower the relapse rate considerably. Clinical trials with as many as 2,000 people (with both low and high dosages) have found 100 percent clearance rates for all participants if artemisinin is taken for 5 to 7 days. There are very few side effects when used properly in short-term treatment.

The constituents of the herb that are antiparasitic are exceptionally systemic in that they spread quickly throughout the body and easily cross the blood-brain barrier. Artemisinin is considered specific for cerebral malaria. Because it infuses the blood, it is carried throughout the body to every cell, all of which need blood to live.

A slightly modified form of artemisinin, or artesenuate, has been found effective for babesia organisms in vitro. Relatively low concentrations of the compound are effective; complete inhibition of *Babesia equi* and *B. caballi* occurred at 0.2 and 1.0 mcg/ml, respectively. (To make artesenuate, artemisinin is modified slightly in order to get patent protection.)

Use of artemisinin in clinical practice, however, has shown only moderate success for this organism; it seems to be effective in about half the people who use it for babesia. Sida and cryptolepis appear to be better alternatives.

A number of clinical trials have occurred with a synthetic form of artemisinin, artemether, in the treatment of schistosoma infections. Schistosoma are a type of blood fluke—and are a major infectious parasitic organism, second only to malaria in numbers of those infected, totaling hundreds of millions worldwide.

Artemether is normally given in a single dose of 6 mg/kg every 2 weeks. It is primarily active against the juvenile form of the parasite rather than the adult. Repeated dosing results in parasite reductions of 90 percent to 98 percent. Artesenuate has been found just as effective.

Artemisinin is also effective against *Neospora caninum*, another type of protozoa that affects both endothelial cells and macrophages. CNS involvement and carditis are common. Artemisinin is effective against a number of other organisms such as *Eimeria tenella*, *Leishmania major* (which infects macrophages), *Toxoplasma gondii*, *Schistosoma mansoni* (liver flukes), and *Clonorchis sinensis* (liver flukes), all parasitical organisms. It is antispirochetal against leptospire organisms, killing them in vitro. Artemisinin does appear to possess broad antiparasitical actions.

ANTICANCER PROPERTIES

Artemisinin is also stimulating interest as an antitumor and anticancer compound. It has shown effectiveness as an anticancer agent both in vitro and in vivo. In vitro studies have found artemisinin effective against human leukemia cells, breast cancer, and colon cancer. Treatment of both bone cancer and cancer of the lymph nodes in dogs was effective with 10 to 15 days of treatment. The use of artemisinin in people with cancer has shown effectiveness as well; Vietnamese doctors have found it successful in curing 50 percent to 60 percent of several different types of cancer patients.

Clinical practice reports indicate the use of artesenuate in the successful treatment of non-Hodgkin's lymphoma (60 mg IM for 14 days), artemisinin for small-cell lung carcinoma (500 mg BID for 4 months), artesenuate (IV) and artemisinin (300 mg BID) for 4 months in the treatment of stage 4 breast cancer with metastases, topical artemisinin in the treatment of multiple skin cancers, oral artemisinin in the treatment of breast cancer with metastases to the spine, and artesenuate in the treatment of stage 4 uveal melanoma.

A number of studies have found the herb to possess anti-inflammatory and antioxidant activity.

Artemisinin is immunostimulatory in vivo. It stimulates phagocytosis, and macrophages become more potent; they are better at phagocytosing malarial-infected erythrocytes.

ARTEMISININ RESISTANCE

There is increasing evidence that using the single compound artemisinin or any of its derivatives is stimulating resistance in the organisms it is being used to treat. Resistant malarial organisms have been found in Cambodia and are beginning to spread worldwide.

A recent study found that malarial organisms go into a dormancy state upon encountering artemisinin and then recover after dosing has ceased.

In consequence, many groups are beginning to use combination therapies to treat susceptible parasites, essentially artemisinin plus a pharmaceutical. It's known as artemisinin combination therapy or ACT.

WHOLE HERB VS. ARTEMISININ

The increasing resistance to artemisinin and its synthetic derivatives is a problem that cannot be solved through multidrug therapy: single constituent pharmaceuticals will *always* end up promoting resistance in disease organisms. A different approach is essential.

As I have already mentioned, there is a conflict between two ideologies in health care and medicine: 1) sustainable, affordable health care that empowers the people who use it; and 2) health care controlled by corporations for their own profit, a model that is designed to keep the people who use it dependent on specialists and corporate manufacturers. There is no way to avoid encountering, or dealing with, this conflict in some form if you explore the use of herbal medicines for your own health.

While the cost of artemisinin is low when viewed from Western, industrialized perspectives, in Africa it is prohibitively high. In 2004 the cost of a course of artemisinin was $2.40, more than most people in Africa can afford. As a result artemisinin forgery has become a lucrative business in Africa. Products that contain no artemisinin are widely available; they do nothing to cure malaria.

A number of NGOs (nongovernmental organizations) such as ANAMED (Action for Nature and Medicine), of which I am an admirer, have begun to address the problem in a simple and direct manner—they are providing artemisia seeds to anyone in Africa who wants them, teaching them how to grow the plant and how to use it to treat malaria. This has resulted in rather predictable responses from Western researchers, physicians, and corporate scientists. They oppose it and sometimes work quite strongly to stop it.

The primary argument being made is that the plant is not very effective against malaria, which of course ignores the reason artemisinin was discovered in the first place—people who used it for medicine had little or no incidence of malaria in their communities. Some researchers go so far as to say the plant does not work at all, *only* the isolated constituent is effective. Jansen (2006) is a perfect example. He comments, "The herbal tea approach to artemisinin for malaria is totally misleading and should be forgotten as soon as possible."[5]

Thankfully, the reaction to such antiquated thinking has been strong.

RITAM (Research Initiative on Traditional Antimalarial Methods), a partnership between the Global Initiative for Traditional Systems of Health at Oxford University and hundreds of international researchers from more than 30 countries who are exploring malaria treatment with traditional plants, responded to Jansen this way: "We believe that this statement is totally misleading and should be forgotten as soon as possible."[6] Their article then explains in depth how most Western researchers, in looking at *Artemisia annua* tea formulations, consistently fail to understand the plant or how it should be used in practice to be effective. It points out, as well, how Hansen's comments are fatally flawed.

Extensive work by RITAM and ANAMED has resulted in comparable tea preparations that are as effective in use as artemisinin.

The artemisinin content in the plant is strongly stable if it is properly stored (out of the sun in foil or plastic bags inside plastic tubs). Even after 1 year in storage, the artemisinin content is nearly identical to that in the freshly harvested plant. (Ceiling-hung plants will begin to degrade after 3 months.) The artemisinin is held in the glandular trichomes of the plant's leaves and flowers, where the essential oils of the plant are also held. These oils protect the artemisinin from degradation, oxidation, fungi, and molds.

Numerous researchers are suggesting that artemisinin combination therapy (ACT) is the best approach to treating malaria as the recrudescence rates are smaller and the parasite has a harder time developing resistance. But the plant already is an ACT substance. Researchers, using identical tiny amounts of *Artemisia annua* and artemisinin, found that these tiny amounts of *A. annua* reduced parasitemia in vivo by 50 percent at day 4, while the artemisinin was no more effective than placebo.

Other researchers, removing the artemisinin from the plant, found it still effective for malaria treatment.

There are other constituents in the plant that have been found to be synergists with artemisinin. Several flavonols have been found to be potentiating synergists with both berberine and norfloxacin in the treatment of MRSA, for instance. They apparently act as a multidrug-resistance efflux pump inhibitor. These same flavonols have also been shown to potentiate the action of artemisinin against the malarial parasite. And both *Artemisia annua* and *Artemisia dracunculus* contain an essential oil, piperitone, that acts as a potentiator of nitrofurantoin against *Enterobacter cloacae*.

The number of synergists and potentiators in the artemisias seems large. The complex combination of multiple antiplasmodium constituents and synergists makes the plant a potent choice for an, essentially, free treatment for those who need it, or want it as the treatment of choice.

There have been a number of clinical trials in the use of the tea (or whole herb or tincture) in treating malaria. Studies have shown that the pharmacokinetics of the herb's artemisinin when taken as a tea are identical to those of artemisinin taken as an isolated constituent:

Clinical trial with tincture:

72 grams of crude extract in divided doses over 3 days in the treatment of 485 cases of *Plasmodium vivax* and 105 cases of *P. falciparum*. Clearance rate was 100 percent, but the patients were not followed for recrudescence.

Clinical trial with whole-herb infusion: 93 percent clearance rate in 254 patients using a 7-day course of whole herb infusion (tea) in the treatment of *P. falciparum*. Recrudescence rate was 13 percent after 1 month.

Clinical trial with capsules: Clinical trial of 165 people infected with *Plasmodium vivax*. Fifty-three were given capsules of *A. annua* that also contained oil (COEA) for 3 days (the oil enhances absorption of the artemisinin). Another 50 received the herb capsules with oil (COEA) for 6 days. Forty-one received capsules without the oil (QHET). Twenty-one received chloroquine. Dosage was 36.8 grams on the first day, 18.4 on subsequent days. Parasite clearance and fever reduction were faster with the capsules than with chloroquine. There was a 30-day follow-up with blood checks every 10 days. About one-third of those who took the COEA herb capsule for only 3 days or who took the non-oil capsules (QHET) experienced recrudescence. Those who took COEA for 6 days experienced about 8 percent recrudescence. There was no recrudescence in the chloroquine group.

Clinical trial with infusion: An aqueous infusion for 5 days in a small trial of five people found 100 percent clearance; no follow-up occurred to check for recrudescence.

Clinical trial with infusion and decoction: A trial using infusions (254 people) and decoctions (48 people) with 5 grams herb in 1 liter of hot water, infused for 15 minutes or boiled for 5 minutes, found both forms effective. Dose was 250 ml (about 8 ounces) four times daily for 7 days in the infusion group and 4 days in the decoction group. Clearance rate was 93 percent and 92 percent respectively. There was a 13 percent recrudescence rate in the infusion group. Recrudescence in the decoction group was not checked.

Early indications are that if the plant is properly prepared and used, it can be as effective as artemisinin or its analogues in the treatment of malaria and other blood parasites. It will be especially effective if combined with other plants described in this chapter, especially sida and cryptolepis.

Localized Antibacterials

Each tree, each shrub, and herb, down even to the grasses and mosses, agreed to furnish a remedy for some one of the diseases [of humankind] and each said: "I shall appear to help man whenever he calls upon me in his need."

—The oral teachings of the Cherokee Nation

Localized nonsystemic antibacterial herbs do not easily cross the GI tract membrane and concentrate in the bloodstream. They are almost always limited to the GI tract itself, the skin, or certain organs of the body. In the latter instance, it is because those constituents that do make it through the intestinal membrane are eliminated from the body through a particular organ (e.g., garlic through the lungs, juniper berry through the kidneys).

The localized antibacterials need to be used with that in mind; they generally do not act as systemics, even if they are being sold as if they do. Nevertheless, they can be exceptionally potent in the treatment of resistant disease organisms if used properly. Here are four of the best of them.

The Top 4 Localized Nonsystemic Herbal Antibiotics

The Berberines
Juniper
Honey
Usnea

The Berberines

For the purposes of this book, most berberine-containing plants can be used as analogues for each other in the treatment of resistant bacterial and fungal infections of the GI tract and skin. I prefer the use of invasive species, however, primarily because they tend to be easily found in the wild, are ubiquitous around the globe, and can be harvested with abandon. They are free to those who know them, and harvesting them does not create the ecological problems that wildcrafting and large agricultural production of plants such as goldenseal and coptis do.

Berberine-containing plants grow nearly every place on Earth. *Phellodendron amurense, Hydrastis canadensis, Mahonia aquifolium, Berberis vulgaris*, and *Coptis chinensis* are only a few of the major species used medicinally.

However, given their prolific natures, I believe that if you are wildcrafting, the *only* genera that should be used as berberine antibacterials are (in the following order) *Phellodendron, Berberis*, and *Mahonia*.

If you are buying, look for *Hydrastis, Tinospora, Corydalis,* and

Coptis, which are established agricultural crops. The latter two genera are major agricultural products in China and are thus sustainable in a nonwildcrafted sense. *Hydrastis* is being grown in the United States, and it is possible to buy organically grown roots. If you do decide to use any of these species, make sure you are getting commercially grown and not wildcrafted plants.

Personally, I prefer the wildcrafted species. In my opinion they are the strongest—domesticated plants have a tendency to get a bit wimpy over time—and I particularly like the idea of using invasive species for invasive diseases. I think it particularly interesting that *Phellodendron* and *Berberis* species are invasive in the same bioregion in which goldenseal was once prevalent. It points up the rather neglected understanding that plants and their constituents perform specific functions in the eco-ranges in which they grow. The loss of a particular medicinal species always leads to ecosystem degradation and weakness. But then, the planet has a long history of engaging in correctives to such damage, invasives being just one of them.

Phellodendron amurense is invasive, especially in the eastern United States, and I believe that it should be the main species used if it is at all available. The plant is a large tree that grows quickly, producing huge amounts of berberine and other alkaloids and synergistic constituents in its inner bark. Branches can be harvested to supply large quantities of medicinal herb with little or no damage to the tree. You can get several years' supply in a short afternoon.

Here is a more inclusive list of the berberine genera, and some of the species, that are known to date.

Hydrastis canadensis, the American goldenseal, is perhaps the best known and most commonly used berberine-containing plant in the United States, but it is rather limited in its range and is endangered in the wild from overharvesting. The root is generally used, which, obviously, kills the plant, contributing to its difficulties in surviving in the wild. It has become a decent agricultural crop in the United States, and organically grown roots are easily found these days. Wildcrafted plants should never be bought. The leaves are weaker and can be used as well as the root, but hardly anyone does. It is the only member of its genus.

Mahonia, a genus comprising 70 or so species, is common throughout the world. Plant classification freaks really want the mahonias included in the genus *Berberis*, which is why you might see *Mahonia aquifolium*, a.k.a. Oregon grape, perhaps the best known of the mahonias, also identified as *Berberis aquifolium*. The lower branches of the mahonias tend to have berberine in them, but the roots are much higher in the alkaloid. Several mahonias are considered invasive in the United States, making them perfect for wild harvesting.

Berberis, a genus of about 500 species of plants, also has a number of species that contain berberine. Barberry, *Berberis vulgaris*, is perhaps the best known. While the branches (especially the lower) contain berberine (scratch the stem—if it's yellow underneath the outer bark, it's got berberine), the roots have a much higher berberine content, by at least a factor of 10. Several species of berberis are considered invasive in the United States, particularly *Berberis thunbergii*, Japanese barberry.

Coptis, a genus of 15 or so species, also has a number of plants whose roots (rhizomes actually) contain berberine. *Coptis chinensis*, a.k.a. goldthread, is probably the best known. The genus is used for a number of reasons, one of which is that it is relatively high in berberine content, up to 9 percent by weight. The root on this genus is tiny (hence "thread"), and it takes a lot of harvesting to get much usable material. The wild species in the United States are at risk and should not be harvested commercially. *Coptis chinensis* is a major agricultural crop in China and is available in bulk, though it is rather expensive.

Phellodendron (*not* the houseplant, which is spelled differently) is a genus of 4 to 10 species (arguments are ongoing) of trees whose bark contains berberine. The best known is probably *Phellodendron amurense*. A great invasive.

Tinospora, a genus of 40 or so twining species of plants, contains berberine. The best known is probably *Tinospora cordifolia*. The bark and stems of this genus are used.

Corydalis, a genus of some 470 species (this genus is sometimes considered to be part of the poppy family), has several species that contain berberine, as well as hydrastine. The medicinal varieties contain a number of opioid alkaloids (try saying that 10 times fast), though in lesser concentration than the opium poppies (about one-tenth as much), and are used in part for their analgesic activity. The best known are probably *Corydalis chaerophylla*, *C. yanhusuo*, and *C. longipes*. The herb is a major agricultural crop in China and bulk purchase is pretty easy.

Argemone is a genus of about 30 species of plants, generally called the prickly poppies. Many of the species contain berberine, the best known of which is the Mexican poppy, *Argemone mexicana*. The aerial parts are used; they contain the berberine (as does the resin), so it is a sustainable-use plant. But the berberine content is rather small and I would not use the plant as a berberine antibacterial myself—even though it has been traditionally used along berberine lines of function; its medicinal functions are more subtle.

Nandina domestica, the only member of its genus, is a suckering shrub, also in the barberry family. It is a rather common ornamental and I think a good choice for a berberine medicinal if you have it in your yard. The lower branches and roots are highest in berberine. Treat it as a *Mahonia/Berberis* species if you are harvesting and making medicine from it; it is pretty much identical.

The genus *Eschscholtzia*, the California poppies, is also reputed to contain berberine, but I can't find much research on it. Berberine and similar alkaloids are also present in a number of other genera such as *Coelocline*, *Archangelisia*, *Chelidonium*, *Toddalia*, and *Thalictrum*.

In this section I will concentrate mostly on *Phellodendron amurense*—and to some extent on *Berberis* and *Mahonia*—however, if you take a look at the traditional uses of the berberines, you will see that they are all used similarly.

Parts Used

Bark, root bark, stems, roots, leaves, resin.

Preparation and Dosage

The alkaloids in the berberine plants, including berberine, are not very water soluble. (So if you see a study showing an aqueous extract of a berberine plant to be not as effective as an antimicrobial, you now know why.) Tinctures need to use a higher alcohol content (generally 1:5, 70 percent alcohol, 30 percent water), and the water needs to be acidic, with a pH of 1 to 6. The addition of 1 tablespoon of vinegar to the tincture mix is recommended if your water is alkaline (hard) or if you don't know. (See chapter 9 for an extensive listing of berberine plants and their alcohol-to-water ratios.)

The berberine plants may be used as a powder for topical application, as a douche, as a wash, as a tincture, in capsules, or as a snuff.

POWDER

Apply to cuts, scrapes, or infected wounds.

TINCTURE

Dried bark of phellodendron: 1:5, 70 percent alcohol, 20–50 drops, up to 4x daily (the taste is exceptionally strong)

In acute dysenteric/diarrheal conditions: Take 1 tsp–1 tbl morning and evening until symptoms subside. Improvement should be seen within 2 days; usually there will be some improvement within 8 hours.

Note: The berberine plants are only about 50 percent active against cholera in clinical trials, as compared with enterotoxogenic *E. coli*, which they completely inhibit. However, if you combine the berberine plants with the root of *any* geranium species, the bark of pomegranate or the peel of the fruit, or the leaf or bark of guava, the cholera organism will be completely inhibited.

As a douche: Add ⅓ ounce tincture to 1 pint water and douche once or twice daily.

As a wash: Add 1 ounce tincture to 2 pints water and wash the affected area morning and evening—especially good for helping acne and infected wounds.

CAPSULES

For non-acute conditions: Take 1 or 2 "00" capsules, up to 4x daily.

In acute dysenteric/diarrheal conditions: Take up to 25 "00" capsules daily for up to 10 days.

SNUFF

Place two thin lines of root powder on a table and snort them vigorously—each line into a different nostril like those cocaine addicts on television, up to 3x daily for up to 7 days.

Side Effects and Contraindications

Caution is advised in pregnancy.

There is a tendency, because of the berberine plants' poor absorption across the intestinal mucosa, to increase the dose of the plants substantially to try to get more alkaloids into the bloodstream. *This is a very bad idea.* Abdominal cramping, nervous tremors, and, most importantly, excessive drying of the mucous membranes will occur at high doses. Do not attempt to use these herbs as systemics.

Herb/Drug Interactions

The berberines are synergistic (or additive) with a number of pharmaceuticals such as fluconazole, ampicillin, and oxacillin. Repeated use of berberine *may* reduce the GI tract absorption of permeability glycoprotein (P-gp) substrates including chemotherapeutic agents such as daunomycin. Berberine intake will *increase* the absorption of cyclosporine A if it is taken after long-term berberine use: One study showed that 3 mg/kg of berberine in six human volunteers taken twice daily for 10 days increased the bioavailability of cyclosporine A by 19 percent. A randomized, clinical trial of 52 renal transplant patients for 3 months found that constant berberine intake significantly increased the amount of cyclosporine A in blood plasma.

Conversely, P-gp inhibitors, such as piperine, will substantially increase (by six times) the uptake of berberine across the intestinal mucosa. Sodium caprate, for example, will do so as well.

(continued on page 268)

Properties of the Berberine Plants

Actions

Analgesic
Antiamoebic
Antibacterial
Anticholeric
Antidiarrheal
Antidysenteric
Antifungal
Anti-inflammatory
Antisecretory
Antiseptic
Antitumor
Astringent
Diaphoretic
Expectorant
Febrifuge
Mucosal anti-inflammatory
Mucosal stimulant
Mucosal tonic

Berberine interferes with adherence of bacteria such as *Streptococcus* spp. to mucous membranes by stimulating the release of lipoteichoic acid from bacteria or by stopping the formation of complexes between the microbial surface and host cells. It inhibits the intestinal hypersecretion (by about 70 percent) induced by cholera, *E. coli,* and other intestinal disease organisms. Berberine targets the assembly of the *E. coli* cell division protein FtsZ. Basically, it is an FtsZ inhibitor, stopping replication of the bacteria.

Some studies have found berberine to be cardioprotective, antimalarial, antioxidative, cerebroprotective, antimutagenic, vaso-relaxing, anxiolytic, and anti-HIV, but these studies are all in vitro; they don't translate well and the berberine would tend to work in most of those instances only if injected.

Active Against

Berberine-containing plants are active against a wide range of microorganisms. Berberine has been the most intensively tested of the plants' alkaloids, though a number of others such as hydrastine, jatrorrhizine, and palmatine have also undergone a fair amount of study. The various antimicrobial alkaloids in the berberines tend to be active against different organisms and are highly synergistic with each other and additionally benefit from other compounds in the plants whose only known functions are to disable antibiotic-resistance mechanisms in microbial organisms. Thus, whole plant extracts, rather than isolated constituents, tend to have a greater range of action and, in my opinion, are much more effective.

This is borne out by numerous studies. As an example, researchers in Italy commented in their research paper, "The crude extract [of *Berberis*

(continued)

Properties of the Berberine Plants—Continued

aetnensis root extracts] was active against Candida species, this activity being higher than that of the alkaloidal fraction and berberine."[7] The berberine-containing plants are very good at what they do—if they are prepared and used properly (i.e., ethanolic extracts or powders used for direct-contact disease treatment rather than systemic disease conditions).

The following list is comprised of microorganisms that have been found susceptible to either individual constituents of the berberine-containing plants or crude extracts of the plants themselves (e.g., *Mahonia*, *Berberis*, *Hydrastis*, *Coptis*, *Phellodendron*). As an example, the ethanolic extract of *Mahonia aquifolium* (as well as two of its constituents) was tested on 20 strains of coagulase-negative staphylococci, 20 strains of *Propionbacterium acnes* isolated from skin lesions of patients with severe acne, and 20 strains of *Candida* spp. isolated from chronic vulvovaginal candidiasis and found active against all of them. The Slovakian researchers comment, "The results indicate a rational basis for the traditional use of *Mahonia aquifolium* for localized skin and mucosal infection therapy."[8] This kind of finding and commentary, at least in cultures other than the United States, is not uncommon.

Aspergillus spp.
Aureobasidium pullulans (black and white strains)
Bacillus cereus
Bacillus subtilis
Blastocystis hominis
Candida spp.
Chlamydia spp. (including *C. trachomatis*)
Corynebacterium diphtheriae
Cryptococcus neoformans
Dengue virus
Entamoeba histolytica
Enterobacter aerogenes
Epidermophyton floccosum
Erwinia carotavora
Escherichia coli
Fusarium nivale
Fusobacterium nucleatum
Giardia lamblia
Helicobacter pylori
Hepatitis B
Herpes simplex 1 and 2
Human cytomegalovirus
Klebsiella pneumoniae
Leishmania spp.
Malassezia spp.
Microsporum spp.
Mycobacterium tuberculosis
Propionbacterium acnes
Pseudomonas aeruginosa
Salmonella paratyphi
Salmonella typhimurium
Shigella spp.
Staphylococcus aureus
Staphylococcus epidermidis
Streptococcus mutans
Streptococcus pyogenes
Streptococcus sanguinis
Trichoderma viride (green strain and brown mutant)
Trichomonas vaginalis
Trichophyton spp.
Trypanosoma cruzi
Vibrio cholerae
West Nile virus
Xanthomonas citri
Yellow fever virus
Zoogloea ramigera

Use to Treat

Internally: Dysenteric diseases of all sorts, especially those caused by resistant bacteria, as well as cholera (better used in combination with geranium root, pomegranate bark or fruit peel, or guava leaf or bark), giardia, bloody stools
Externally: Topically for infected wounds from bacterial and fungal organisms; conjunctivitis and other eye infections, especially trachoma
Mouth, throat, vagina: As a tincture or spray, or as a douche, for bacterial, fungal, and yeast infections of the mucous membranes of the throat, mouth, vagina

Finding Berberine Plants

Phellodendron amurense bark, *Coptis chinensis* root, and *Corydalis yanhusuo* root are available in bulk from 1st Chinese Herbs. *Berberis vulgaris* and *Mahonia aquifolium* root bark and organically grown *Hydrastis canadensis* root are available from Pacific Botanicals. *Tinospora cordifolia* is available from Banyan Botanicals. *Argemone mexicana* seeds grow easily and are available many places if you Google them. The "resin" is often sold as a psychoactive (sigh), which makes it easily found at usually ridiculous prices. What this "resin" should in fact be is the dried latex, but it generally is not for, as most confess, it is very time intensive to gather. Usually the "resin" is a concentrated extract of the plant. It will work as a berberine, but there are much cheaper alternatives. The latex itself is actually fairly high in berberine and was once a staple of regular practice botanical medicine in the United States but is nearly impossible to find now. The dried plant is a bit hard to find as well.

Glutin, a fraction isolated from gluten, *increases* the transport of berberine alkaloids across the mucosa. Eating gluten-rich foods *may* increase the amount of berberine-type alkaloids moving across the intestinal mucosa. Gum arabic inhibits the crossing of most alkaloids other than berberine. Coptis interferes with the movement of constituents from radix scutellariae (*Scutellaria baicalensis*) across the intestinal membrane.

Habitat and Appearance

I will primarily look at just three plants here: *Phellodendron, Berberis,* and *Mahonia.*

PHELLODENDRON

Phellodendron amurense is a rather impressive deciduous tree (*deciduous* simply means "falling" because it loses its leaves in the fall); it is a native of Manchuria. It was introduced into the United States as an ornamental in the 1870s and escaped into urban fringe forests in New York State and Pennsylvania. It easily moves into multiple forest types and densities. It is now considered invasive in Illinois, New York, Pennsylvania, Massachusetts, Connecticut, and Virginia.

The tree grows to 60 feet tall (largest found was 90 feet) with a fairly short, wide trunk from which the tree begins branching almost immediately, giving it a widely spreading full canopy to 40 feet in diameter. The trunk has a deeply ridged and corky outer bark. The name *phellodendron* means "cork tree" (*phellos* meaning "cork," *dendron* meaning "tree"). So the plant is sometimes referred to as the corktree or the Amur corktree (from the region in Manchuria from which it comes). The female tree produces clusters of grape-like fruits (each containing two to five seeds) that possess a strong odor so that often only the male plants are cultivated, usually as a sterile cultivar, the so-called macho hybrid (rather oxymoronic).

The fruits have a high sugar content and are good food sources for birds and other animals, who routinely spread the seed far and wide. The leaves are edible and sometimes used in salads, soups, stews, and as a tea. The tree's primary use in the United States has been as a shade tree and ornamental. The bark has been used as a cork source (though a poor one); the tree is often used for lumber in China; the berries and inner bark are the source of several dyes; the fruits are used in insecticides, soaps, and lubricants. The inner bark is what is used medicinally. It is a good tree for bees and helps restore damaged soils when planted along with *Pinus sylvestris*.

BERBERIS

Both *Berberis thunbergii*, Japanese barberry, and *B. vulgaris*, common barberry, are introduced plants. Both are invasive here and there, Japanese barberry the most so. It is considered an invasive throughout the upper Midwest and Northeast—20 states and the District of Columbia altogether. Both it and common barberry outcompete the only native barberry, *Berberis canadensis*, which is slowly disappearing. Nor do wildlife like to browse the introduced species. *Berberis* species are abundant in nearly every state, except Texas, Florida, Nevada, Arkansas, Louisiana, Mississippi, and Oklahoma.

Japanese barberry forms dense stands in woodlands, canopy forests, wetlands, pastures, and meadows. The leaves are prickly (hence "barb" berry) and look a bit like holly leaves, and whitetail deer studiously avoid the plant. The plant grows up to 15 feet in height. The fruits are edible and were often used for jams.

MAHONIA

Mahonias are very similar in appearance. *Mahonia aquifolium* is mostly found on the East Coast, from Georgia up into Canada, and on the West Coast from California up into Canada and eastward into Montana. *Mahonia repens* is widely spread from the Mississippi River west, from Texas into Canada and a bit around the Great Lakes. *Mahonia fremontii* is in the southwest, Colorado, New Mexico, Arizona, Utah, Nevada, and California. *Mahonia bealii* is located throughout the Southeast. It is strongly present in most states except the extreme Northeast and the central plains into Louisiana and Mississippi.

Mahonias and the barberries, one or the other, grow in nearly every state in the United States. If you add in the phellodendrons, you can find a berberine plant just about anyplace. And, of course, all three genera are common in much of the world. The *Berberis* genus is very prolific, with a lot of diversity, in Africa, South America, and Asia. The mahonias are prolific in eastern Asia, North America, and Central America and have been widely planted throughout Europe. *Phellodendron* is widely dispersed in Asia, Russia, Europe, and North America.

Cultivation and Collection

Phellodendron tolerates a great many soil types and transplants easily. It does take a while to recover from transplanting, so it is usually planted in spring. Most people buy saplings for planting, but the seeds germinate easily (better with stratification) and sprout well; the plant is a strong grower. The seeds are highly allelopathic, killing off competing plants and protecting their growing zone. The tree spreads fairly easily once established—if you don't get the sterile cultivar. ("Macho"—how can it be macho? I don't get it.)

The root system is fairly shallow, so it needs room to spread. The tree loves disturbed areas and full sun, and it will tolerate most soils (sand, loam, clay, acidic, alkaline) and likes them well drained, occasionally wet. It is highly tolerant of drought and cold, resistant to nearly all pests, and likes it in Zones 3 through 7, which includes most of the United States except for the extreme South, Southwest, and Pacific coastline. The tree takes 7 to 13 years to set seed.

The inner bark may be harvested for medicinal use at any time, but when harvested in spring (April 4 through 20 in China), the inner and outer bark is more easily removed. Cut limbs are the best source of the bark unless for some reason you need to cut a whole tree. In regions where purists are trying to exterminate *Phellodendron* as an alien invader, you may be able to obtain whole trees from which to harvest considerable amounts. The outer bark is removed and abandoned and then the inner bark peeled off, cut into slices, and dried. Sometimes, no one knows why, the Chinese fry it with salt during the drying process (studies have found no difference in the strength of the resulting herb). In China they dry it in the sun, but I prefer it in a shady, dry location in the herb room myself.

Japanese barberry is shade tolerant, is drought and cold resistant, loves disturbed ecosystems, loves sunlight, and can seemingly grow just about anyplace. The plant spreads by seeds (which are themselves spread by birds and animals eating the fruit and excreting the seeds over a wide range), root and branch cuttings, live branches touching the ground, and root spread. Any root left in the ground will resprout. It is a prolific seed producer; the seeds have a 90 percent germination rate. It forms dense stands wherever it takes root in the wild and is very hard to eradicate. Ticks infected with *Borrelia* (Lyme disease) love the thick stands of the plants and are often densely present in them.

The plant's wood is very strong, so it has to be cut into small (1 inch or less) segments while still fresh. Don't do it later unless you have a dedicated wood chipper to use for your medicinals (or a meth addict friend with an axe—well, better stick with the chipper). Scrape your fingernail along the bark of the sections you intend to harvest. When the outer bark scrapes off, the inner bark should be yellow; if not, don't use it. The roots are tough to dig but have the highest alkaloid content. Use a tough, indestructible shovel (no wooden handles), long-handled clippers, a pickaxe, sweat, determination, and profanity. The outer bark of the roots is the most potent, but many people use the whole thing, chopped small and then cut and sifted, to make tinctures. It's easier.

Harvest the plant in autumn. With a good-sized plant, the roots and lower branches should last you a very long time. Dry well in the shade, and store in plastic bags inside plastic tubs, in a dark, dry location.

Mahonias are handled identically to barberries for medicine making, harvesting, and cultivation.

Plant Chemistry

The chemistry of the various berberine-containing plants differs a bit even though they are all used similarly. Over time, familiarity with the individual species allows a much more sophisticated use of the plants. This section will only highlight some of the major plant constituents in some of the species, beginning with the berberine content.

Coptis teeta has about the highest percentage of berberine of all plants—from 8 percent to 9 percent in the rhizome. *C. chinensis* runs 4 percent to 8 percent. *Berberis aristata,* as far as I can tell, has the most berberine in its genus, about 5 percent in the roots and 4 percent in the lower stems. *B. vulgaris,* the most commonly used species, has 1 percent to 1.5 percent berberine in its roots, about one-tenth of that in its stems, even less in the leaves. *B. croatica* is about the same. *Hydrastis canadensis* root contains about 3.4 percent berberine and 2.5 percent hydrastine. The leaves contain about 1.5 percent berberine and 0.5 percent hydrastine. The older the *Hydrastis* plants, the more they contain. Fall plants are stronger.

Phellodendron amurense bark runs about 3 percent to 4 percent berberine. *P. wilsonii* and *P. sachalinense* are reputed to contain the most berberine, followed by *P. chinense.*

Phellodendron species contain berberine, oxyberberine, epiberberine, caffeic acid ethyl ester, isovanillin, ferulic acid, dimethoxylariciresinol, methyl-beta-orsellinate, limonin (about 1 percent of the plant) and various other liminoids (obakunone, nomilin, etc.), 12-alpha-hydroxylimonin, gamma-fagarine, cathin-6-one, 4-methoxy-N-methyl-1-quinoline, palmatine, oxypalmatine, lyoniresinol, beta-sitosterol, stigmasterine, amurenlactone A, amurenamide A, phellodensins, various phellodenols, magnoflorine, jatorrhizine, various coumarins, phellodendrine, phellodendric acid, various quercetins, platydesmin, skimmianine, chilenine, and pteleine.

The five major alkaloids in the plant are considered to be berberine (about 80 percent of total alkaloids), palmatine, jatrorrhizine, phellodendrine, and magnoflorine.

The other berberine-containing plants have just as complex a chemistry, though their alkaloids tend to be a bit different. They all do similar things.

Traditional Uses of the Berberines

The plants are used around the world in very similar ways, the main differences being that both *Corydalis* and *Argemone* species contain either opioid or opioid-like constituents, making them very useful for pain relief in addition to their other functions.

Although the different berberine-containing plants will have unique applications when you get more sophisticated in their use, for my purposes here—the treatment of resistant GI tract infections with presenting dysentery or severe diarrhea (bloody or not), resistant infections of the mouth and throat, and skin infections—all the plants work similarly. From a look at their traditional uses, you can see that healers for the past several thousand years in every geographical region have found similar uses for all the berberines.

Hydrastis canadensis: As a bitter tonic, mucous membrane tonic; for skin disorders including infection and inflammation, eye and ear infections, mouth ulcers, throat and mouth infections, fever, diarrhea, dysentery, catarrh, vaginal discharges, liver congestion and gallbladder problems, menstrual irregularities, ulcerative colitis, cancer.

***Mahonia* spp.:** As a bitter tonic, mucous membrane tonic; for liver and blood stagnation, skin problems including inflammation and infections, GI tract infections, ulceration, fever.

***Berberis* spp.:** As a bitter tonic, mucous membrane tonic; for skin inflammation and infection, GI tract problems, cholera, dysentery, diarrhea, fever, cancer, liver stagnation, poor blood, gout.

***Coptis* spp.:** For abdominal problems, GI tract problems, dysentery, cholera, enteritis, typhoid, respiratory tract infections, UTIs, gynecological inflammations, ear/nose/throat infections, jaundice, fever, blood problems, eye inflammation, insomnia, abscesses, skin problems.

***Corydalis* spp.:** As a bitter tonic, analgesic, mucous membrane tonic; for liver stagnation, spleen stagnation, stagnant blood, menstrual irregularities, ulcers.

***Phellodendron* spp.:** As a bitter tonic; for GI tract problems, dysentery, jaundice, vaginal inflammation and discharges, urinary tract infections, pain, swelling in knees and feet, boils, sores, abscesses, ulcers, eczema, canker sores, burns, fever, night sweats.

***Argemone* spp.:** As a sedative, laxative; for jaundice, skin diseases, cough, venereal disease, vaginal discharge, arthritis, kidney pain, postpartum difficulties, dropsy, swelling of the legs, malaria, fever.

Many of the other berberine-containing plants have been used similarly.

AYURVEDA

The phellodendrons are not that common in India, but the barberries are and have been used for millennia. Five species are commonly used, the main ones being *Berberis vulgaris* and *Berberis aristata*. They are used just as all berberine-containing plants are. See Traditional Uses of the Berberines, page 273.

TRADITIONAL CHINESE MEDICINE

Phellodendron, known as *huang bo* or *huang bai,* is considered to be one of the 50 fundamental herbs of traditional Chinese medicine (TCM). It has been used for millennia and appears in medical texts as early as 300 BCE. It is considered bitter and cold, affecting urinary bladder, kidney, and large intestine meridians. It is used to clear heat and dry dampness, to reduce fire and release toxins. See Traditional Uses of the Berberines, page 273, for specific TCM uses. Normal dosage in China is 3–10 grams of the dried herb (1⁄10–1⁄3 ounce). The plant has also been a part of traditional Korean and Japanese medicine for a very long time, used for similar diseases and conditions.

Coptis, Corydalis, Mahonia, and *Berberis* species have all been a part of TCM for millennia and are used in similar ways.

WESTERN BOTANIC PRACTICE

Phellodendron has been unknown until now. *Hydrastis*, *Berberis* species, and *Mahonia* species were all used for a very long time, in just the same ways all berberine plants are.

Scientific Research

All the berberine plants, and berberine (in vitro studies), are highly active against a wide range of microorganisms, especially bacteria. There are literally scores if not hundreds of such studies on the compound.

Part of the problem with berberine as a systemic is that it does not move across the GI tract membranes very well; it tends to be limited to where it can touch for its activity. Researchers have been trying for years to find a way to make it broadly systemic but have not succeeded. Most of the pharmacokinetic studies have focused on injectable forms of berberine or other, similar, alkaloids. Oral administration of crude plant preparations has shown some movement of alkaloids, e.g., berberine and palmatine, into blood plasma in rats, but the amounts are tiny, 0.31 ng/ml as compared to 18.1 ng/ml if pure berberine is injected. Tiny amounts of berberine have been found in the pancreas, heart, kidney, spleen, lung, testes, and uterus. This does have some tonic and stimulatory effects on those systems, which is reflected by the plant's traditional uses. The tiny systemic amounts do provide *some* systemic antimicrobial help, just not very much and certainly not enough to treat a resistant systemic disease.

In human volunteers (China), normal dosing produced about 0.020 ng/ml in plasma, very large doses got it up to 3.0 ng/ml in the blood, still not enough for systemic treatment of serious diseases, and this was from ingesting pure berberine. Oral intake of goldenseal (product contained 77 mg hydrastine, 132 mg berberine) produced only 0.1 ng/ml of *both* constituents (combined total) in blood plasma of human volunteers. Berberine (and presumably many of the other alkaloids in these plants) just doesn't transfer well across the GI tract membranes; however, the amounts that do are very quickly expressed into the urine for excretion, into the mucous membranes for excretion by that route, or routed to the liver, where they are expressed into the bile. The amounts expressed in the urine (about 5 percent) are what account for the use of berberine plants in the treatment of urinary tract infections (for which they do work to some extent). The amounts concentrated in the liver and then expressed into the bile (0.5 percent) are what account for the traditional uses of the herbs for sluggish liver and as a bile stimulant. Berberine is metabolized in the liver and the metabolites excreted into the bile, which then expresses them into the GI tract. The gut bacteria play a role then in the enterohepatic circulation of the metabolites. These metabolites remain more prominently in the body than berberine itself, however still at fairly low levels.

The particular substance, pervasive in the intestinal epithelium (and hepatocytes), that keeps berberine from circulating widely in the body is permeability glycoprotein, a.k.a. P-glycoprotein. P-glycoprotein distributes a great many substances across the mucous membranes of the intestinal tract, including herbal constituents. However, it is also responsible for transporting substances the body identifies as toxic out of the body, often through urine and bile—the berberine-plant alkaloids are some of them. Because P-glycoprotein (or its directors) identifies berberine-like alkaloids as toxic, they are not allowed to cross the intestinal barrier to circulate in any concentration in the bloodstream.

However, the tiny amount of alkaloids that do circulate in the bloodstream increases the level of the active immunoglobulin A antibodies (IgA) in the mucous membranes—though this action is much, much higher in the intestines because the herb is actually able to touch the membranes there. IgA is one of the most potent antibodies in the human body, and it infuses the mucous membranes in order to fight infections that seek to gain entry there. In this instance the body is identifying the berberine alkaloids and their metabolites as an infectious agent and producing IgA antibodies in response. Stimulation of the mucous membranes and the IgA antibodies helps prevent infections. This is the main source of the immune-modulating and immune-potentiating actions of the berberines and is why the herbs, if used properly, help prevent and can effectively treat viral and bacterial infections of the mouth, throat, and sinuses. Synergistically, berberine also interferes with the adherence of bacteria, e.g., *Streptococcus pyogenes*, to epithelial cells, thus reducing disease incidence.

The berberine plants are, however, most specific for intestinal infections from pathogenic organisms. That is where their great strength lies. Berberine reduces the intestinal secretion of water and electrolytes caused by infectious intestinal bacteria such as cholera and *E. coli* organisms, inhibits cholera and other bacterial entertoxins, reduces smooth muscle contraction and intestinal motility (thus reducing cramping), delays intestinal transit time, reduces inflammation in intestinal tissues, and is directly bactericidal to cholera and other dysenteric/diarrheal organisms. Berberine specifically inhibits bacterial adherence to mucosal or epithelial surfaces, thus stopping the infection.

Because berberine is so widely antimicrobial, many people have used berberine plants (and many companies have touted them) as systemic antibacterials. They are not and are only partially effective for colds and flu, their other main use. (They are active against some viruses and do potentiate mucous membrane function, which helps the membranes fight off microorganisms.) Goldenseal is the primary berberine plant used medicinally in the United States and it is ridiculously overused, usually for the wrong things. There are much better plants for colds and flu.

Many of the berberine-containing plants have been found to contain multidrug-resistance (MDR) reversal activity, usually inhibiting efflux pumps in resistant bacteria. *Berberis* species and *Hydrastis canadensis* contain 5'-methoxyhydnocarpin-D (5'-MHC) and pheophorbide A, which inhibit the NorA efflux pump in *Staphylococcus aureus*. This is part of what makes the plants so effective in treating resistant organisms, especially MRSA. There are numerous other compounds in the berberine plants that show this kind of MDR inhibition.

The MDR inhibitors in the berberine plants have been found to be synergistic with the alkaloids in the plants. They have also been found to be synergistic with pharmaceuticals, increasing their activity and effectiveness in treating resistant organisms and lowering the necessary dose for antibacterial, antifungal, and antiamoebic action.

In this section I am only going to look in any depth at research on the phellodendrons and berberine as an isolated constituent.

PHELLODENDRON

An in vivo trial in the treatment of both acute and chronic induced inflammation using an ethanol extract of *Phellodendron* and *Coptis* (in a 2:1 ratio) found the tincture to be as potent in its effects as celecoxib and dexamethasone in reducing inflammation. In vitro studies on human osteoarthritis cartilage found that the plant significantly inhibited collagen and chondrocyte destruction by inhibiting proteoglycan release and type II cartilage degradation; down-regulating aggrecanases, matrix metalloproteinase (MMP) activity, and phospho-ERK 1/2, JNK, and p38 MAP kinase signaling; and up-regulating TIMP-1 activity. Another found potent antioxidant activity by the plant.

Eighty people (45 completing) were enrolled in an 8-week, placebo-controlled, randomized, double-blind study of the effects of a *Phellodendron amurense* bark and *Citrus sinensis* peel combination capsule (740 mg, twice daily) on primary osteoarthritis of the knee in both overweight and normal-weight persons. Overweight participants lost an average of 5 percent of body weight, and lipid levels, blood pressure, and fasting blood glucose levels normalized. There was significantly less inflammation and fewer symptoms of osteoarthritis in all those who used the herb combination.

A clinical trial with 28 participants (premenopausal women), double-blind, placebo-controlled, and randomized, testing a combination extract of magnolia and *Phellodendron* bark found no weight gain in the extract group but gains in the placebo group. The extract group had lower cortisol levels in the evening (the placebo group, higher) and lower levels of stress.

A combination blend of *Phellodendron* and magnolia, in a randomized, parallel, double-blind, placebo-controlled, clinical trial with healthy, overweight women (40 participants, 26 completing) found the extract effective in reducing temporary, transitory anxiety.

Phellodendron has been found effective in treating periodontal disease.

Extracts of *Phellodendron* (Nexrutine) fed to TRAMP mice for 20 weeks significantly inhibited prostate cancer cell proliferation and progression. There have been a number of studies that found similar antitumor activity of the plant for the prostate. It's strongly active on the prostate gland in vitro, inhibiting contractility. Dietary berberine and dietary *Phellodendron* extract were found to inhibit cell cycle progression and lung tumorigenesis in mice.

In vivo studies with hyperuricemic mice found a decrease in uric acid levels in mice ingesting a high-dose *Phellodendron* extract. Other studies found that the plant constituent phellodendrine suppresses autoimmune responses in mice and guinea pigs. Unlike prednisone and cyclophosphamide, the extract did not affect antibody production.

Phellodendron extracts prevent ethanol-, aspirin-, stress-, and pylorus-ligated-induced ulcers in mice. Extracts of *P. wilsonii* were highly protective of mouse liver in CCl4-induced hepatotoxicity. Other species provided only moderate protection.

During in vitro studies *Phellodendron* was found to be antioxidant, antitumor, anti-inflammatory, antimicrobial (plaque), anti–herpes simplex 1, and antibacterial against a wide range of bacteria.

Clinical (and a few other) studies with other berberine-containing plants:

123 people with acute bacillic dysentery were treated with a decoction of Sankezhen (any of four *Berberis* species used in China: *soulieana, wilsoniae, poiretii,* or *vernae*). Of them, 113 were cured, 4 improved. In another trial with 94 people, 88 were cured.

A trial used tablets prepared from *Berberis poirettii* decoction in the treatment of 228 cases of chronic bronchitis. Of them, 12.3 percent experienced cure, 39 percent marked effects, 38 percent improved. (A tincture would have worked better.)

An in vivo trial with goldenseal found that the plant was helpful in treating liver cancer in rats. The plant's constituents do possess some antitumor actions, and their concentration in the liver was found to be useful in the treatment of liver cancer, primarily as a supportive therapy.

Berberis vulgaris, when used instead of antibiotics in chicken feed, substantially increased the birds' weight, just as antibiotics do.

BERBERINE (AND OTHER BERBERINE-PLANT ALKALOIDS)

Quite a number of the in vivo studies of the effectiveness of berberine as an antimicrobial use injectable forms of the compound. I am omitting most of these here. They don't in any way indicate the actions of the compound when used as an herbal preparation. Injection is one of the ways researchers are trying to make the compound systemic. There has been some success at this, but there is a rather high toxicity when the isolated constituent is used that way, a toxicity that does not occur when crude extracts of the plants are used.

I am also skipping most of the in vitro studies, which are voluminous. Berberine's antimicrobial actions have already been mentioned throughout this section. Here are just a few clinical results of berberine's use.

A clinical trial with children suffering from giardia (ages 5 months to 14 years) was conducted in India. Berberine, administered orally, 10 mg/kg/day, was effective in eradicating the infection, comparable to quinacrine hydrochloride, furazolidone, and metronidazole.

Four hundred adults presenting with acute watery diarrhea were treated in a randomized, placebo-controlled, double-blind trial of berberine. Berberine combined with tetracycline was potently effective. Berberine alone reduced diarrheal stools and cyclic adenosine monophosphate concentrations in stools by 77 percent; another study found that berberine reduced diarrheal stools in cholera and/or enterotoxigenic *E. coli* (ETEC) up to 50 percent and that it was more potently effective in treating ETEC than cholera; another trial in a randomized, controlled trial of 165 adults with either ETEC or cholera found that in those with cholera berberine significantly reduced the mean 8-hour stool volume; however, with ETEC berberine completely inhibited diarrhea in half the participants within 24 hours.

Clinical (human) trials—placebo-controlled, randomized, double-blind—with 63 men with enterotoxigenic *E. coli* diarrhea found 400 mg of berberine sulfate to have dependable effectiveness, surpassing pharmaceuticals. In the 8 hours following treatment those in the berberine group experienced significant decrease in stool volume. Within 24 hours 42 percent of the participants in the berberine group stopped having diarrhea, versus 20 percent in the placebo group.

Another trial in the treatment of giardia in India found that berberine improved gastrointestinal symptoms and reduced giardia-positive stools. Berberine was found as effective as metronidazole at only half the dose.

In a clinical study with 51 people of an aqueous berberine preparation versus sulfacetamide in the treatment of *Chlamydia trachomatis* eye infections, berberine was found to be slightly less effective than the drug. However, the drug did not completely eradicate the organism and relapses occurred. In the berberine group there were no relapses of those cured, even after 1 year. Other clinical studies have found similar outcomes. The crude extracts of berberine plants have consistently been found more effective than berberine.

Palmatine was used to treat 1,042 cases of gynecological infection, upper respiratory infection, surgical infection, tonsillitis, enteritis, and bacillary dysentery with good effect. In the treatment of 200 cases of vulvovaginal candidiasis, 171 were cured, 24 improved.

Numerous in vivo studies have found berberine to be tonically antitumor for a number of different kinds of cancers, from breast to bladder to gastric to liver. It down-regulates metalloproteinases 1, 2, and 9 and is a potent COX-2 inhibitor.

Berberine, in vivo, oral administration, has been found to reduce insulin resistance in rats and to lower blood glucose levels and correct blood lipid metabolism disorders. In essence it suppresses intestinal disaccharidases, benefitting diabetic states while also improving glucose metabolism through the induction of glycolysis and increasing insulin sensitivity.

It has also been found to be immunomodulatory (rather than stimulatory). It does increase IgA antibodies in mucosal tissue, but it also reduces the overactivity of various aspects of the immune system. In other words if the immune system is ramped up by an autoimmune dynamic or hyperactivated by something like phytohemagglutinin or phorbol dibutyrate plus ionomycin, berberine modulates the response, suppressing the overactivity.

Juniper

Family: Cupressaceae

Species Used: There are 50 or 59 or even 67 species (taxonomists have to use their fingers and toes to count) in the *Juniperus* genus; all of them can be used similarly.

Parts Used

Usually the berries and needles, but the bark, wood, and root are all active.

Preparation and Dosage

The constituents in the junipers are readily soluble in alcohol but vary in water depending on what part of the plant you are using. The berries must be tinctured in alcohol or eaten whole to be effective. The needles will work to some extent in water (but are better in alcohol—the monoterpenes just aren't that water soluble, as numerous studies have found), the bark not so well.

Use: The berries for urinary tract infections. The berries or needles for upper respiratory or GI tract infections. The heartwood, roots, bark, berries, or needles for skin infections and infectious dysentery. The essential oil for airborne and upper respiratory infections.

TINCTURE

Berries: 1:5, 75 percent alcohol, 5–20 drops, up to 3x daily.

INFUSION

Chopped or powdered needles prepared as a standard infusion, covered, 4–6 ounces, 3–6x daily.

DECOCTION

A strong decoction of the herb has been traditionally used in many cultures to sterilize brewing equipment, cooking utensils, surgical instruments, hands, counters, etc. The decoction is also effective as a wound wash to either prevent or cure infection. Use 1 ounce herb per quart of water, boil 30 minutes, then turn off the heat and let steep overnight.

BERRIES

In whole form, for gastric problems: eat 1–5 berries per day for 2 weeks.

POWDER

Add any part of the plant to wound powders or use alone to prevent or cure infection in wounds.

STEAM

Any part of the plant, but usually the needles or berries. Use in sweat lodge or sauna directly on the stones or boil 4 ounces of needles in 1 gallon water, pour the resultant tea on stones, and inhale steam. Or just inhale the steam as it boils.

ESSENTIAL OIL

For sinus and upper respiratory infections, 8–10 drops in water in a 1-ounce nasal spray bottle, 4–6x day; shake well before use. Or use the essential oil in a diffuser for helping prevent and cure upper respiratory infections. Moderate amounts can be mixed in water for use as steam inhalant or in a sweat lodge for upper respiratory infections.

Side Effects and Contraindications

There has been a long-standing assertion in scores of herbals that the use of this plant may cause kidney irritation and that it is highly

Properties of Juniper

Actions

Antibacterial
Anticatarrhal
Antifungal
Anti-inflammatory
Antimicrobial
Antineoplastic
Antinociceptive
Antioxidant
Antirheumatic
Antiseptic
Antiviral
Carminative
Digestive
Diuretic
Hypoglycemic
Hypolipidaemic
Radical scavenger
Stomachic

Active Against

Alcohol extracts of juniper show activity against 57 strains of 24 bacterial species in the following genera:

Acinetobacter
Bacillus
Brevundimonas
Brucella
Enterobacter
Escherichia
Micrococcus
Pseudomonas
Staphylococcus
Xanthomonas

They have been shown to inhibit, as well, 11 *Candida* species. They are also active against biofilm formation. Some antimicrobial specifics:

Acinetobacter baumannii
Actinomyces bovis
Aspergillus fumigatus
Aspergillus niger
Bacillus brevis
Bacillus cereus
Bacillus megaterium
Bacillus subtilis
Caenorhabditis elegans
Candida spp.
Clostridium perfringens
Cryptococcus neoformans
Enterococcus faecalis
Escherichia coli
Fusobacterium necrophorum
Geotrichum candidum
Hansenula anomala
Helicobacter pylori
Klebsiella oxytoca
Klebsiella pneumoniae
Leishmania donovani
Listeria monocytogenes
Micrococcus flavus
Micrococcus luteus
Microsporum gypseum
Mycobacterium spp. (including *M. tuberculosis*, even resistant strains such as H37Rv, and seven non-tuberculosis types)
Plasmodium falciparum
Proteus mirabilis
Proteus vulgaris
Pseudomonas aeruginosa
Rhodotorula spp.
Salmonella typhi
Serratia marcescens
Shigella dysentariae
Shigella sonnei
Staphylococcus aureus (including resistant strains)
Staphylococcus epidermidis
Staphylococcus intermedius
Streptococcus durans
Streptococcus faecalis
Streptococcus mutans
Streptococcus sanguinis
Trichophyton mentagrophytes
Trichophyton rubrum
Yersinia enterocolitica

Juniperis also active against various cancer cell lines, SARS coronavirus, and herpes simplex 1.

contraindicated in kidney disease. (Guilty of this myself.) I have used the plant for more than 2 decades and have never seen any problems. The phytomedicalist Kerry Bone and others have tracked back the emergence of this belief; it began in the latter part of the nineteenth century, apparently from the administration of large doses of the essential oil to animals. Recent studies with rats have found, contrary to popular belief, a kidney-protecting effect from the use of the plant. This bears out the long use by the Eclectics of the berries in the treatment of active kidney disease and inflammation. I no longer consider the herb contraindicated in kidney disease, nor do I feel that kidney irritation can occur from normal use.

The only side effect I have ever seen from use was a mild diarrhea when the essential oil (15 drops in 1 ounce of olive oil) was used in the treatment of an ear infection. The mix was applied three times daily with a cotton swab. The diarrhea stopped upon discontinuance of the herb.

The essential oil is not really for internal use other than as a steam inhalant or for aromatherapy. Neither the plant itself nor the berry appears to produce any side effects, nor have I ever heard of any.

Caution should probably be exercised by diabetics in any long-term use of the plant as it affects blood glucose levels and may alter insulin requirements. It should probably not be used long term with pharmaceutical diuretics. *However,* almost no one uses the plant long term for healing; usually it is a short-course herb for UTI.

Herb/Drug Interactions

None noted.

Habitat and Appearance

Generally, there are two main types of junipers. The first is a typical sort of evergreen tree (sometimes shrubby looking) growing up to 50 feet tall. The second is a low, spreading shrub, usually with nasty, prickly needles that will easily penetrate clothing and skin. It is often intentionally planted along walkways and near the front doors of houses. And of course, to make things difficult, many of the tree species start out with needles very much like the low-spreading shrubs and only develop their scale-like needle structure as they age.

The trunk and branches of both types tend to have a reddish look to them, the outer bark peeling off in strips all on its own, giving the plant a rather shaggy, disreputable look. The needles on the shrubby species, primarily *Juniperus communis*, are exceedingly sharp, a bit blue-green in color, and somewhat similar to the needles on pines, firs, and spruce species. The needles on the tree species are more similar to those on some types of true cypress and cedar species, having an overlapping, scale type of growth, really not much like those of the pines, spruce, and firs.

Both species are readily identifiable due to the presence of their "berries," which are actually small cones that form after fertilization of the flowers. Like everyone else, I just call them berries. (Yes, I know tomato is a fruit, but no one cares.) The berries are green when first formed, then turn purplish during the winter, after a good frost.

Juniperus communis is a circumpolar species of the northern hemisphere. It and its high-altitude relations (*J. sibirica, J. montana*) are generally found from 8,000 feet up to timberline. The tree species grow lower, up to about 8,000 feet, and are widely spread throughout the world; various species can be found in Africa as far south as Zimbabwe, and also in Australia and South America. The genus has been

Finding Juniper

It probably grows someplace near you. Go and pick the blue/purplish berries and use them, or buy them . . . they are available from herb suppliers everywhere.

Alternatives: Any evergreen species, especially thuja, cedar, pine, fir, and spruce in that order. Thuja, cedar, and pine have shown significant antibacterial activity in laboratory study against antibiotic-resistant bacteria, as has fir and, to a lesser extent, spruce. This tends to bear out their long traditional use for healing infectious disease. Dosages for all the evergreens are comparable.

widely planted as ornamentals throughout the world. All of the species can be used for medicine.

Cultivation and Collection

Given that the berries of the junipers do contain seeds, there is no doubt that the trees propagate that way. Information on starting them from seed, however, is very hard to find. Everyone apparently plants seedlings—I just can't find out where the seedlings come from (storks maybe or perhaps Hogwarts). In any event, the seedlings need a well-drained soil in which to grow.

You can gather the needles, bark, roots, or heartwood at any time. First-year berries (they are green) should be gathered after the first frost, second-year berries (they are bluish-purple) at any time. Basically, the berries should be purplish before you use them for medicine—the frost is what does it.

Plant Chemistry

There are some 80 to 100 different compounds that have been identified in the junipers so far. Generally, alpha-pinene, junipene, eicosane, hexadecane, stenol, heptacosane, aromadendrene, germacrene, alpha-copaene-8-ol, ledol, elemol, trans-caryophyllene, epoxy caryophyllene, amorphene, and limonene are the major constituents. There is also totarol, ferruginol, longifolene, trans-communic acid, cedrol, alpha-cedrene, beta-cedrene, alpha-cedrol, 3-carene, terpinen-4-ol, beta-pinene, sabinene, myrcene, mycene, thujone, caryophyllene, cadinene, elemene, linalool, piperitone, gamma-terpinene, trans-pinocarveole, rho-cymene, alpha-terpineole, gamma-cardinene, beta-carophyllene, bornyl acetate, germacrene B, germacrene D, verbenol, camphene, tricyclene, beta-eudesmol, humulene, borneol, nerol, geraniol, carvacrol, and so on.

The constituents differ not only in species, but in species' location and in their age. Century-old trees have markedly different chemical profiles than those a decade old. The primary constituents in all species are monoterpene hydrocarbons, which are highly bioactive, strongly antimicrobial compounds.

Traditional Uses of Juniper

Juniper, and all the evergreens, have been used in every culture on Earth for purifying and cleansing—physically, emotionally, and spiritually. They have been used in sweat baths and saunas throughout time to help prevent or cure illness.

One of the often overlooked attributes of the evergreens is their vitamin C content. All animals except the higher primates synthesize their own vitamin C. The new spring growth of the evergreens is lighter in color, less astringent, and decidedly more citrus-tasting than older growth (it has a definite lemon-lime flavor). This new growth has traditionally been used in the human diet in scores of cultures to treat scurvy.

AYURVEDA

There are five species of juniper used in India, *Juniper communis* being the most common. Called by a variety of names, depending on which local language is being used, it is *hapusha* in Sanskrit. The berries are the main part of the plant used for medicine, though the leaves and wood are sometimes used as well.

Juniper is considered aromatic, carminative, stimulant, emmenagogue, digestive, stomachic, strongly antibacterial, and diuretic. It is used for scanty urine, chronic Bright's disease, hepatic dropsy, coughs and pulmonary disease, fever, gonorrhea, leukorrhea, catarrh, arthritis, amenorrhea, tuberculosis, diabetes, and improving digestion and appetite.

TRADITIONAL CHINESE MEDICINE

There are 23 primary species of juniper in China with numerous subspecies. Most of them are designated by a phrase ending in *bai* (or beginning with *bai*, depending on whether you read left to right or right to left); e.g., *chui zhi bai* for *Juniperus recurva*, or *bei mei yuan bai* for *Juniperus virginiana*. The junipers *are* used in Chinese medicine; it's just that none of my sources have much about it. "Used similarly to thuja," says one fairly rare book, "see that listing." The book then stops at the letter "N." And, of course, I haven't been able to find volume two anyplace. Irritating. And wouldn't you just know it, none of my other Chinese herbals list thuja either. Increasingly irritating.

However, the tiny amount I can find lists juniper as traditionally used for treating bleeding from coughs, for colds, for hemorrhage, as a general tonic, and for convulsions, detoxification of the blood, hepatitis, and sweating. It is used in the treatment of chronic obstructive pulmonary disease in situations where there is phlegm overproduction and congestion, blood stasis, and spleen deficiency.

WESTERN BOTANIC PRACTICE

Junipers were extensively used by indigenous cultures in the Americas for the exact same conditions as those in China and India. Additionally, they used them for diarrheal conditions, colds and flu, ulcers, throat infections; as an aromatic for lung conditions; for vaginal infections and scanty menses, especially after childbirth; as a primary tuberculosis medicine, a wash for skin infections, an anthelmintic, and a general disinfectant to prevent disease or to clean rooms after disease.

The Eclectic physicians in the United States used the berries as a potent diuretic, for dropsy, for ascites, as a specific for infected mucous discharges from the urethra, and for cystitis, pyelitis, pyelonephritis, and renal hyperemia. They were also used for leukorrhea, gleet, gonorrhea, scorbutic diseases, skin infections, eczema, psoriasis, and skin parasites. They were used similarly in Europe. Juniper is still official in German medical practice.

Scientific Research

There has been little scientific study on juniper, other than some rather extensive explorations of its constituents and their antimicrobial activity. A few in vivo studies do exist.

In vitro studies have found that extracts of the heartwood of various juniper species are comparable in their antimicrobial effects to streptomycin. Leaf extracts are comparable in potency to amphotericin B. Other in vitro studies found that leaf extracts were very active against resistant staph and bacillus bacteria, as potent as ampicillin and erythromycin in their zones of inhibition. Juniper inhibits the NorA efflux pump in staph organisms, making them more susceptible to the antibacterial compounds in the plant.

In vivo studies: Tacrolimus, a drug used for immunosuppression after organ transplants, can cause, among other things, severe kidney damage. Tacrolimus-induced kidney damage in rats was completely reversed by the use of juniper oil. The renal cell membranes incorporated vasodilatory prostanoids, the herb elevated PGF2-alpha urinary excretion, and the precipitous fall in inulin clearance usually caused by the drug was completely prevented. (This bears out the Eclectic use of the herb in treating kidney disease.) Additionally, the kidneys and livers of mice injected with CCl4 who had previously been given an oral extract of juniper were strongly protected from injury. The researchers commented that *J. phoenicea* leaf extracts "show a remarkable effect in enhancing liver and kidney functions and may thus be of therapeutic potential in treatment of hepatotoxicity and nephrotoxicity."[9]

Juniper berry oil is high in 5,11,14-eicosatrienoic acid, a polyunsaturated acid similar to that found in fish oil; it is highly resistant to peroxidation. Hepatic reperfusion injury in rats fed the oil as a regular part of their diet was significantly minimized. (This bears out the traditional tonic use of the herb for treating digestive/liver problems.)

Juniper extracts showed potent anthelmintic activity against pinworm infections in mice; they are strongly anti-inflammatory to induced edema in mice and antinociceptive to induced pain; they significantly lower blood glucose levels in induced-diabetic mice while also increasing zinc levels in the liver.

Juniper extracts, and various compounds in juniper species, are potently active against a wide range of *Mycobacterium* organisms, bearing out the plant's traditional use for treating TB.

Juniper also contains, as do nearly all evergreens, a rather amazing constituent called totarol. Like many of the constituents in juniper (longifolene, alpha-pinene), totarol is strongly antibacterial. Totarol is antimicrobial against a wide range of microorganisms, including the mycobacteria, enterococci, staphylococci, streptococci, *Pseudomonas,* plus a variety of other Gram-negative organisms, and a number of parasitic organisms. It is potently synergistic with the other antibacterials in juniper; studies have found that it potentiates a wide range of pharmaceutical antibiotics as well. It is highly active at tiny doses and is a main part of the synergistic potency of the plant as an antimicrobial, antioxidant, antitumor, hepatic protector, and cholesterol-lowering herb. The constituent is also highly effective in the treatment of skin diseases such as severe acne. It is a fairly strong NorA efflux pump inhibitor.

A number of compounds in the plant, especially the berries, most especially terpinen-4-ol, substantially increase the output of urine without reducing either potassium or electrolyte levels in the body. Kidney filtration rate is also enhanced. The reasons why the highly antibacterial monoterpenes in the plant work so well is that the body immediately works to excrete them through the urinary passages. This has the effect of disinfecting the whole system. If you have a resistant UTI, this is the one plant you want to be sure to use for it.

Honey

Any organic wildflower honey can be used effectively in the treatment of antibiotic-resistant skin and wound infections. There is some evidence that large-scale agricultural honeys and single-plant honeys are less potent than wildflower honeys. There are a few exceptions. Manuka honey from New Zealand, produced mainly from the flowers of *Leptospermum scoparium,* is very potent (which is why you will see it for sale all over the Internet at indecent prices—about four times the cost of locally produced wildflower honeys).

The belated recognition of the potency of honey in treating resistant bacterial infections of the skin, especially those acquired in hospitals, has led to significant study, clinical use, and trial of honeys in medical practice since the first edition of *Herbal Antibiotics* in 1999, primarily in the UK. Predictably, a pharmaceutical honey has been produced (which is, of course, tremendously expensive compared to local honeys). Called Medihoney, it is the only honey allowable for use in the medical system in the UK. (A brand called Revamil is used in the Netherlands.) The USFDA has also accepted the use of a pharmaceutical honey by clinicians in this country, again very expensive—though, of course, almost no U.S. hospitals are using it. Nevertheless, *any* wildflower honey will do. The more plants the bees collect nectar from, the more potent it will be. If it is organic, it will tend to be relatively free of agrochemical pollutants. Also important.

Other bee products such as propolis and royal jelly are also highly effective against resistant organisms. Studies have found them stronger in some instances than honey, but they are more difficult to apply. Royal jelly, when added to honey, increases its effectiveness.

Preparation and Dosage

Honey can be applied directly to wounds or used internally for immune stimulation, overall health improvement, and treatment of colds, flus, and respiratory infections.

DIRECT APPLICATION

For burns (first, second, and third degree): Direct application full strength, covered by sterile bandage, changed once or twice daily.

For ulcerations, bedsores (even to the bone): Same as for burns.

For infected wounds: Same as for burns.

For wounds: Same as for burns.

For impetigo: Dilute honey enough to use as a wash, then apply 2x daily.

For seborrheic dermatitis: Same as for impetigo.

INTERNAL USE

As a preventive: Take 1 tablespoon, undiluted or in tea, 3x daily.

For acute conditions: Take 1 tablespoon honey each hour, or 1 tablespoon in tea 6–10x daily.

Best colds and flu tea: 2 tablespoons ginger juice, juice of 1/4 lime, pinch cayenne pepper, 1 tablespoon honey, hot water.

Side Effects and Contraindications

External use: None.

Internal use: Mild to severe anaphylaxis in rare instances for those with allergic reactions to bee stings.

Traditional Uses of Honey

I have used honey in healing for over 20 years now; there is nothing comparable for treating wounds of any sort, no matter how infected or bad they are. It is *the* premier wound healer on this planet.

Honey is the nectar of the flowers of plants, gathered by the bee, and stored in its stomach for transport to the hive. Natural honeys are from a profusion of wildflowers, whatever grows locally. With natural

Properties of Honey

Actions

Potent antibiotic against all known forms of resistant bacteria that infect the skin and wounds. In addition:

Antiallergenic
Antianemic
Anticarcinogenic
Antifungal
Anti-inflammatory
Antiviral
Expectorant
Immune stimulant
Laxative
Tonic

Promotes healing for wounds, moist wounds, peptic ulcers, and bacterial gastroenteritis; reduces plaque; good for gingivitis; facilitates debridement; soothes inflamed tissues; acts as a wound barrier; and stimulates skin and muscle regeneration.

Active Against

Acinetobacter spp.
Alcaligenes faecalis
Aspergillus niger
Bacillus stearothermophilus
Bacillus subtilis
Burkholderia cepacia
Candida spp.
E. coli O157:H7 (25 strains)
Enterobacter cloacae
Enterococcus faecalis (essentially any vancomycin-resistant enterococci)
Extended-spectrum beta-lactamase (ESBL) bacteria
Haemophilus influenzae
Helicobacter pylori
Herpes simplex
Klebsiella oxytoca
Klebsiella pneumoniae
Listeria monocytogenes
Malassezia spp.
Micrococcus luteus
Morganella morganii
Mycobacterium spp.
Proteus spp.
Pseudomonas aeruginosa (152 isolates)
Rubella virus
Salmonella enteritidis
Salmonella typhimurium (49 strains)
Serratia marcescens
Shigella dysentariae
Staphylococcus aureus (58 isolates and all MRSA strains tested)
Staphylococcus spp. (coagulase-negative species)
Stenotrophomonas maltophilia
Streptococcus spp.
Trichosporon spp.

Honey is also highly effective against bacterial biofilms.

(continued)

Properties of Honey—Continued

Use to Treat

Use for prevention and treatment of all infected skin wounds: cuts, abrasions, leg and skin ulcers, gangrene, diabetic ulceration of the foot, all fungating wounds (skin ulceration with necrosis and bad smell), necrotizing soft-tissue infections, postsurgical wound infections, burns (first through third degree), cellulitis, furunculosis, abscesses, necrotizing fasciitis, conjunctivitis, radiation burns and wounds, gingivitis, dental plaque, and helicobacter infections of the stomach and duodenum. Use it prophylactically at the exit sites of medical devices to prevent infection. To prevent infection from catheter insertion, the catheter should be coated with honey before insertion. May be used similarly with all medical equipment that is being inserted into the human body.

Finding Honey

There is almost always someone in every local area that produces local wildflower honey. Many grocery stores carry it. However, recent research on store-bought honeys in the United States has found that up to 75 percent of them cannot genuinely be considered "honey." Many manufacturers remove all pollen from the honey. Sometimes it is then adulterated with corn syrup. Researchers found, however, *all* honey from farmers' markets, food co-ops, and natural food stores to be the real thing. Good honey should *always* contain a bit of pollen, which will make it appear slightly cloudy to the eye.[10]

honeys it is exceedingly uncommon to have a honey gathered from a single species of plant such as the alfalfa or clover honeys of today unless that plant species exists in great abundance (as heather does in

Scotland). As such, natural bee honeys generally possess the essence of a multitude of wild plants—all of them medicinal. Honeybees have a strong attraction to many strongly medicinal plants: vitex, jojoba, elder, toadflax, balsam root, echinacea, valerian, dandelion, wild geranium; in fact almost any flowering medicinal herb, as well as the more commonly known alfalfas and clovers. The nectar from a multitude of medicinal plants is present in any wildflower honey mix and so are whatever chemical constituents were present in the nectars. In addition to the plants' medicinal qualities, the plant nectars are subtly altered, in ways that modern science has been unable to explain, by their brief transport in the bees' digestive system. Before regurgitation the nectars combine in unique ways with the bees' digestive enzymes to produce new compounds. Honey, often insisted to be just another simple carbohydrate (like white sugar), actually contains, among other things, a complex assortment of enzymes, organic acids, esters, antibiotic agents, trace minerals, proteins, carbohydrates, hormones, and antimicrobial compounds. One pound of the average honey contains 1,333 calories (compared to white sugar at 1,748 calories), 1.4 grams of protein, 23 mg of calcium, 73 mg of phosphorus, 4.1 mg of iron, 1 mg of niacin, and 16 mg of vitamin C, along with vitamin A, beta-carotene, the complete complex of B vitamins, vitamin D, vitamin E, vitamin K, magnesium, sulphur, chlorine, potassium, iodine, sodium, copper, manganese, and high concentrations of hydrogen peroxide and formic acid. Honey, in fact, contains over 75 different compounds. Many of the remaining substances in honey (comprising 4 percent to 7 percent of the honey) are so complex that they have yet to be identified.

Scientific Research

In the years since the first edition of *Herbal Antibiotics* was published, honey has become a significant medical treatment for surgical wounds, wound healing, and burns in hospitals, especially in the UK. It has become, in fact, a major part of standard-practice medicine there—in part because of the spread of resistant organisms, against which honey is reliably effective. Many clinical trials (more than 30) have been conducted on its use. Here are a few of them, from the UK and elsewhere.

Thirty-two children with pyomyositis abscesses were split into two randomized treatment groups. The abscess cavities were packed twice daily with either honey- or Eusol-soaked gauze. Honey-treated wounds healed faster, and length of time in the hospital was shorter, than those treated with Eusol.

Eighty-eight people were enrolled in a nonrandomized, open-label, side-by-side comparison of various forms of second-intention healing of donor site for split-thickness skin grafts. Honey-impregnated gauzes showed faster epithelization time and a lower level of pain than the other methods used.

A trial with 60 patients with chronic complicated surgical or acute traumatic wounds found that honey was easy to apply, kept the wounds clean, stopped infection, and was exceptionally safe.

One hundred and five people participated in a single-center, open-label, randomized, controlled trial in the treatment of honey for wounds. The honey-treated group's wounds healed significantly faster, in 100 days compared to 140 for the control group.

One hundred and eight people with venous leg ulcers engaged in a multicenter, open-label, randomized, controlled trial of honey treatment compared with IntraSite Gel. There was increased incidence of healing, effective desloughing, and lower infection rates in the honey-treated group. Other trials have found similar outcomes.

Fifteen people with pressure ulcers were treated with honey and 11 with ethoxy-diaminoacridine plus nitrofurazone dressings. Honey group healing was approximately four times that of the pharmaceutical group.

Only one of 20 patients in a honey group developed intolerable oral mucositis when receiving radiation, a better outcome than with lignocaine. Other studies have replicated this.

Thirty infected diabetic foot wounds were treated with honey for 3 months. Complete healing was achieved in 43 percent of wounds treated, and decrease in size of ulceration and healthy granulation were observed in another 43 percent. The bacterial load in all ulcers was significantly reduced after the first week of honey dressing. Failure of treatment occurred in 6.7 percent. A number of other studies have been conducted on the treatment of diabetic foot ulcers and all have found comparable outcomes. For example: 60 people with limb-threatening diabetic infections were split into three groups: 1) full-thickness skin ulcer; 2) deep-tissue infection and osteomyelitis; 3) gangrenous lesions. All ulcers in group 1 healed and 92 percent of those in group 2 healed. All people in group 3 healed after surgical excision, debridement of necrotic tissue, and treatment with honey ointment (which also included royal jelly).

Seventy-eight people (ages 10 to 50) with burns on less than 50 percent of the body were split into two groups, one receiving honey dressings, the other silver sulfadiazine (SSD). Average healing duration in honey-treated patients was 18 days, with SSD it was 33 days. Wounds in all who received treatment within 1 hour of the burn and were treated with honey became sterile in less than 7 days. None in the SSD group did. All honey-treated wounds became sterile within 21 days, but only 36 percent of those in the SSD group did within that time span. Outcomes were significantly better for the honey group. There was faster healing, no infection, less scarring and postburn contractures, and significantly decreased need for debridement irrespective of when the patients was admitted for treatment.

A randomized, double-blind, clinical trial among goldmine workers in South Africa was carried out using honey to treat shallow wounds and abrasions. Honey was found to be just as effective as IntraSite Gel in healing. The cost of the honey was approximately 49 cents (South African rand) versus 12.03 for the pharmaceutical.

In a clinical trial using honey to treat labial herpes, the duration of attacks, degree of pain, occurrence of crusting, and mean healing time with honey were found to be 35 percent, 39 percent, 28 percent, and 43 percent better respectively than with acyclovir treatment. With genital herpes the results were 53 percent, 50 percent, 49 percent, and 59 percent better respectively.

Thirty people (20 male, 10 female) with seborrheic dermatitis and dandruff were treated with a topical application of raw honey. The patients had presented with scaling, itching, and hair loss. Diluted raw honey (90 percent honey diluted with warm water into a manageable wash) was used every other day for 4 weeks and left on for 3 hours before rinsing with warm water. Half the patients acted as controls. In all the people using honey, itching was relieved and scaling disappeared, all within 1 week, and hair loss was reduced. Within 2 weeks skin lesions healed and disappeared. The honey-treated patients were treated prophylactically for 6 months afterward with one application of honey per week. None of the 15 patients treated with honey relapsed.

In a clinical trial of 139 children, honey was found to be more effective than dextromethorphan and diphenhydramine in alleviating nighttime cough due to upper respiratory infections. (Other studies have found the drugs and honey to be relatively equal in their effects. Parents, though, have generally reported honey to be better than the pharmaceuticals.)

Honey as a consistent additive to food has shown remarkable results in medical trials. Of one group of 58 boys, 29 were given 2 tablespoons of honey each day (one in the morning and one in the evening), and the other 29 boys were given none. All received the same diet, exercise, and rest. All were the same age and general health. The group receiving honey (after 1 year) showed an 8.5 percent increase in hemoglobin and an overall increase in vitality, energy, and general appearance.

Honey has been effectively used clinically for the treatment of ulceration to the bone the size of a human fist and third-degree burns. Complete healing has consistently been reported without the need for skin grafts and with no infection or muscle loss. Additionally honey has outperformed antibiotics in the treatment of stomach ulceration, gangrene, surgical wound infections, surgical incisions, and the protection of skin grafts, corneas, blood vessels, and bones during storage and shipment.

Honey is also exceptionally effective in respiratory ailments. A Bulgarian study of 17,862 patients found that honey was effective in improving chronic bronchitis, asthmatic bronchitis, bronchial asthma, chronic and allergic rhinitis, and sinusitis. It is effective in the treatment of colds, flu and respiratory infections, and general depressed immune problems.

Results have been good in clinical practice as well. The department of pediatric oncology at Children's Hospital at the University of Bonn regularly uses honey in the healing of wounds impaired by chemotherapy and has found it highly successful.

There have been a number of clinical reports of the use of honey by physicians in the treatment of various wounds:

Treatment of eight patients with leg ulceration used honey. Ulcer size decreased by 60 percent, odor was eliminated, pain reduced.

A chronic wound in a patient with dystrophis epidermolysis bullosa was treated. The wound, despite many treatments, had never closed in 20 years. A honey-impregnated dressing closed and healed the wound in 15 weeks.

Treatment of a patient with longstanding venous leg ulcer resulted in total healing. The honey was effectively antibiotic, anti-inflammatory, and deodorizing.

Six patients with chronic venous leg ulcers who underwent split-skin grafts experienced healing in 22 days without complications.

Two nursing-home patients with pressure ulcers were treated with honey. There was a rapid healing of the ulcers, and pain and odor were significantly reduced.

Twenty-eight cases of Fournier's gangrene were treated. Honey was found to accelerate wound healing in the six patients in whom it was used.

A woman with extensive phlegmonous and necrotic lesions in the abdominal integuments after a traumatic rupture of the colon was successfully treated with honey. Complete wound healing was achieved.

A man with pyoderma gangrenosum and ulcerative colitis (in the tropics) had his skin lesions successfully treated with honey.

Seven people with MRSA-infected wounds were treated with honey after antibiotics failed to eradicate the infection. All were successfully treated.

There have been scores of in vivo studies on the wound-healing actions of honey, with some 600 animals. In the treatment of auricular burn, induced wounds (incision, excision, burn, dead-space wounds), surgical wounds, bacterial infection of burns, burn contraction, and bite wounds, honey was found to be exceptionally effective. Intraurethral honey application healed urethral injury in Wistar male rats. It promotes angiogenic activity in rat aorta. The immune systems of rats fed fennel honey, propolis, and bee venom were more protected against induced staph infection than those of controls. Intraperitoneal honey administration prevents postoperative peritoneal adhesions. Honey promotes intestinal anastomotic wound healing in rats with obstructive jaundice. Following bowel resection, oral honey was effective in stimulating healing and reducing infection.

Honey has been found in vitro to be immune stimulating, skin regenerating, anti-inflammatory, antibacterial, antiviral, antifungal, antioxidant, free-radical scavenging, immunomodulatory, and antimutagenic. Antibacterial activity has been found effective with as little as a 4 percent honey solution. Full strength is better.

Salves made with honey, beeswax, and olive oil have been found effective against staph and *Candida* organisms.

Note: Raw wildflower honey should be used, *not* the clover or alfalfa honey readily available in grocery stores. Alfalfa and clover crops are heavily sprayed with pesticides *and* they do not have the broad activity available in multiple-plant honeys. Further, large commercial honey growers may often supplement their bees' food with sugar water, which dilutes the honey's power. Pure wildflower honey should lightly burn or sting the back of the throat when taken undiluted.

Usnea

Family: Parmeliaceae, but some people insist the usneas are in their own family, the Usneaceae. Most sources consider that to be unacceptable as well as completely wrong. (Fisticuffs at 10:00 P.M.)

Common Names: *Old man's beard or a number of similar phrases to do with hair or beard*

Species Used: There are 600 or so species of usnea. *Usnea barbata* and *U. longissima* are the most common, but any *Usnea* species will do. I prefer the smaller, tufted species (generally *Usnea hirta*) rather than *longissima*; I feel they are stronger in their actions; however, due to the larger size of *longissima*, it is the most commonly harvested species. (The others take hours.) *Usnea barbata* is also fairly good-sized, but there is currently some potential for that species to be banned for use in the United States even though it is a very safe plant (see Side Effects and Contraindications, page 301).

Part Used

Whole lichen.

Preparation and Dosage

It has taken some time to learn how to properly prepare *Usnea* for use. Ryan Drum, an herbalist in Washington State, was most responsible for providing understanding of how to generate the best immune-stimulating activity of the plant.

In essence, the polysaccharides in the inner cortex of the lichen contain the immune-potentiating compounds. These are much more efficiently extracted by heat. Given that the plant possesses a unique synergism—both immune-potentiating and antibacterial, antiviral, and antimicrobial actions—it makes sense, if you are using the plant to treat disease (rather than infected wounds or vaginal infections), to make sure the immune fractions of the plant are extracted along with the antibacterial fractions.

Additionally, while the polysaccharides are water soluble, many other compounds, including usnic acid, are not. The plant needs to be tinctured for optimum outcomes if you are treating disease conditions.

The plant appears rather delicate, but it is not. The plant must be ground well in a grinder or pestle before tincturing. Once it is ground, you will find that you now possess a greenish powder and a bundle of white threads. The white threads are the inner cortex, the green powder the outer sheath.

WOUND POWDER

If you are treating wounds with *Usnea,* run the ground herb through a fine mesh or strainer. You can place the resulting powder directly on the wound or mix with other powdered herbs for a stronger blend. (You will have a bunch of white threads left over.)

TINCTURE

Again, the immune-stimulating polysaccharides are most efficiently extracted with heat. To do this, when you are making your tincture, heat the herb first in the water you are going to use for tincturing. The best way is in a slow cooker (or, failing that, on low heat, covered, overnight in the oven).

Use a tincture ratio of 1:5 (1 part herb to 5 parts liquid). (See chapter 8 for more on this.) The liquid should be composed of half

Properties of *Usnea*

Actions

Analgesic
Antibacterial
Antifungal
Anti-inflammatory
Antimitotic
Antineoplastic (cancer)
Antioxidant
Antiparasitic
Antiproliferative (cancer)
Antiprotozoal
Antiseptic
Antiviral
Drug synergist (potentiates clarithromycin against *H. Pylori*)
Immunostimulant
Inhibitor of biofilm formation

Active Against

Primarily Gram-positive bacteria, and very strongly so, both resistant and nonresistant strains:

Bacillus megaterium
Bacillus subtilis
Bacteroides spp.
Clostridium spp.
Corynebacterium diphtheriae
Enterococcus faecalis
Enterococcus faecium
Listeria monocytogenes
Micrococcus viridans
Mycobacterium tuberculosis
Propionbacterium acnes
Staphylococcus aureus
Staphylococcus simulans
Streptococcus faecalis
Streptococcus mutans
Streptococcus pyogenes

A number of these bacteria cause diseases of the GI tract, others of the skin.

Usnea species have been found active, in a number of in vitro studies, against a few Gram-negative bacteria: *Helicobacter pylori*, *E. coli*, *Yersinia enterocolitica*, and *Proteus mirabilis*. Interestingly, the first three of these cause infections in the GI tract, for which *Usnea* will be useful as it is not a highly systemic herb. The latter bacteria generally cause urinary infections.

Usnea is active against a number of viruses: herpes simplex, polyomavirus (a tumor virus), Junin virus, Tacaribe virus, and Epstein-Barr.

It is active against a number of parasitical disease organisms: *Trypanosoma cruzi*, *Echinococcus granulosus* (and its cysts), and *Toxoplasma gondii.* And some yeasts: *Malassezia* yeasts, *Microsporum gypseum*, *Trichophyton mentagrophytes*, *T. rubrum*, and several *Candida* species.

Usnea and usnic acid are active against a number of cancer cell lines: lung and breast, malignant mesothelioma cells, and vulvar carcinoma cells.

(continued)

Properties of *Usnea*—Continued

Use to Treat

Resistant Gram-positive bacterial skin infections, vaginal infections (as a douche), resistant Gram-positive bacterial or TB infections of the GI tract and throat, fungal skin infections, resistant bronchial and pulmonary infections caused by Gram-positive bacteria or TB, and conjunctivitis (as eyedrops).

Finding *Usnea*

It grows in nearly every forest or orchard if you just look for it. It is widely available on the Internet through herbal suppliers.

water and half pure grain alcohol. So if you have 5 ounces of herb, you will use 25 ounces of liquid—12.5 of water, 12.5 of alcohol.

Put the powdered herb in the slow cooker, add the 12.5 ounces of water, and stir well. It will turn into a kind of mush. Cover and then cook on low heat for 48 hours. Let cool enough to work with it without burning yourself, then pour into a heat-tolerant jar (Mason or equivalent), add the alcohol when the mix is still warm but not hot, and then put on the lid and shake well. Let macerate for 2 weeks, then decant and strain out the herb. Bottle and store out of the light.

Tincture dosage: 30–60 drops, up to 4x daily; or in acute conditions, ½–1 tsp, 3–6x daily.

As a douche: Add ½ ounce tincture to 1 pint water, and mix well. Use as douche or skin wash. Douche twice daily, upon rising and before retiring, for 3 days.

As a wash: For impetigo (staph or strep infections of the skin), put the tincture, or a 1:1 dilution of the tincture with water, directly on the site of infection (using a cotton ball or cloth). Wash the site upon rising and before bed.

As a nasal spray: Combine 10 drops of tincture with water in a 1-ounce nasal spray bottle. Use as needed for bacterial infections of the nose and sinuses.

TEA

Combine 1 tsp herb with 6 ounces hot water; let steep 20 minutes.

For disease prevention or immune stimulation: Drink 2–6 ounces, up to 3x daily.

In acute conditions: Drink up to 1 quart a day.

Note: Usnea is only partially water soluble. To make the strongest tea or decoction: Grind the herb first, then add enough alcohol to wet the herb and let it sit, covered, for 30 minutes to an hour. Then add hot water and let steep for 15 to 30 minutes.

Side Effects and Contraindications

Should not be used internally during pregnancy. May cause contact dermatitis.

Usnea has been found to readily absorb heavy metals in potentially toxic amounts. This has been noted as particularly problematic in extreme northern latitudes. Generally, the amount of usnea taken internally will not contain sufficient amounts of heavy metals to present a problem. In order to avoid problems, harvest usnea at least 300 feet from roads, factories, and polluted areas.

Note: There has been concern expressed in a number of forums about the toxicity of usnic acid. The problem, once more, has arisen through the improper use of an isolated constituent for weight loss. This has led to calls for the banning of usnea as an herb in the United States.

As usual, the promoters of the isolated constituent for weight loss were engaging in practices that are highly questionable ethically. They sold, and heavily hyped, the isolated constituent of usnea, usnic acid, as a weight-loss product. Unfortunately usnic acid in isolation and in large doses is very toxic to the liver. Several people died, others needed liver transplants. As a result the National Toxicity Program recommended a review of the toxicity of not only usnic acid but also *Usnea barbata*. Unfortunately, given the bias of the FDA, the odds are high that *Usnea barbata* will also be found to be unsafe for general use—when it in fact is not.

Usnic acid should never be used in isolation. The usnea lichens, however, are extremely safe for herbal use. More on the controversy can be found in "Safety Issues Affecting Herbs," by S. Dharmananda (at itmonline.org/arts/pas.htm).

Herb/Drug Interactions

Usnea is synergistic with clarithromycin, increasing its effectiveness.

Habitat and Appearance

Usnea grows on trees throughout the world, on every continent. Generally prefers conifers (pine, spruce, juniper, firs), deciduous hardwoods (oak, hickory, walnut, apple, pear, and so on), and the odd variant such as coconut palms.

Collection

Usnea is an extremely prolific though slow-growing, long-lived, gray to yellow-green lichen growing on trees throughout the world. The whole lichen may be harvested at any time. Again, I prefer the small, tiny tufted species that grow in the forests around where I live. They take longer to harvest, but they are not endangered and, I feel, are more potent than *U. longissima* and *U. barbata*.

Endangered status: While *Usnea longissima* is prolific in some areas, in others (California, northeast United States, Europe, Scandinavian countries) it is endangered. Logging and development have destroyed its main habitat, old-growth forests. It is also very sensitive to pollution and climate change. *U. longissima* is the *Usnea* species most often sold by herbal companies and most commonly wildcrafted because of its size, which ranges up to 3 feet in length. This species should *not* be sold by commercial companies nor bought from them by anyone. It should be harvested only for personal use from regions where it is in abundance. Again, *any* species of *Usnea* will do.

Lichen Chemistry

Usnic acid is the main constituent that everyone talks about; it is a potent chemical, highly antibacterial. *Usnea* species contain anywhere from 0.22 percent to 6.49 percent usnic acid. *U. longissima* is reported to have the most usnic acid content. However, many of the other constituents of the usneas are strongly antibacterial; hirtusneanoside and vulpinic acid are a couple of them.

In addition to usnic acid, usnea contains vulpinic acid, protolichesterinic acid, a number of orcinol derivatives, longissiminone A and B, glutinol, ethyl hematommate, friedelin, beta-amyrin, beta-sitosterol, methyl-2,4-dihydroxy-3,6-dimethylbenzoate, barbatinic acid, zeorin, ethyl orsellinate, 3-beta-hydroxy-glutin-5-ene, oleanolic acid, methylorsellinate, benzaldehyde, dibenzofuran, anthraquinone, hirtusneanoside, menegazziaic acid, stictic acid, glyceryl trilinolate, numerous polysaccharides including isolichenin, raffinose, numerous phenolic compounds, usnaric acid, thamnolic acid, lobaric acid, stictinic acid, and a lot of other stuff. About 50 percent of the plant is water-soluble polysaccharides.

One of the more interesting developments in the medicinal chemistry of lichens is the recognition that lichens often harbor diverse fungi that themselves are highly bioactive. Some of the fungi are harbored on the outside surfaces, others are lichenicolous—they fruit from the lichen thalli. But some of the most interesting are endolichenic fungi—they live within the lichen thalli. One lichen, *Letharietum vulpinae,* has more than 1,000 fungal strains living on and within it. Usneas also contain numerous fungal strains, and these strains also possess bioactivity when used medicinally. An associated fungus from *Usnea cavernosa,* for example, has been found to contain some unusual compounds: corynesporol, dehydroherbarin, and herbarin. Dehydroherbarin potently inhibits the migration of cancer cell lines in vitro and, along with herbarin, possesses weak antiamoebic and antimicrobial activity.

Again, plants (or lichens as in this case) are exceptionally complex; their full chemical range is unlikely to ever be completely understood. Nevertheless, they are potently synergistic in their chemical actions. Some of the actions attributable to usnea are likely from associated fungal strains.

Traditional Uses of Usnea

Commonly called old man's beard, a name derived from its appearance, usnea is a lichen that grows on living and dead trees throughout the world. It is quite common in North America, Europe, Asia, and Africa (less so in South America and Australia), and this wide availability and its strong antibacterial properties make it a significant herb in treating resistant bacteria.

Usnea ranges in size from a small tuft to large hanging strands resembling hair. It may be a gray-green in the smaller species and a mild yellow-green in the larger hanging strands. As a lichen, the herb is in actuality a symbiote composed of two plants intertwined. The inner part of the plant (the cortex) is a thin white thread (a filamentous fungi) that, when wet, stretches like a rubber band. The outer part—the sheath or thallus—(an algae) gives the herb its color and grows round the inner rubber-band-like cortex. The algae (cyanobacteria in some types of lichen) is a photobiont, providing photosynthesis for the symbiotic organism. The filamentous fungi (a mycobiont) provides water and minerals.

The distinctive method of identifying usnea is wetting it and stretching it to see if it is springy and, when it snaps apart, looking for the distinctive white thread of the inner plant. This inner band is strongly immune stimulating; the outer sheath is where most of the plant's (yeah, I know, it's a lichen) other actions (e.g., antibacterial) come from.

Usnea has been traditionally used throughout the world for skin infections, abscesses, upper respiratory and lung infections, vaginal infections, and fungal infections. The lichen (*U. longissima* in this case), sometimes soaked in garlic juice or a strong garlic decoction (sometimes not), is an older medical method of treating large gaping wounds in the body (Spanish moss was also used this way). The moss absorbs blood and provides, along with the garlic, antibacterial, anti-inflammatory, antiseptic, astringent, analgesic, and wound-healing actions directly inside the wound.

Usnea is used for abscesses in veterinary practice in Canada.

AYURVEDA

There are some 30 species of usnea that grow in India, among them *Usnea complanata*, *U. ghattensis*, and *U. emidotteries*. They have been used in traditional practice, but I can find little on the particulars.

TRADITIONAL CHINESE MEDICINE

Generally called *songluo* (sometimes *haifengteng*), usnea species, primarily *diffracta* (sometimes *longissima*), are used to clear heat in the body and to clear the liver of sthenic heat. Usnea is used for the treatment of cough due to hot phlegm, conjunctivitis, headache, carbuncle, and lymph node TB. It is considered to be antipyretic, mucolytic, detoxicant, anti-inflammatory, and analgesic.

WESTERN BOTANIC PRACTICE

Of ancient use in Europe but unknown in the United States until relatively recently. Indigenous cultures in the Americas used the usnea lichens primarily for wound dressings.

Scientific Research

Most of the scientific studies have focused on usnic acid—essentially trying to develop pharmaceutical drugs given the constituent's strong antibacterial activity. Nearly all the work has been in vitro. There have been no clinical trials using the herb and very few in vivo studies. There have been a few clinical trials in China using either usnic acid or its sodium salt, sodium usnate.

In clinical trials with sodium usnate in the treatment of pulmonary and intestinal TB, clinicians found that there was rapid improvement of cough, anorexia, fever, and diarrhea.

Microscopic examinations after 14 days were negative for the tubercule bacillus. In one trial with 30 cases of pulmonary TB using sodium usnate, 24 were cured, 1 had marked improvement, 5 improved. Average treatment length was 71 days, dosage was 30 mg three times daily.

In another trial, 203 cases of chronic bronchitis were effectively treated with either usnic acid or sodium usnate. The compounds showed strong antitussive, expectorant, and antiasthmatic effects.

In the treatment of surgical suppurative wounds, sodium usnate stimulated the separation of necrotic tissue and the growth of new tissue. It was strongly disinfectant and anti-erosive, stimulating the healing of second- and third-degree burns, cervical erosion, and cracked nipples. It was found effective in the treatment of trichomonas vaginitis.

In veterinary practice a 1 percent alcohol solution of usnic acid was used effectively for treating suppurative conjunctivitis, endometritis, mastitis, and suppurative wounds in cows and horses.

Usnic acid, at a dose of 20 mg once or twice daily for 6 days, then 10 mg daily for an additional 25 days, stopped the development of experimental TB in guinea pigs. It stopped the development of pathological tissues in spleen, liver, and lungs of guinea pigs who had usnic acid added to their diet.

Two studies focused on the gastric-mucosa-protective actions of two of the plant's constituents: usnic acid and diffractaic acid. Diffractaic acid inhibited gastric mucosal lesions, oxidative stress, and neutrophil infiltration. Usnic acid prevented indomethacin-induced gastric ulcers in mice and was found to be highly antioxidant. A water extract of *U. longissima* also prevented that form of induced gastric ulcer in rats and was found to be a strong antioxidant. A methanol extract of *U. longissima* prevented pulmonary thrombosis in rats, and prevented platelet aggregation in vitro. In other studies, the anti-inflammatory activity of various usnea species has been found to be as strong as, and sometimes superior to, that of phenylbutazone and hydrocortisone hemisuccinate, the analgesic action as strong as that of noraminophenazone, and the antipyretic activity as strong as (or stronger than) that of aminophenazone. Usnea is active in both acute and chronic inflammation in rats and significantly accelerates skin wound healing, again in rats. The methanolic extract of *U. ghattensis* was found to be hepatoprotective in rats against ethanol-induced toxicity.

Usnea possesses antioxidant actions, is a strong superoxide and free radical, and is active in preventing lipid peroxidation. *Usnea barbata* extracts inhibit prostaglandin E2 synthesis and COX-2 expression in vitro and appear to be protective of keratinocytes when exposed to ultraviolet B. Usnea possesses strong wound-closure activity in vitro. Both usnic and diffractaic acid have shown antipyretic and analgesic actions in vivo.

Usnea and usnic acid, in vitro and in vivo, inhibit cancer cell formation and proliferation in breast and pancreatic cell lines and in induced colorectal cancer in rats. Crude extracts of *Usnea fasciata* showed up to 90 percent inhibition of sarcoma 180 and Ehrlich tumor cells in vitro.

In general, there has been little clinical research on the effectiveness of traditional uses of usnea. In clinical practice, however, I have found the herb very effective for topical use in the treatment of resistant bacteria, as a douche, and for urinary tract infections.

Antivirals

A large number of structurally unique antiviral compounds from medicinal plants (herbs) have been identified. The advantages of natural compounds are fewer side effects in comparison to orthodox medical drugs, and the production of synergistic effects for a more positive treatment outcome.

—Kaio Kitazato et al., "Viral Infectious Disease and Natural Products with Antiviral Activity"

There has been very little work in the popular press (especially in the West) on herbal antivirals—and most of what has occurred is embarrassingly poor. There are a number of reasons for this.

The field of antivirals itself, whether medical or herbal, is in relative infancy, which partly explains the problems in the literature. The general overemphasis on bacteria as disease-causing agents in the public (and medical) mind, irrespective of culture, also contributes to the problem. Then, there is the nature of viruses themselves and the difficulty of actually creating effective pharmaceutical antivirals. There are, in fact, very few pharmaceutical antivirals compared to antibiotics—generally people only hear of two: ribavirin and Tamiflu (oseltamivir). This is a much reduced pharmaceutical armamentarium compared to the scores of antibiotics that are common in most people's vocabularies; *penicillin* is, I suspect, a word known to most of the world's population.

Most of the scientific research (at least in the past and especially in the West) on viral treatment has been focused not so much on finding effective antivirals but on vaccines. And researchers have been pretty successful at this over the past 50 years—the eradication of smallpox is one of the great triumphs of technological medicine, as is the polio vaccine. So, we have vaccines now for an increasing number of viral diseases: smallpox, polio, measles, hepatitis B, influenza strains, and so on.

Thus, the focus of most medical viral research, in contrast to bacterial research, has been on vaccines. In consequence, few people ever think of *antivirals* as a specific entity that might be useful in medicine; *antibiotic* is a word that everyone has heard of, has used, and knows. The word *antiviral* is not. Nevertheless, antivirals do exist in great quantity in the world. In plants.

Viruses are an intimate part of life on this planet and every life form, including plants, has experienced viral infections during the billions of years there has been life here. Plants, the finest chemists on Earth, have created, just as they have in their dealings with infective bacteria, a wide range of compounds in response to viral infection. Similarly to plant antibiotics and bacteria, while *all* plants have created a variety of compounds to protect them from viruses, some, when used as medicines, tend to be a great deal more effective than others. The trick is to find which are the most effective, the most reliable, the most potent.

The strongest herbal antivirals are more easily revealed *if* the medicinal plant world is examined through a number of lenses and then, afterward, those findings are cross-correlated. The lenses I used for this book are:

- The history of the plants' uses in community medicine in whatever cultures have access to them—what some people call indigenous or traditional practice
- The history of the plants' uses in developed medical systems such as traditional Chinese medicine, Ayurveda, or Western botanic practice
- Contemporary uses of the plants among community herbalists;
- Outcome experiences among contemporary peoples who are using the plants for healing
- Scientific study of the plants' medicinal actions as viewed through in vitro, in vivo, and human clinical study[11]

- A factor that I have found a primary indicator of strong medicinal action—the invasive status of the plant. For, interestingly enough, many of the strongest antibacterial and antiviral plants are invasives.[12]

And while I am not yet using this as a primary identifier, it is becoming evident that many of the most potent antivirals are also synergists. This is a relatively new category of herbal medicines—in the West at any rate. Synergists are plants that, when used with other medicinal substances (herbs, supplements, pharmaceuticals), through a variety of mechanisms, *increase* the potency of those substances against microbial pathogens. A number of the herbs in this book are very potent synergists.

The plants that show strong activity when viewed through a majority of these lenses end up on the list. It is then the final factor comes into play: access. There are some truly magnificent antiviral and antibacterial plants in Africa, South America, and China that simply are not to be had in the Western world, no matter how actively they are sought—unless you travel to those places. The plant medicines in this book tend to be somewhat easy to find and that is important. It's no good to know of a great antiviral if you can't find any of it to use as medicine.

Many of the antiviral herbs in this book are broad-spectrum antivirals, that is, they are active against a wide range of viruses. I tend to think of these as the most potent antivirals in a general sense (e.g., Chinese skullcap). There are others with a more narrow range but that are very antiviral for specific viruses (e.g., ginger, elder). *All* of them have shown potent activity in historical use across long timelines. *All* of them have been found effective in contemporary usage. Nevertheless, these are not the only antiviral herbs there are. These are just the ones that I have used with success, the ones that have shown up the most strongly in this examination of them, in this particular year, for these particular viruses.

Again, there are *a lot* of great herbal antivirals out there; over time, more will be understood and discussed *and* used as medicine. So, don't think these are the only ones to use; they are just the ones that I have used the most, that have the deepest historical use, that have the greatest presence in the literature, and that have the best research on them.

The Top Seven Antiviral Herbs

Chinese skullcap
Elder
Ginger
Houttuynia
Isatis
Licorice
Lomatium

In this section I include the top seven antiviral herbs, five honorable mentions, one truly important supportive herb for nearly all viral infections, and two very useful antiviral supplements. Here they are.

Chinese Skullcap

Family: Lamiaceae or is it the Labiatae, or are those synonyms? (I feel another taxonomic rant coming on.)

Species used: *Scutellaria baicalensis* is the primary species used in China and the one meant when Chinese skullcap is talked about (and the one this monograph will focus on). It most definitely does not mean the American skullcap, *Scutellaria lateriflora*—or any of the other American species. For reasons I will discuss in this monograph I strongly suggest you *not* use *S. lateriflora* as a substitute for treating viral infections. Note that *Scutellaria macrantha* is a synonym for *S. baicalensis*.

Common names: Legion for the many different skullcaps, however for *S. baicalensis*: English—Chinese skullcap, baikal skullcap, scute (really hate that one—"you are so *scute*"), golden root (really like that one). Chinese—huang qin. (Ban zhi lian is the Chinese for *S. barbata.*)

Part Used

The root and the root only—generally only from plants older than 3 years. There is reason to believe that the increase in pharmacological action of

Chinese skullcap over the usual American species used as medicinals is due to the difference between using the root in Chinese practice and the leaf in American practice. As far as I know there has been virtually no examination of the root as a medicinal in any of the Western species.

There are, as well, no *substantive* studies on the difference between roots and leaves of any species of skullcap as regards their chemical compounds. The few I have seen that touch on it do show substantial differences between the leaf and the root and this really does need to be explored, especially if American herbalists are insisting that the American skullcaps are interchangeable with the Chinese. (And some of them are.) However, as some researchers have commented, "The results showed that the components and relative contents of the essential oils among flowers, stem, leaves, roots, and seeds have significant differences."[13] This is, of course, true of nearly all plants on Earth and one of the most basic understandings of herbal medicine.

Preparation and Dosage

Medicinals prepared from this plant are a bit hard to find in the United States, though not impossible. (I know only a few sources for Chinese skullcap root tinctures, but hundreds for the American leaf tinctures.)

TINCTURE

If making it yourself, again, use the root. After harvesting the root, cut it into easy-to-use pieces, let it dry in a cool, shaded location, then powder the root pieces and tincture them. The ratio should be 1:5 (one part herb, five parts liquid), with the liquid being 50 percent alcohol, 50 percent water. Take 1/4–1/2 tsp 3x daily. In acute conditions, double that. Remember: If using for CNS damage or encephalitis, you want to flood the brain and CNS with the compounds over a long enough time period to sharply reduce the inflammation and protect and restore the neural structures of the brain. I think the tincture best for this purpose.

For sleep: The plant and root are high in melatonin, so they can help with sleep. If you are using it for that, take just before bedtime, 1/2 tsp of the tincture.

Exploring *Scutellaria* Species

The Chinese do use another skullcap species, *Scutellaria barbata*, which is considered much weaker but still specific for certain conditions. There is, however, an important distinction about the medicines made from these various skullcap species. The most studied species, and the one considered the strongest, is *S. baicalensis* and with that species the Chinese use the root *only*. (See Part Used, page 310, and Western Botanic Practice, page 323.) With *S. barbata* and the various American species the aerial parts are used. This difference, aerial part versus root, makes *all* the difference in the medicinal impacts of the plants. The leaves just aren't as strong, especially for viral infections. After several millennia of use, the Chinese consider all other skullcaps to be inferior to *S. baicalensis* in their medicinal effects. And I assume (makes an ass of u and me) that they must have tried the roots of the other species and found them not as strong; nevertheless, what if they didn't . . . ? Perhaps we in the West should do a little experimenting with some roots of our own.

Now, that being said, there are 200, or 300, or 350 species in the genus *Scutellaria* . . . taxonomists are absolutely positive about those figures. Many of the various skullcaps are used similarly as medicines in the regions in which they grow; most of them contain the same constituents. However, there has been very little study on species other than *S. baicalensis*. As illustration, there are over 600 journal articles on PubMed on *S. baicalensis* (and its major constituents), but only 88 on *Scutellaria barbata*, just 24 on *Scutellaria lateriflora* (the main American species), a mere eight on *S. viscidula*, six on *S. indica*, four on *S. racemosa*, three on *S. galericulata*, and one each on *S. regeliana*, *S. incana*, *S. taiwanensis*, and *S. austrotaiwanensis*. There's even less on the others.

Some studies have shown that *S. baicalensis*, *S. barbata*, *S. lateriflora*, and *S. racemosa* have similar constituents in their roots—but then the roots of those other species are almost never used in medicine making,

Fresh leaf tincture: If you want to use the aerial parts of the plant, get or make a 1:2 tincture of the fresh leaves and stems. Tonic doses run from 10–30 drops up to 6x daily, but I have taken up to 1/2 ounce of the tincture at a time (of the American skullcaps anyway) without side effects; there apparently are none even at high doses.

so there is no way to know if in practice they are as potent as the Chinese skullcap root. (If you try roots other than those of *S. baicalensis*, let me know how they work. Let's start something here.)

S. lateriflora, a.k.a blue skullcap, mad dog skullcap, Virginia skullcap, hoodwort (along with *S. galericulata*, i.e., marsh or common skullcap), is the species most commonly used in the United States. *S. racemosa* is more common in South America, and *S. barbata* is the other main species used in traditional Chinese medicine. Constituent studies have found that those three varieties all contain baicalin, baicalein, scutellarin, wogonin, melatonin, and serotonin—the constituents considered to be the most active in Chinese skullcap. Other studies, on the roots of *S. viscidula* and *S. amoena*, found very similar constituents in *them*. It does seem that most of the species contain baicalein, baicalin, and wogonin at the very least—though the amounts in differing species have not been *comparatively* studied to any degree.

However, one study that did examine the constituent levels in the roots of *Scutellaria planipes* and compared them with *S. baicalensis* found that the root constituents were very similar in nature, degree, and number, and were equally active as antibacterials and antiallergics. Another study (Chinese) showed that the root of *Scutellaria rivularis* stimulated the production of monoclonal antibodies to encephalitis virus E protein, just as the root of *S. baicalensis* does.

So . . . it may turn out that many of the skullcaps can be used interchangeably with *S. baicalensis* as medicines—but *only* if the roots are used, which they generally aren't. Again, I think the roots of various skullcap species should be explored to find out if they can be used interchangeably with the Chinese variety. So, if you are using the American skullcaps, try harvesting some of the root of whatever species you are growing, and make it into medicine and find out how it works. (Then e-mail me.)

POWDER

The Chinese dosages are large, as usual, generally 3–9 grams at a time. Most of the clinical studies and trials used similar dosing. If you are using capsules, this is the dosage range you should be exploring, divided into three equal doses every 4 hours or so. Capsules are pretty much impossible to find, but you can get the powdered herb fairly easily. I would use 1 tsp of the powdered root 3–6x daily.

Note: The herb reaches peak levels in the plasma and body organs in about 1 hour and only lasts in the body for about 4 hours, so you really do need to dose about every 3 to 4 hours.

AS A WASH

The fresh juice of the plant can be used as an eye wash for eye infections, as can the cooled infusion or decoction of the root.

Side Effects and Contraindications

Side effects from skullcap are rare, mostly gastric discomfort and diarrhea. It should not be used during pregnancy. Caution should be exercised if you are taking pharmaceuticals as it can increase the bioavailability of the drugs, thus increasing their impacts. It may interact additively with blood-pressure-lowering drugs. Type 1 diabetics should exercise strong caution with the herb as it can affect insulin and blood sugar levels.

Herb/Drug and Herb/Herb Interactions

Lots. Chinese skullcap is a synergist, perhaps as efficacious as licorice, ginger, and piperine, and should probably be added to that category of herbs. Among other things it inhibits the NorA efflux pump, which inactivates some forms of antibiotic resistance. Like the other synergists I know of, it is also a strong antiviral, which is beginning to stimulate speculation. Nevertheless, the herb strongly affects pharmaceuticals and herbs taken along with it.

Baicalein, one of the major compounds in *S. baicalensis*, is synergistic with ribavirin, albendazole, ciprofloxacin, and amphotericin B.

S. baicalensis is strongly inhibitive of CYP3A4, a member of the cytochrome oxidase system. And this inhibition is dose dependent; the more you take, the more it is inhibited. CYP3A4 is a type of enzyme, strongly present in the liver, and is responsible for catalyzing reactions involved in drug metabolism. Many of the pharmaceuticals that are ingested are metabolized by the CYP3A4 system, meaning that some portion of the drug is inactivated, usually by being altered to another molecular form. With pharmaceuticals, the normal dosage range you are given is adjusted to take this metabolization into account. If you are using Chinese skullcap, then less of the pharmaceutical is going to be metabolized. In some cases this will make the impacts of the drug stronger, with the bioavailable dose higher. With other drugs it is the metabolites created by CYP3A4 that are active in the body. In this circumstance, since the herb inhibits CYP3A4, the metabolites of the pharmaceutical you are taking will be reduced in degree and have *less* effect in the body. Acetaminophen, codeine, cyclosporin, diazepam, erythromycin, and so on are all affected in one way or another. The herb does affect the amount of antibiotics that enter the system.

To make things more complicated, one of the herb's constituents, oroxylin A, is a strong P-glycoprotein inhibitor. P-glycoprotein is strongly present in the blood-brain barrier, the lining of the GI tract, renal tubular cells, capillary endothelial cells, and the blood-testes barrier. It reduces the amount of substances that cross over those barriers in order to protect what is on the other side. (This is why berberine is mostly confined to the GI tract.) P-glycoprotein inhibitors allow more of a substance to cross barriers that are high in P-glycoprotein. That means that if you are taking skullcap, any substance taken with it will end up in higher levels in the bloodstream, thus increasing its impacts in the system.

This means that Chinese skullcap will act through two different mechanisms to increase drug and herb uptake in the body.

Also, because cancer cells use P-glycoprotein as a form of efflux pump in order to eject drugs designed to kill them from the cancer cells, Chinese skullcap will increase the effectiveness of anticancer drugs by inhibiting P-glycoprotein-mediated cellular efflux. Paclitaxel uptake, for example, was increased over twofold when administered with oroxylin A.

All this applies equally to herbs and supplements that you take along with skullcap. If you are using this herb along with licorice, which is also a potent synergist, through its own mechanisms (as is ginger), everything else you take will be much more potent and pronounced in the body. (This is one reason why licorice and skullcap are considered such important medicines in Chinese practice and why they are commonly added to many herbal combinations.) *Keep this in mind.*

Habitat and Appearance

This plant likes to grow in wettish, sandy, and rocky-type seashore or creekish locations in the wild, from sea level to 6,000 feet in altitude. It is native to east Asia: China, Mongolia, Japan, Korea, Siberia, Russia. (Many of the skullcaps like it wet and tend to grow along streambeds and creeks.)

It's a perennial growing up to a foot in height (hardy to zone 5). It flowers in August, seeds are ready in September. The plants are hermaphrodites and are pollinated by insects.

And I have to admit, Chinese skullcap is beautiful, the lanceolate leaves a vibrant green, the flowers the most delicious purple. The flowers are supposedly shaped like little skullcaps—people used to wear similar, though larger, ones in the Middle Ages . . . so they say. But *they* also said that the Earth was flat and that pharmaceuticals were safer than herbs and that there was no one on the grassy knoll.

I think Chinese skullcap the most beautiful of the skullcaps. Richo Cech, at Horizon Herbs, describes it like this: "The purple flowers are like schools of dolphins breaking through green waves in a summer sea." Beautifully put and very apt.

It is commonly grown in the United States as a garden plant due to its resistance to drought and cold. It can survive nearly anything. (And so can you if you use it as medicine.)

Cultivation and Collection

Sow seeds outdoors in late spring (or in a pot or cold frame in early spring). The seeds generally sprout within 10 to 20 days. Separate

(continued on page 320)

Properties of Chinese Skullcap

Actions

Chinese skullcap is a broad-spectrum antiviral. It inhibits hemagglutinin and neuraminidase, inhibits viral replication, suppresses viral gene expression, reduces viral RNA in infected cells, inhibits viral fusion with cells, protects cell membranes from virus-initiated cytokines, reduces the expression of the viral matrix protein gene, interferes with viral entry by interacting with viral envelope proteins and cellular CD4 and chemokine receptors, regulates the innate antiviral immunity of the host by modulating cytokine production at the time of viral insult, lowers host cell membrane fluidity thus inhibiting the formation of virus-induced membrane pores in host cells (which in itself stops viral entry into host cells), inhibits viral release from infected cells, inhibits viral cytokine cascades, increases apoptosis in infected cells, stimulates innate resistance to viral infection, promotes the development of monoclonal antibodies to encephalitis virus E protein, and is directly virucidal.

***S. baicalensis* is also:**

Anodyne
Antianaphylactic
Antiangiogenic
Antibacterial
Anticholesterolemic
Anticonvulsant
Antidiarrheal
Antidysenteric
Antifungal
Antihypertensive
Anti-inflammatory
Antimetastic
Antioxidant
Antispasmodic
Antitumor
Astringent
Cholagogue
Diuretic
Expectorant
Febrifuge
Hemostatic
Hepatoprotective
Nervine
Neuroprotective
Sedative (mild)

Active Against

This plant is a major broad-spectrum antiviral with a wide range of activity against viruses. It is active against:

Adenovirus (3 and 7)
Avian infectious bronchitis virus
Coliphage MS2
Coxsackie B virus (3, 4, and 5)
Epstein-Barr virus
Hepatitis A
Hepatitis B (resistant and nonresistant)
Hepatitis C
Herpes simplex viruses
HIV-1
Human T cell leukemia virus
Influenza A (H1N1, H3N2—resistant and nonresistant)
Influenza B
Measles virus

(continued)

Properties of Chinese Skullcap—Continued

Active Against—Continued

Mosaic virus
Parainfluenza viruses (in general)
Polio virus
Porcine reproductive and respiratory syndrome virus
Respiratory syncytial virus
SARS coronavirus
Sendai virus (parainfluenza type 1)
Vesicular stomatitis virus

Chinese skullcap is synergistic with other antivirals (as is licorice, they should be used together if possible). It does have a fairly wide range of action against bacteria and some other microbes, but the effects are variable; by this I mean it is not primarily a major systemic antibacterial as cryptolepis is, for example. Many of its antibacterial and antiviral effects tend to be not direct, that is, through antimicrobial actions, but sideways through the stimulation of the body's own immune responses, reduction of cytokine cascades, or protection of host cells. Antibacterially, the herb does have some really potent effects against some bacteria, particularly staph organisms, resistant and nonresistant. It is also nicely active against mycoplasma and some others such as klebsiella organisms. In general, the herb can be used as a primary adjunct to any treatment of resistant bacterial disease as it is synergistic with both herbs and pharmaceuticals, will markedly reduce cytokine cascades along a rather broad range, and has its own antibacterial actions to add to the mix.

The entire list of organisms it is active against includes:

Actinomyces viscosus
Angiostrongylus cantonensis
Bacillus subtilis
Bacteroides melaninogenicus
Bordetella pertussis
Candida albicans
Chlamydia trachomatis
Corynebacterium xerosis
Diplococcus pneumoniae (a.k.a. *Streptococcus pneumoniae*)
Enterococcus faecalis
Escherichia coli
Helicobacter pylori
Klebsiella pneumoniae
Lactobacillus plantarum
Micrococcus sedentarius (a.k.a. *Kytococcus sedentarius*)
Microsporum audouinii
Microsporum canis
Mycobacterium smegmatis
Mycobacterium tuberculosis
Mycoplasma hominis
Neisseria meningitidis
Proteus vulgaris
Pseudomonas fluorescens
Salmonella spp.
Shigella dysenteriae
Shigella flexneri
Staphylococcus aureus (resistant and nonresistant strains)
Staphylococcus epidermidis
Staphylococcus hominis

Streptococcus hemolyticus
Streptococcus mutans
Streptococcus sanguis
Toxoplasma gondii
Trichophyton violaceum
Ureaplasma urealyticum
Vibrio cholerae

Use to Treat

Viral infections, especially pandemic influenzas and encephalitis, respiratory infections, pneumonia, infections that affect the central nervous system (essentially *any* infection that has accompanying meningitis or encephalitis such as viral encephalitis or meningitis, mycoplasma, Lyme, viral and bacterial CNS infections, and so forth), impaired brain function, fevers, intermittent fevers, GI tract disorders with accompanying inflammation, diarrhea and dysentery, hepatitis, nephritis, urinary tract infections, nervous irritability, epileptic seizures, convulsions, and sleep disruptions. You can also use Chinese skullcap as supportive therapy in cancer.

Note: The root tincture of this plant is extremely specific for reducing inflammation in the brain, reducing the cytokine cascades initiated by viral and other microbial agents in the CNS, and alleviating CNS impacts of those microbes. It should be used in any treatment of viral or bacterial CNS infection.

Other Uses

Some cultures use the leaves as a steamed vegetable; the dried leaves are common as a tea.

Finding It

The best root tinctures come from Elk Mountain Herbs (elkmountainherbs.com) and Woodland Essence (woodlandessence.com). The powdered root can be purchased from 1stChineseHerbs.com (1stchineseherbs.com). You can get really good seed from Horizon Herbs (horizonherbs.com).

the sprouts when large enough to handle. Grows easily in sunny locations in ordinary garden soil that remains a bit moist. Soil needs to be well drained in sun or partial shade. It is hardy to zone 5 and survives dips as low as –10°F. It will survive drought pretty well once established.

You can harvest the aerial plant at flowering and make a fresh plant tincture (if that is how you are going to use it). But, again, the roots are more potent. They should be harvested after 3 years of growth (or more), cut to usable lengths, and dried carefully in the shade (though the Chinese do it in light sun). Once well dried, they should be stored in plastic bags in a plastic tub in a coolish location in the dark. Spring roots are more potent (as usual). Good-quality organic freshly dried roots should be yellowish, even a bright yellow, in color. Most of the imported Chinese roots tend to be a bit oxidized, the yellow color fading a bit. Poorly prepared or severely oxidized roots will be greenish or even black in color. Don't bother with them.

You can, if you wish, and if you are a fan of the aerial tinctures of the skullcaps, harvest the root *and* aerial parts of the plants and make a tincture from both, separately.

Plant Chemistry

More than 295 different compounds have been found in *S. baicalensis* so far. The six most important are presumed to be baicalein, wogonin, oroxylin A, baicalin, wogonoside, and oroxylin-A 7-O-glucuronide. All are strongly anti-inflammatory, antiviral, and antitumor in action. Some of the other important compounds are considered to be scutellarin, naringenin, apigenin, luteolin, melatonin, and serotonin. All are strongly biologically active. All are synergistic with each other.

Until relatively recently it was supposed that melatonin was not present in plants, only in animals. (Wrong, as such definitive pronouncements often are.) A number of plants are now known to produce melatonin (and serotonin). Chinese skullcap has some of the highest levels (7 mcg/g) so far discovered (some rice family plants have more). Studies have found that the melatonin in plants is strongly present in the plasma of animals that ingest them and that it does bind to melatonin-binding sites in the brain, creating specific effects. (One being helping with sleep cycle normalization.) Melatonin is highly active in the brain; it detoxifies hydroxyl radical, hydrogen peroxide, nitric oxide, peroxynitrite anion, peroxynitrous acid, and hypochlorous acid.

Melatonin is an upstream antioxidant; many of its metabolites, created when our bodies process it or when the plant compound detoxifies oxidants, are also potent antioxidants. It is also synergistic with a number of antioxidant enzymes and other antioxidants such as vitamin C, vitamin E, and glutathione. Melatonin is active at both the micro and macro levels, exerting antioxidative effects at the level of cells, tissues, organs, and organisms. It is a very unique substance, much different than other antioxidants—and not well understood even now. Not only does it work to repair other biomolecules but under in vivo conditions it is four times more potent than vitamin C and E in protecting tissues.

Melatonin is intimately involved in the regulation of people's circadian rhythms, including their healthy sleep cycle. Part of the reason that the sleep cycle is interrupted as people age (and during inflammatory infections in the CNS) is that the oxidative events in the brain are higher and the levels of melatonin (and its regulatory effects) are much lower. Using plants high in melatonin (which is more effective than using melatonin supplements) can normalize the circadian rhythms, including the sleep cycle, and reduce inflammation in the brain and CNS.

The constituents of Chinese skullcap do enter the plasma in substantial amounts. Baicalein is strongly concentrated in the lungs, brain, and hippocampus, wogonin in the liver, kidneys, and lungs. Baicalin concentrates in the brain, specifically in the striatum, thalamus, and hippocampus. Many of their metabolites are strongly present in those locations as well. These all provide potent CNS protection and amelioration of existing infection dynamics.

Traditional Uses of Skullcap

Outside traditional Chinese medicine and American Eclectic practice the uses of the skullcaps among people around the world are fairly uniform.

The Tibetans, for instance, use five species, including *S. barbata*, but their usages are interesting. Usually the juice of the plant or root is used for wounds, fevers, indigestion, and gastric troubles. Essentially this is showing both antiviral, antibacterial, and fever-lowering actions (and yeah, GI tract actions).

The indigenous tribes of the United States used eight different skullcaps including *S. lateriflora*. Again, the usage range is interesting. The usage range is a bit broader than the Tibetan and includes, for the aerial parts, decoctions and infusions for sore eyes, chills and fever, colds, coughs, heart troubles, and as laxatives. Indigenous tribes also used root decoctions and infusions as emmenagogues and abortifacients to expel afterbirth, as antidiarrheals, to treat the nerves and breast pain, as kidney medicine, to prevent smallpox, to prevent colds and flu, and to keep the throat clean. Again, the range of broad uses shows antiviral and antibacterial uses, fever-lowering actions, GI tract dynamics, female reproductive tract action, and a tiny bit of nervine action.

What is interesting about this is that the nervine use of the plants among traditional cultures is almost entirely absent. Given the historical American use of the plant, for centuries, is the leaves as a primary nervine agent and that there is pretty much no indigenous use (out of millennia of their contact with the plants) of skullcaps along that line, well, it's intriguing.

The indigenous uses, when examined in depth, do however show a difference in action between plant and root, and the root actions tend to mirror those of the Chinese skullcap.

AYURVEDA

Several skullcaps are listed in my older Ayurvedic herbals, but there is nothing on use.

TRADITIONAL CHINESE MEDICINE

Skullcap is one of the 50 fundamental herbs of Chinese medicine and has been in use for more than 2,000 years. It is one of the most widely used herbs in Chinese medicine.

It is considered bitter and cold and to dispel heat (fever reducer, anti-inflammatory), to expel damp heat (e.g., lung infections), to be a detoxicant, to stop bleeding, and to prevent abnormal fetal movements (which I think, in part, is an indication of its effectiveness for fetal mycoplasma infections). It is specific for fever, cough, pneumonia, hemoptysis, jaundice, hepatitis, dysentery, diarrhea, bloody stool, vexation, insomnia, headache, enteritis, acute conjunctivitis, uterine bleeding, abnormal fetal movements, hypertension, carbuncle, and furuncle. And, again, there is nothing in traditional use that emphasizes its nervine actions.

Most of the scientific studies on the plant have been conducted in China.

WESTERN BOTANIC PRACTICE

The Europeans tended to use *S. galericulata,* the American Eclectics *S. lateriflora,* and it is probably from the Europeans that the Americans got their usage range for the plant. Both were used similarly primarily as tonic, nervine, and antispasmodic herbs. The Eclectics considered their species specific for chorea (involuntary movements), convulsions, tremors, intermittent fever, neuralgia, to help sleep, and for nervous afflictions such as delirium tremens and hysteria with involuntary muscle movements. It was used in all cases of nervous excitability, restlessness, and wakefulness, especially after acute or chronic illness. It was considered to be a cerebrospinal specific. The usual dose was half an ounce of the recently dried herb in half a pint of boiling water. The herb was considered to lose its effectiveness if kept too long in the dried state.

The English use was similar with the addition of uses for nervous headaches, headaches from coughing, St. Vitus' dance (has *nothing* to do with rock and roll), hiccups, and tertian ague.

This is in fact the usage range still employed by American herbalists, and very few of them, unless using the Chinese skullcap, use the root. In current American practice skullcap is considered to be a mild, soothing, and reliable nervine, less stimulating than pasque flower and without the druggy feeling that accompanies valerian if used for sleep.

Scientific Research

There are a lot of studies on Chinese skullcap: in vitro, in vivo, and human and clinical trials and studies. The compounds in the root are, not surprisingly, synergistic with each other. All that have been studied are potently antiviral, anti-inflammatory, antioxidative, and free radical scavenging. Wogonin is the most potent nitric oxide (NO) inhibitor, oroxylin is the most potent in inhibiting lipid peroxidation, baicalein appears to be the most potent antiviral compound. Together they produce effects beyond the individual constituents. (In one study the bacteriostatic effect of the root decoction was compared with that of both baicalin and debaicalin. The root decoction was the strongest.)

The root has strong cytokine impacts, reducing NO, iNOS, IL-3, IL-6, IL-17, COX-2, PGE2, NF-κB, IkappaBalpha (IκBα), IL-1α, IL-2, IL-12, TNF-α, VEGF, TGF, IFN-γ, and tends to upregulate IL-10. It inhibits the production of IgE thus suppressing the expression of histamine. It has especially strong impacts in the spleen. It attenuates the activity of c-Raf-1 kinase, MEK1 and MEK2, ERK-1 and ERK-2, p38 MAPK, and JNK.

IN VITRO STUDIES

Flavones from the root are strongly neuroprotective. Baicalein strongly inhibits the aggregation of neuronal amyloidogenic proteins and induces the dissolution of amyloid deposits. Wogonin stimulates brain tissue regeneration, including the differentiation of neuronal precursor cells. Baicalin promotes neuronal differentiation of neural stem/progenitor cells by modulating p-STAT3 and bHLH (basic helix-loop-helix) protein expression.

Wagonin is neuroprotective against cerebral ischemic insult, and at tiny micromolar concentrations completely suppresses the activity of NF-κB, and inhibits the migration of microglial cells to ischemic lesions, thus reducing inflammation at the site of injury. It inhibits the movement of the cells in response to the chemokine MCP-1.

Baicalein attenuates the induced-cell death of brain microglia in mouse microglial cells and rat primary microglia cultures by strongly inhibiting NO through the suppression of iNOS. The compound inhibits NF-κB activity in the cells as well.

Four compounds in the root inhibit prostate cancer cell proliferation.

Baicalin suppresses IL-1ß-induced RANKL (receptor activator of NF-κB ligand) and COX-2 production at a concentration of 0.01 mcg/ml. The longer the constituent is applied, the stronger the effect. Used on human periodontal ligament cells it shows highly protective effects.

Baicalein inhibits IL-1ß- and TNF-α-induced inflammatory cytokine production from human mast cells via regulation of the NF-κB pathway. It inhibits NF-κB and IκBα phosphorylation.

Baicalin promotes repair of DNA single-strand breakage caused by hydrogen peroxide in cultured fibroblasts.

The plant inhibits aromatase, thus reducing the conversion of androgens into estrogens.

There are scores of other in vitro studies such as these, all showing potent anti-inflammatory and cytokine-modulating actions of the herb and its constituents.

IN VIVO STUDIES

In rats, oroxylin A markedly enhances cognitive and mnestic function in animal models of aging brains and neurodegeneration. Baicalein is anticonvulsive, anxiolytic, and sedative in rats.

Flavonoids from the stems and leaves of *Scutellaria baicalensis* improve memory dysfunction and reduce neuronal damage and levels of abnormal free radicals induced by permanent cerebral ischemia in rats. Other studies have found that the compounds can enhance and improve learning and memory abilities and reduce neuronal pathological alterations induced by a variety of chemicals in mice.

S. baicalensis reduces symptoms associated with chronic cerebral hypoperfusion (and chronic lipopolysaccharide infusion), including spatial memory impairments, hippocampal MAPK signaling, and microglial activation.

Baicalein protects mice hippocampal neuronal cells against damage caused by thapsigargin (TG) and brefeldin A (BFA). The constituent reduces TG- and BFA-induced apoptosis of hippocampal cells, reduces the induced expression of endoplasmic reticulum stress-associated proteins, and strongly reduces the levels of MAP kinases such as p38, JNK, and ERK. It reduces ROS accumulation and levels of MMPs. It strongly protects the mitochondria from oxidative damage.

A number of in vivo studies have found baicalein to reduce both edema and intracranial hypertension during brain infection due to pertussis bacteria. It also inhibits the neurotoxic action of kainic acid in the rat brain.

Scutellaria baicalensis (in combination with bupleurum) is strongly neuroprotective against iron-reduced neurodegeneration in the nigrostriatal dopaminergic system in rat brains, showing it to be useful for treating CNS neurodegeneration.

When mice, subjected to transient global brain ischemia for 20 minutes, are treated with baicalein (200 mg/kg once daily), neuronal damage is minimal compared to controls, and MMP-9 activity in the hippocampus is inhibited. Pretreatment with baicalein prevents the damage.

Wogonin is also strongly protective in the brain. In rats damaged by either four-vessel occlusion or excitotoxic injury (systemic kainate injection), wogonin confers protection by attenuating the death of hippocampal neurons. It inhibits the inflammatory activation of the microglia by inhibiting iNOS, TNF-α, NO, IL-1ß, and NF-κB. In vitro studies have found that lipopolysaccharide-activated macrophages are protected similarly.

An ethanol extract of *S. baicalensis* has been shown to prevent oxidative damage and neuroinflammation and memory impairments in artificial senescence mice (mice that get old very fast artificially—to study aging). The hippocampus and the mitochondria are strongly protected and neuroinflammation sharply reduced. Expressions of COX-2, iNOS, NO, PGE2, Bax, cleaved caspase-3 protein are all reduced. Bcl-2 was increased. The effects are dose dependent and are most effective at 100 mg/kg (that would be 7 grams for a 150-pound person, just in the dosage range usually used in China).

Baicalin reduces the severity of relapsing-remitting experimental autoimmune encephalomyelitis induced by proteolipid protein in a mouse model of multiple sclerosis. All the histopathological findings decrease in the mice given the extract.

Baicalin has a protective effect against induced encephaledema in neonatal rats; glutamate and glutamic acid levels decrease, reducing excitotoxicity, and GABA (gamma-aminobutyric acid) increases.

Baicalin, administered to mice infected with influenza virus, increases survival time, eliminates the virus from the lungs, reduces hemagglutination titer and infectivity in the lungs, and reverses pneumonic pathological changes.

Baicalin protects rat brains from pertussis bacilli-induced brain edema. It is 20 times more potent than deferoxamine in reducing lipid peroxidation, and is markedly better at reducing edema, chelating iron, and activating SOD.

Baicalin reduces intracranial hypertension from pertussis bacilli in rabbit brains better than tetramethylpyrazine. The pathologic alterations in the brain are significantly reduced by the use of baicalin.

Baicalin, given to pregnant rats, increases the lung surfactant phospholipids in the fetus and accelerates fetal lung maturation.

Baicalein has been found to be antidepressant in animal models of depression. It reverses the reduction of extracellular ERK phosphorylation and the level of BDNF (brain-derived neurotrophic factor) expression in the hippocampus of CMS (chronic mild stress) model rats.

Oral administration of baicalein in mice infected with Sendai virus results in a significant reduction of viral titers in the lungs and a reduction in the death rate.

Oral administration of baicalein in mice infected with influenza A virus shows significant effects in preventing death, increasing life span, inhibiting lung consolidation, and reducing lung virus titer in a dose-dependent manner. Amounts as low as 1.2 mcg/ml of baicalin (the metabolite of baicalein) result in significant inhibition of the virus. (Note: Plasma levels of baicalin from the ingestion of skullcap root are significantly higher than this after dosing with 3–9 grams per day.)

Baicalein is highly synergistic with ribavarin against H1N1 influenza. The combination produces much better outcomes in mice infected with influenza A than ribavirin alone.

Baicalein and wogonin inhibit irradiation-induced skin damage by suppressing increases in MMP-9 and VEGF through the suppression of COX-2 and NF-κB.

In mice infected with hepatitis C virus and treated with *S. baicalensis,* the serum virus content of the mice decreases after treatment with the herb.

S. baicalensis treatment inhibits passive cutaneous anaphylaxis and reduces histamine release in rats receiving intradermal injections of anti-DNP (dinitrophenol) IgE. It is also effective in reducing IL-6 and TNF-α in mouse models of pelvic inflammatory disease. The herb is both anti-inflammatory and antinociceptive.

S. baicalensis extract stimulates the formation of red blood cells and their precursors under conditions of cyclostatic myelosuppression and sleep deprivation.

There are many more studies than these; this just gives a very good overview of the range of actions of the plant and its constituents.

HUMAN STUDIES

The root decoction has been used in a number of clinical situations in China to effectively treat scarlet fever, chronic bronchitis, and epidemic cerebrospinal meningitis. (Details are unfortunately sketchy.) The herb is almost always used in combination, so individual studies are few. But there are some here and there:

Sixty-three people with bacterial meningitis were split into two groups; 32 were treated with both an antibiotic and baicalin, 31 were treated with an antibiotic alone. The inflammatory cytokines in the CNS were markedly lower in the baicalin group, mortality was significantly reduced, and the symptom picture was markedly improved.

Sixty patients with pulmonary infection were treated with either piperacillin sodium or injection of *Scutellaria baicalensis*. Before treatment there was no difference in clinical data. Treatment outcomes were similar in both groups.

In 63 children with upper respiratory infections (51 upper acute, 11 acute bronchitis, 1 tonsillitis) 51 benefited from using the decoction of the root; temperature normalized in 3 days.

A decoction of *S. barbata* was used with 14 women with metastatic breast cancer in a trial at the Memorial Cancer Institute (Hollywood, Florida), as supportive therapy to normal chemo and radiation. The study authors commented that the herb was safe, well tolerated, and showed promising clinical evidence of anticancer activity.

A 12-week randomized trial of *Scutellaria baicalensis* and *Acacia catechu* in Alabama in the dietary management of knee osteoarthritis found that the placebo group had a much higher incidence of respiratory infections than the herbal group. (No mention is made in the study abstract of the herbal compound's effects on osteoarthritis.) However, another study in Arizona, in a randomized, short-term, double-blind event, found that the same mixture (code-named flavocoxid) was as effective as naproxen in controlling signs and symptoms of osteoarthritis of the knee. There was, again, a higher incidence of other effects in the nonherbal group, including more edema and musculoskeletal discomfort.

Russian studies with the root found that it increased the relative number of T lymphocytes in lung cancer patients receiving antineoplastic chemotherapy. Another Russian study with 88 lung cancer patients found that ingestion of a powdered extract of *S. baicalensis* root was accompanied by increased hemopoesis and an increase in immune markers.

There have been a number of combination therapies using *S. baicalensis* in China in the treatment of minimal brain dysfunction, bacillary dysentery, eye infections, and leptospirosis. All showed good outcomes.

Baicalin has been used effectively in treating meningitis, infectious hepatitis, hepatitis B, and acute biliary tract infections. In one study, baicalin was used in the treatment of bacterial meningitis. Sixty-two people with the condition were separated into two groups; one received an antibiotic, the other baicalin. The levels of TNF-α, NO, IL-1 in both plasma and cerebrospinal fluid were monitored. The cytokines were significantly lower in the baicalin group, and mortality was significantly reduced as well.

S. baicalensis has also been found to ameliorate irinotecan-induced gastrointestinal toxicity in cancer patients.

The tincture of *S. baicalensis* was used effectively in treating 51 cases of hypertension. Blood pressure levels dropped with accompanying symptom improvement.

Elder

Family: Caprifoliaceae or maybe Adoxaceae, the literature isn't clear.

Species used: There are five or maybe 30 species of elders. Taxonomists are not sure . . . again. They used to be in the Caprifoliaceae or honeysuckle family (the taxonomists, not the elders) but DNA scientists got involved again and decided that, no, *this* is not a honeysuckle, as anyone looking at a taxonomist can plainly see. It is an Adoxaceae. The suffix *-aceae*, by the way, indicates the members of a plant family, and the prefix *adox-* is the descriptive of that family. *Adox* comes from the ancient Greek and means "not according to right reason, absurd, opposed to common sense." The taxonomists are, however, pretty sure that the elders are in the genus *Sambucus*.

Roughly, there are two forms of elder, the red and the blue. (The red are smaller, conservative, and somewhat toxic, the blue are larger, more progressive, and people friendly.) Some people (i.e., taxonomists) say, inevitably, that there are really *only* two species of elders: *Sambucus nigra* (the blue/black berry group) and *Sambucus racemosa* (the red berry group). So, *Sambucus canadensis* is not really *Sambucus canadensis* anymore but *Sambucus nigra* ssp. *canadensis*. Because of the (reputed) higher toxicity of the *S. racemosa* group, the blue species are the ones usually used for medicine. (Though, to be clear, indigenous peoples use every species irrespective of berry color for both medicine and food. And the medicinal uses are very similar, irrespective of color. Please see the preparation section for more on this.)

And just to make it more complicated, there are two species that have white berries (red, white, *and* blue—they are a patriotic genus): *S. australasica* (okay, okay, the berries on this one *are* kind of yellow, hence the name *yellow* elderberry) and *S. gaudichaudiana*, the Australian white elder.

The most commonly used medicinal species is *Sambucus nigra*, which grows throughout North America, Europe (into the Scandinavian countries), western Asia, northern Africa, New Zealand, Australia, many Pacific islands, and so on. It's an invasive, making it dear to my heart.

Even though the other blue-fruited species are not quite as widely established, being, I guess, less invasive, most, if not all, of them can be used as medicine: *S. australis* (southern elder, found in South America and Australasia), *S. canadensis* (American elder, found in eastern North and Central America to Panama), *S. cerulea* (blue elderberry, found in western North America), *S. ebulis* (European dwarf elder, found in central and southern Europe, northwest Africa, southwest Asia), *S. javanica* (Chinese elder, found in southeast Asia, Malaysia, the Philippines), *S. lanceolata* (Madeira elder, found on Madeira island), *S. melanocarpa* (found from the western United States into Canada), *S. mexicana* (Mexican elder, found in the Sonoran desert), *S. neomexicana* (New Mexico elder, found from the western United States up into Canada), *S. palmensis* (Canary Island elder),

S. peruviana (Peruvian elder, found in South America), *S. simpsonii* (Florida elder, found in the southeastern United States), *S. velutina* (velvet elder, found in southwestern North America). The only blue/black berry species I know personally are *S. nigra, S. cerulea, S. mexicana,* and *S. canadensis*. I've used them all for medicine at one time or another. They seem pretty interchangeable to me.

No matter where you live, you will probably be able to find an elder someplace near that you can use as medicine. However . . . I will talk mostly about *Sambucus nigra* with a bit on the others here and there.

Synonyms: The genus and its various species are in flux due to taxonomitis, and synonym accusations are flying everywhere. For sure, *S. cerulea* and *S. caerula* are probably the same plant, but then again, maybe they are really *S. mexicana,* or maybe *S. nigra,* or something.

Common names: Legion. Everyplace the plant grows, it has a local name. The plants have been used in food, medicine, and crafts since people have been. In the West, elder—reputedly from the fact that if you use the plant as medicine, you will become one. Some say that the plant itself is an elder to the plant communities around it, a gateway to the depths of the plant world.

Parts Used

Most commonly the berries and flowers but the leaves, bark, and root all have a long tradition of medicinal use. You will often see warnings not to use the inner bark, leaves, or root of this plant, but that is a rather recent phenomenon (since 1910 or so). Historically, they have all been used with good effect. (The secret is in the preparation.)

This particular genus, like some others such as comfrey, is suffering from a certain, unfortunately common, form of phytohysteria known as "this-plant-will-poison-you-because-someone-got-sick-from-it-once." So, *don't use herbs!* Most of us who are members of the neo-herbal renaissance have suffered its effects in one form or another. Nevertheless, I have used most parts of this plant for medicine and found them all beneficial. It just depends on what you are needing, why, how you prepare it, and the dose.

More on this next. Kind of a rant actually.

Preparation and Dosage

Most people these days are working with the berries only (a very few American herbalists use the flowers medicinally, but not normally as a primary treatment approach). Usually what is used, especially in Germany—and probably because of German approaches everyplace else—is a standardized liquid extract (or standardized lozenge) or some other variation of the berry juice: expressed juice, syrups, a tea, or a juice decoction. Dosage usually being a cup of the tea or a glass of the juice or a couple tablespoons of the syrup for influenzal infections for reducing fever. I don't agree with this limitation on the medicinal use of the plant but then I tend to be grumpy.

Rant: In reading articles about elder it is common to continually be exposed to the phytohysterical pronouncement that the plant is poisonous. Well, it is not. The various parts of the plant are emetic (and purgative if you take enough) *if used fresh*. That simply means that you will feel nauseated and possibly vomit if you take too much. The flowers are the least likely to cause any nausea or vomiting and thus are considered safe by most phytohysterians everywhere. The berries may cause some degree of vomiting and nausea if you take too much at once (see the discussion of side effects on page 337 for an amusing anecdote) or if you are especially susceptible to the compounds in the plant. But they are fairly safe in that respect, so the hysteria alert level is only Orange with the berries. The rest of the plant, however, is in the Red alert level range, and from reading about it, I am pretty sure the plant could kill off most of the Western hemisphere with just a few drops of the leaf tincture.

Here is a sampling. This first one is from *HerbalGram* and runs mild on the Panic Index:

> Improperly prepared elder preparations can induce toxic effects in humans through poisonous alkaloid and cyanogenic glycosides that are found in the roots, stems, leaves, bark, and unripe berries. Effects of cyanide, also known as hydrocyanic acid (NCN [sic, this should be HCN]), on humans include nausea, vomiting and diarrhea, as well as central nervous system and respiratory depression, and general lethargy.[14]

Here's one, however, that tips the needle into the Red, and it is not uncommon: "One word of caution: don't eat raw elderberries. They are poisonous! In the raw form, they produce cyanide."[15] I can just hear the exclamation points on that last word, can't you? There's about eight of them! Then there is this one: "Elderberries must never be eaten raw. All parts of the plant contain the toxin hydrocyanic acid which is destroyed by cooking."[16] (That last bit is the important part, and I will get back to it in a minute.)

The hysteria about the red berry varieties is even more pronounced because the HCN in them is in higher quantities. Nevertheless, they can be used as well . . . if you treat them just as the black berry varieties, discussed below, are. Essentially you *heat* them.

The cyanogenic compounds in elder, which are also strongly present in cherries and apples, for example, *can* poison you . . . if you take them as isolated compounds. But the "poisoning" they are talking about here merely consists of nausea, weakness, dizziness, and vomiting—the usual things that happen when you eat something that disagrees with you. The plant is *not* a poisonous plant the way hemlock is (see Socrates for more on this); it's an emetic (vomit) and in large doses a purgative (poop) and the word "poisonous" really should not be used to describe it.

The plant uses these compounds to protect itself from predators, especially vegetarians. When plant-eating animals forage too much on elder, they get dizzy and weak, and if that does not stop them and they keep at it, they eventually wander away to vomit. At that point, they pretty much forget about eating altogether, which is the point. If the plant were poisonous, it would just kill the animals, but it doesn't. In fact, it likes to be foraged a bit; it helps the growth and health of the plant (and the health of the animal). However, the compounds in the plant that cause vomiting occur in just the right amounts to stop foraging when the limit of the plant's tolerance is reached. The cyanide compounds in plants such as elder are normally held separately in different parts of the plant. When the animal chews the leaves, the crushing of the leaves, bark, and so on frees the compounds and combines them, making, in the case of cherry, cyanide gas. Both this and HCN slow (or even paralyze) respiration by inhibiting an enzyme in the mitochondria of cells, cytochrome c oxidase. This is what makes the eater dizzy and a bit breathless. It is also why cherry bark is such a good herb for coughs, or why it has antitussive actions (this is basically what *antitussive* means). In essence, it paralyzes the lungs, which is how it stops hacking coughs. If understood properly, elder can also be used as a potent antitussive herb for unremitting coughs.

Raw kidney beans (and a few other beans) are also considered poisonous unless they are cooked sufficiently by briskly boiling for at least 10 minutes—after having been soaked for 5 hours. (Slow cookers that never reach high temperatures can increase the toxicity fivefold.) But you never see the same kind of phytohysteria about kidney beans as you do with elder. People are simply told to cook them sufficiently to avoid the problem. So, let's stop it all right here and begin talking about what is true for this plant.

Boiling the plant (that is, the leaves, berries, bark, or root), beginning with cold water and raising the heat, for 30 minutes will reduce the cyanide (or HCN) content to nearly nothing. (With cassava, for instance, the fresh leaves contain 68.6 mg/kg of HCN. Boiling them, beginning with cold water, for 30 minutes reduces this to 1.2 mg/kg, making them safe for use. If you start with hot water, the reduction is only to 37 mg/kg.) The longer the boil, the lower the cyanide compound content.

This is why, in the Asian traditions, they use the stems, leaves, and roots (of the *red* species no less) with impunity. To treat broken bones 1/2 to 1 ounce of the leaves is boiled in 3 cups of water until reduced to 1 cup, which is then consumed. And this is continued for 2 weeks. The root is used similarly for arthritic conditions. The boil time on this is long, much longer than 30 minutes. They are producing what is called a concentrated decoction.

The many chemical compounds contained in the plant are much stronger in the leaves, stems, and roots, and by this I am talking about not just the HCN content but the antiviral compounds, the antibacterial compounds, the anti-inflammatory compounds, and so on. The best medicines are going to come from a much more sophisticated preparation process of the plant than any I have so far read of. To elucidate . . .

The leaves, like peach leaves, are a very reliable nervine. That is, they relax the nervous system. That is why the herb was used for epileptic fits and various dementias and uncontrollable movements by both European and American herbalists for centuries. Dosage of the fresh leaf tincture runs from 5–10 drops, taken no more than each hour (though some people can take much higher doses—in fact up to 1 teaspoonful every hour).

Because the fresh stem, leaf, and root can cause nausea, they also cause sweating. This helps lower fevers and is very useful during viral infections. A tincture of the stem can be used to initiate sweating if you take just enough to cause that and not enough to start vomiting. This varies for each person but in general, the dosage range is similar to that of the fresh leaf tincture. (I haven't yet worked with the root and so can't comment on it. However, the Asians use it, as a concentrated decoction, for arthritic inflammation and, given its constituents, it would be very good for that.)

The flowers are best if they are prepared as a hot infusion, covered. That is, put 1 ounce of the flowers, dried or fresh, in a quart of hot water, cover, and let sit until cool. This retains the essential oil compounds of the flowers in the liquid, and they have unique antiviral qualities themselves. You can drink as much as you wish of it.

The berries are fine, but the seeds possess HCN and this is what makes some people vomit. So nearly all sources recommend cooking them first. The following is a very good recipe.

Elderberry Syrup for Colds and Flu

INGREDIENTS

- 1 cup dried elderberries (or 2 cups fresh)
- 2 quarts water
- 20 cups sugar (yes, yes, I know)

To make:

If you are using dried elderberries, soak them overnight in the refrigerator in the water. In the morning, put the pot on the stove and bring the contents to a boil. Once boiling, reduce the heat to a simmer, and cook until the liquid is reduced by half. (Hours.) Do *not* skim the surface of the liquid; this keeps the resins in the syrup, which you want to do. When the liquid is reduced by half, remove from the heat, let cool, then strain through a wire strainer, mashing the remaining liquid out of the berries with a strong spoon. Throw the berries away, return the liquid to the pot, set it over medium heat, and add the sugar, stirring until it is completely dissolved. Let cool.

The amount of sugar in the syrup will stop it from spoiling. Bacteria cannot live in high-sugar-content solutions such as honey. If you don't want this much sugar, you can use half as much, but you should add 20 percent alcohol to keep the mix from going bad.

To use:

Dosage for adults is 2–4 tablespoons every 2 to 4 hours during the early stages of a cold or flu infection. This is what is called a concentrated decoction and it is pretty good, if used at the first signs of infection.

If the flu gets established, use this syrup along with the influenza protocol in chapter 2 or, at the very least, the fresh ginger juice tea on page 118. If you'd prefer an elderberry-only treatment, you can add the syrup to 8 ounces of an infusion of the leaves and drink every 3 hours or so. I would also use 8 ounces of the flower infusion and 5–10 drops of the leaf tincture on the same time schedule.

If you are using the fresh juice, which many do, it will be less strong than the syrup, so you will need more. Just test it to make sure you are not easily nauseated.

It is possible, with practice, to create a mixture based on this type of formulation that would be a powerful treatment for respiratory viral infections, one much more sophisticated than just the syrup. It would be strongly antiviral, strongly anti-inflammatory, and potently analgesic. For example:

Antiviral Elder Recipe

INGREDIENTS:

- 1 cup dried elder leaves
- 1/2 cup dried elder stems
- 2 1/2 quarts water
- 1 ounce elderberry syrup (see recipe on page 335)
- 1 ounce fresh elder leaf tincture
- 1 ounce elder stem bark tincture

To make:

Powder the dried leaves and stems as finely as possible in a blender or grinder. Place in a pot with the water and bring to a boil. Reduce the heat to a simmer and cook until the liquid is reduced by two-thirds. Remove from the heat and let cool. Press the decoction through a cloth to remove the plant matter. Add the elderberry syrup and tinctures to the liquid and stir well.

To preserve this, you may need to add sugar to the stem/leaf decoction after you press it. If so, reheat, add enough sugar to bring the sugar content up to 65 percent or so, and let cool before adding the rest of the ingredients. However, you can also refrigerate it, or add enough alcohol to bring the alcohol content up to 20 percent, in order to preserve it.

To use:

Take 2–4 tablespoons every 2 to 4 hours, less if you feel nauseated. Start slow and work up.

Caution

I have seen people eat handfuls of ripe elderberries or drink copious amounts of the fresh-juiced berries without nausea *and* I have seen one person eat a small handful of ripe elderberries or drink a small amount of the juice and vomit explosively. *There seems to be a wide range of sensitivity to the HCN in the plant.* And there is HCN in the fresh tinctures that has not been removed by heating. If you are going to use the antiviral elder recipe above—or any of the fresh leaf and stem tinctures—I recommend that you test your sensitivity by beginning with small doses and working up until you find your nausea level. The majority of people appear able to take the herb with impunity.

Also note that the fresh juices of the leaves, the stems, and the roots are potently emetic. If you need to vomit, for whatever reason, they can be used in small doses for this purpose.

Plants harvested near roadways and industrial sites have been found to have much higher levels of heavy metals than those in other locations. Careful where you harvest.

Side Effects and Contraindications

Sometimes . . . diarrhea, nausea, vomiting, depending on the dose, what part of the plant you are using, how it is prepared, and your individual biological response to the medicinal. There are few reports of side effects from these plants except for that.

From individual reports, *S. mexicana* berry appears to be a bit more nausea-inducing than the other varieties of blue/black berry species. There is one report of a group of people drinking juice pressed from "the berries, leaves, and stems" (Juice from the leaves and stems? Are these crack babies?), and 11 of them, within 15 minutes, experienced weakness, abdominal cramps, nausea, and vomiting. Eight of them were taken (by helicopter for god's sake!) to the hospital, where the physicians remarked on the dangerousness of self-medicating and the natural world in general (especially the intersection of the two). "All recovered quickly." Well, I guess so. Look, it will just make you vomit and only then if: 1) you take too much, or 2) you have an individual reaction to the plant, or 3) you take too much of the fresh or raw leaves, stem, root, or, sometimes, the uncooked berries. Once the stuff is out of your system, that's it. No more trouble.

Because the individual response to the herb varies so widely, you should start with low doses and work up. Some people can take large amounts—that is, handfuls of raw (or dry) berries all day long, or large doses of the leaf tincture, while with others, 10 ripe, raw or dried, berries will cause nearly immediate vomiting.

Herb/Drug and Herb/Herb Interactions

None have been noted, but speculation abounds that elder may exert additive actions when combined with laxatives or diuretics or decongestants or various jams and jellies (producing sugar overload, just an FYI on that one). A couple of reports say that, in rats, the herb interferes with the impacts of phenobarbital and morphine, reducing their effects.

Alternatives: Poke root, *Phytolacca americana*, has a number of similarities to elder including its medicinal actions and the hysteria about being poisonous. The plant (all parts: leaves, roots, berries) contains a tremendously potent antiviral compound, pokeweed antiviral protein (PAP), that is broad-spectrum against a wide range of viruses (and other antiviral compounds as well). Used in its purified form, it has inactivated the HIV virus in mice, making them HIV free. The poke plant itself could very well be a potent broad-spectrum antiviral, and it should be examined in some depth for this use. As well, the root is a very strong lymph system herb, one of the few that I know of besides red root, so it also helps clear the lymph system of viral and bacterial debris and potentiates the actions of the nodes, spleen, and so on. I suspect that poke, as a medicinal plant, can be prepared identically to elder in order to use the plant as a reliable antiviral. Because the plant also has major impacts on the spleen and lymph system, that would make it a primary plant to use for viral encephalitis.

Eating Fresh Berries

Because the fruits contain potently active antioxidants, if you juice the berries in the presence of oxygen (essentially in your kitchen or herb room), many of the constituents will combine with oxygen as the cell walls are broken, reducing the potency of the compounds. Eating the berries fresh eliminates this problem.

Habitat and Appearance

Most people describing elder say it is a largish shrub, occasionally a small tree. But all the elders I have known look like trees to me and pretty much to everyone I know who has seen a live one. (Well, okay, *S. canadensis* is more bush-like; it does stay pretty small. And, well, *S. neomexicana* is pretty bush-like, too, I guess.) I have seen *S. cerulea* up to 40 feet tall, and sources say others in this genus can reach 50 feet. I just can't get the descriptive "small" from that. But I guess when they were young . . .

The branches of the tree/bushes have leaves that are pinnate, meaning for every leaf on one side of the stem, there is another opposite, and in spite of the fact that everyone I know calls these leaves they are really leaflets, I guess; the whole stalk that has leaves on it is a pinnate leaf, or something. Anyway, once seen never forgotten. The leaflets usually are a bit serrated along the edge. However . . . one species, black lace elder, a developed species, has leaves a bit more "lace-like." It's an ornamental, if you like that sort of thing, but not really a member of the medicinal group, historically speaking. I don't know if it is usable medicinally.

The flowers form an umbel (flattish umbrella-like cluster), often the size of an adult hand or larger. They produce black or blue or purplish or black/blue/purplish berries when ripe (except for the red/white/yellow berry species, which I am not going to go into here). In some species, the flowers are usually white (occasionally pink) and possess a marvelous smell. All the ones I use usually smell heavenly. But in some species they reputedly smell fetid. The flowers are upright on the stems in very prolific clusters. The berries, when ripe, are heavy and hang down from the weight.

The bark is very rough and corrugated when older. I've never harvested the root, so don't know what it looks like (yet). It is reported to be a potent emetic, so, if you need to vomit . . . and we all need to sometime or another . . . that's the ticket.

S. nigra grows in pretty much any kind of terrain: from floodplains to forest gaps to suburbs to industrial wasteland. The only limit seems to be highly shaded areas; it needs some sun to be happy. I have seen various *Sambucus* species growing from sea level to over 9,000 feet in altitude, in wet locations, in dry locations, in hot, rarely cold climates, in extremely cold climates (in Canada, for example), in wilderness, and in cities. It's a great invasive medicinal.

Cultivation and Collection

Richo Cech, of Horizon Herbs, my go-to guy for reliable information on growing medicinals, recommends that you take the dried berries, soak them overnight, "smash them, and remove the seeds. Sow in outdoor conditions, in pots or flats, and expect germination in the spring. . . . The best conditions for germination are cool, moist shade. . . . Elderberries will not grow properly in sterile soil. Sow seeds in very rich and composty soil medium. . . . Once germinated, the seedling grows very rapidly into a handsome bush or small tree. Grow out in a shaded place in pots for a year before transplanting to final location." The flowers appear in about 3 years and are normally pollinated by beetles and flies of various sorts with a few bees thrown in for good luck.

The flowers are collected in full bloom (June/July), the berries when ripe (August/September), and either dried out of the sun and stored in plastic or glass containers in coolish, dark locations or used fresh in tinctures, cordials, cough syrups, and so on. The leaves can be picked at any time and tinctured fresh or dried for use later, with the same storage conditions. The inner bark is treated similarly.

Plant Chemistry

The elders contain several hundred identified compounds including fairly high levels of phosphorus, vitamins A, B_6, and C, and most if not all the amino acids. They are also heavy in polyphenols and anthocyanins. The main anthocyanins are cyanidin 3-glucoside (Cy3G), cyanidin 3-sambubioside, cyanidin 3,5-diglucoside (Cy3,5dG), and cyanidin 3-sambubioside-5-glucoside. These have a wide range of effects; cyanidin 3-glucoside, for example, is a rather potent anticancer agent. They are all highly antioxidant. Fruits of the plants contain from 360–1,300 mg/100 g and from 270–660 mg/100 g of CY3G and Cy3,5dG, respectively.

As with all plants, there are variations in chemical profiles even among different plants of the same species. Nevertheless, all elders (red and black berry types) contain very similar chemical profiles. All elders are particularly high in compounds with a wide range of antiviral activity. To elucidate further . . .

They contain a unique group of compounds called ribosome-inactivating proteins (RIPs). There are two known types of these proteins, types 1 and 2. Until recently the main ones known were type 2 RIPs such as ricin and abrin. All are extremely toxic. In contrast, those in elder are *not* toxic, putting them in a unique chemical class of their own.

S. nigra bark contains a complex grouping of type 2 RIPs such as nigrin b, basic nigrin b, SNA, SNA 1′, and SNLRP. The berries contain nigrin f and nigrin s. Leaves of the dwarf elder, *S. ebulis*, contain type 2 RIPs ebulin 1 and ebulin r1 and r2 as well as type 1 RIPs called ebulitins. The fruits contain a type 2 RIP called ebulin f. These ebulins are strongly antiviral with low toxicity and represent a novel antiviral mechanism in plants—they essentially use these compounds to protect themselves from plant viruses. As researchers have noted, "Biochemical and molecular studies have shown that the elderberry tree expresses a complex mixture of type-2 RIPs and/or lectins in virtually all tissues . . . [and] the antiviral activity of RIPs against plant viruses is well-documented."[17] But these compounds also have activity against a wider range of viruses such as HIV and influenza.

The plants are also very high in flavonoids that have been found to bind to H1N1 virions, inactivating them. Once the viruses are bound, they can't infect host cells. Elder flavonoids have a very strong affinity for influenza viruses, somewhat like a magnet and iron filings. The degree of inhibition of these flavonoids is similar to that of Tamiflu.

Specific compounds such as apigenin, beta-sitosterol, betulin, caffeic acid, chlorogenic acid, cyanin, ferulic acid, glycyrrhetic acid

(continued on page 345)

Properties of Elder

Actions

In my opinion this herb is a narrow-spectrum antiviral but a fairly good one in its range. (I am starting to suspect its range is much greater than any of us realize, however.) Currently, I think it the least strong of the herbs listed in this section, but I suspect that is because of the failure to commonly use the leaves and bark as antivirals. The flowers and berries are most commonly used, and they appear to be the weakest parts of the plant. Nevertheless, the berries do possess some good activity against, primarily, influenza viruses (and some other enveloped viruses, especially respiratory) *and* the plant is a moderate invasive and broadly available throughout the world. If you have nothing else handy for a severe respiratory infection, use it. For some people it works very well, especially if you use the herb *right at the beginning of an influenza infection*, just when that tingle in the bones begins.

As an antiviral, elder inhibits viral replication, inhibits neuraminidase, reduces hemagglutination, binds influenza viruses thus inhibiting them from infecting host cells, contains nontoxic type 2 ribosome-inactivating proteins, is directly virucidal, inhibits maturation of viruses, is a depurinating agent—with depurinating activity against both viral nucleic acids and infected host cell ribosomes—and protects against viral infection if taken prophylactically.

It is also antibacterial (directly and through anti-quorum-sensing activity), antifungal, analgesic, anti-inflammatory, antinociceptive, anticancer, antiangiogenic, antiteratogenic, diaphoretic, diuretic, prostaglandin synthesis inhibitor, antipyretic, antioxidant (the berries have more antioxidant strength than vitamins C and E), and a moderate immune stimulant.

Active Against

As an antiviral, elder is primarily active against enveloped viruses (see Plant Chemistry, page 340). The flowers, berries, leaves, and bark all have a range of activity against microbial pathogens; however, the berries have been the most exhaustively tested. Still, in spite of the hysteria about using the bark and leaves, they are also potently antimicrobial though more needs to be done in looking at just *what* range of microbes they are active against and *how* they are to be prepared for use. I suspect the antimicrobial actions are consistent among the different parts of the plant, but no one has really explored that to any extent. However, a look at the plant chemistry reveals that all parts of the plant contain compounds specifically active against enveloped viruses; these are not just confined to the berries and flowers. And *the compounds are much stronger in the leaves, bark, and roots.* Given the historical importance of the plant and its common use as a medicinal throughout the world, there is just too little research on it. This section contains *only* those microorganisms that some part of the elder plant has been tested against:

Elderberries: influenza A (H1N1—various strains; H5N1—KAN-1; H3N2—various strains), influenza B (three different strains), animal influenza (three different turkey and swine strains), HIV (four serotypes), feline immunodeficiency virus (FIV), herpes simplex viruses, tobacco mosaic virus, various mycoviruses, *Haemophilus influenzae*, *Staphylococcus aureus* (resistant and nonresistant), *Streptococcus pyogenes*, group C and G streptococci, *Branhamella catarrhalis*, *Helicobacter pylori*, *Bacillus cereus*, *Pseudomonas aeruginosa*, *E. coli*, *Salmonella poona*, *Shigella* spp., *Mycobacterium phlei*

Elder flowers: influenza A and B, *Staphylococcus aureus* (resistant and nonresistant), *Bacillus cereus*, *Salmonella poona*, *Pseudomonas aeruginosa*, *Mycobacterum phlei*

Elder leaves: tobacco mosaic virus, lymphocytic choriomeningitis virus, Columbia SK virus, *Bacillus cereus*, *Serratia marcescens*, *E. coli*, *Epidermophyton floccosum*, *Microsporum canis*, *Microsporum gypseum*, *Trichophyton mentagrophytes*, *Trichophyton rubrum*

Elder stem bark: respiratory syncytial virus, lymphocytic choriomeningitis virus, Columbia SK virus, *Candida albicans*, *Trichosporon beigelii*, *Malassezia furfur*, tobacco mosaic virus

A combination formula made from *Sambucus nigra*, *Gentiana lutea*, *Primula veris*, *Verbena officinalis*, and *Rumex* spp. (called Sinupret in Europe) was found to be broadly antiviral, showing activity against influenza A, parainfluenza, human rhinovirus B, Coxsackie virus, adenovirus C, and respiratory syncytial virus.

Use to Treat

Influenza and other respiratory infections. Most commonly this usage includes only the berries as a concentrated decoction or syrup (or, more weakly, an infusion of the flowers). However, a concentrated decoction of berries, stem bark, and leaves gives the most potent antiviral combination of all.

The leaves, root, and stem bark, decocted, for internal inflammations, broken bones, and arthritic complaints. The leaves, decocted, for liver disease and inflammation. But again, see the preparation section on page 331 for more on this.

(continued)

Properties of Elder—Continued

The leaves and bark for topical fungal infections. All parts topically for herpes sores and skin inflammations.

The leaf tincture in small doses as a nervine relaxant, an internal anti-inflammatory, and an analgesic for pain.

The root tincture if you really, really need to vomit explosively. (Really, it's much better than ipecac.)

A number of cultures use elders (e.g., *Sambucus ebulis*) as a primary, first-use anti-inflammatory, feeling that it is especially useful when compared to pharmaceutical anti-inflammatories. A brief look at the Iranian usage range gives a good overview of the plant's capacities.

In Iran the root is particularly valued as an anti-inflammatory (the leaves as well) and is used topically to reduce swellings from bites, stings, and infected wounds. There is also judicious use of the root and leaf internally as nonsteroidal anti-inflammatories for rheumatoid complaints along with the topical use. (Normally they are decocted prior to internal use; see the preparation section.) The leaves are widely used in Iranian herbal practice to reduce swellings in the liver and kidneys, as a diuretic, and as a liver protectant. The undecocted root (tincture or infusion) is commonly used, in tiny doses, as a tea for dropsy (essentially reducing leg edema through diuresis). Larger amounts are used as a purgative, to induce vomiting in case of poisoning or to realign the stomach mucous membranes (similarly to the American physiobotanical uses of lobelia in the nineteenth century).

Other Uses

The flowers as fritters or as adjuncts in wine and beer, the bark for dye, the berries for wine, beer, jellies, jams, and pies (black *and* red varieties), and the odd whistle here and there from the stems.

Finding It

Not hard. Decent tinctures that have moved outside the elder*berry* box are rare though.

(present in some species), isoquercetrin, kaempferol, linoleic acid, linolenic acid, lupeol, malic acid, oleanolic acid, oleic acid, palmitic acid, quercetin, rutin, sambucine, shikimic acid, stigmasterol, tannic acid, tyrosine, undecylenic acid, and ursolic acid are also antiviral, some strongly so.

These compounds are active across a range: herpes simplex viruses, Coxsackie B1 and 3, enterovirus 71, HIV (and SIV), influenza, chikungunya virus, Epstein-Barr, hepatitis B, hepatitis C, hepatitis E, Japanese encephalitis, West Nile encephalitis, vesicular stomatitis virus, poliovirus, adenovirus-3, porcine circovirus, porcine epidemic diarrhea virus, rhinoviruses, Junin virus, cytomegalovirus, respiratory syncytial virus, tobacco mosaic virus, SARS and other coronaviruses, dengue, fowlpox, rotavirus, canine distemper virus, murine norovirus, feline calicivirus, and Ebola.

The compounds in elder are particularly active against enveloped viruses. These include the influenza viruses, herpesviruses, pox viruses (shingles/chicken pox), hepatitis B and D, the flaviviruses (West Nile, dengue, tick-borne encephalitis, yellow fever, Japanese encephalitis, and so on), coronaviruses (upper respiratory and GI tract infections and SARS), paramyxoviruses (mumps, measles, respiratory syncytial virus, parainfluenza), rhabdoviruses (vesicular stomatitis virus), bunyaviruses (hantavirus), filoviruses (Ebola, Marburg), and retroviruses (HIV). Various parts of the plant *have* been tested against some of the viruses in these groups and have been found active against them. Further, historical use in a number of cultures includes some of these disease categories. It seems as if the plant may in fact be a broad-spectrum antiviral for all enveloped viruses.

Many of these compounds act synergistically. The result is a fairly potent grouping of compounds that deeply affect influenzal and other enveloped organisms. As only one example . . .

Palmitic acid is a rather novel CD4 fusion inhibitor that blocks HIV entry and multiplication, while a number of other compounds are directly virucidal against the virus and still other compounds such as astragalin stimulate immune function and response. Palmitic acid also stimulates viral clearing responses against influenza viruses. But it, at the same time, induces a long-term memory (up to several years) in the body's CD8 T cells of that response against influenza viruses *and* inhibits the production of mature viral particles while, again, numerous other compounds in elder are directly virucidal for the organisms, and others inhibit viral binding to host cells, and others stimulate specific immune responses.

The elders also contain cyanogenic glycosides such as sambunigrin and ebuloside—and these compounds are higher in leaves, stems, and roots, respectively, which is why people rather frantically say you should not use those parts of the plant for medicine. These are the compounds that raise the phytohysteria levels among those who understand medicinal plants . . . not.

The particular compounds that cause these effects have very specific medicinal actions as well and very useful ones at that. As usual the dose is the thing (eat 5 pounds of sugar and tell me how you do) *and* the preparation. Again, please see some details on this in the Preparation and Dosage section on page 331. There is more to this than meets the stomach lining.

Traditional Uses of Elder

This plant has been used by people as medicine since people have been on every continent on which it grows.

The genus name, *Sambucus*, comes from ancient Latin, Greek, and Aramaic roots and is the name of an ancient musical instrument, a.k.a. panpipes, made from the hollow stems of the plant. The plants used to be (or maybe still are) in the Caprifoliaceae family. *Caprifolia* itself is from the ancient Greek as well and means "goat leaf." It was the ancient name for a honeysuckle. But the meaning goes deeper than that as the ancient god of wild woods, fields, and music, Pan, possesses, in part, a goat shape. The elders were felt to be a primary plant of the god Pan. The plant was felt to cure nearly all the ills of humankind (thus allowing one to *become* an elder). That is, it is a *pan*acea.

The word *pan* is also from the ancient Greek, meaning "all, wholly, entire, altogether, by all, of all"—and yes, I have read philological treatises on the topic, so tear thy hair not oh ye reasonless reductionists.

AYURVEDA

Sambucus nigra and *S. ebulis* both exist in Ayurvedic practice but not in any depth. *S. ebulis* has a minor role, the roots used in dropsy.

S. nigra use is more extensive; the flowers, berries, roots, leaves, and stem bark are used, the flowers and leaves used fresh. The inner bark is a hydrogogue, cathartic, and antiepileptic. The flowers are diaphoretic, sudorific, and laxative. The berries increase renal function, the root is an aperient.

TRADITIONAL CHINESE MEDICINE

I don't find anything on this genus in my research library, which is extensive in some respects, though it seems as if there should be something since the plant grows in that region. But, after way too much searching of journals on the Internet, I did begin to find some information here and there. Still, it took a bit of serendipity and some cleverness to find it. Despite this, the genus doesn't seem to be considered a major medicinal in any sense of the word. The usage range is odd as well. It doesn't overlap well with the genus use in the Americas or in Europe, in spite of the fact that constituent studies find very similar compounds in the Chinese species.

Three members of the genus, all red berry species, have been used in China for millennia (they just don't seem very excited about it).

Sambucus formosana (one site lists the Chinese name as mao gu xiao) appears to be the least used member of the genus, and I can find little on it. It, like *S. chinensis*, has been used to treat liver disease. One site lists this species name as a synonym of *S. chinensis*, another site as a synonym for *S. javanica.* (There are apparently taxonomists *everywhere.*)

I do find a bit more on *Sambucus chinensis* (in traditional Chinese medicine known as lu-ying, in English as Chinese elder), but it did take some searching. (At least one site lists this plant name as a synonym for *S. javanica.*) Syrups of the berries *and* the leaves are used (decoctions again). The herb is considered to be warm and bitter and is used for dispelling blood stasis and dispelling wind rolling. Lu-ying's primary uses seem to be for the treatment of hepatitis and liver injury, for inflammations, and as an analgesic. It is also used to induce sweating, as a diuretic, for bruises, rheumatism, dislocations, nephritis, edema, beriberi, and urticaria.

Assuming this species name *is* a synonym, then the use data expands a bit (but . . . the plant under the name *Sambucus javanica* is listed by a number of sources as *not* growing in China even though it is called Chinese elder—are taxonomists even human? Have they no mercy?). The whole plant would be then anodyne, antiphlogistic, depurative, diuretic, emetic, and purgative. The leaves and root are used for pain and numbness, bone diseases, and rheumatic problems. The fruit is used as a depurative and purgative. A decoction of the berries is used to treat injuries, for skin diseases, and for swellings. A decoction of the leaves is used as a diuretic and an anodyne (pain reliever).

In Indonesia *S. javanica*'s leaves are primarily used for pain relief. One-half to 1 ounce of leaves is boiled in 3 cups of water and reduced to 1 cup, and the decoction consumed for 14 days. (Note: No emetic warnings are shouted.) For beriberi, 1–2 ounces of fresh root, stems, and leaves is treated similarly, the cooled decoction consumed for 14 days. (Again, no emetic warnings occur.) For jaundice, the roots only are used, as a concentrated decoction. (Another site lists multiple synonyms for this plant, including *Ebulis chinensis*, though, upon examination, that also seems to be the name of an Argentine mussel. So, no, taxonomists have no mercy.)

Sambucus williamsii is also listed as a species long in use in traditional Chinese medicine. On that I do find a bit more usage, over centuries, for inflammation, broken bones, and joint diseases. There are actually some good studies on the actions of the plant leaves in healing broken bones and osteoporosis (see the Scientific Research section on page 350). This use for broken bones and bone loss is interesting and potentially opens up a whole new range of action for this genus.

S. javanica is also used for this; it makes sense to explore it further. The action appears specific to the leaves (concentrated decoction).

Sambucus williamsii is also considered anodyne, carminative, diaphoretic, diuretic, and emetic. The leaf is also used to treat (and alleviate, i.e., break) ague fits (essentially intermittent fevers with sharp swings into both extremely hot and cold states, i.e., fits). The flowers are diaphoretic and diuretic. The juice of the stem is used as an emetic. A decoction of the root for arthritis inflammations.

Still, there is so little on the genus compared to so many others; it doesn't appear to have a major place in traditional Chinese medicine.

WESTERN BOTANIC PRACTICE

Elders have been used in European medical practice for more than 2,500 years for inflammatory conditions, for sore throats, as a purgative, as an emetic, and for wounds. The leaves were a major ingredient in salves for the treatment of wounds, bruises, and sprains. Used internally, they are expectorant, diaphoretic, and diuretic. The berries were used for rheumatism, erysipelas, colic, diarrhea, epilepsy, and dropsy.

The use of the various *Sambucus* species by the indigenous peoples of the Americas was extensive, for both red and blue berry species. *S. canadensis* bark was used as an emetic, laxative, blood purifier, for wounds to prevent infection, for skin inflammations, for jaundice, as a wash for pain, as a poultice for headaches, as a laxative for children, and to treat measles, diphtheria, and mumps. The leaves were used in ointments for wounds and burns, and a leaf infusion to wash skin sores to prevent infection, as a diuretic, for dropsy, and for jaundice. The berries for rheumatism, as a wine as a tonic, and for fevers. The flowers to sweat out fevers, for colds and pulmonary troubles, and to treat colic in infants. The root as an emetic, for liver troubles, as a poultice for swollen breasts, and as a poultice for a baby's unhealed navel.

And so on and on and on.

The various species (*S. cerulea, S. mexicana, S. neomexicana, S. nigra, S. velutina*, and so on) were all used pretty similarly. In essence: for fevers and colds, as an emetic, as a purgative, for skin inflammations, for rheumatism (arthritic complaints) and sore joints, to treat wounds, as a diuretic, and for liver troubles.

The American Eclectic botanical physicians had a similar range of use.

There has been very little new exploration of this plant as a primary medicinal by contemporary American herbalists, probably due to phytohysteria contamination.

Scientific Research

There hasn't been nearly enough study on this plant. However, the pharmacokinetics of this plant, at least of the anthocyanins, are good.

Anthocyanins are a group of water-soluble pigment compounds that exist in plants, in all their tissues, but we notice them primarily in the fruits. They create the various colors of the fruits: red, purple, or blue. They are a kind of flavonoid. Closely related compounds called anthoxanthins are what are contained in the white and yellow berry species of elder. These kinds of compounds have been extensively studied as medicinals and they do have a wide range of actions: anticancer, antiaging, neuroprotective, anti-inflammatory, antioxidant, antibiotic, analgesic, and blood sugar regulating. The anthocyanins in elder are particularly potent and are the compounds in elder that have been most extensively studied.

They reach peak presence in the body within 30 to 60 minutes after ingestion. They are high in the urine and GI tract mucosa, and in the liver and bloodstream to a lesser extent. The half-life is about 2 hours. They are absorbed in the small intestine and can be found in the body (and urine) as intact glycosides, methylated forms, and glucuronidated derivatives.

There have also been some studies of the pharmacokinetics of ursolic acid, which is present in fairly high quantities in the plant. Ursolic acid has anticancer properties, is potently anti-inflammatory through its downregulation of MMP-9 and inhibition of COX-2, stimulates anabolism (increasing muscle mass and decreasing fat accumulation), thus reducing muscle atrophy, and is cardioprotective, analgesic, antibacterial, antiviral, antidiabetic, and antioxidant. Once ingested, it is widely present in blood plasma, reaches peak concentration in 1 hour, and reaches its half-life in 4 hours.

Elder is a potent COX-2 inhibitor and inducer of quinone reductase. (*S. racemosa* inhibits ornithine decarboxylase.) It also tends to act in the body as a cytokine modulator; it increases the body's production of IL-10 if it is taken during an infection, downregulating the levels of other cytokines as necessary, but if taken early in the disease process, it inhibits viral upregulation of IL-10 and increases antiviral cytokine production and activity. One study found that ethanol leaf extracts of *S. ebulis* reduce TNF-α and its associated induction of VCAM-1 (vascular cell adhesion molecule-1). Intracellular adhesion molecule-1 (ICAM-1) levels were also reduced in that study. Elder modulates the production of interferon gamma (stimulating it if necessary, lowering it if it is too high) and hematopoietic growth factor GM-CSF by monocytes and lymphocytes. In vivo studies with mice have found that elderberry extracts enhance the immune system through increased levels of T cells, B cells, interferon, and IL-2. (There are some reports that show that Sambucol, a proprietary elderberry extract, stimulates TNF-α production. This perplexes scientists but in fact the herb tends to modulate cytokine production, raising it if necessary, lowering it if it is too high.)

Normally, when herbs or their compounds are tested by scientists in their labs, they do it in vitro (lab/test tube), in vivo (animal), or with human clinical study or trial. Unknown to most people there is a fourth category, in planta (i.e., in plants). This will, I suspect, be a growing category for research as time goes by. Most of the studies on elder and its constituents have been in vitro, and many of those findings have already been scattered throughout this monograph. Here are a few from the other categories.

IN PLANTA

Elder has been found to be directly virucidal against tobacco leaf virus, to inactivate the virus through depurination, and to be host protective if later challenged by viruses.

IN VIVO

Sambucus ebulis protects mice from the teratogenic effects of albendazole. TheraMax, a proprietary blend of green tea and elderberry (*Sambucus nigra*), is effective against seven of eight strains of influenza A and B (in vitro); when used on mice infected with mortal doses of influenza viruses, it significantly slowed the arrival of death, curtailed weight loss, and improved lung hemorrhage scores. *Sambucus ebulis* leaves were found to possess potent wound healing activity when used as an ointment on mice. *Sambucus williamsii* extracts (part of plant not stated but it was apparently the leaves or stems) exerted protective effects on ovariectomy-induced bone loss in rats. It improved trabecular bone mass and cortical bone strength, decreased urinary calcium excretion, increased serum calcium levels, increased tibial bone mineral density, and exerted beneficial effects on the microarchitecture of the trabecular bone. A methanolic extract of the stems of *Sambucus sieboldiana* (*S. racemosa* subtype) was found to possess antiosteoporotic activity. It inhibits bone resorption in ovariectomized rats.

In a particularly interesting study, mice were given Sambucol, an extract of elderberry. It caused a shift in immune response in the face of microbial challenge. In mice then infected with leishmania parasites, Sambucol delayed the onset of the disease by upregulating Th1 cytokines. However, when given to mice challenged with malarial parasites, the incidence of cerebral malaria increased substantially. In essence it exacerbated the Th1 dominant cytokine cascade during malarial infection, leading to a worsening of symptoms. The berries appear to *possibly* act as a Th1 activator, while the leaves act as a Th1/Th2 modulator. (So, don't take the berry syrup if you have malaria.)

HUMAN STUDY

Sixty patients, aged 18 to 54, suffering from influenza symptoms for 48 hours or less, were enrolled in a randomized, double-blind, placebo-controlled study of the effectiveness of elderberry syrup. Participants received 15 ml ($^1/_2$ ounce) of an elderberry syrup or placebo for 5 days. Symptoms were relieved on average 4 days earlier in the elderberry group.

Sambucol, in a placebo-controlled, double-blind study, was used to treat a group of individuals in Panama during an influenza epidemic. Those using the elderberry extract experienced a significant improvement in symptoms, including fever, in 2 days. A complete cure was recorded for most within 2 to 3 days. Serum examination showed high hemagglutination inhibition titers to influenza B.

Ginger

Ginger is a decent antiviral *only* if you are using the fresh rhizome, not the dried root. Specifically: the juice of the fresh root (though an alcohol tincture of the fresh root *will* work, it's just not as good). In Chinese medicine the dried root and the fresh root are considered different medicines with *very* different actions—because they are. The plant's constituents alter considerably with drying as many of the volatile oils are lost; other constituents morph as they dry. For more information on ginger as an antiviral and a synergist, see page 437.

Houttuynia

Family: Saururaceae.

Species used: *Houttuynia cordata* almost always. There are two species in this genus but the most recent one, *Houttuynia emeiensis*, was only discovered in 2001. Some taxonomists consider this second species identical with *Houttuynia cordata*, the species used for millennia in the East and first identified by the West in 1783. Some insist it is different. There has been some intense name-calling as a result. (Taxonomists are like our children.) The two species are used interchangeably, but the newest one grows in a very limited range and is not widely available.

There is reportedly a wide range in the taste of *Houttuynia cordata*, which a number of sources attribute to chemical variations in the species depending on where it is grown. The Chinese/Vietnamese chemotype is reported to possess a taste/smell similar to coriander; the Japanese chemotype, according to one anonymous reporter, has "a strange lemon or orange odour that is often compared with ginger." To those who hate the taste, every species apparently tastes like rotten fish. To those who like it, heaven itself has become food, and, they insist, the plant never has smelled or tasted like fish.

One of the plant's closer relatives is yerba mansa (*Anemopsis californica*), which grows in similar terrain, has a very similar flower, and has a somewhat similar range of medicinal actions. Yerba mansa was once named *Houttuynia californica* in the nineteenth century, which does lead, occasionally, to some confusion.

Synonyms: *Houttuynia foetida, Polypara cochinchinensis, Polypara cordata, Gymnotheca chinensis*, and, sometimes, if one group of taxonomists wants to make the other group really mad: *Houttuynia emeiensis*.

Common names: It's pronounced "hoo-TY-nee-ah" big fella, and, yes, you may yell that loudly at square dances, hootenannies, and cattle roundups. Other names: heart-leaved houttuynia, lizard tail, Chinese lizard tail, chameleon plant (as opposed to the specific variety called 'Chameleon'), heartleaf, fishwort, fishmint, bishop's weed, doku-dami (Japan), and yu xing cao (China). The Chinese name literally means "fishy-smell herb" because, well, it smells like fish.

Parts Used

The aerial parts are used for medicine, the roots and leaves as pot herbs everywhere they grow (well, except in the United States).

Preparation and Dosage

The fresh plant is much more antibacterial/antiviral (as is the tincture) and is traditionally pounded to make juice for oral administration internally, on wounds, or as eyedrops. The remaining mashed plant can be used as a paste applied topically to wounds and bites; the decoction (allowed to cool) can be used for an external wash. The Japanese use a tea, taken regularly, as a tonic medicine. I prefer a tincture of the fresh plant leaves.

FRESH PLANT TINCTURE

The tincture should preferably be made 1:2, that is, one part herb to two parts liquid. The liquid should be pure grain alcohol if you can get it. So, if you have 16 ounces of plant leaves, you would add 32 ounces of alcohol, let it macerate for 2 weeks, decant, and press out the liquid.

Contrariwise, you can make it 1:5 from the dried leaves. That is, one part dried leaves, five parts liquid. In this instance the liquid should be half pure grain alcohol and half water, essentially a 50 percent alcohol liquid. So, if you have 1 ounce of leaves, you would use 5 ounces of liquid and then continue as above.

As for dosage:

For viral infections: 1/4–1/2 tsp up to 6x daily, depending on how acute the condition is.

For mycoplasma and bartonella: 1/2 tsp 3x daily.

The tincture can taste nasty, very fishy to some, so put it in something with a strong taste to cover it (fish soup?). Otherwise it can be hard to get it down—for some. I don't find it all that bad myself. It is not great but is only mildly fishy to my incredibly sensitive ("Hey! Are you looking at me?") taste buds.

There are a few companies selling the tincture for absurd prices, which, given that the plant is an invasive and very easy to grow, I find obscene.

DECOCTION

Traditionally the herb (sometimes the root) is used, either dried or fresh, to make a decoction. For dried, 15–30 grams (about 1/2–1 ounce) of the dried plant is decocted (that is, briefly boiled), allowed to cool, then consumed. Fresh, 30–50 grams of the fresh herb is decocted similarly. Examination of the decocted herb has, however, revealed that it loses much of its antibacterial/antiviral actions upon being boiled (which is why the Chinese tend to boil it really, really briefly). If decocted intensively, the plant works well to stop diarrhea but is relatively inactive antimicrobially.

POWDERS AND CAPSULES

You can also find the powder, sometimes concentrated at 5:1, sometimes just the regular old powdered herb, from some Chinese herb companies. You can encapsulate the powder if you cannot take the taste of the tincture. I have been unable to locate any pre-encapsulated forms on the market. The herb really isn't that popular in the West at this point.

If you do encapsulate it yourself, use "00" capsules. I would begin with two capsules 3x daily and see how it goes, adjusting the dose depending on how it works for you. Contrariwise, you can work with the powder directly. I would begin with 1/2 tsp 3–6x daily and see how it works. (I normally only use the tincture.)

I have never been sure of how to dose the 5:1 concentrated powders that the Chinese often make; presumably you would take one-fifth the dose of the nonconcentrated form, but that is just a guess.

Side Effects and Contraindications

Fishy-smelling breath (according to several former spouses). The taste can be terrible to the point of gagging (some say). Other than the nausea from the taste there are no reported side effects in the literature from oral ingestion of the plant.

It does have emmenagogue actions (though oddly enough the herb is not traditionally used for starting menstruation), so it should not be used in pregnancy. However, a few individual reports from China say it can, very rarely, cause congestion in the vagina (but I am not really sure what that means unless it is an overproduction of mucus, as in "congested" lungs or nasal passages; it certainly can't be congestion as in "traffic congestion," as in "traffic on I-80 is backed up to the State Street Parkway so take an alternate route").

The Chinese sometimes use it as an injectable, and there have been some severe anaphylactic reactions to that. So . . . don't inject it.

Herb/Drug and Herb/Herb Interactions

None have been noted in the literature or in any anecdotal reports that I can find.

Habitat and Appearance

Houttuynia is a creeping perennial. The stem is a sort-of trailing viney thing that creeps along the ground and from which sub-stems sprout vertically to about 14 inches in height at most. When thickly growing, it can look a bit like a small bush. The leaves are heart-shaped, alternate, from 1 to 3 inches wide, and 1 to 3 inches long. The (original, non-cultivar) plant leaves actually look quite a lot like those of the common violet. The noncultivar flowers are pretty, four-petaled, greenish-white with an upraised spike sort of like a tiny cattail (a.k.a. the terminal spike).

There are a number of cultivated varieties that have been mucked about with to give color variations. They may be mottled green and red, green and yellow, green-leaved with a rim of red, magenta and green, and orange or even mixes of all of those. There is even a nearly black-leaved variety. And of course the flowers have been altered as well, with some of the varieties sporting red blooms. These varieties have the usual ridiculous names associated with them: 'Chameleon',

'Flame', 'Joker's Gold', 'Sunshine', 'Variegata', and so on. They are common in gardens throughout the world.

The roots are more correctly creeping rhizomes that run just under the soil in a tangled mat something like a writhing mass of spaghetti noodles. They are sort of golden in color.

The original native range of the plant was wide, from Nepal and India through China and Indochina into Japan, and south into Vietnam, Thailand, and Java. But it's a good hitchhiker and spread, in its original form, throughout the Pacific islands, Australia, and New Zealand as ships sailed here and there over the centuries. Once it was introduced as an ornamental it went everywhere and is now common throughout Europe and North America. It has an especially strong presence in eastern Europe, the UK, and Russia.

The plant will grow from sea level to 7,500 feet, and it likes it wet, that is, if it is growing wild. Its standard terrain is ravines, streamsides, forests, wet meadows, slopes, thicket and field margins, trailsides, roadsides, and ditch banks.

It tends to prefer moist loamy soils, shallow water, and low light conditions (dappled sun/shade) either in forests or not. It is particularly fond of growing on the margins of ponds and waterways—really any type of wettish to boggy location that is coolish and shaded. It is highly tolerant of cold and is hardy to about 0°F but can tolerate dips to –30° F. (Horizon Herbs grew it in unheated greenhouses in February in the state of Oregon just fine.) It is hardy in zones 4 through 11, essentially most of the United States. In spite of its natural preferences, the plant can tolerate full sun (though it may scorch—it really does like a bit of shade) and is drought resistant. Few animals will eat it; rabbits (reportedly) detest it (they have the second kind of taste buds—*bunny* buds).

Cultivation and Collection

Houttuynia is an invasive, which makes it of particular interest to me. Like many invasives it is potently medicinal and a decent edible, if you like the flavor. I consider it another plant that should be planted by everyone who wants healing independence and wide availability of potent medicinal plants for themselves and their families. Once it's planted you will have both food and medicine forever. Just don't let your neighbors catch you—practice the confused look you developed in high school for the time someone brings up the fact the plant is killing off the *real* American plants and that you, yes *you*, have a duty to stop it.

The plant is banned from importation in New Zealand (too late) and a number of other places (still too late). The plant is reportedly invasive in Texas, Louisiana, Alabama, Florida, North Carolina, and Pennsylvania.

Houttuynia is a hermaphrodite—another reason many Americans are uncomfortable with the plant. Thus, it can self-seed—there doesn't have to be a mommy *and* a daddy. There are some 1,000 seeds per 0.04 gram of seed weight, and every plant produces a lot of seed. Any and all portions of the root will grow as well. It is just reproductively irritating no matter how you look at it.

Once established it just doesn't let go. There are numerous humorous reports on the Internet of people planting it as a ground cover and having it take over their gardens, yards, and lives. Digging it out is difficult as every piece of overlooked root, no matter how small, will, well, root and produce a new plant, something every eradofanatic discovers the next spring. From one killed plant, a thousand rise to take its place. Often the Internet stories end with the writers adding rather glumly that their houses are for sale.

Plant sex, destroying American suburbs everywhere.

Reportedly the growing condition that will produce the strongest growth is a clay, loam soil, 5.9 pH, with 78 percent moisture content. Still, houttuynia can be grown in much drier conditions than it normally likes as long as you keep it watered. It will tolerate sandy, loamy, and clay soils. It can even grow in water up to 2 inches deep. It flowers in June (usually). It grows extremely quickly.

Houttuynia is reportedly very hard to grow from seed, but those who have done it say that you should sow the seeds in a greenhouse in spring, keeping the soil moist, then separate them into individual pots when they are big enough. Transplantation can occur any time after that.

The more variegated the plant, the less hardy, the less medicinal, the less invasive. Most of the variegated species will tend to relapse into the more basic unvariegated state if you let them. Gardeners are warned to pick off and dispose of any green leaves that show up to keep this from happening. I would suggest the opposite approach.

In China, the plant is traditionally harvested after flowering and then dried in the sun. It is usually used as a decoction, 15–30 grams of the dried plant or 30–50 grams of the fresh. It is usually not decocted for long in order to prevent the heat loss of volatile oils. The more it is heated, the worse its antimicrobial actions become. The primary reason it is heated is to get rid of the fishy smell—about 1 minute does it, so they say. However, in spite of all that, the Chinese consider the fresh plant the strongest form of the herb.

If you are making tinctures, use the fresh plant picked just at flowering. If you want to dry the plant, bundle and hang it, and when it is completely dry, store it in plastic bags out of the sun, preferably in plastic tubs, well sealed.

Note: Houttuynia hyperaccumulates lead and arsenic, so don't harvest it from around mines.

Finding It

If you are going to grow it for medicine, try to get the original, unmucked- about-with plant if you can, not the highly variegated varieties ('Chameleon' is the worst to use for medicine). Horizon Herbs sells the plants and they are pretty good ones—horizonherbs.com. You can get the seeds from suppliers here and there but the plants are reportedly hard to grow from seed; the easiest way to grow the herb is from divided rootstock. If you want a very good fresh tincture at a decent price, try Woodland Essence (woodlandessence.com). The dried herb (in both powder and cut form) is available from 1stChineseHerbs.com.

Properties of Houttuynia

Actions

As an antiviral, houttuynia inhibits viral replication, interferes with the function of the viral envelope, is directly virucidal, stops virion release from infected cells, and prevents viral infection if taken prophylactically. It is also:

Analgesic
Anthelmintic
Antibacterial
Anticancer
Antifungal
Anti-inflammatory
Antileukemic
Antimicrobial
Antioxidant
Antitussive
Astringent
Depurative
Diuretic
Emmenagogue
Febrifuge
Hemostatic
Hypoglycemic
Immunomodulatory
Larvacidal
Laxative
Ophthalmic

Active Against

Moderately broad-spectrum antiviral. It is active against influenza virus A (H1N1 strains), SARS-related coronavirus (FFM-1, FFM-2), dengue virus serotype 2, avian infectious bronchitis virus (a coronavirus), enterovirus 71, enteric cytopathic human orphan (ECHO) virus, herpes simplex virus 1, herpes simplex virus 2, HIV-1, cytomegalovirus, porcine epidemic diarrhea virus, and pseudorabies herpesvirus. Studies have found it ineffective against polio and Coxsackie viruses.

The herb also has a good range of action against bacteria and other microbes. It is active against:

Aedes aegypti larvae
Aspergillus spp.
Candida albicans
chromomycosis fungus
Colletotrichum capsici
Corynebacterium diphtheriae
Cryptococcus neoformans
Diplococcus pneumoniae (a.k.a. *Streptococcus pneumoniae*)
Epidermophyton rubrum
Fusarium oxysporum
Haemophilus influenzae
Hymenolepis diminuta
Leptospira spp.
Malassezia pachydermatis
Microsporum ferrugineum
Microsporum gypseum
Mycobacterium tuberculosis
Mycoplasma hominis (30 strains)
Neisseria catarrhalis (a.k.a. *Moraxella catarrhalis*)
Proteus vulgaris
Salmonella choleraesuis (a.k.a. *S. enterica*)
Salmonella enteritidis
Sarcina ureae
Shigella flexneri
Shigella schmitzii (a.k.a. *S. dysenteriae*)
Shigella shigae (a.k.a. *S. dysenteriae*)
Shigella sonnei
Sporotrichum spp.
Staphylococcus albus
Staphylococcus aureus
Streptococcus hemolyticus
Tinea imbricata
Vibrio cholerae

There are a number of Internet sites insisting that the herb is active against trichophyton and gonococci, but intensive searching has failed to turn up any relevant documents supporting it. Every site I can find simply repeats the same thing—all apparently from the same initial site, wherever that is. It is reported that James Schaller, M.D., found the herb effective, in vitro and in vivo, against bartonella species, but I can't find any actual data on that to support it.

Use to Treat

Respiratory viral infections—especially SARS and influenza, ECHO infection, neurological enterovirus infections, neurological encephalitis infections, and dengue fever.

The herb is also excellent for mycoplasma infections, any serious infections in the lungs especially with abscesses, infections in the urinary passages and kidneys, genital infections, dysentery and any bacterial diarrheal conditions, various diseases of the eye (fresh juice or tea applied topically), and skin infections with pus or boils. It is especially indicated if any of these conditions are accompanied by foul-smelling discharge.

Other Uses

As food. The young shoots and leaves are very tender (later in the year the leaves become somewhat bitter) and are a major food source in all the plant's native regions. There are varying reports on the taste and smell. Some say that the leaves have a slight orange smell and taste, others that it is reminiscent of coriander, others insist it is actually a slight fishy smell and taste, and still others report that it is more akin to rotten fish. From all accounts this is another of those plants like cilantro—you either love it or hate it. If you hate it, the taste is rank (in varying degrees of rankness depending on your level of hate). However, if you love it, it is wonderful with delicate shadings of flavor. (Taxonomists are now arguing that there are two species of taste buds, one that . . .)

The leaves, for those who like it, are used in salads or are steamed as a pot herb or even blended with rice as a main dish. The rhizomes are washed and cut in 3- to 4-inch lengths and added to stir-fry. Both are sometimes used as a main ingredient in meat and other dishes. The leaf tea (dokudami cha) is common in Japan as a medicinal drink.

Plant Chemistry

Houttuynoside A, various houttuynoids (A through E), houttuynin, lauryl aldehyde, caprylic aldehyde, quercetin 3-rhamnoside, quercetin 7-rhamnoside, n-capric acid, cordarine, quercitrin, isoquercitrin, decanoyl acetaldehyde, alpha-pinene, beta-pinene, linalool, camphene, myricene, limonene, caryophyllene, afzerin, hyperin, chlorogenic acid, beta-sitosterol, stearic acid, oleic acid, linoleic acid, myrcene, 2-undecanone, hyperoside, p-cymene, eucalyptol, beta-ocimene, nonanal, fenchyl alcohol, menth-2-en-l-ol, trans-pinocarveol, verbenol, camphor, beta-terpineol, pinocarvone, isoborneol, pelargol, terpinen-4-ol, myrtenal, alpha-terpineol, verbenone, trans-carveol, piperitone, isopulegol acetate, bornyl acetate, isobornyl acetate, benzyl isobutyrate, undecanal, alpha-terpinyl formate, dihydrocarvyl acetate, neryl acetate, undecyl alcohol, geranyl acetate, 4-acetamido-l-hexanol, beta-caryophyllene, beta-farnesene, lauryl alcohol, beta-chamigrene, valencene, methyl undecyl ketone, alpha-bulnesene, dodecanoic acid, nerolidol, spathulenol, caryophyllene oxide, viridiflorol, juniper camphor, methyl tridecyl ketone, phytone, heptadecanol, phytol, phytol acetate, a variety of aristolactams, piperolactam, aporphines, splendidine, lysicamine, 4,5-dioxoaporphines, norcepharadione B, noraritolodione, various amides, and so on. The herb is reportedly high in potassium, magnesium, and sodium.

A significant number of these compounds possess antiviral and/or antibacterial actions. The whole herb was found to be more effective than any of the isolated constituents, showing a profound synergism in its chemical actions. One study found *Houttuynia emeiensis* to be more potent in its antibacterial effects than *H. cordata*. (Several taxonomists were found fighting in the parking lot just afterward.)

Traditional Uses of Houttuynia

There is a lot of indigenous and local use of the plant throughout its native range, both for food and medicine. The tribes of the Kameng district of Arunachal Pradesh (which is in northeast India) use 1½ ounces of the fresh root, boiled as a decoction until reduced by half. The dose is half a glass of the decoction twice daily for a week in the treatment of dysentery, diarrhea, and cholera.

In Nepal the fresh juice of the root is used for indigestion, topically for skin diseases, and as eyedrops for eye infections. The juice of the leaf is dripped into wounds to prevent infection, to kill maggots in the wounds, and to accelerate healing.

In Thailand the herb is used to treat venereal and skin diseases and as a diuretic and urogenital antiseptic.

It is used in Japan as a tonic tea, for chronic earache, as a lotion, and as a liquor. Its name in Japanese, dokudami, literally means poison-blocking. It is considered to be an herb for detoxification of the blood to increase overall health of the body. Usually 4–12 grams (1/7 to a bit less than 1/2 ounce) are used to make the tea. The lotion is made by soaking the dried plant in shochu liquor (about 25 percent alcohol) for 10 days, straining it, then adding glycerin. It is then used on the skin for healing. The liquor is made by putting the dried plant in a bottle, adding shochu to about three-quarters the level of the bottle, then adding honey to top it off. After 3 months, the herb is filtered out and the liquor stored in the refrigerator. It is drunk as a tonic. Essentially this is what we herbalists in the United States would call a cordial.

The greatest depth of use has been in traditional Chinese medicine.

AYURVEDA

In spite of tribal use, I can't find much on the plant as a part of formal Ayurvedic practice. It is apparently used in combination formulas for the treatment of AIDS (as an antiviral adjuvant) throughout the country, but that is about all I can find.

TRADITIONAL CHINESE MEDICINE

In traditional Chinese medicine yu xing cao is considered to be slightly cold, pungent, and specific for the lung channel. It has traditionally been used for removing toxic heat, eliminating toxins, reducing swelling, discharging pus, and relieving stagnation. It is specific for promoting drainage of pus, lung abscess with purulent expectoration, heat in the lung with cough, lung abscesses, cough with thick sputum, dyspnea, edema, carbuncles and sores, dysuria, leukorrhea, acute dysentery, and acute urinary infections. It is considered latent-heat clearing, anti-pyretic, detoxicant, anti-inflammatory, and diuretic. The fresh juice is used for snakebite and skin infections. Common medicinal use in China is for chronic nephritis, inflamed pelvis or cervix (pelvic inflammatory disease), gonorrhea, rheumatism, anal prolapse, hemorrhoids, inflamed respiratory tract (including pneumonia and bronchitis with or without edema), prevention of postoperative infections, inflammation and pus in the middle ear, measles, tonsillitis, chronic sinusitis, nasal polyps, inhibiting anaphylactic reactions, and various cancers.

Again, the fresh leaf is considered to be more efficacious than the dried.

WESTERN BOTANIC PRACTICE

Very little use in the West until recently. Few American herbalists use it. Most understand it not at all. It has achieved some prominence from those treating Lyme and its coinfections, usually bartonella.

Scientific Research

Most of the scientific studies have occurred in China, often with injectable forms of the herb. Numerous others have been conducted in India and Thailand. Few have occurred in the United States. (The herb tastes funny.) In general, the studies found that the effects were dose dependent, in other words, the more they gave, the better the outcome. Since the herb has shown no toxicity from oral ingestion (up to 16 grams per kilogram in mice, a huge dose), that would indicate that largish doses can be used very effectively.

In vitro studies found that the herb (water extract) significantly increases IL-2 and IL-10 cytokines. IL-10 is also known as cytokine synthesis inhibitory factor; it is an anti-inflammatory cytokine. It essentially downregulates other cytokines and blocks NF-κB activity. It is specific for counteracting the effects of mast-cell-initiated allergic reactions, which is why the herb is good for stings and bites and anaphylactic reactions. The herb also stimulates the production of CD4+ lymphocytes. It is especially active in the spleen.

Herpes simplex virus (HSV) 1 and 2 depend on NF-κB activation for replication. In vitro studies found that houttuynia suppresses HSV infection by inhibiting NF-κB activation. The herb's inhibition of NF-κB has also been found to significantly reduce chemotaxis during infection, reducing cellular migration. The herb also inhibits hydrogen peroxide impacts on cells and lipid peroxidation by 80 percent.

In vitro research found that the herb is active against 21 staph aureus strains (but is not very active in stopping biofilm formation in that organism).

In vitro study found that while the herb is strongly active against enterovirus 71, its activity is much higher in cells pretreated with the herb than if it is administered postinfection.

In vitro the herb inhibits the production of lipopolysaccharide-induced COX-2 and PGE2 in mouse macrophages. The herb reduces Th2 cytokines, specifically IL-4 and IL-5. It inhibits HMC-1 cell migration. It also inhibits DNA topoisomerase 1 activity.

Houttuynia liquid extract protected and restored white blood cell counts in mice X-rayed and administered cyclophosphamide. It normalized connective tissue growth factor and increased levels of adiponectin in streptozotocin-induced diabetes in rats.

Eight hundred mg/kg of the herb reduced the numbers of *Hymenolepis diminuta* flatworms in rats by nearly 75 percent and the egg count by nearly 60 percent. In comparison the drug praziquantel showed 87.5 and 80 percent effectiveness.

Water extracts of the herb significantly reduced NO levels in *Salmonella*-infected macrophages and extended life spans of *Salmonella*-infected mice given a lethal dose of the bacteria from 7 days (no herb) to 23 days. The effects were dose dependent.

The herb is strongly inhibitive of avian infectious bronchitis in vitro and was found to protect chicken embryos from infection by the virus and to protect 50 percent of mature chickens from infection.

The herb, as a water extract, was used to treat bleomycin-induced pulmonary fibrosis in rats. The herb significantly decreased SOD, malondialhehyde, hydroxyproline, interferon-gamma, and TNF-α. The morphological appearance of the lung was markedly improved.

A number of studies found that the herb strongly inhibited induced-oxidation events in rats. It specifically inhibited NF-κB, TNF-α, NO, COX-2, and PGE2. It also inhibited passive cutaneous anaphylaxis (PCA) in mice, inhibited IgE-mediated systemic PCA, reduced antigen-induced release IL-4 and TNF-α, inhibited degradation of IkappaBalpha. It specifically inhibited antigen-induced phosphorylation of Syk, Lyn, LAT, Gab2, and PLC gamma-2. Further downstream it also inhibited Akt and MAP kinases ERK-1, ERK-2, JNK-1, and JNK-2 but not p38.

Extracts of the herb protected rat kidneys when rats were injected with streptozotocin. TGF-ß1 and collagen type 1 levels in renal tissues decreased, and BMP-7 increased.

Water extracts of the herb showed antiobesity effects in mice by inhibiting glycerol absorption and corn oil-induced increases in triglyceride levels. The herb inhibited oleic acid increases in blood plasma.

Cows with bovine mastitis were treated with a form of houttuynin, a compound from houttuynia. In acute mastitis 88 percent were cured and 53 percent showed microbiological clearance. In cows treated with combination penicillin/streptomycin, the rates were 90 percent and 55 percent, respectively. In subacute conditions the houttuynin results were 94percent and 48 percent. In the pharmaceutical group, they were 94 percent and 44 percent. (This finding is significant because of the degree of mycoplasmal infection in dairy herds, a major cause of bovine mastitis.)

A modified form of houttuynin both protected mice from and corrected induced membranous glomerulonephritis in mice. It inhibited the expression of NF-κB and MCP-1.

A water extract of the herb protected rat primary cortical cells from beta-amyloid-induced neurotoxicity, specifically through modulating calcium influx and protection of mitochondria.

Researchers in Korea are interested in a class of food herbs they are calling phytobiotics, among which is houttuynia. In one study, researchers found that adding it to chicken feed instead of antibiotics resulted in similar effects on weight, disease reduction, and health as pharmaceuticals without the negative side effects, including antibiotic resistance. Lipid oxidation in the meat was significantly reduced. In another study, the mortality of chicks challenged by *Salmonella* was significantly reduced when the herb was included in their feed. PGE2 synthesis decreased, CD4+ increased, the CD4+:CD8+ ratio balanced, and immune function in all chicks was enhanced.

Many of the human studies with the herb used an injectable form and found it highly effective for treating bronchopulmonary complaints including pneumonia. Oral dosing of a compound formula that included *Platycodon grandiflorum* was also effective. Both oral and injectable forms were found prophylactic for leptospira infections. Used alone or in combination with *Artemisia annua* the herb was an effective treatment for leptospirosis.

Cotton impregnated with the water extract (or oral tablets) was used in treating chronic cervicitis with lesions. Applied once every day for 5 days (243 people participating) the cure rate was 81 percent.

Of 100 cases of chronic suppurative otitis media treated with ear drops of the distillate of the herb, 95 were cured. Thirty-one of 33 cases of atrophic rhinitis benefited from nose drops of the solution. Irrigation with the extract was effective in treating chronic maxillary sinusitis. And in other studies houttuynia (water extract) was used to irrigate nasal passages after endoscopic sinus surgery for those with chronic sinusitis and/or nasal polyps. The herbal extract was found to be more effective than two other irrigants used.

A clinical trial in China in the treatment of chronic-relapsing ulcerative colitis found the herb cured 20 of 21 and gave improvement in the other. Stool normalization, cessation of diarrhea, reduction of blood in stool, and abdominal pain disappearance all were faster in the herbal group than in those being treated with pharmaceuticals. (Again this is an important study as this kind of condition is relatively common in chronic mycoplasma infection.)

The herb's constituents move fairly rapidly into the bloodstream and maintain a high presence. The absorption half-life after oral ingestion is 3.5 hours. The herb's constituents are present in the highest amounts in the lungs, heart, liver, kidneys, and serum, in that order.

Elimination of constituents, metabolized or not, in the urine and feces is very low; the main route of excretion is the lungs (breath). Radioactively labeled houttuynine was found in rat tissues for up to 48 hours. The highest levels were in the bronchi (especially at 1 and 4 hours postinjection) and in descending order in the gallbladder, liver, ovaries, intestine, spleen, kidneys, and lungs. Oral dosing found the highest levels in the bronchi after 24 hours.

Isatis

Family: Brassicaceae. (This family is the home of all cruciferous vegetables such as cabbages, broccoli, and brussels sprouts and the reason why the tincture of this plant tastes kind of like spoiled broccoli/cabbage. So, if you combine it with houttuynia . . . well, let's just say you are in for a treat.)

Species used: There are somewhere between 30 and 80 species in this genus. Well-degreed taxonomists speak authoritatively, and rather insistently, of just how many species really are in this genus—few of them cite the same figures, or the same plants. As yet, I cannot find a definitive work on the genus. So, there's 30, or 48, or 79—a bunch of plants anyway. (Taxonomist: a person who is taxing, that is, someone "not easily borne, wearing, burdensome, onerous.")

The most commonly used species is *Isatis tinctoria* (worldwide), but *Isatis indigotica* is fairly prominently used in China (as is *tinctoria*), *Isatis costa* is used in Pakistan, *Isatis cappadocica* in Iran, and still others here and there. All the species seem to contain similar chemistry; all (at least all the sources I have read say so) have been used to produce the indigo dye that the genus is known for.

Synonyms: Some taxonomic compulsivists list *Isatis indigotica* as a synonym for *tinctoria,* but chemical examination of the two continually reveals significant differences (not that *that* will deter them).

Common names: Isatis, woad, dyer's woad.

Parts Used

Root and leaves.

Preparation and Dosage

Isatis has traditionally been used as a decoction in China, where the longest history of use has occurred. The use of isatis tinctures is fairly new, although the Chinese and Japanese have been testing the activity of alcohol extracts for several decades. The plant is rarely used as a single tincture but is normally combined with other herbs. If you are going to use it as a single, you might consider using it as a decoction as the Chinese have traditionally done. (I do not think that capsules or tablets are an effective form for the herb; there is no clinical data on them and I have not seen good effects in practice from their use.)

In traditional Chinese medicine the roots and leaves are considered to be different medicines and are used for slightly different things (see the section on traditional Chinese medicine on page 379). Most people in the United States who do make tinctures are using the root; nevertheless, the leaves are exceptionally potent and are considered to be more specific for upper respiratory infections than the root—they are the most antiviral part of the plant.

I agree with a number of practitioners who have found the leaf better for acute conditions, and the root for chronic. The root seems to be better at modulating immune dynamics, increasing immune response, and moderating inflammation—just helping to tone down and even out everything while increasing immune potency. It, as well, does have a number of the potent antiviral compounds in it, so I like to include it, with the leaves, in formulations. It is also the most antibacterial part of the plant. The best tincture formulation, in my opinion, comes from a mixture of the root and leaves: one part root, two parts leaves. The roots are sometimes hard to dig if you are wildcrafting them, however the aerial parts can easily be wildcrafted and both root and leaves can be bought online.

The leaves need to be dried before tincturing; do not use them fresh unless you are making dye. In addition, they need to be heated (as does the root) to better extract the polysaccharides. (The Chinese do things for thousands of years for a reason.) Also: You need soft water, that is, acidic, anywhere from a pH of 1 to 6, in order to more effectively extract the bioactive alkaloids from the plant. Most of the constituents are soluble in water, so you won't need much alcohol, mostly just enough to bring out a few alcohol-soluble constituents and to stabilize the tincture so it won't go bad when stored. Studies have found that high-alcohol-content extractions are not as effective as water extracts for treating virus infections; alcohol/water combinations are better than pure alcohol or pure water for extracting the constituents needed to treat bacterial infections.

TINCTURE

Use an herb:liquid ratio of 1:5, with the liquid being 25 percent alcohol. Use two parts leaves, one part root. (Tastes terrible.)

Take (for example) 5 ounces dried root (grind it well) and 10 ounces dried leaves (also ground well). That makes 15 ounces of herb. You will need five times that of liquid, that is, 75 ounces. Of that liquid, 25 percent (one-quarter of it) will be alcohol, the rest will be water. You will need, then, 56 ounces of water, 19 of alcohol.

Add the ground-up herbs to a cooking pot, mix in the 56 ounces of water, bring to a boil. *If you do not have soft water, or if you do not know, you will need to add 1 tablespoon of vinegar as well to help extract the alkaloids.* Cover the pot and boil for 30 minutes. Then let it cool to room temperature. You can put the covered pot in the sink with cold water to speed this up. (Don't let it tip over; just an FYI on that one.)

When the mix is cool, pour it all into a large jar with a lid, and add the 19 ounces (liquid measurement) of alcohol. Put the lid on and let it sit for 2 weeks. Shake it every once in a while.

When done, pour off the liquid, and squeeze the marc (the herbs) to extract as much liquid as you can. Then throw the pressed herbs away (in the compost or garden of course). Bottle and label. As for dosage:

As a preventive: 30 drops up to 6x daily.

In acute conditions: 1 tsp up to 10 times daily.

Note: Again, I would not normally use this herb as a single, but only in combination with other herbs such as lomatium or licorice.

DECOCTION

The Chinese dosage is quite high, as usual, compared to Western approaches. Root decoctions: 10–30 grams (1/3–1 ounce) of the root boiled for 30 minutes; 1 cup drunk 3x daily for a max of 3 weeks. Leaf decoctions: 9–15 grams; 1 cup drunk 3x daily (in acute conditions 60–120 grams).

CAPSULES OR TABLETS

Again, I am not convinced this is a useful way to take this herb; all indications from the research are that the herb is most effective if heated in water and a decoction made. Nevertheless, if you must: 200 mg 3x daily. In acute conditions: 2 grams daily. Again, the leaves are better for viral influenzas.

Side Effects and Contraindications

Leaf: Occasionally nausea, rarely vomiting. Root: Rarely allergic reactions, urticaria, cyanosis of the face, dyspnea—but these were from intramuscular injections; there is no evidence of this from oral ingestion.

However, caution should be exercised in long-term use. Normally, you would not take isatis for longer than 3 weeks. This should be sufficient to deal with anything you have, especially if you have combined the herb with other antivirals. You should avoid using the herb as a single medicinal if you are presenting with a subjective feeling of cold without fever. The herb *may* induce a deep chill with overuse (longer than 3 weeks). Under some circumstances, longer use can lead to feelings of weakness, light dizziness, and an odd feeling in the bones. Stopping the herb will correct the condition within a few days. Isatis should not be used by people on dialysis or those experiencing renal failure—high doses or long-term use may negatively affect the kidneys.

Herb/Drug Interactions

Synergist with antibiotics and viral vaccines, increasing the activity of both. The herb may interfere with tests for measuring total bilirubin content.

Habitat and Appearance

Isatis is native to southeastern Russia and China but has hitchhiked widely with people and is now common throughout Europe, northern Africa, Japan, the United States, and Canada. Isatis is mainly a northern hemisphere plant. It was a major agricultural crop a great many places, planted widely for several thousand years, due to its use as an indigo dye for cloth—but it escaped. (Italy has now begun growing it again as an important agricultural crop—a source of natural, nonpolluting indigo dye.)

Isatis is invasive nearly everyplace it gets transplanted—yet another potent invasive medicinal for emerging infections. The plant is especially invasive in the western United States, up into Canada, and around the Great Lakes region. It can be found wild in California, Colorado, D.C., Idaho, Illinois, Montana, Nevada, New Jersey, New Mexico, New York, Oregon, Utah, Virginia, Washington, West Virginia, Wyoming, British Columbia, Ontario, and Quebec. It is considered invasive in Canada and at least eight western states. A few isatis plants even traveled as passengers on the first Chinese space mission—one giant leap for plantkind.[18]

Like many of the potent antimicrobials that we need for resistant infections, this one is growing all around us, insisting we notice it. Nevertheless, as an invasive, it has been targeted as a plant to be terminated with extreme prejudice. Plant purists (phytoaryans) of various stripes exist in many locations and spend a great deal of their time working to eradicate isatis. They tend to exhibit phytohysteria at the simplest provocation and will speak badly of the plant if you bring it up in conversation—forgive them, for they know not what they do.

Isatis is a biennial (usually) though it can annualize if the climate forces it to or even straggle on as a perennial for a while. The plant begins as a basal rosette and looks something like a cross between the dandelion rosette and that of broccoli. It does have some small, rounded teeth on the first-year leaves that the second-year leaves don't have, but there isn't the same kind of toothiness as that belonging to dandelion leaves. The leaves in first-year rosettes are up to 7 inches in length with a cream-colored midrib. They are broadest at the tip and taper to a point at the base. I think the plant looks more broccoli-like in color and texture the second year; the stalk it sends up reminds me quite a lot of that pile of semi-edible stuff you have left after you take the broccoli heads off for cooking, or at least a well-watered plant does. (Unfortunately, to my tongue, the tincture tastes not like broccoli but a bit like spoiled cabbage or broccoli—interfering with my enjoyment in taking it . . . a lot—and I work to mask it with other herbs such as yerba santa. It helps. A little.) Isatis growing in more semiarid locations tends to get a bit woody and darker in color as it ages, the stem being, like the ripe seeds, a bit purplish/brown in color. The second-year leaves clasp the stem rather than having a slender stem (petiole) attachment.

The flowering stalk that it sends up the second year, to my eye, looks a bit like broccoli when it has gone to seed—the agriculturally grown isatis more so. The flowering stalk can be from 1 to 4 feet in height; it puts out clusters of yellow flowers that look to my eye a great deal like those of St. John's wort. They are bright yellow. It flowers in May/June and begins to set seed immediately. The flowers continue growing up compounded racemes, the seeds following closely behind, developing from the earlier flowers that have already matured. It takes about 8 weeks from the beginning of flower-stem growth to the setting of the first seeds.

If environmental conditions don't support seed production the second year, the plant can continue as a rosette for several years until they do. That plant, not surprisingly, tends to be bigger, both roots and rosette.

The seed pods (each containing one seed) are flattish and remind me of rolled oats, in spite of their green color when young. They turn a dark purplish-brown when ripe. The pods hang off the flowering stalk in their thousands, lined up like paratroopers about to exit a plane over enemy-controlled territory. Each plant can put out as many as 500 seeds a season; later generations tend to spread out from that first plant in a sort of expanding zone of conquest, extending from a common center. It doesn't take long to dominate the landscape. The seeds can remain viable for years in the soil. Once freed from the seed pod, *every* seed will germinate. (It can't be bargained with. It can't be reasoned with. And it absolutely will not stop. Ever.)

The plant loves alkaline, semiarid soils and it does very well in them. It spreads rapidly in such soils, and doesn't need disturbed soils to extend into a new locale; it crowds out normal vegetation just fine. The plant seeds produce potent chemicals that inhibit competing plants; even its own seeds won't germinate until the chemicals are leached out of the soil after the parent plant dies the second winter.

Isatis is especially invasive in ecologically disturbed areas (even if they appear sound to the eye), especially where there has been overgrazing by cattle. The rate of spread is intense, one site in Montana reporting an increase from infestation in 2 acres to over 100 in 2 years. It reduces cattle grazing capacity by about 40 percent on infested range—part of its ecological function. Even sheep and goats don't like to eat it, and that is saying something. It is intensely bitter the older it gets.

Radishes are also a member of the Brassicaceae family and the root of isatis is indeed sort of radish-like, a bit like a cross between a daikon radish and a carrot, except for the color. The first-year root tends to be a bit fuller, more plump, and the root bark (tannish-brownish with a hint of gold) a bit lighter in color. The plants send out lateral roots in the upper foot of soil to tap surface water as well as sending down a taproot to drink from deeper sources. The second-year roots go much deeper, up to 5 feet (3 feet is more common). The root bark the second year is a bit darker. When sliced the inner bark is a light cream, the

(continued on page 376)

Properties of Isatis

Actions

As a broad-spectrum antiviral, isatis is directly virucidal, inhibits viral replication, inhibits virus attachment to cells, inhibits hemagglutination, inhibits viral neuraminidase (equivalent to Tamiflu in potency), inhibits RANTES. It potentiates the effectiveness of viral vaccines and is an immune stimulant, anti-inflammatory, antipyretic, antinociceptive, antiallergenic, tyrosinase inhibitor, antioxidant, antifungal, antibacterial, antiparasitic, antileukemic, antitumor, potent urease inhibitor, potent cross-class serine protease inhibitor, butyrycholinesterase inhibitor, lipoxygenase inhibitor, antiendotoxin, and dioxin antagonist (including against TCDD or 2,3,7,8-tetrachlorodibenzodioxin, the most potent).

Active Against

Isatis is a very broad antiviral herb. It is active against influenza viruses A and B (various strains of H1N1 as well as H6N2, H7N3, H9N2), SARS coronavirus, Coxsackie virus (B2, B3, B4), rubella virus, avian infectious bronchitis virus, respiratory syncytial virus, human adenovirus type 3, measles, mumps, varicella virus (chicken pox/shingles), Epstein-Barr, hepatitis B, herpes simplex virus 1, cytomegalovirus, hemorrhagic fever with renal syndrome (HFRS) virus, porcine reproductive and respiratory syndrome virus, swine pseudorabies virus, Newcastle disease virus, goose parvovirus, and porcine parvovirus.

It has some antimicrobial actions as well, against *Staphylococcus aureus*, *Toxoplasma gondii*, *Plasmodium falciparum*, *Leishmania* spp., *Pseudomonas aeruginosa*, *Trichophyton schoenleinii*, *Aspergillus niger*, *Candida albicans*, *Trichophyton simii*, *Macrophomina phaseolina*, *Bacillus pasteurii* (a.k.a. *Sporosarcina pasteurii*), leukemic and liver cancer cells, and possibly other cancers. Alcohol/water extracts of *Isatis microcarpa* (dried) leaves are active (in vitro) against *Bacillus subtilis*, *B. sphaericus*, *Staphylococcus aureus*, *Pseudomonas* spp., *E. coli*, *Salmonella* spp., *Aspergillus niger*, *A. flavus*, *Fusarium oxysporum*, *Alternaria tenuis*, and *Microsporum fulvum*. Water extracts of the root are active against *Staphylococcus* spp., *Bacillus subtilis*, *E. coli*, *Salmonella typhi*, *Streptococcus* spp., and *Haemophilus influenzae*.

The isothiocyanates in the plant, especially phenethyl isothiocyanate, are potently inhibitory of *Clostridium difficile*. (Some monographs on isatis list a number of other organisms against which the herb is supposedly effective, e.g., *Neisseria* spp. The data they cite comes from Chinese texts that don't identify which plants were tested—see the section on traditional Chinese medicine on page 379.)

Use to Treat

The herb is strongly specific for influenza (all strains irrespective of source), SARS, all primary respiratory virus infections, viral pneumonia, meningitis, pseudomonas lung infections, scarlet fever, sore throat, laryngitis, tonsillitis, Epstein-Barr (especially with acute-onset sore throat), gastroenteritis, hepatitis, bacterial conjunctivitis (as eyedrops), leukemia, chicken pox, shingles—generally, any viral infection including encephalitis.

Isatis is strongly active against paramyxoviruses, which include respiratory syncytial virus, mumps, measles, and Newcastle disease. Although not tested against other members of this group (rinderpest, canine distemper, metapneumovirus, Hendra virus, Nipah virus, morbillivirus), it is being used in veterinary practice with good effect for canine distemper, rinderpest (before eradication), and Newcastle disease. It seems to be broadly active against this group. The herb is widely used in China for viral hepatitis, but I have located only two tiny studies on its activity in this regard.

The herb is also widely used for encephalitis in China with apparently good results. I can find nothing testing the antiviral activity of the herb against any encephalitis viruses. However, the herb is strongly active against the rubella virus, which is a member of the Togaviridae family of viruses, which also includes a number of encephalitis viruses. There are some clinical studies of the herb being used for encephalitis B (Japanese encephalitis virus) in China with very good outcomes (see Scientific Research on page 380). And the herb is high in kaempferol, common in many plants, that is specifically, and strongly, active against the Japanese encephalitis virus. Its history of use in China for these viral diseases strongly supports the herb's use in these conditions. I would use it as an adjunct for *any* encephalopathy of viral origin.

Other Uses

The plant has a very long history as a dye plant for making an indigo dye for cloth. There is a very good description of how to make the dye from fresh plants at woad.org.uk/html/extraction.html ("How to Extract Woad Dye in 10 Easy Stages," by Teresinha Roberts, June 5, 2012), though by googling the Internet you will get a number of good sites. The same dye was sometimes used for tattooing and also body painting the Picts and the Brittanni in that Mel Gibson movie.

core darker, the same color as the outer bark. The roots are fleshy, generally 1 to 3 inches in diameter, and, unless garden-grown, hard to dig up except for the top layers. They like tough soil.

Finding It

Plant it, you won't regret it (though antiphytoimmigrants probably will if they find out). It will supply potent medicine for you and your family indefinitely as it reseeds easily once established. Or if you live in the right region you can wildcraft it; the invasive plant societies will love you for it. Seeds are available from Horizon Herbs (horizonherbs.com).

You can get bulk isatis root, powder, cut and sifted, or concentrated from 1stChineseHerbs.com. They carry the leaf as well. You can also get a very nice tincture of the root from Sage Consulting & Apothecary (sagewomanherbs.com).

Cultivation and Collection

Isatis *loves* semiarid, alkaline, average-to-poor soils with enough water to ease its thirst but not to overhydrate it. However, if you garden-raise it and water it well, it will grow fleshy and fat and look much more like a broccoli plant than otherwise. The plant has very low nitrogen requirements. It propagates easily from seeds sown in sunny locations. Sow in fall or spring. It seeds itself readily once established. Survives to –30°F. Doesn't like the shade; needs sun. Will grow from sea level to 7,000 feet or so. Tolerates salty air and soil. *Isatis tinctoria* is often one of the earliest plants to emerge in spring (self-motivated, early riser).

Usually, *only* the leaves and roots are used medicinally. The stems are discarded, the flowers ignored, the seeds overlooked. The seeds are most likely highly medicinal but for some reason no one has explored their medicinal uses. (They contain a large amount of diverse fatty acids and are very high in the anticancer compounds glucobrassicin, neoglucobrassicin, and glucobrassicin-l-sulfonate. They also contain the glucosinolate precursors to the anti-inflammatory compound tryptanthrin.) The leaves and roots have somewhat different actions, so harvest and store them separately. (See the Preparation and Dosage section on page 368 for more.)

The root should be harvested in the fall of the first year or the spring of the second. Clean and slice the roots while they are still fresh, as you would carrots. Layer them on a tray and dry out of sunlight in a warm location.

Harvest the leaves from the first-season and second-season plants prior to flowering (if possible). The plant will releaf as it is harvested. When the plant is cut or the leaves damaged, later leaves can produce up to 65 times as much glucobrassicin. The leaves contain a number of important chemical precursors when they are harvested fresh; *they need to be dried at heat* for the chemicals to convert to their final form. The most important end-product chemicals are tryptanthrin and indirubin. Tryptanthrin is a potent anti-inflammatory compound that strongly inhibits prostaglandin and leukotriene synthesis—it is also potently antiparasitic against toxoplasmal, malarial, and leishmanial parasites. It is found in much higher levels in dried leaves than in fresh. Indirubin is potently anti-inflammatory as well, although in different ways. It is strongly cytotoxic to leukemia cells and is very virucidal. Indirubin is three to five times higher in the dried leaf than in the fresh.

Traditionally, the leaves are harvested, then allowed to dry in the sun for several days, then brought inside to finish drying. The most tryptanthrin is produced when the plants are dried at around 100°F.

Bag both leaves and roots, separately, in plastic when completely dry. Store in plastic tubs out of the sun. Leaves will last several years, roots much longer. If you can't store this way, replace the leaves yearly, the roots every other year.

A Eurasion rust fungus has been imported by the phytopolice to try to kill the plants off. Check any plants you harvest and skip those with the rust fungus present. You will know it when you see it: The leaves look sick, turning brown, spotted, shriveling.

Plant Chemistry

More than 65 nonvolatile plant compounds have been identified in the leaves of isatis: alkaloids, flavonoids, fatty acids, porphyrins, lignans, carotenoids, glucosinolates, and cyclohexenones. And another 70 volatile compounds as well: aliphatic hydrocarbons, acids, alcohols, aldehydes, esters, aromatic aldehydes, ethers, furans, isothiocyanates, thiocyanates, sulfurated compounds, nitriles, terpenes, sesquiterpenes—the usual suspects. The isothiocyanates account for about 40 percent of the total volatile fraction.

Isatis also contains indican, isatin, isatisine A, indirubin, bisindigotin, kaempferol, indigotin, epigoitrin, isatinones A and B, trisindoline, salicylic acid, syringic acid, benzoic acid, gamma-linolenic acid, indolin-2-one, anthranilic acid, 3′-hydroxyepiglucoisatisin, epiglucoisatisin, various flavone C-glucosides, various sphingolipids, mannitol, various glucopyranosides, indolinone, indigo, alpha-linolenic acid, cytidine, hypoxanthine, uridine, xanthine, guanosine, L-pyroglutamic acid, sinigrin, uracil, beta-sterol, daucosterol, o-aminobenzoic acid, glucobrassicin, neoglucobrassicin, glucobrassicin-l-sulfonate, along with several hydroxycinnamic acids and, as usual, a whole bunch of other stuff. There is 20 times more of the cancer-preventing glucobrassicin in isatis than its relative broccoli.

Traditional Uses of Isatis

Isatis has been used for millennia in Asia as a medicinal and has been cultivated since neolithic times elsewhere for its use in textiles, body paints, inks, and medicine. It was widely cultivated throughout Europe until the early twentieth century when chemical dyes replaced the need for natural indigo sources. The name of Glastonbury, a town in Somerset, England, is thought to mean "place where woad grows." Many archaeological sites from the neolithic contain isatis remnants, including the French cave of l'Audoste, in Bouches du Rhône, and the Iron Age settlement of Heuneburg in Germany. Isatis seed impressions have been found on many examples of ancient pottery. Egyptian mummy wrappings were sometimes dyed with the plant. Dye shops with the remains of isatis plants have been found in ancient Viking settlements. The author of the Lindisfarne Gospels used a woad-based pigment (isatis) for his blues. Deep blue dye plants were very rare in the ancient world and the color was highly prized.

Since woad is biodegradable and renewable it is beginning to be commercially grown again to make both ink and dye (for inkjet printers and small craft dyers).

AYURVEDA

Isatis is traditionally used in Ayurvedic practice but I can find little on it. Used as a digestive tonic and for GI tract problems.

TRADITIONAL CHINESE MEDICINE

Isatis has been used for millennia in China. The leaves of the plant are referred to as daqingye, the root as banlan'gen; they are considered to be close but somewhat different medicinals with slightly different actions. However there is a problem in extrapolating from Chinese studies of the herb (a point rarely made when citing the Chinese studies). The problem is that four different plants (all from different genera) are referred to as daqingye in Chinese medicine, and two different ones as banlan'gen. While the plants are used interchangeably with each other, the problem is that the early Chinese clinical trials with the plants did not differentiate species in a number of instances. Later studies are much better.

The leaves (daqingye) are used as a bitter, cold herb, anti-inflammatory, detoxicant, for reducing fever, and for removing heat from the blood. It is considered specific for fever, colds and flu, maculae, papulae, pharyngolaryngitis, parotitis, encephalomeningitis, encephalitis B, erysipelas, and carbuncle. It is considered good for headache and sore throat. The root is considered to be bitter, cold, with latent-heat-clearing properties, antipyretic, detoxicant, and anti-inflammatory, and for clearing heat from the blood. It is used for erysipelas, macular eruption due to pathogenic heat, loss of consciousness, hemoptysis, pharyngitis, mumps, and conjunctivitis.

The Chinese used the leaf decoction to good effectiveness in treating the SARS outbreak there several years ago. It is now widely used for influenza and viral pneumonia, hepatitis, mumps, encephalitis, and gastroenteritis.

WESTERN BOTANIC PRACTICE

Isatis has a long history of use in Europe, at least as far back as the fifth century BCE. Hippocrates recommended the plant for treating wounds, ulcers, and hemorrhoids. Galen and Pliny recommended it as well. In the late Middle Ages it was used for snakebites, wounds, and inflammation. The American Eclectics didn't use it much, mostly as a vulnerary and styptic. It has only just recently emerged into Western awareness as a medicinal, mostly for its antiviral properties. As yet, it is still little understood by American herbalists in spite of its being an invasive in the United States, and those who do use the plant generally use it the wrong way. They use the root as the main medicinal instead of the leaf, which is more active, especially against viral infections. Most use the plant as tablets or capsules even though it is not very active in those forms—water extracts, for example, are significantly more effective in stimulating immune responses than both high-concentrate alcohol extracts and the herb in solid form.

Many American herbalists, regrettably, don't know the plant at all.

Scientific Research

There have been a number of good clinical trials in China on the use of the herb for various things; I am not going into any depth on the ones that don't make a distinction as to which plant was used. Trials where the plant (leaf) is not clearly identified were conducted with upper respiratory infections, influenza, mumps, measles, infectious hepatitis, and infectious lymphocytosis. Trials where the root is not identified occurred with chicken pox, encephalitis B, hepatitis, mumps, influenza, infectious mononucleosis, herpes simplex, herpes zoster, pityriasis rosea, verruca plana, cerebral meningitis, diphtheria, and fulminant conjunctivitis.

Given the many later studies (in

vitro, in vivo, human) that show that isatis is active against many of these organisms and/or conditions, there is good reason to believe that it was isatis that was used in some or all of the studies.

Isatis tinctoria leaf was used to treat patients with encephalitis B (Japanese viral encephalitis). Headache and other symptoms were sharply reduced, and the mortality rate was decreased in both mild and serious cases—in critical patients, Western intervention was needed along with the herb in order to prevent death.

Sixty people with rubella were randomly assigned to two groups. One received a combination formula of isatis root, milkvetch root, and basket fern, while the control group received ribavirin—both for 20 days. The isatis formula and ribavirin were effective for both groups; the isatis group responded more quickly to treatment.

Twenty healthy people experienced induced contact dermatitis; they were then treated with a variety of isatis extracts as well as pure tryptanthrin. The isatis extracts were more effective than the tryptanthrin in resolving the dermatitis.

A randomized, double-blind, parallel study was conducted with 200 people suffering from bacterial conjunctivitis. Isatis root eyedrops were used (versus levofloxacin) to treat them. The drops were administered six times daily; 90 percent were cured.

Twenty patients with head or neck cancer were split into two groups in order to test isatis root for the treatment of radiation-induced mucositis. The first group received normal saline, the second gargled, then swallowed an isatis root decoction. Those receiving the decoction had significantly reduced severity of mucositis and anorexia and less swallowing difficulty. This study echoes other reports that the root decoction heals ulceration in and regenerates mucous membranes.

Purified extracts from isatis—indirubin and meisoindigo (an indirubin metabolite)—were used to successfully treat chronic myelogenous leukemia.

In vivo trials with isatis leaf in rats found that the herb was highly effective in treating chronic pseudomonas lung infection (similar in its dynamics to cystic fibrosis). The herb reduced the incidence of lung abscesses, decreased the severity of macroscopic pathology in lung tissue, and altered the inflammatory response in the lungs from an acute inflammation dominated by polymorphonuclear leukocytes to a less-intense chronic type inflammation dominated by mononuclear leukocytes.

In vivo trials with mice found that isatis enhanced the protectiveness of viral vaccines (foot and mouth disease). In other trials, extracts of isatis leaf reduced induced inflammation in mice. Both topical and oral ingestion were effective; purified tryptanthrin extracts were not effective. (Unusual extracts were tested: supercritical CO_2 and dichloromethane.) An in vivo study with mice found that dichloromethane extracts of isatis leaf were effective as an anti-inflammatory in the treatment of arthritis. And extracts of isatis leaf were found to inhibit allergen-induced airway inflammation and hyperreactivity in mice.

Isatis root extracts were found to be highly protective of mice after total-body irradiation, modulating inflammation and reducing tissue damage.

And when endotoxins from Gram-negative bacteria were injected into rabbits, administration of an extract from isatis root (o-aminobenzoic acid) reduced fever and destroyed 84 percent of the endotoxins. Deaths dropped from 70 percent to 20 percent.

Isolated fatty acids (compound K) from *Isatis tinctoria* leaf prolonged survival of cardiac allografts in alloantigen-primed mice. Compound K, when combined with tacrolimus, significantly inhibited heart transplant rejection in mice.

An isolated constituent of isatis, indirubin, and an indirubin metabolite, meisoindigo, are used as a combination therapy in the treatment of myelogenous leukemia in China. They have been found to be antiproliferative and cytotoxic to cancer cells, and in clinical use they have extended survival times considerably, inducing hematologic remission.

Scores of studies have been conducted on the antiviral, antibacterial, antifungal, and cytoinhibitory actions of both the leaf and root. Crude extracts of isatis (and various isolated constituents) have been found more effective than ribavirin in their antiviral actions on Coxsackie viruses. They are as effective as Tamiflu (in vitro) in inhibiting viral neuraminidase. (Neuraminidases are enzymes that are essential for viral entry into the host cells.) Tamiflu acts as it does because it inhibits the enzyme that allows influenza viruses to enter cells to replicate.

Several compounds in the plant have been found to be potent urease inhibitors. Urease is an enzyme found in many bacteria, yeast, and fungi. A urease inhibitor is, in essence, an antimicrobial against microbes that need that enzyme to function (such as some of the mycoplasmas).

Tryptanthrin (especially), gamma-linolenic acid, and an indolin-2-one derivative are highly anti-inflammatory, inhibiting COX-2, 5-lipoxygenase (5-LOX), the expression of inducible nitric oxide synthase (iNOS), human neutrophil elastase, and the release of histamine from mast cells. Indirubin is a potent inhibitor of cyclin-dependent kinase 5 (CDK5), glycogen synthase kinase 3ß, and inflammatory reactions in delayed-type hypersensitivity.

Licorice

Licorice is an unusual medicinal. It is potently antiviral, moderately antibacterial (but fairly strong against a few bacterial species such as *Staphylococcus* and *Bacillus* spp.), moderately immune potentiating, and a very potent synergist.

Since licorice should also be considered a primary synergist plant, you can turn to page 423 for more information. *It should rarely be used alone or in large doses for extended periods.*

Lomatium

Family: Apiaceae, the carrot family.

Species used: There are 70 or maybe 80 species in this genus—trying to pin a taxonomist down is like gluing feathers on a donkey so it can fly. They are indigenous to the United States (lomatiums, not taxonomists) and grow from the Mississippi River region throughout the West, Southwest, and Northwest. A number of them can be used medicinally but information on the genus and its medicinal uses is very sparse. *Many of the species are exceptionally rare and are endangered so be highly conscious if you are wildcrafting. Only harvest if the species is very common in your area or is not endangered.* The most commonly used lomatium is *Lomatium dissectum,* but several others can be used identically and grow in enough abundance, here and there, to be harvested and are (usually) not considered endangered: *L. ambiguum, L. bicolor, L. cous, L. foeniculaceum, L. grayi, L. macrocarpum, L. nudicaule, L. orientale, L. simplex, L. triternatum.*

L. dissectum, L. cous, L. bicolor, L. foeniculaceum, L. macrocarpum, and *L. orientale* have the widest range, some of them extending into Iowa, Minnesota, and Missouri. *L. nudicaule,* though confined to the Northwest, has a particularly long history of medicinal use and is considered by some to be stronger than *L. dissectum.*

There are, just to make things harder, two varieties of *L. dissectum, L. dissectum* var. *dissectum* and *L. dissectum* var. *multifidum.* The former is more prevalent east of the Cascade mountain range, the latter west. The former likes more rain and lower altitudes, the latter likes it semiarid and grows as high as 7,000 feet. I have generally used *multifidum;* it appears to be somewhat stronger in its medicinal effects. Almost no source you order from will be able to tell you which variety of *dissectum* they are selling you.

Synonyms: The *Lomatium* genus used to be the genus *Leptotaenia.* It was reclassified during World War II—shortly before it was inducted.

Lomatium dissectum, for example, used to be *Leptotaenia dissecta*. For some reason *Lomatium dissectum* was also once called *Ferula dissoluta, ferula* meaning "rod" and *dissoluta* meaning "debauched, unrestrained by convention or morality," ergo, debauched rod (there's a really good joke here but . . .). In any event, it appears that botanists and taxonomists are closely related, perhaps from an ancient debauchery.

Common names: Lomatium, biscuit root, cough root, Indian consumption plant, desert parsley, Indian parsnip. *Lomatium dissectum* is sometimes known as fernleaf biscuitroot.

Biscuit root, desert parsley, and lomatium are the general common identifiers and will usually be combined with a descriptive to create a particular species' common name in a geographical area, e.g., northern Idaho biscuit root, Bradshaw's desert parsley, California lomatium.

Parts Used

The root is normally what is used, but the seeds are highly active. They often contain considerably more constituents than the root and may be used instead (though hardly anyone does).

Preparation and Dosage

Lomatium is generally used as a tincture (at least these days).

TINCTURE

Fresh root: 1:2 herb:liquid ratio. Chop the wilted root as finely as possible with a very sharp knife, place in a jar, add the tincturing medium (70 percent grain alcohol, 30 percent water), cover, and let macerate 2 weeks. Dosage: 10–30 drops up to 5x daily. In acute conditions, take 10–30 drops each hour.

Dry root: Same as for the fresh root, except powder the root and use an herb:liquid ratio of 1:5.

Fresh seeds: Same as for the fresh root.

Dry seeds: 1:3, 50 percent alcohol. Dosage: 1 dropperful 3–5x daily or once per hour in acute conditions.

Common influenza tincture blend: Combine equal parts of lomatium, red root, licorice, and pleurisy root (*Asclepias tuberosa*) tinctures. In acute conditions with debility (bedridden, lingering loss of energy, failure to thrive, pneumonia) take up to 1 tsp 6x daily. You should make up 16 or so ounces to keep on hand. When the flu hits you won't want to make it. (I do, however, prefer the more extensive formulation described in chapter 2; see page 122.)

INFUSION OR DECOCTION

You can try it, it worked for the indigenous peoples. I have tasted and used the tea myself and its impact on the tongue is nearly as strong as that of the tincture. Somehow, in spite of not being water soluble, the aromatics are indeed getting into the tea. (It is prepared by pouring hot water over the root and leaving it covered for an hour or so. This does help keep the aromatics in there.)

Add 1 tsp of the powdered root to 6 ounces hot water, cover, and let steep.

Influenza decoction blend: Robin Seydel's influenza blend (via Northwest herbalist Ryan Drum): Combine 1 ounce each of lomatium seeds, lobaria lichen, licorice root, Oregon grape root, echinacea blossoms, red clover blossoms, and rowan berries. Grind all the herbs into a powder (or as close as you can get). Add to 1 quart hot water, and boil for 2 to 4 minutes. Remove from the heat, cover, and let steep for an hour. Then strain, add lemon juice and honey to taste, and drink hot, 1 quart per day.

STEAM INHALANT

Pour boiling water over some of the freshly chopped root or seeds (which should be in a hot-liquid-tolerant container). Drape a towel over your head and the container, and breathe in. This works a treat for influenzal infections. Take the tincture, too.

Side Effects and Contraindications

Pregnancy and a nasty rash. (Actually, that should be "Nasty rash and pregnancy"—you won't get pregnant from taking the tincture.)

From what is known, the plants are exceptionally nontoxic. Injections of isolates of the plants at 2.5 percent of the weight of mice were not toxic in any way—no observable differences at all. *However*, the plant is contraindicated in pregnancy *and* about 1 percent of people using the herb get a rather nasty rash. The rash appears to be associated only with *Lomatium dissectum*; the use of other species has apparently not produced it.

As far as anyone knows, this *is* an allergic reaction to the plant but it is a rather unusual one—there is no itching, no discomfort other than the visual. Herbalist Michael Moore reports that he found it occurring *only* with the fresh root tincture and only then if the tincture was taken as a single, i.e., not blended with anything else.

The rash usually begins within 8 hours of taking the tincture. It can cover the whole body—warm baths often make it worse. The rash is a deep to dark red, even purplish. It can cover the entire body (most people stay home to avoid encountering the human subspecies *Homo staris*). There is rarely, if ever, any itching or discomfort. It's just there. *Nothing* will make it better, not steroids, not Benadryl, not calamine lotion, not Pepcid, not herbs, not herbal washes, not doctors or hospitals. So save your money and skip the emergency room visit—besides physicians don't know squat about plant medicines, or their side effects. (Though they are often highly prejudiced against them.) It's grin-and-bear-it time. The rash will disappear within a week or so after its initial occurrence.

To avoid the rash, use lomatium as part of a mixture, not singly, and use the dried root, not the fresh root, for tinctures. Oh, and don't spend a lot of time looking in the mirror.

Herb/Drug Interactions

None known.

Habitat and Appearance

The lomatiums are called desert parsleys for a reason; their leaves and stems often look very similar to those rarely purchased parsley bunches you see in the grocery store and sometimes buy and use a tiny bit of for an experimental recipe before the rest decays into a dessicated phytomemory (often found months later) in the bottom of the vegetable drawer in the refrigerator. Some of the species are small, like that parsley bunch, while others are much larger; *L. dissectum* is one of the giants.

Like most of this family, *L. dissectum* begins as a fernlike bunch of basal leaves that, as the plant matures, sends up a rather substantial flowering stalk. The fernlike leaves of this species may be up to a foot long, with a dozen or so leaves spreading out from the root core. The flowering stalks can be from 2 to 5 feet in height. They are usually leafless. The plant flowers in early spring, the seeds mature in late summer or early fall.

The roots are 3 or so inches in diameter and up to 2 feet long (*L. nudicaule*: 6 inches in diameter, up to 3 feet long); they're big. Herbalist Michael Moore describes the root in his typical fashion:

> The root is fleshy, thick at the top, lumpy, and irregular, like a mutant cross between a carrot and rutabaga, with odd parts left over. The skin is pearly grey, with many oil glands spread throughout the variously cream- and yellow-colored flesh.[19]

Most lomatiums grow in well-drained, sandy or rocky soil—basically a certain kind of deserty-sandy-dryish-hard-to-get-to, hard-to-dig-in, old volcanicy or decomposed granity terrain and soil. There are a few exceptions—such as *L. nudicaule*. But herbalist Ryan Drum comments that *that* particular plant was most likely brought to the island on which he lives in Puget Sound by the Salish who settled there. The plant only grows near old Salish settlements on extensive beach sand flats with few other plant competitors, a terrain similar to the deserty homeland it was transplanted from.

The lomatiums are semiarid plants of the Great Plains, deserts, high mountains, and northwest United States. That's where you will find them.

Properties of Lomatium

Actions

Analgesic
Antibacterial
Antifungal
Antimicrobial
Antiseptic
Antispasmodic
Antiviral
Expectorant
Mucous membrane tonic

Active Against

There have been few studies on the activity of the lomatiums against microorganisms and virtually none on their activities against viruses. The two most comprehensive studies occurred in 1948 and 1949 in the United States. Both focused on the antibacterial activities of extracted aromatics of the root, one isolated through steam distillation, the other through ethyl acetate extraction and filtration. The range of activity was fairly broad. Fractions of the steam distillate were found active against the following:

Achromobacter lacticum
Agrobacterium spp.
Aspergillus spp.
Bacillus spp.
Candida albicans
Clostridium spp. (mildly)
Coccidioides immitis
Corynebacterium diphtheriae
Diplococcus pneumoniae
Eberthella typhosa
Escherichia coli (mildly)
Fusarium spp.
Haemophilus influenzae
Histoplasmosis capsulatum
Micrococcus tetragenus
Microspermum trichoderma
Mucocus capsulatus
Mucor culmorum
Mycobacterium spp.
Mycoderma spp.
Neisseria spp. (mildly)
Pestallotia funera
Proteus spp.
Pseudomonas spp.
Pythium debaryanum
Rhizoctonia spp.
Serratia marcescens
Shigella spp.
Staphylococcus spp.
Streptomyces griseus
Trichophyton spp.
Zooleal spp.

In the ethyl acetate extracts study, several different forms were used at varying degrees of strength. They were found active against the following:

Bacillus subtilis
Corynebacterium diphtheriae
Diplococcus pneumoniae
Escherichia coli (mildly)
Micrococcus aureus
Neisseria catarrhalis
Proteus vulgaris (mildly)
Pseudomonas aeruginosa (mildly)
Serratia marcescens (mildly)
Streptococcus pyogenes
Vibrio comma (a.k.a. *V. cholerae*)

The ethyl acetate extracts were not active against *Klebsiella pneumoniae*, *Salmonella schottmuelleri*, or *Aerobacter aerogenes*.

Both studies found the steam and ethyl acetate isolates much more active against Gram-positive organisms than Gram-negative (as usual). Even at concentrations of 10^{-3} the Gram-positive organisms were completely inhibited. Some of the Gram-negative organisms were, however, highly susceptible to the isolates, e.g., *Vibrio comma*, *Neisseria catarrhalis*.

There have been no in-depth studies on the antiviral properties of lomatium, however a few researchers looking a bit more broadly report the plant roots to be active against rotavirus and HIV as well as *Bacillus subtilis*, *Staphylococcus aureus*, *Colletotrichum fragariae*, *Mycobacterium tuberculosis*, *Pseudomonas aeruginosa*, *Trypanosoma cruzi*, and *Propionbacterium acnes*.

In spite of the lack of viral studies, I, and many others, have found the plant highly active against most viral and bacterial respiratory infections, including pneumonia. I haven't found anything better for serious, debilitating influenza, avian flu, swine flu, West Nile, or incapacitating pneumonia. In some instances the people were bedridden, very weak and debilitated; in others, ER physicians had diagnosed them with severe pneumonia. In all cases focused treatment (i.e., high, frequent doses) worked well, though in the more debilitated instances, it took weeks to turn it around. Normally, people begin to show improvement within a day or two.

Use to Treat

Upper respiratory viral infections, all influenza strains, SARS, viral encephalitis, pneumonia. Lomatium is most effective, in my opinion, if combined with other herbs such as red root, licorice, pleurisy root. Nevertheless, it is very potent by itself and can be used as a single (however, see the section Side Effects and Contraindications on page 386). The taste is intense though you can get used to it.

Clinicians have reported good success in using the plant for other viral infections, for instance, Epstein-Barr and cytomegalovirus (in chronic fatigue-like situations), hepatitis C (lowering viral load), and HIV. Some (Michael Moore) have used it in the treatment of shigella and other bacterial infections with good success.

There is a tendency to look at the plant as a systemic antibacterial due to the early studies. I think the plant is better thought of as a systemic antiviral, especially for respiratory infections, most especially the emerging influenza strains. See Western Botanic Medicine (page 395).

(continued)

Properties of Lomatium—Continued

Other Uses

The roots of many lomatiums, before they attain maturity, are highly edible (though the taste may take some getting used to). The roots have traditionally been eaten fresh, steamed, roasted, boiled, in soups and stews, canned, or dried to crispy, and very tasty, sticks (if the roots are small enough). Larger immature roots or the sweeter varieties were peeled, pounded into cakes, and dried in the sun, hence the "biscuit" part of the common name. Lewis and Clark compared the taste of the dried cakes to bread. Most lomatium species were apparently used similarly.

Finding It

You can order the sliced and dried roots rather easily online. I prefer Pacific Botanicals for most herbs that I have to order in bulk; their quality is supreme.

Cultivation and Collection

The lomatiums don't cultivate easily, though a few agricultural groups are insisting they are indeed growing the plant and at least one commercial company describes its tincture as being from organically grown roots. Still, germination of the seeds is reportedly difficult. The plant *could* grow in similar terrain any place on Earth, but it would take work to get it to take in a new location. Transplanting may be a better option.

If you are wild-harvesting, you need to be aware of a couple of things. The first is the terrain: Lomatium likes it tough. *Lomatium dissectum,* and its variants, likes to grow around impossibly difficult rocky outcrops and the roots are tenacious. Find some in soil and skip the rocky ones. The second is the *nature* of the root itself: It appears in different forms depending on its age, the time of year, and which species it is from. Michael Moore comments:

> In the spring the roots ooze milky aromatic sap; by fall the sap is more resinous and balsamic; but in any case, the sticky bitter aromatic sap and the soft, fibrous flesh (not at all woody) differentiate this big Lomatium from the others of the genus. The Lomatium clan is huge, with eighty closely related species in the western states. For many years the large size of a few of these plants (most Lomatiums are quite small) caused botanists to classify them apart in the genus Leptotaenia. The larger Lomatiums, by whatever name, are an amorphous group, and I have found several strikingly varied stands whose roots are typical of *L. dissectum* in their morphology and constituents, which act like *L. dissectum* when tinctured, have identical constituents as measured by TLC (think-layer chromatography), but don't particularly look like *L. dissectum*. I have found these plants in such varied locations as Modoc County, California, northwestern Wyoming, and the front range of Colorado. . . . Most of the other large Lomatiums that grow in the range of *L. dissectum* have sweet, starchy parsniplike roots and could not be confused with this bitter, aromatic, oily- and waxy-rooted giant.[20]

Moore lists the species that he has found to be usable as *L. dissectum, L. multifidum, L. eatonii*, and *L. occidentalis*. Ryan Drum comments that *L. nudicaule* is just as good if not better. *Lomatium grayi* and *L. dissectum* overlap in their range and the two are often confused.

In any event, the root you are harvesting must be strongly aromatic, bitter, and oily if it is to be antiviral. Normally this is seen *only* in mature plants. If it is not, then it probably won't work as a medicinal though it will work as a rather good food source.

You can harvest the roots at any time of the year. They are easier to identify in the spring, a bit easier to dig after spring rains.

Dry the roots for a few days, then cut them up (they are a bit too resinous if you don't let them dry a little first). *Make sure you cut them up.* Generally they are sliced into wheels as you would slice a carrot. If you dry them whole, you will need a chainsaw to reduce their size later. (Just an FYI on that one.) Once the root circles are well dried store them in well-sealed plastic bags inside a well-sealed plastic tub out of direct sunlight in a coolish location. They will last several years. At least.

Moore likes the spring roots for making a fresh root tincture, and the fall roots for dried root tincture. I tend to prefer spring roots in this family; they are much bigger in my experience and, I feel, more potent. That is because the roots of all perennials grow throughout the winter, albeit very slowly. By spring they are full of stored nutrients and tend to be juicy and fat. By fall they have used those stores to send up stalks and set seed. Fall roots are stringier, a bit dryish and beef-jerkyish.

The big lomatiums are perennials; it takes them years to mature—often as much as a decade before they can be harvested. *Many sources put the minimum period of growth before the plants can be harvested for medicine at 20 years.* Some of the lomatiums in the wild are very old indeed—several hundred years; old-growth plants are not just trees.

Ryan Drum notes that the young *L. nudicaule* roots are sweet and starchy, very tender and highly edible, much like a plant candy. Only the older plants, when matured, will present with the typical oily, resinous, aromatic medicinal constituents needed in this species. Numerous other sources indicate that the same is true of *L. dissectum* and its variants—the plants need somewhere near a decade at minimum before they begin generating their volatile, and potently antiviral, oils and become useful for medicine.

If you harvest a root and it is sweet and starchy, then eat it but don't use it for medicine. However, all indications are that the seeds can be used no matter how old the plant is; they possess a similar chemistry to the root. This is borne out in part by the traditional uses of the seeds of *L. nudicaule* by the Salish in northwestern Washington State. They used *only* the seeds for medicine (the root was a food staple), and their traditional uses of the seeds are for the same range of problems that the roots are now used for in conventional practice.

Plant Chemistry

One of the main problems with scientific studies on the lomatiums (there haven't been many) is that researchers rarely make any distinctions between older plant roots that are highly aromatic and younger plant roots that are not. (It took highly schooled plant specialists *decades* to realize that some plants they had listed as perennials—or biennials—were in fact unique monocarpic plants, *Frasera speciosa* being an example. That plant may take anywhere from 20 to 100 years before it sends up a stalk and flowers, and once it does, it dies. These specialist guys, they are a bit slow. And no, they didn't think to look at any of the Native American data on that plant.)

Comparison studies on the lomatiums should only occur with plants of similar ages; the differences in the percentage of compounds found in various subspecies of *Lomatium dissectum* could easily be from differences in the age of the roots tested. The current chemistry studies, which are nice to have, are nevertheless suspect in some of their conclusions about the species studied due to the failure of the researchers to indicate the age of the plants or to be certain the plants were of a similar age before comparisons.

Nevertheless, many members of the *Lomatium* genus (and the carrot family of which it is a member) have a number of similar chemistries, e.g., apiol, a calcium antagonist widely present in the carrot family and strongly present in the seeds and roots of *Lomatium californicum* and *Ligusticum hultenii*. The antiasthmatic and antispasmodic compound Z-ligustilide is common in many of the lomatiums as well.

Most of the chemical studies on the lomatiums have been conducted by butterfly researchers since butterflies are strongly attracted to this genus (the researchers are looking for the exact chemical attractants so they go deep). The nearest to a comprehensive look at the chemistry of the main medicinal species has occurred with the essential oils of two variants of *Lomatium dissectum*. The roots, seeds, and stems all were found to contain a number of terpenoid hydrocarbons, among other things.

The seeds of *Lomatium dissectum* var. *dissectum* were found to contain 113 compounds; the seeds of *Lomatium dissectum* var. *multifidum* contained 138. The leaves and upper stems of variety *dissectum* contained 137 compounds; those of variety *multifidum* contained 173. The root of variety *dissectum* had 68 compounds; oddly, the study doesn't reveal the number of root compounds of variety *multifidum*.

Variety *dissectum* is particularly rich in esters, specifically the 2-methylbutyrates; the primary compounds found are: phellandrene, limonene, beta-caryophyllene, palmitic acid, E-beta-ocimene, linolenic acid, octanol, octyl acetate, myrcene, 4-methylpentyl 2-methylbutyrate, alpha-bisabolol, cuparene, Z-S-hexenol, decyl acetate, longifolene, palmitoleic acid, Z-ligustilide, and E-2-methyl-3-octen-5-yne. The roots of the two closely related forms of *Lomatium dissectum* have very similar chemistries but they do differ, e.g., *Lomatium dissectum* var. *multifidum* has about 20 percent longifolene (a major constituent of many pines) in its complex of essential oils, while *Lomatium dissectum* var. *dissectum* has only about 3 percent.

Studies with other lomatiums have found similar compounds. The best in-depth look at species other than *dissectum* comes from Philip S. Beauchamp, et al. They identified over 200 constituents in the plants. While all of the plants did not have the same constituents, they were similar in their compounds. The principal components of the six species (*brandegei, eastwoodiae, graveolens, howelii, junceum,* and *parryi*) are (in order or prominence): alpha-pinene, beta-pinene, camphene, alpha-phellandrene, alpha-terpinene, beta-phellandrene + limonene, Z-beta-ocimene, gamma-terpinene, p-mentha-2,4(8)-diene, linalool, dehydrosabina ketone, terpinen-4-ol, cryptone, alpha-terpineol, methyl chavicol, citronellol, methyl thymol, linalyl acetate, lavandulyl acetate, citronellyl acetate, beta-bourbonene, benzyl-2-methylbutyrate, beta-elemene, italicene, dodecanal, beta-caryophyllene, gamma-elemene, alpha-humulene, 7-epi-e,2-dehydrosesquicineole, gamma-muurolene, germacrene D, beta-selinene, bicyclogermacene, germacrene A, alpha-cadinene, germacrene B, epi-alpha-cadinol, alpha-muurolol. There are a number of highly antimicrobial tetronic acids in the root.[21]

Other species (*californicum, dasycarpum, grayi, lucidum, macrocarpum, nuttallii, rigidum, suksdorfii, utriculatum*) contain large amounts of similar constituents: falcarindiol, coniferyl ferulate, ferulic acid, Z-ligustilide, senkyunolide, trans-neocnidilide, apiol, suksdorfin, osthol, chromones, sibiricin, macrocarpin, beta-phellandrene/

limonene, decanal, dodecanal, bornyl acetate, germacrene D, alpha-humulene, bicyclogermacrene, alpha-pinene, beta-pinene, peucenin 7-methyl ester, beta-caryophyllene, Z-3-hexenol, palmitic acid, linoleic acid, E-2-hexenal, sabinene, terpinen-4-ol, myrcene, various coumarins, glycosides, and flavonoids. Z-falcarinol levels are particularly high in most lomatium species' roots.

The chemistry of the lomatiums, as with most plants, is complex and poorly understood. The seeds and aerial parts do have a great many more compounds than the roots, the seeds appearing nearly as active as antimicrobials as the roots. However, the roots do possess a number of compounds unique to them and are generally, in traditional practice and conventional herbal circles (though not in indigenous), considered to be the most potent antiviral parts of the plants.

Again: Only as the plant roots age do the major aromatics become highly concentrated in the roots; the seeds possess them from the beginning.

Traditional Uses of Lomatium

I have spread what would normally be in this section throughout this monograph. Read on.

AYURVEDA

Unknown.

TRADITIONAL CHINESE MEDICINE

Unknown.

WESTERN BOTANIC MEDICINE

All the lomatiums were known to the indigenous cultures that lived among them. All of them used the plants similarly: roots for food, seeds and roots for medicine (among other things). Lewis and Clark knew of the plants' uses for food, as they used them on their trek across the country once they were introduced to them. They almost certainly would have known of the plants' uses as medicine. Many of the trappers who lived in the region would have known as well. They didn't seem to have written about them, however. Lomatium only came to the awareness of the medical community during the influenza epidemic of 1918–1919.

The Washoe tribe in Nevada used the plant to treat members of the tribe who had fallen sick with the disease. A report on their use of the plant was printed in the *Bulletin of the Nevada State Board of Health,* in January 1920, by a physician, Ernst Krebs. If you have read, in depth, the description of just what the 1918 influenza virus did in the bodies of those it infected and then compare the outcomes in practice from lomatium during the pandemic, the effects of the herb are considerable.

> The Indians gather this root in the late fall, November being considered the proper month for gathering. The root is used in the fresh or dry state. It is cut up and a decoction is made by boiling the root in water, skimming off the top and giving large doses of the broth. A pound of root is considered about the proper dose to treat a case of fever for 3 days, which is the longest time needed to break up a fever due to influenza or pulmonary disease, although the Washoes used it as a panacea. Whether a coincidence or not, there was not a single death in the Washoe tribe from influenza or its complications, although Indians living in other parts of the State where the root did not grow died in numbers. It was such a remarkable coincidence that the root was investigated by a practicing physician who saw apparently hopeless cases recover completely without any other medication or care of any kind.
>
> A preparation was prepared and employed in a great many cases among the whites, from the mildest to the most virulent types of influenza, and it proved itself to be a reliable agent in preventing pulmonary complications. Other physicians were induced to give it a trial with the same results. It is beyond the experimental stage, as its therapeutic action in this direction is established and beyond any doubt. The cases in which it has been used run into the hundreds. There is probably no therapeutic agent so valuable in the treatment of influenzal pneumonia and, as far as being tried, in ordinary lobar pneumonia if started early. Its action on coughs is more certain than opiate expectorants and its benefit is lasting. It acts as a powerful tonic to the respiratory mucus membranes. It is a bronchial, intestinal and urinary antiseptic and is excreted by these organs.[22]

Interestingly, the aromatic constituents in the root are only mildly soluble in water, are better soluble in alcohol, and are lost when boiled (making a decoction). Given the traditional indigenous preparation methods, there are obviously a number of other compounds in the root, water soluble and heat resistant, that are, inescapably, strongly antiviral.

For a while, the reports of the efficacy of the plant stimulated study of its actions, but the emergence of pharmaceutical antibiotics stopped research on the plant until Michael Moore began speaking about it in the early 1970s. It is now considered (among many herbalists) to be *the* primary antiviral medicine in the U.S. herbal community.

Scientific Research

Most of this section has been spread throughout the rest of this monograph, so, just a couple of notes here:

The lomatiums contain a large number of chemically unique coumarins (pyranocoumarins, furanocoumarins, prenyloxycoumarins, prenyloxyfuranocoumarins, and so on) that have been found in a number of studies to be powerfully antiviral against both RNA and DNA viruses ("remarkable" is how one research team put it). The compounds penetrate the viral coat and inhibit ribonucleoprotein-complex-associated activity among other things. They have been found exceptionally potent against influenza viruses (H1N1, etc). *Ferula assa-foetida,* once considered a close relative of *Lomatium dissectum* (formerly *Ferula dissoluta*), is especially rich in the same compounds; they are more potent against influenza viruses than amantadine. (Specifically, they inhibit the M2 ion channel.) The compounds in lomatium are in fact some of the most potent M2 ion channel inhibitors known.

Lomatiums also have high levels of longifolene, which is an exceptionally active antimicrobial. It is as active as the pharmaceutical nifurtimox against *Trypanosoma cruzi,* which causes Chagas' disease. It is primarily active against Gram-positive bacteria.

Honorable Mentions

There are a few other herbs that are showing potent antiviral actions that I think warrant closer examination over time. They are *Ampelopsis brevipedunculata, Forsythia suspensa, Sophora flavescens, Strobilanthes cusia,* and boneset (*Eupatorium perfoliatum*) and red root (*Ceanothus velutinus*). The only ones I will offer any depth on here are boneset and red root. (And, yes, there are *lots* of other plants with antiviral actions; this is just a beginning. And yes, I do know about *Ocimum sanctum.*)

AMPELOPSIS BREVIPEDUNCULATA

Ampelopsis brevipedunculata, a.k.a porcelain berry, is an invasive, especially in the eastern United States, and is native to Asia. It's a woody vine that grows to 25 feet in length with an extensive root system. It mimics kudzu root in a lesser, porcelain berry sort of way, covering whatever it can as it spreads. It is on the lists of most phytoaryans; it is considered armed and dangerous, to be exterminated with extreme prejudice.

The herb is active against a number of viruses, including enterovirus 71, hepatitis, and varicella zoster. The stem, roots, and leaves are all used, though the stem and roots are the most commonly used for treating viral diseases. A water/ethanol extract of the roots and stems was found to be the strongest medicinal plant compound, of any tested, for treating four strains of enterovirus 71. The plant is traditionally used in Japan and parts of Asia as a major anti-inflammatory, hepatoprotective, and analgesic.

It has a number of immune modulation effects and has proved effective in treating liver fibrosis. It protects the liver from various toxic substances, is active against breast cancer cells, is a fairly potent antioxidant, is decidedly anti-inflammatory, and is analgesic. Because the plant is an invasive, its use really should be further explored.

FORSYTHIA SUSPENSA

Forsythia suspensa is one of the 50 fundamental herbs in Chinese medicine. It is a weeping forsythia, a large shrub, and quite pretty. It has escaped cultivation and is moderately invasive throughout the United States.

It is called either qing qiao or huang qiao in Chinese medicine, depending on whether the green or fully ripe yellow fruit is used as medicine. The unripe fruit is considered to be the strongest. (Rarely, the stem bark and leaves are used.) The dried fruit, whatever its ripeness, is used for fever, headache, restlessness, delirium, lymph gland enlargement, erysipelas, boils, and inflammations.

The herb is highly active against influenza A viruses, avian infectious bronchitis virus, cytomegalovirus, and respiratory syncytial virus. A number of the compounds in the plant have a fairly wide range of antiviral action (ursolic acid, oleanolic acid, quercetin, rutin, pinoresinol), and the plant really should be tested further. Studies on the leaves have found them to be stronger in their impacts than the flowers.

It is anti-inflammatory, antioxidant, vasorelaxive, antibacterial (against staph, *Helicobacter pylori, E. coli*), antiemetic, cytoprotective, and diuretic (antiedema).

SOPHORA FLAVESCENS

Sophora flavescens is also an herb used in traditional Chinese medicine, in which it is called ku shen. It is used for the treatment of viral hepatitis, viral myocarditis, gastritis, enteritis, cancer, and various skin diseases. The root is usually used. The plant is considered specific for jaundice, dysentery, leukorrhea, itching, scabies, eczema, and dysuria when used in combination with other plants.

The herb has been found active against a range of viruses: hepatitis B, respiratory syncytial virus, Coxsackie B3, HHV-6, coronavirus, influenza A (H1N1), rotavirus, herpes simplex virus 1 and 2, HIV, and various cancers. It is a potent neuraminidase inhibitor and also has some antibacterial (staph, enterococci, resistant and nonresistant) and antifungal (*Aspergillus niger*) actions.

STROBILANTHES CUSIA

Strobilanthes cusia is a plant that deserves more attention as an antiviral in that it contains many of the same compounds (e.g., tryptanthrin, indigo, indirubin) as isatis. (One of the plant's common names is actually Assam indigo and it was once used, as isatis was, as a source of indigo dye.) And, not surprisingly, it is a pretty good antiviral, too. In Chinese medicine it is called da-chang-yeh. The roots and leaves are used.

The plant is active against a number of viruses including influenza A (H1N1) strains, hepatitis B, herpes simplex virus 1, Sindbis virus, eastern equine encephalitis virus, Getah virus, and tobacco mosaic virus. Studies *in planta* found it increased innate resistance in plants to virus infections.

The plant contains some fairly potent compounds that target the subgenomic RNA of alphaviruses and alphavirus-like RNA viruses. This viral group, when it infects people, causes rashes and arthritis and encephalitis.

The plant has also shown antiplasmodial and antifungal activity.

In Chinese medicine, the plant is used for influenza, epidemic cerebrospinal meningitis, encephalitis B (Japanese viral encephalitis), viral pneumonia, and mumps. It is used for sore throats, aphthae, inflammatory diseases of the skin, and to reduce fever. The plant is considered antinociceptive, anti-inflammatory, and antipyretic.

Because the plant has so many of the same potent antiviral compounds as isatis and because it is widely grown throughout the world as an ornamental, its antiviral actions should be studied in more depth. One hope: Because the plant is in a different family, maybe it won't taste like isatis, i.e., spoiled cabbage.

Boneset

There have been extremely few studies on boneset; most of them are very old and what newish ones there are mostly quote nineteenth-century texts. Recently Mareike Maas, in Germany, has been doing some very good in-depth research on the plant, much of which is very hard to get in English. Her work is showing that the plant has a much wider range of antiviral actions than was formerly understood. I suspect the plant is going to be a more useful antiviral than previously thought.

Family: Compositae.

Species used: There are 36, or 60, or pi? species in the *Eupatorium* genus, taxonomists being troublesome again. Nearly all are native to the Americas, *Eupatorium cannabinum* being an exception. Many of the species in the genus are medicinal, and some do have a very similar range of action. However, this is the one I know best, so *Eupatorium perfoliatum* it is.

Common names: Boneset, common boneset, throughwort, agueweed, feverwort, sweating plant—but no one has used those last three names since 1885. (And it's pronounced A-gyew-weed, not aaagh-weed, big fella.)

Parts Used

Aerial parts, in flower or just before flowering, depending.

Preparation and Dosage

The herb is bitter and about as much fun to drink as a tea made from earwax. Honey helps considerably . . . and if you have the kind of flu where you can't taste anything. Generally, the herb is taken as tea or tincture but few take the tincture directly on the tongue. Too bitter.

TEA

Cold tea: Combine 1 ounce of herb with 1 quart boiling water, and let steep overnight. Strain and drink throughout the day. The cold infusion is better for the mucous membrane system and as a liver tonic. If you want to help fevers, you need to take the tea hot.

Hot tea: Combine 1 tsp herb with 8 ounces hot water, and let steep 15 minutes. Take 4–6 ounces up to 4x daily. Boneset is only diaphoretic when hot and should be consumed hot for active infections or for recurring chills and fevers.

TINCTURE

Fresh herb in flower: Use a 1:2 herb:liquid ratio, with 95 percent alcohol. Dosage: 20–40 drops in hot water up to 3x daily.

Dry herb: Use a 1:5 herb:liquid ratio, with 60 percent alcohol. Dosage: 30–50 drops in hot water up to 3x daily.

For acute viral or bacterial upper respiratory infections: Take 10 drops of tincture in hot water every half hour up to 6x daily.

For chronic conditions: When the acute stage has passed but there is continued chronic fatigue and relapse, take 10 drops of tincture in hot water 4x daily.

Side Effects and Contraindications

For some reason the phytohysteria surrounding elder is not present with this herb. Boneset is an emetic when taken in large doses, so an early sign that you may be taking too much is *nausea*. Generally, the cooler the tea the less nausea. However, the tea really must be taken hot to help fevers. The herb *may* be contraindicated in pregnancy but no one really seems to know why. *Sometimes* some people have an allergic reaction to plants in this family (chamomile, feverfew, ragwort, tansy), so if you are allergic to those, careful with this one.

Herb/Drug Interactions

None noted.

Habitat and Appearance

The plant is pervasive in the eastern half of the United States and Canada, from Texas, Oklahoma, North Dakota, and so on eastward. However, every place I've seen it grow has been wettish, humid, with good soil.

Boneset grows up to 3 feet tall, they say. I've never seen it get that big, but most of my experience of the plant has been in the tiny state of Vermont. Two feet seems about average, just as with hominids. The plant grows in a straight stalk, the leaves going north-south, then east-west, then north-south again. The leaves continue on through the stalk, hence throughwort; it basically looks like the opposing leaves were glued together at the wide end and the stalk just punched through them. Once seen, never forgotten.

Cultivation and Collection

The plant is a perennial and likes full or partial sun in moist to wet conditions, on the edges of swamps, along streams, in wet meadows, in marshlands, basically anyplace mosquitoes like to breed except maybe old tires. It spreads by seed; there are a lot of sources on the Internet.

If collected at flowering and allowed to dry, the plant will usually go to seed as it dries. It should only be collected in flower (August or September) if being tinctured fresh and *right now*. If you are going to use it as a tea, it should be picked just prior to flowering, hung upside down in a shaded place, and allowed to thoroughly air-dry. If you pick it in flower and try to dry it then, it will go to seed as it is hanging there, like a bat, upside down, waiting to come suck your blood late in the night, and there will be a mess.

Finding It

Fields and streams in the eastern United States, the Internet, herb stores here and there. Horizon Herbs sells the seeds.

Plant Chemistry

Methylglucuronoxylan, astragalin, eufoliatin, eufoliatorin, eupatorin, euperfolin, euperfolitin, euperfolide, euccannabinolide, eupatoriopicrin, hyperoside, rutin, polysaccharides, a number of guaianolides, and a bunch of other stuff. Many of those are sesquiterpene lactones, common in the eupatoriums. There are a number of caffeic acid derivatives in the plant, at least five flavonoid glycosides, and a number of

Properties of Boneset

Actions

Analgesic
Antibacterial (mild)
Anti-inflammatory
Antiviral
Cytotoxic
Diaphoretic
Emetic (mild)
Febrifuge
Gastric bitter
Immunostimulant (increases phagocytosis)
Mucous membrane tonic
Peripheral circulatory stimulant
Smooth muscle relaxant

Active Against

There hasn't been a lot of testing of this plant as an antimicrobial. It is mildly active against some Gram-positive bacteria such as *Staphylococcus aureus* and *Bacillus megaterium*. It is stronger in its actions against malarial parasites (*Plasmodium* spp.), making it essentially a midlevel anti-plasmodial herb. It has pretty good activity as an antiviral against influenza A (H1N1). Although not tested for it, I do believe this species is active against some, if not all, serotypes of dengue.

The eupatoriums do have a range of action against viruses, but there has been much too little work on them. *Eupatorium patens* is active against dengue-2, HSV-1, and HSV-2; *Eupatorium articulatum* against HSV-1 and vesicular stomatitis virus (VSV); *Eupatorium glutinosum* against

dicaffeoylglucaric acid derivatives that are considered unusual. (And if David Hoffmann is reading this that means: depsides of hydroxycinnamic acids with hexaric acids.) These unusual compounds are particularly high in the flowers.

Traditional Uses of Boneset

AYURVEDA

Nope, but there are other eupatoriums used in this system.

VSV; *Eupatorium bunifolium* against herpes simplex viruses. Most of these eupatoriums have been used similarly to boneset.

Note: Because of the common name *boneset* some people think this eupatorium good for setting bones. Others, however, insist that the name came from a common, ancient name for dengue, breakbone fever, and that the herb has never been used for setting bones and, more, indigenous peoples never used it for that either. (Feelings run high.) I have taken various sides in this over the years but did think it highly amusing a number of years ago when a well-respected indigenous herbalist (from the United States) who had used the herb for over 50 years (and who had learned its use from *her* teacher when she was very small) informed a rather self-satisfied group of herbalists that she used the herb primarily for setting broken bones (as a compress/poultice) and had done so all of her life. (So, now, I read fiction novels and don't think about why it is called what it is called.)

Use to Treat

Influenza, dengue fever, malaria, all viral infections with intermittent fever (hot, then cold, then hot, then . . .), and aches and pains. Comment: I consider the plant a useful adjunct botanical for intermittent viral infections (flu, malaria, dengue), not a primary treatment botanical. It will really help lower fevers. It will help with the aches and pains of viral infections. It *will* make you sweat (if taken hot as a tea, as it should be).

TRADITIONAL CHINESE MEDICINE

No, but there are other eupatoriums used in this system.

WESTERN BOTANIC PRACTICE

The plant, indigenous to North America, has been used by native peoples for millennia, specifically for intermittent fevers and chills, with pain in the bones, weakness, and debility. The American Eclectics used it for intermittent (i.e., malarial), typhoid, and remittent fevers, for general debility, pneumonia, cough, epidemic influenza, colds, catarrh, and pains accompanying those conditions. It was one of their primary remedies.

Scientific Research

The sesquiterpene lactones in boneset have a large range of actions. They are highly immunostimulatory and very active against cancers. One study found the herb itself to be potently cytotoxic, in essence comparable to the strength of the pharmaceutical chlorambucil.

The specific lactone active against the malarial parasite is considered to be a dimeric guaianolide. It has a range of antiplasmodial actions but is strongest against *Plasmodium falciparum*. The action is mild (compared to herbs such as cryptolepis) but if the plant is added to a traditional antimalarial that is strong, such as cryptolepis, the effects are mutually supportive. A homeopathic formulation of boneset was found to significantly inhibit plasmodial replication (60 percent inhibition). And an in vivo study with mice found that the homeopathic preparation of the herb did inhibit plasmodial parasites but not completely.

South and Central American healers have been using homeopathic preparations of boneset to try to minimize the impacts of dengue fever outbreaks. In Rio in 2008, a homeopathic preparation containing phosphorus (30c), *Crotalus horridus* (30c), and *Eupatorium perfoliatum* (30c) was given to nearly 160,000 people. The incidence of the disease, compared to the same time period the year before, fell by 93 percent. In comparison, in areas not using the homeopathic preparation the disease incidence increased 128 percent. (Note: A few other, much smaller studies using the homeopathic of eupatorium alone for treating the common cold and dengue fever—though the people who were ill were not actually tested for dengue [the researchers guessed based on symptoms]—did not find any usefulness from the preparation.)

Clinical trials have shown that boneset stimulates phagocytosis better than echinacea, is analgesic (at least as effective as aspirin), and reduces cold and flu symptoms. In mice it has shown strong immunostimulant activity and cytotoxic action against cancer cells.

The herb is a decent anti-inflammatory. It is anti-inflammatory for lipopolysaccharide-stimulated macrophages, primarily by inhibiting NO and iNOS expression. CSF-3, IL-1α and ß, and the chemokines CCL2, CCL22, and CXCL10 are all inhibited. TNF-α is moderately inhibited. Indications are that it inhibits NF-κB.

Again, despite boneset's long use and potent reputation, little research has occurred with the plant.

Antiviral Supplements

While there are a number of supplements that do help during viral infections (vitamin C, vitamin B complex), zinc seems the most crucial, while monolaurin has shown some good antiviral activity in vitro and users report help from its addition to viral protocols.

ZINC

Zinc has been found active against a number of viruses (alphaviruses) and supportive in treatment for others (influenza, HIV). Studies have found that zinc supplements can triple the survival rate for children with pneumonia, for example, and that it significantly reduces the duration of the common cold.

Dosage: 10–25 mg daily depending on age and weight; 25–40 mg daily during acute episodes.

MONOLAURIN

Monolaurin is one of the major constituents of coconut oil and one of the factors in "the coconut oil miracle." It has been found, in vitro, to be active against measles, HIV, HSV-1 and HSV-2, hepatitis, Epstein-Barr, infectious bronchitis virus, rubella virus, Newcastle virus, dengue (four serotypes), lymphocytic choriomeningitis, vesicular stomatitis virus, visna virus, cytomegalovirus, influenza viruses, pneumonovirus, and respiratory syncytial virus. Caveat: Most of these in vitro studies are hard to find; many of the assertions come from people connected with products, or are merely repetitions of other sources. There are very few in vivo studies, and even fewer with people. However, the constituent is considered safe (it's on the FDA's Generally Recognized as Safe list), and it has shown some very good effects against HIV in in vivo studies. I have seen some people experience good healing with it.

Dosage: 2–4 grams per day.

Supporting Lymph Function

During many viral infections, especially those that affect the lungs, the lymph system can become overloaded, the nodes severely inflamed, the spleen enlarged. Herbs that stimulate lymph action are very important to use. My favorite one is red root.

Red Root

Family: Rhamnaceae.

Species used: *Homo dissertationus* has determined that there are 50 or 60 or 4^3 species of *Ceanothus* in the Americas, from Canada to Guatemala. The genus doesn't grow anyplace else, at least not *natively*, though it is an ornamental throughout most of the world in one species shape or another.

Most species can be used medicinally; the most common are *C. velutinus*, *C. cuneatus*, *C. integerrimus*, *C. greggii*, and *C. americanus*. All species are apparently identical in their medicinal actions. My personal favorite is *Ceanothus fendleri*, a.k.a Fendler's ceanothus, which grows in my region and which I have been using for more than 25 years. The important part is the color of the bark—see Cultivation and Collection on page 410.

Common name: Red root mostly, but in the old days it was supposedly called New Jersey tea (so they say; I never heard anyone say that phrase, at least when referring to something that does not inebriate).

Part Used

The root or inner bark of the root.

Preparation and Dosage

Red root can also be used as a tincture tea, strong decoction, gargle, or capsules (but really, I think the tincture is best).

TINCTURE

Dry root, in a 1:5 herb:liquid ratio, with 50 percent alcohol. Dosage: 30–90 drops up to 4x daily.

TEA

1 teaspoon powdered root in 8 ounces water, simmer 15 minutes, strain. Dosage: Drink up to 6 cups daily.

STRONG DECOCTION

1 ounce herb in 16 ounces water, simmer slowly for 30 minutes, covered. Dosage: 1 tablespoon 3x or 4x per day.

GARGLE

In cases of tonsillitis or throat inflammation gargle with strong tea 4–6x per day.

CAPSULES

Take 10–30 "00" capsules per day if you must.

Side Effects and Contraindications

No side effects have been noted; however red root is contraindicated in pregnancy.

Herb/Drug Interactions

Should not be used with pharmaceutical coagulants or anticoagulants.

Habitat and Appearance

The various species in this genus seemingly grow everywhere in North and Central America, from Canada to Guatemala, from sea-level coastal scrublands to pine forests at 9,000 feet or higher. They can grow in hot, humid locations and semiarid desert areas. They are widely divergent in appearance, too, from tiny deciduous ground covers (up to 12 inches tall) to large evergreen bushes (to 9 feet tall) to "small" trees to 25 feet in height. Their foliage ranges from tiny leathery leaves to large broad softies. Some species' branches have "spines," some don't. They do all have leaves though, so identification should not be a problem.

The flowers grow in tufted clusters and are intensely fragrant. (Yummy to my nose—at least with *C. fendleri.*) The seed capsules are identical on all species I have seen, three-lobed triangular things that, again in all species I have seen, turn a reddish color, the exact color of the root bark (and tincture), when mature. That and the flowers, once you have seen them, are the easiest ways to identify the genus.

Cultivation and Collection

This genus has been intensively cultivated, and there are scores if not hundreds of cultivars and hybrids. Adding to the confusion, the plants mix with abandon in the wild and . . . well, basically they just have sex whenever and with whomever they wish and the result is a very variable genus. In any event, you can get a large number of types if you wish to grow the species yourself. The genus should grow in just about any geographical location, and it has made a home in other places than the Americas by masquerading as an ornamental; it is common in the UK and the EU. It will soon (I hope) escape into the wild, where it will be found to be invasive, for in ceanothus habitat, there are some two million seeds produced per acre once the plants establish themselves. They are propelled under great force out of the capsules (to extend their range) and can remain viable for centuries. I really love these guys.

The plants are propagated by seed or cuttings. The seeds need to be scarified first (show them horror films?) and then stratified. They are usually soaked in water for 12 hours followed by chilling for 3 months—mimicking winter.

The roots/inner root bark should be harvested in the fall or early spring—whenever the root has already had a good frost. The inner bark of the root should be a bright red, and this color should extend through the white woody root as a pink tinge after a freeze. The root must look like this to be actively medicinal. If you get the roots in the late spring, summer, or early fall, they will be white throughout with just a hint of pink in the inner bark. They just will not work like that. It takes that cold snap to stimulate the production of the chemical constituents that you need the plant for.

Caution: The root is extremely tough when it dries. It should be cut into small 1- or 2-inch pieces with plant snips while still fresh or you will regret it. Really. Trust me on this one thing.

Store the cut and dried roots in plastic bags in large plastic bins in a cool place and they will last you for years.

Properties of Red Root

Actions

First and foremost red root is a lymph system stimulant and tonic. It is anti-inflammatory for both the liver and spleen. It is also an astringent, mucous membrane tonic, alterative, antiseptic, expectorant, antispasmodic, and exceptionally strong blood coagulant.

Finding Red Root

North and Central America, the Internet, herb stores. In gardens nearly everywhere. It is commonly planted throughout the UK and the EU—though the herbalists in those regions, for the most part, have not yet cottoned on to that fact. It will grow well in those regions, or . . . you can sneak into a garden some night and dig some. Just be really, really quiet.

Alternatives: Poke root (*Phytolacca*) is an excellent alternative. Dosage however should be one-third that of red root. As well, poke itself contains some fairly potent antiviral compounds in the fruit, root, and so on. The pokeweed antiviral protein has been shown to cure mice of HIV infection and is apparently active against a wide range of viruses. I have a feeling about poke . . . it may turn out to be a much more important medicinal than we have thought it to be.

Cleavers will have some of the same effects but the dosage should be four times that of red root. The fresh juice of the plant is best. Cleavers, additionally, strongly inhibits elastase (by about 60 percent) and is useful for bacteria that use elastase as part of their infection strategy.

Plant Chemistry

Betulin, betulinic acid, bacteriohopanetetrol, ceanothic acid, ceanothenic acid, ceanothine, ceanothamine, ceanothane, americine, integerressine, integerrenine, integerrine, methyl salicylate, a lot of tannins, flavonoids, flavonol glycosides, flavonones, dihydroflavonols. The leaves have a somewhat different profile, but I won't include it here as the root is what we are dealing with. The plant is fairly high in protein, iron, copper, zinc, magnesium and very high in calcium. The roots are nitrogen fixers and possess nitrogen-filled nodules.

Traditional Uses of Red Root

Red root is an important herb in many disease conditions in that it helps facilitate clearing of dead cellular tissue from the lymph system. When the immune system is responding to acute conditions or the onset of disease, as white blood cells kill bacterial and viral pathogens they are taken to the lymph system for disposal. If the lymph system clears out dead cellular material rapidly, the healing process is enhanced, sometimes dramatically. The herb shows especially strong action whenever any portion of the lymph system is swollen, infected, or inflamed. This includes the lymph nodes, tonsils (entire back of throat), spleen, appendix, and liver.

AYURVEDA

Nope.

TRADITIONAL CHINESE MEDICINE

Not remotely.

WESTERN BOTANIC PRACTICE

Red root has a very long history in the Americas. The indigenous cultures used the plant for a wide range of complaints from arthritis to influenza, primarily as an astringent. The early American herbalists picked it up and the Eclectics then developed the use of the plant considerably, using it as an astringent, expectorant, sedative, antispasmodic, and antisyphilitic. It was used specifically for gonorrhea, dysentery, asthma, chronic bronchitis, whooping cough, general pulmonary problems, and oral ulcerations due to fever and infection. Its primary use, however, was for enlarged spleen and, to some extent, enlarged liver.

Scientific Research

There hasn't been much study on the plant, however, and really nothing looking in depth at its actions on the lymph system, including the spleen, though there are some nice hints here and there.

In recent years there has been a minor amount of exploration on the antimicrobial actions of red root. Several of the root compounds have been found active against various oral pathogens including *Streptococcus mutans, Actinomyces viscosus, Porphyromonas gingivalis,* and *Prevotella intermedia.* The flowers are active against *Staphylococcus aureus* and a couple of candida species; the roots probably are, too.

Betulin and betulinic acid, which are fairly prominent in the root, have a broad range of actions, in vivo and in vitro: antiplasmodial, antiviral, anti-inflammatory, anthelmintic, antioxidant, antitumor, immunomodulatory. Ceanothane is a fairly strong antistaphylococcal, antiplasmodial, and antimycobacterial. These various actions are going to have some effect on bacterial and viral diseases but exactly what and how much is not clear.

There is some evidence that red root's activity in the lymph nodes also enhances the lymph nodes' production of lymphocytes, specifically the formation of T cells. Clinicians working with AIDS patients, who have historically low levels of T cells, have noted increases after the use of red root. It is especially effective in reducing inflammation in the spleen and liver from such things as excessive bacterial garbage, white blood cell detritus in the lymph, and red blood cell fragments in the blood in diseases like babesiosis. There is evidence, clinical, that it has broad action throughout the lymph system and helps reduce not only the spleen but also the appendix when inflamed and that it stimulates lymph drainage as well in the intestinal walls.

A number of human trials have occurred using the herb as a tincture extract (usually 10–15 ml per person). The trials focused on heavy bleeding including excessive menstruation, and the plant was found to be a powerful coagulant and hemostatic in all studies. A marked reduction of clotting time was noted.

In one study, a single oral administration of 3.5–7.0 ml of a hydro-alcoholic (tincture) extract of ceanothus (species *americanus*) resulted in an interesting effect: At low doses accelerated blood clotting occurred within 10 to 20 minutes after administration. However, at higher doses coagulation *decreased* 1 hour after administration. This raises interesting speculations about the herb's range of actions.

In vivo studies have shown marked hemostatic activity and hypotensive action. In vitro studies have also found a strong reverse transcriptase inhibition and a broad antifungal activity.

Synergistic Herbs

Sometimes it seems as if doses of supposed active constituents are too low to have an effect, and in the absence of clinical proof this has led sceptics to dismiss these medicines as mere placebos. . . . It is still routine to investigate and extract medicinal plants with a view to finding the single chemical entity responsible for the effect, and this may lead to inconclusive findings. If a combination of substances is needed for the effect, then the bioassay-led method of investigation, narrowing activity down firstly to a fraction and eventually a compound, is doomed to failure, and this has led to the suggestion that the plants are in fact devoid of activity. . . . When activity is thought to be lost through purification, synergy should be suspected.

—Dr. Elizabeth Williamson, "Synergy and Other Interactions in Phytomedicines" (*Phytomedicine* 8, no. 5 [2001])

All investigations have shown that most of the extracts and individual constituents thereof exert multivalent or pleiotropic pharmacological effects (this multivalance of pharmacological activities can generate additive or overadditive, potentiated synergistic effects). . . . The synergistic effects that have been measured exceed the effects of single compounds, or mixtures of them at equivalent concentrations, by a factor of two to four, or more.

—Dr. Hildebert Wagner, "Natural Products Chemistry and Phytomedicine in the 21st Century" (*Pure and Applied Chemistry* 77, no. 1 [2005])

Synergy, in its simplest definition, means that the combination of two (or more) things produces outcomes greater than the sum of the individual parts and, additionally, that those outcomes *cannot* be predicted from a study of the individual parts themselves. Individual plants, because of their complex chemistry, are highly synergistic organisms by themselves. If plants are used in combination, the complexity, and resultant synergy, increases substantially.

Within older healing traditions such as traditional Chinese medicine (TCM) and Ayurveda, the inherent synergistic nature of plant medicinals and plant combinations is an integrated aspect of healing.

Those systems, over millennia, developed their own language and understanding of plants as synergists. A similar understanding, using our own Western terminology and perspectives, has been lacking in our medical approaches—herbal or otherwise.

Medical technologists (usually from the younger generations) have slowly begun to move away from the dogma of monotherapy—that is, the use of a single compound to treat disease. It's not that they inherently wanted to or that they innately understood that the system in which they were trained was flawed. Their change, as it is with most of us, was driven by events occurring in the outside world that they could no longer ignore; mainly, the emergence of multidrug-resistant microorganisms and AIDS.

AIDS (along with cancer), because of its spread, its disease dynamics, and its amazing adaptability, has forced a shift from a monotherapy frame to that of a multitarget paradigm of therapeutics. Multitarget therapies not only focus on killing the disease organism—which with AIDS and cancers are often futile—but also focus deeply on activating the natural defense, protective, and repair mechanisms in the body. In other words they also stimulate immune responses to disease and, as well, the body's own highly elegant repair mechanisms.

The emergence of multidrug-resistant bacteria has also been a factor in challenging the monotherapy paradigm. As fast as new pharmaceuticals were developed for resistant organisms, new resistance emerged. Physicians learned, eventually, that if they combined therapies, for example if they used antimalarial drug combinations, the development of malarial resistance could be delayed. (Not stopped, mind you, just delayed.) But that recognition opened up the understanding that complex drug therapies were much more effective against the disease and, as well, could slow down and, presumably if they were elegant enough, stop resistance development altogether. The use of artemisinin combination therapy (ACT) is a product of that understanding. At a very crude, simplistic level these approaches by medical technologists are beginning to mimic the actions of plant medicines, as well as older systems of healing such as TCM.

Changes in Western Monotherapy

Western herbalists have never been completely captured by the monotherapy paradigm, though they have often been strongly influenced, and sometimes fully seduced, by it. Medical (and naturopathic) herbalists, for example, since they often tend to mimic a medical reductionist model, generally lean much more strongly toward monotherapeutic thinking. They often lose sight of plant complexities in the search for "active" constituents and standardized herbs.

Community herbalists, like their counterparts in all third- (and some second-) world countries, tend to be more cognizant of plant complexities and subtleties, in part simply because they haven't been trained to believe they know some ultimate truth about the nature of plant medicines or reality as a whole. Most of them consider plants to be an expression of the general intelligence and livingness of Nature. They never have felt plants to be insentient substances that can be analyzed and completely understood by science and then used however human beings wish.

All Western herbalists, no matter their orientation, do know that plants are much safer than pharmaceuticals, that they tend to produce more complex effects in the body than pharmaceuticals, and that they need to be part of a more complex treatment regimen, one that also includes immune regeneration and support for the body's natural repair mechanisms. Herbalists just naturally tend to be more multitarget-therapy oriented than the majority of physicians. And most Western herbalists, not all, understand that whole-plant extracts are often more effective than isolated constituents and that plant combinations are often more effective than single-plant extracts.

In spite of this, Western herbalists as a group have nearly no understanding of synergy in plant medicines. Those few that do have some sense of it tend to speak of it in such vague terms that the concept is virtually useless. Part of the problem is simply that the concept hasn't had any developed presence in the herbal literature. It is hard to think about something you have never heard about.

Another very common problem is the fear of sounding too "New-Agey" or "airy-fairy"—translation: not "scientific" enough. Herbalists, like all other people on the planet, do want to be accepted by their culture; the pervasiveness of such a widespread reductionist paradigm has had the (often intended) effect of causing people to censor their own thoughts. Thus the long-term herbal mimicry of the monotherapy paradigm in both the United States and Europe that has had such a tenacious and negative influence on the field.

Medical herbalists often lose sight of plant complexities in the search for "active" constituents.

More deeply problematical, the majority of Western herbalists simply have not spent much time developing *their own* particular in-depth understanding of plant medicines, nor have they trusted themselves enough to support the modern development of *their own* unique system—a system that has very old roots in numerous indigenous cultures in the Americas, the older European cultures (Greek and Roman, for instance), and that of community herbalists nearly everywhere. Instead, most have mimicked older systems (TCM, for instance) or taken on the trappings of the newer system of technological medicine. They have spent decades trying to force their unique Western system, a system of which they have some sense every day of their lives, into those forms. (The American herbalist Michael Moore was a major exception to that trend.) Square peg into round hole living. It is time to *own* our own unique system, without embarrassment, without pretending or trying to be what we are not.

There are many aspects to our emerging Western herbal paradigm that need to be developed in depth; one of those is the understanding of plant synergy. The following information is an early beginning, however brief or incomplete, in attempting to address it.

Understanding Plant Synergies

In the sense I am using the concept here, plant synergists act to increase the activity of other plants used for healing while affecting the body itself through a number of other, supportive actions. They do this through a wide range of mechanisms:

- They act to reduce toxic side effects of primary constituents.
- They increase depth and broadness of constituent penetration by among other things increasing intracellular transport.
- They enhance constituent activity by acting at different points of the same signaling cascade.
- They decrease the effective dose needed for cure.

Certain plant compounds alter the pharmacological actions of others and change their physicochemical properties, influencing biochemical parameters such as solubility, bioavailabilty, and activity. Some compounds enhance immune responses while others attack microbial organisms, weakening them and making them more susceptible to the heightened immune system. And still others specifically work to reduce viral and bacterial defenses to antimicrobial plant constituents so that the plant's antibacterial and antiviral compounds are more effective.

Plants suffer bacterial and viral infection, just like we do. One of the things they do to deal with bacterial infections is produce antibacterial substances such as berberine. Correspondingly, all bacteria, to differing degrees, have learned to deal with antimicrobial substances, most simply, to protect themselves from antimicrobial attack. One way they do this is to utilize multidrug-resistance pumps. MDRs act to pump antibacterial substances that get into a bacterial cell out again. In response, plants, over time, innovated chemical constituents that would deactivate MDRs.

Berberis fremontii (also known as *Mahonia fremontii*), one of the berberine-containing plants, for example, contains a compound,

5′-methoxyhydnocarpin (5′MHC), that is a potent MDR inhibitor of the efflux pump found in some Gram-positive bacteria, especially staphylococci. The plant then, when used medicinally, acts synergistically. One compound, 5′MHC, inactivates the MDR in the staph organisms, and another, berberine, kills the bacteria. (And yet another compound in the plant, porphyrin pheophorbide A, acts synergistically with both of them to kill MRSA organisms.) Sublethal doses of berberine, in numerous experiments, when combined with 5′MHC, become decidedly lethal. The compound 5′MHC itself has no antibacterial activity at all. Not surprisingly 5′MHC is common among the berberine-containing plants.

Because of the nature of this book, I am going to primarily explore plants that contain potent efflux inhibitors that deactivate those particular bacterial resistance mechanisms and, as well, plants that allow more effective penetration of plant compounds into the body. The field is still new; there isn't a lot to work with yet, but I hope that this section will give you a good idea of the complexity that is possible when looking at synergists. I hope it will stimulate you to deepen the work yourself, for all of us are going to need to know these things.

Something to keep in mind: Herbalism is and always will remain an art. Analytical knowledge, while important, has to be combined with a *feeling* for the craft, for the plants, for the people who come to us for help, and . . . for the bacterial organisms themselves. From this comes art . . . and the ability to truly reason while at the same time developing a genuine capacity to heal.

As I've said before, we need both feeling *and* thinking for this craft to flourish inside us, and behind it all, a deep and abiding love for the plants and the earth from which they, and we, come.

To begin I'll just look briefly at a few of the synergists that have promise for the future, then I will get into several in more depth and explore how to use them for the treatment of resistant bacterial infections.

A Quick Look at Some Synergistic Plants

Most of the current synergy research taking place is looking at plants and plant compounds that can reverse drug resistance. Unfortunately, for my purposes anyway, most of the resistance-modifying studies that have taken place are looking at reducing the resistance of various forms of cancer to pharmaceuticals. I am not covering those here but am focusing solely on those that have been found to modify resistance in bacteria. MRSA is the bacteria upon which most study of medicinal plants' ability to modify resistance has occurred.

In the list that follows, most of the plants were tested by using an antibiotic on a resistant organism, then adding the plant to the mix and seeing what happened. Once the herb, or its constituent(s), were combined with the antibiotic, the antibiotic either became effective or was so at much reduced levels, usually by a factor of four to eight, though in the case of thyme, the effectiveness threshold of tetracycline against MRSA went from 4 to 0.12 mg/L. Further tests were then conducted to find out just which bacterial efflux pumps were inactivated by the plant.

> Plant synergists increase the activity of other healing plants while supporting the body itself.

Dalea versicolor and ***Dalea spinosa*** both contain substances that are mildly antibacterial but others that specifically inhibit a particular efflux pump (NorA) in multidrug-resistant *Staphylococcus aureus*. They also inhibit the Bmr efflux pump found in *Bacillus subtilis*.

Ipomoea murucoides, Mexican morning glory, contains a number of compounds that are also potent inhibitors of the NorA efflux pump in resistant staph. These are, to date, the most potent inhibitors of NorA found, increasing the effectiveness of antibiotics sixteenfold.

Geranium caespitosum also has a potent efflux inhibitor active against MRSA. It potentiates the activity of the plant antimicrobials berberine and rhein as well as the antibiotics ciprofloxacin and norfloxacin. Other geraniums act similarly; these plants are exceptionally good to combine with berberine in the treatment of GI tract infections such as *E. coli* and cholera.

Cymbopogon citratus, lemongrass, while having only mild antibacterial activity itself, is an exceptionally potent synergistic activator of antibiotics against MRSA.

Rauwolfia serpentina and ***R. vomitoria*** are active against the Bmr efflux pump in *Bacillus subtilis*, the NorA and Tet(K) pumps in MRSA, the PmrA pump in *Streptococcus pneumoniae*, and an ABC transporter that is associated with ciprofloxacin resistance.

Epicatechin gallate and **epigallocatechin gallate**, both in green tea (*Camellia sinensis*), have been found to be highly potent efflux inhibitors for both MRSA and *Staphylococcus epidermidis*. They inhibit both NorA and Tet(K) efflux pumps.

Rosmarinus officinalis (rosemary), ***Thymus vulgaris*** (thyme), and ***Lycopus europaeus*** (gypsywort, bugleweed) have been found effective against the Tet(K) efflux pump in *E. coli* and MRSA and the Msr(A) pump in MRSA.

Prosopis juliflora (and other *Prosopis* species—the mesquites), a very good medicinal tree and intense invasive, contains a number of potent piperidine alkaloids, one of which has been found to be a very potent inhibitor of the NorA pump in MRSA.

Extracts of myrrh gum (***Commiphora***), gotu kola (***Centella asiatica***), wild carrot (***Daucus***), licorice, and bitter orange (***Citrus aurantium***) are all effective in inhibiting the AcrAB-TolC efflux transporter that is present in a number of Gram-negative bacteria. (They are especially effective against multidrug-resistant *Salmonella enterica* var. *typhimurium.*) This efflux mechanism is a homologue of the MexAB-OprM efflux transporter that is widely present in resistant Gram-negative organisms. Both pumps affect a wide range of antibacterials. When used with pharmaceuticals, these plants reduced the MIC (minimum inhibiting concentration) by factors of 4 to 32.

Thymus vulgaris, thyme, inhibits the MexAB-OprM efflux pump and its gene expression. MexAB-OprM is heavily involved in the removal of tetracycline, beta-lactams, fluoroquinolones, chloramphenicol, novobiocin, macrolides, ethidium bromide, aromatic hydrocarbons, and homoserine lactones. Thyme essential oil, in tiny doses, 1 or 2 drops, when taken directly by mouth will enter the bloodstream immediately. If combined with herbs such as cryptolepis, it will potentiate their action against Gram-negative bacteria. Remember: *Tiny* doses.

The problem with most of these plants (gotu kola and licorice are exceptions) is that they are not highly systemic; that is, they are only moderately, if at all, present in any quantity in the blood. This makes their use as systemic synergists difficult—though of course they can be used topically and directly in the GI tract.

The next two are *most likely* systemic, though I don't know them well enough to say, and the final one *is* systemic and could be used to a limited extent as a systemic synergist for some resistant bacteria.

Caesalpinia benthamiana (syn. *Mezoneuron benthamianum*) and ***Securinega virosa*** are two fairly important but relatively unknown (to Western herbalists) medicinal plants. The first has a wide activity against both Gram-negative and Gram-positive bacteria and is used to treat dysenteric diseases, and early indications are it may be systemic in nature. The second plant has some similar actions, especially in its wide use for dysenteric diseases. Both are efflux inhibitors. They definitely warrant further study.

Punica granatum (pomegranate), the final plant in this list, is synergistic with ampicillin, chloramphenicol, gentamicin, tetracycline, and oxacillin against 30 different MRSA and MSSA (methicillin-sensitive *Staphylococcous aureus*) strains. The plant extracts inhibit ethidium bromide efflux mechanisms in a number of different types of bacteria. There is also some evidence, not conclusive, that it is effective against the MexAB-OprM efflux pump in Gram-negative bacteria.

Pomegranate is systemic in that many of its constituents are circulated widely in the blood (peak in 1 hour, lasting about 4 hours), but how effective it would be to use it in practice, I don't know. The plant has not been considered to be a synergist in any culture that uses it and really not much as an antibacterial in any of the healing systems I have looked at. It has been used for millennia in Ayurveda but primarily as an astringent (juice) somewhat like cranberry juice, or for intestinal worms (bark/root).

However, recent research is showing some interesting activity in the plant in the treatment of high blood pressure, the prevention of normal cellular degeneration that accompanies aging, reducing DNA damage, and reducing stress levels in the body.

An In-Depth Look at Three Plant Synergists

I will now explore three synergistic plants in detail: licorice, ginger, and black pepper and its primary constituent, piperine.

Licorice

Family: Leguminosae

Species Used: There are 18 or 20 or 30 species in the genus *Glycyrrhiza* (this gets tiresome—make up your minds). They are native to Europe, North Africa, Asia, Australia, and North and South America. All species have been used medicinally, but the two most common are *Glycyrrhiza glabra* (the European licorice) and *Glycyrrhiza uralensis* (the Chinese). Russian licorice, *G. echinata,* is often used in that region; the American licorice *G. lepidota* is rarely used these days in spite of its wide native range but was frequently used as a medicinal by the indigenous peoples in the Americas. (And, yeah, they used it just the same way.)

In this section I will refer to both the European and Chinese species herein as "the plant" or as "licorice," sometimes as "it." They are used pretty much interchangeably. If I talk about another species' actions, I will list it by name.

Licorice is an unusual medicinal. It is potently antiviral, moderately antibacterial (but fairly strong against a few bacterial species such as *Staphylococcus* and *Bacillus* spp.), and moderately immune potentiating. But one of its real, and generally overlooked, strengths is that it is a very potent synergist. In fact, it should be considered one of the primary synergists in any herbal repertory.

Parts Used

The root, though the leaves do have similar but much milder actions.

Preparation and Dosage

Used as tincture, as tea, in capsules. Again: This herb is best used with other herbs in a combination formula.

One of the primary things to keep in mind when using licorice is that the higher the glycyrrhizin content, the more antiviral the herb will be. If using the herb as an antiviral, you *should not* use deglycyrrhized licorice.

There is a lot of variety in the glycyrrhizin content of licorice roots. It varies depending on species as well. In the Japanese pharmacopoeia the glycyrrhizin content of the root has to be at least 2.5 percent, i.e., 25 mg per gram of root. In the Chinese (as well as under WHO guidelines) it has to be 4 percent, that is, 40 mg per gram of root. Unfortunately, in the United States growers don't test the glycyrrhizin (a.k.a. glycyrrhizic or glycyrrhizinic acid) content of their harvested roots. So there is no way to know how much is in there. I rarely am a fan of such testing, but in this case I think it warranted for two reasons: 1) It will be easier to create proper dosages of the herb in practice and 2) it makes it easier to determine the likelihood of side effects and how to dose the additives that, if taken with the herb, will reduce or eliminate the chance of those side effects.

Glycyrrhiza uralensis generally has less glycyrrhizin than *G. glabra*, though tests have shown that Mongolian varieties of *G. uralensis* run higher, from 27–58 mg/g, though the low end is more common. I would not use *G. uralensis* for treating viruses unless that was all you had; in fact, most species roots run under 25 mg/g. *G. glabra* really is the way to go on this one.

Because the Chinese actually have to create 4 percent product by law, I would tend to buy imported roots if you really want to make sure you have at least that level of glycyrrhizin. They do sometimes import bad product into the United States, but assuming they have not in this case, if you buy from a Chinese herb supplier like 1stChineseHerbs.com, you would theoretically be getting around a 4 percent root.

To begin, the roots you use must be 3 years or older (4 years if you are using *G. uralensis*). The glycyrrhizin content of younger roots is very low compared to the older roots.

There are a number of beliefs about how the root should be prepared. Some people feel that an infusion or decoction, or even a concentrated decoction, of the root (with the later addition of 20 percent alcohol to stabilize it) produces the best extract. I am not so sure. Studies in China and Japan have found that the glycyrrhizin is best extracted in a water and alcohol blend, not in water. In fact a mix of 50 percent alcohol and 50 percent water produced the most efficient extraction in all the studies I have read. So, I am going to take a wild guess and go with that here.

TINCTURE

Use the dried root, in a 1:5 herb:liquid ratio, with the liquid being 50 percent alcohol and 50 percent water. In general, the glycyrrhizin extracts better in lower-pH water (somewhat acidic), so you might want to add a tablespoon of vinegar to your water.

Dosage: 30–60 drops up to 3x daily. In acute conditions: ½ tsp (2.5 ml) 3–6x daily, blended with other herbs, and generally for a maximum of 6 weeks at this dose and only if you take the additional supplements described under contraindications (page 427).

A company called Standard Process makes a standardized tincture, 1:1. Average dosage is 2.5 ml daily, which will give 75 mg glycyrrhizin. Dosage for acute viral infections would be 2.5–5 ml 3x daily (see the discussion of WHO, EU, and Japanese guidelines below). Note: This brand is not easily found, but you can find it if you google "licorice high grade 1:1." Some sources sell it by the 500-ml bottle, that is, about 16 ounces. It will last awhile; the pricing is actually reasonable on that size. If you actually do want a reliable product as regards glycyrrhizin content, I would suggest this one.

INFUSION

Combine ½ to 1 tsp of powdered root with 8 ounces water, simmer for 15 minutes, uncovered, then strain. Drink up to 3 cups a day. In acute conditions, drink 1 cup every 2 hours.

DECOCTION

The traditional preparation in Japan (standard now in the Japanese pharmacopoeia) is as follows: 6 grams powdered root in 500 ml (about 16 ounces) water; bring to a boil, uncovered, and let boil moderately until the liquid is reduced to 250 ml. (This will be fairly mucilaginous.) Then add enough water to bring the volume up to 1,000 ml. Drink throughout the day. Tests in Japan found that this preparation will have about 50 mg/g of glycyrrhizin. (I assume here that the powdered root they used conformed to the Japanese standard of 2.5 percent glycyrrhizin.)

CAPSULES OR POWDER

Take 4,000 mg (i.e., 4 grams) daily in three divided doses. Note: ¼ tsp of the powder is about 2,000 mg. *However*... Chinese doses run high, as they tend to do, up to 9 grams daily. Oddly, the WHO monograph lists the dosage range as 5–15 grams daily, somewhat higher. Assuming that you are getting a 4 percent glycyrrhizin content in the root, that will give you 200–600 mg of glycyrrhizin daily, which is the WHO suggested limit. The European Union standards suggest that people not consume any more than 100 mg of glycyrrhizic acid per day. In Japan glycyrrhizin intake is suggested to be kept to 200 mg per day. So, as usual, you have a range to choose from. *If* you are struggling with a severe viral infection for which this herb is specific, especially if it is severe encephalitis, there is no reason, keeping the contraindications in mind, to not use the higher WHO dose during limited treatment of 4 to 6 weeks' duration. Again, please keep in mind the side effects and contraindications.

Note: You can get licorice root standardized to either glycyrrhizin or glycyrrhic acid content if you look for it. Douglas Labs makes a 500-mg capsule standardized to contain 12 percent glycyrrhizin per capsule. This will give you 60 mg glycyrrhizin per capsule. For acute viral infections, if you are using this brand, take 1 or 2 capsules 3x daily. Note: Make *sure* you don't accidentally buy the deglycyrrhized stuff; they make both kinds. It is a fairly easy brand to find online.

There are a number of different brands that have licorice root standardized for anywhere from 12 percent to 25 percent glycyrrhizic acid. I would take these similarly during acute viral infections, looking to get up to 600 mg daily of glycyrrhizic acid.

Side Effects and Contraindications

Generally, licorice is nontoxic, even in high doses. However, long-term use, especially if you use the herb as a single (rather than in combination), and most especially if you use large doses, can cause a number of rather serious side effects. Even the use of a tea over several years will do it, and every now and then, due to the rather good range of effects the herb has, someone does. (This makes antiherb proponents *very* excited.)

Note: *This herb should rarely be used in isolation or in large doses or for long time periods*—that is, longer than 4 to 6 weeks. (However, see the next paragraph on page 428.) The side effects can be severe: edema, weak limbs (or loss of limb control entirely), spastic numbness, dizziness, headache, hypertension, hypokalemia (severe potassium depletion)—especially in the elderly. Additional problems are decreases in plasma renin and aldosterone levels, and at very large doses decreased body and thymus weight and blood cell counts. Essentially, this complex of symptoms is a condition called pseudoaldosteronism, which licorice can and indeed does cause if you take too much of it for too long. However . . .

Taking licorice along with some other supplements *can* reduce or even eliminate the tendency of the herb to produce pseudoaldosteronism. There is an intravenous form of glycyrrhizin commonly used in China that contains 40 mg aminoacetic acid (glycine), 2 mg L-cysteine, 1.6 mg sodium sulfite, and 4 mg monoammonium glycyrrhizinate (glycyrrhizin) per 2-ml vial. Normal dosing is 40–60 ml IV and up to 100 ml. The oral therapeutic dose is as high as 200 mg daily. This combination eliminates pseudoaldosteronism as a side effect. You can add both glycine and L-cysteine to your protocol to limit the potential for pseudoaldosteronism if you are taking large doses of licorice for extended periods. (Glycine, minimum 2,000 mg daily; L-cysteine, minimum 500 mg daily.) The addition of potassium (5,000 mg daily) will also help prevent the hypokalemia. Again: Licorice should be taken in combination with other herbs—this reduces the tendency for side effects by itself. And, if you do need to take largish doses of licorice, even with other herbs, for severe viral infections, please add these supplements to your regimen and carefully monitor for side effects.

Because of licorice's strong estrogenic activity, it will also cause breast growth in men, especially when combined with other estrogenic herbs. Luckily all these conditions tend to abate within 2 to 4 weeks after licorice intake ceases. Caution should be used, however, in length and strength of dosages.

A number of studies have found that large doses of licorice taken long term during pregnancy have detrimental effects on the unborn children. Low doses are apparently safe. Again, this plant should not be used in large doses or for lengthy periods of time *especially if you are pregnant.*

The herb is contraindicated in hypertension, hypokalemia, pregnancy, hypernatremia, and low testosterone levels. However, for short-term use in those conditions (10 days or less), in low doses combined with other herbs, it is very safe.

Herb/Drug Interactions

The plant is highly synergistic. It is also additive. It should not be used along with estrogenic pharmaceuticals, hypertensive drugs, cardiac glycosides, corticosteroids, hydrocortisone, or diuretics such as thiazides, spironolactone, or amiloride.

Habitat and Appearance

The *Glycyrrhiza* genus is a member of the pea family with the usual pea-type leaves—a bunch of oval leaflets running along a central stem. The plants are perennials, can grow to 6 feet in height, and bush out to 3 feet. The plants produce spikes of the usual pea-family flowers during the summer. They range in color from yellowish to blue to purple in the various species. The plant sends out both roots and rhizomes, the roots thick and fleshy, up to 4 inches in diameter, going as deep as 3 feet. The creeping rhizomes spread out from the primary root up to 26 feet in length, often sending up shoots of new plants far from the original. The roots and rhizomes of the cultivated species are light in color, the wild species darker. The inside of most of the species is yellowish, and, in the European and Chinese species at least, quite sweet. The American species is not very sweet, though a lot of sources say it is (I have eaten it; still waiting for that sweet taste to emerge on my tongue). The American species, though low in sweetness, possesses many of the same medicinal actions as the more prominent medicinal species. I've not encountered any of the other less common species in practice.

The licorice flowers mature into clusters of spiky brown seed capsules each about the size of a grape (at least in the American species—the only one I have seen).

The genus ranges from semi-arid desert to lush, wet climes such as Yorkshire, England, and from sea level to 8,500 or so feet in altitude. When wild, the plants often like growing along waterways in sandyish soil. The American species is endemic throughout Canada and most of the United States excluding the Southeast. The European species is cultivated many places in the Americas but has escaped and can be found here and there in California, Nevada, and Utah. I can't find a record of any wild species in mid- to southern Africa (even though it is most likely grown there), but the genus seems to have spread pretty much everywhere else. If you look around, you will probably find a licorice native in your eco-range someplace.

Cultivation and Collection

The plants grow fairly easily from root cuttings; the seeds are more demanding. The seeds need to be stratified for several weeks, then scarified and soaked for 2 hours in warm water before sowing if you want an easy germination. Treated seeds will germinate at about an 80 percent rate, and untreated at around 20 percent. Once started, the plants are pretty intent on remaining and spreading wherever they want to. Make sure you want it where you plant it—you won't be able to get rid of it if you change your mind. A few places here and there consider it an invasive, because, well, it is.

Both the European and Chinese varieties warrant planting in the wild and letting them go; they are well able to look after themselves if released from captivity. As they are a major medicinal, the more they spread, the better off we will be.

The plants like a free-draining friable soil with a pH between 6 and 7, but they can take on a greater range than that and do quite well. They are drought tolerant and like the sun but do need a bit of water; they often grow wild along streambeds, where they are very tenacious.

It takes a few years for the plants to establish themselves (2 to 3 years is a good minimum period of time), but once they do, you will be able to harvest from them pretty much forever. You will rarely, if ever, be able to dig up the entire root system of an established plant, and it will continue to grow and spread from what is left. Commercial growers generally achieve somewhere between 15 and 50 tons per hectare of roots once the plants have matured. The older the plants and the deeper the dig, the bigger the yield. The plants produce a lot of root mass. You can get enough medicine for an entire family from just one established plant, pretty much forever.

Properties of Licorice

Actions

Adrenal cortex stimulant
Adrenal tonic
Analgesic
Antibacterial
Anticancer/tumor inhibitor
Antihyperglycemic
Anti-inflammatory
Antioxidative
Antispasmodic
Antistressor
Antitussive
Antiulcerative
Antiviral
Cardioprotective
Demulcent
Estrogenic
Expectorant
Gastric secretion inhibitor
Hepatoprotective
Immunomodulant
Immunostimulant
Laxative (gentle)
Mucoprotective
Prevents biofilm formation
Protects from effects of radiation exposure
Smooth muscle relaxant
Stimulates pancreatic secretions
Synergist (potent)
Thymus stimulant

Licorice is a fairly potent synergist. It is specifically called for in treating resistant Gram-negative infections as it is most potent against that family of efflux mechanisms. In general, it increases the action of other herbs and pharmaceuticals, and if added to a mixture prior to tincturing, it will enhance the extraction. It also acts as a detoxicant, and, most important, licorice is an inhibitor of one of the main efflux mechanisms in Gram-negative bacteria. As an antiviral, it prevents viral replication across a wide range of viruses, inhibits viral growth, inhibits neuraminidases in numerous influenza strains, inactivates virus particles, and inhibits RANTES secretion. As an immunostimulant, it stimulates interferon production, enhances antibody formation, and stimulates phagocytosis.

It takes about 4 hours for licorice's glycyrrhizin to reach maximum serum concentration after oral ingestion; then it is slowly excreted, and eventually eliminated at 72 hours after ingestion. It stays in the body a long time.

Active Against

Arboviruses
Arthrinium sacchari
Bacillus coagulans
Bacillus megaterium
Bacillus stearothermophilus
Bacillus subtilis
Candida albicans
Chaetomium funicola
Clostridium sporogenes
Cytomegalovirus
Enterococcus faecalis

(continued)

Properties of Licorice—Continued

Active Against—Continued

Enterococcus faecium
Enterotoxigenic *Escherichia coli*
Enterovirus 71
Epstein-Barr virus
Haemophilus influenzae
Helicobacter pylori
Hepatitis B and C
Herpes simplex
HIV-1
Influenza A (various strains, H1N1, H2N2, H9N2, novel H1N1 [WT], oseltamivir-resistant novel H1N1, and so on)
Japanese encephalitis virus
Klebsiella pneumoniae
Mycobacterium tuberculosis
Newcastle disease virus
Plasmodium spp.
Pseudorabies virus
Respiratory syncytial virus
Salmonella paratyphi
Salmonella typhi
Salmonella typhimurium
Sarcina lutea
SARS-related coronavirus (FFM1, FFM2)
Shigella boydii
Shigella dysentariae
Staphylococcus aureus
Streptococcus lactis
Streptococcus mutans
Streptococcus sobrinus
Toxocara canis
Trichophyton mentagrophytes
Trichophyton rubrum
Vaccinia virus
Varicella zoster virus
Vesicular stomatitis virus
Vibrio cholerae
Vibrio mimicus
Vibrio parahaemolyticus

Use to Treat

Use in cases of respiratory viral infections and oral bacterial problems (for gums and mucous membranes). Use as an adjunct for bacterial infections, especially of the GI tract and respiratory tract, especially if there is cramping or ulceration. But primarily, in the context of this book, use licorice as a synergist in systemic bacterial infections.

Note: Licorice should be used in combination rather than alone. See Side Effects and Contraindications (page 427). I would not recommend that this plant be used as a single medicinal.

Other Uses

As a sweetener. *Glycyrrhiza glabra* is also a potent plant remediator for reclaiming saline-heavy soils.

Finding Licorice

You can buy very good quality European licorice from Pacific Botanicals, my preferred source. 1st Chinese Herbs has the Chinese variety. Seeds can be had from Horizon Herbs or Richters, an international seed merchant.

Note: Some of the licorice in commerce comes from eastern Europe, which possesses some of the highest levels of soil and air pollution in the world. It makes no sense to buy potentially contaminated herbs to use for their broad-spectrum immune and liver actions. Organically grown licorice is much better. If you buy both and compare them, you will find a significant difference in quality.

The plant roots and rhizomes should be harvested in the fall or early spring and dried out of the sun. The larger roots should be cut into smaller sections before being dried.

Plant Chemistry

There are hundreds of compounds in licorice, many of which have been intensively studied. The main one is glycyrrhizin, which makes up to 24 percent of the root by weight. Also: glabrin A and B, glycyrrhetol, glabrolide, isoglabrolide, scores of isoflavones, coumarins, triterpene sterols, saponins, and so on and on and on.

Traditional Uses of Licorice

Licorice has been used as a food plant and medicinal for between four and five millennia. The genus name, *Glycyrrhiza,* is Greek in origin, *glykys* meaning "sweet" and *rhiza* "root." The root's main constituent, glycyrrhizin, is 50 times sweeter than sugar. All the species have been used in medicine in any geographical region they grew and by any culture that had access to them.

AYURVEDA

Variously known as *mulethi, yasti-madhu, jasti-madhu, madhuka, mithiladki,* and so on. The plant is considered cooling, tonic, demulcent, expectorant, diuretic, and a gentle laxative. It's used for treating poisoning, ulcers, and diseases of the liver, bladder, and lungs. Any inflammation in the mucous membranes anywhere in the body. For cough, sore throat, hoarseness, fever, and as a general tonic in debility from long-term disease conditions, especially those that are pulmonary or of the GI tract.

Licorice is considered a synergist, a specific additive to other herbal formulations.

TRADITIONAL CHINESE MEDICINE

Known as *gancao* in Chinese medicine, licorice has been used in China for 3,000 years or so. The herb is considered sweet and mild, to regulate the function of the stomach, and to be qi tonifying, lung demulcent, expectorant, latent-heat cleansing, antipyretic, detoxicant, anti-inflammatory and spleen invigorative and is a synergist in many herbal formulations. The herb is used in pharyngolaryngitis, cough, palpitations, stomachache due to asthenia, peptic ulcer, pyogenic infection, and ulceration of the skin.

WESTERN BOTANIC PRACTICE

The ancient Egyptians used the plant as a major medicinal; the plant has often been found in their tombs. The Greek Theophrastus, in the third century BCE, noted the plant's use for asthma, dry coughs, and respiratory problems. The Romans called the plant *liquiritia,* which eventually was corrupted to the word *licorice*. It was a primary medicine in ancient Rome for coughs. It was used throughout Europe as a primary medicinal, and although harvested in the wild originally, it has been a main agricultural crop for more than 1,000 years.

The American Eclectics used it intensively, as did most medicinal practitioners in the Americas. The Eclectics used it for coughs, catarrhs, irritation of the urinary passages, diarrhea, and bronchial diseases. It was an early agricultural medicinal, grown by most people in their medicinal gardens. The indigenous tribes of the Americas used the indigenous species similarly; that is, for sore throat, chest pains, swellings, coughs; as an antidiarrheal; for stomachache, fevers, toothache, skin sores, spitting blood; and as a general tonic.

Scientific Research

The medicinal species have been intensely studied for years. This look will be brief, as a full monograph would run to hundreds of pages.

As an immune stimulant: A double-blind, repeated (within subject), randomized trial with *Echinacea purpurea, Astragalus membranaceus*, and *Glycyrrhiza glabra* found that licorice significantly increased CD25 expression on T cells. It also increased CD69, CD4, and CD8 expression on T cells.

Postoperative sore throat: Forty adults about to undergo elective lumbar laminectomy were split into two groups. One received water, the other water with licorice. The use of licorice gargle performed 5 minutes before anesthesia was effective in reducing or eliminating the incidence and severity of postoperative sore throat in patients.

Tuberculosis: A randomized, double-blind, placebo-controlled study with 60 people with sputum-positive pulmonary tuberculosis was conducted. They were split into two groups, one taking placebo, the other licorice—in addition to their regular therapy. Sputum conversion was seen in 80 percent of the licorice group, and 70 percent in the placebo group. Fever was relieved in all in the licorice group, and 80 percent in the placebo group. Cough was relieved in 96 percent of the licorice group, and 81 percent of the placebo group. GI side effects were seen in 20 percent of the placebo group, and none of the licorice group. ALT and AST levels were raised in 6 percent of the licorice group, and 30 percent of the placebo group. Elevated uric acid in serum was observed in 3 percent of the licorice group, and 16 percent of the placebo group.

Hepatitis: A single compound, an interferon stimulator, from licorice was used to treat patients with subacute hepatic failure. The survival rate was 72 percent compared to 31 percent in those who received traditional therapies.

Atopic dermatitis: A licorice gel was used to successfully treat atopic dermatitis in a double-blind clinical trial, 30 people in each group. The gel significantly reduced erythema, edema, and itching over the 2-week trial.

Aphthous stomatitis: Bioadhesive patches containing licorice were used to control the pain and reduce healing time in recurrent aphthous ulcer. Licorice patches caused a significant reduction in the diameter of the inflammatory halo and necrotic center compared with placebo. (There have been three of these trials, all successful.)

Pharmaceutical side effects: In a comparative trial, licorice, when used along with spironolactone in the treatment of polycystic ovary syndrome, significantly reduced the side effects from spironolactone when used alone.

Peptic ulcer: Licorice was found in a trial with 100 people with peptic ulcer (86 of whom were unresponsive to conventional treatment) to be effective: 90 percent experienced good effects, 22 were cured, 28 were significantly improved.

Hepatitis A: In 13 cases of infectious hepatitis treated with licorice, the icterus index normalized in 13 days, urinary bile pigments were negative in 10 days, marked reduction of hepatomegaly took 9 days, pain over the liver disappeared in 8 days.

Hepatitis C: Glycyrrhizin has been used in Japan for more than 60 years in the treatment of hepatitis C. In several clinical trials it has been found to significantly lower AST, ALT, and GGT concentrations while reversing histologic evidence of necrosis and inflammatory lesions in the liver.

Lichen planus: In a clinical trial, 66 percent of people with lichen planus who took glycyrrhizin were cured.

Oral herpes: Glycyrrhizic acid cream, applied six times daily in people with acute oral herpetic infections (HSV1), resolved pain and dysphagia within 24 to 48 hours.

There have been a number of trials using licorice in combination with other herbs. It reduced risperidone-induced hyperprolactinemia in patients with schizophrenia. Reduced hyperuricemia in vegetarians. Was effective in the treatment of advanced pancreatic and other gastrointestinal malignancies. Was successful in the treatment of 138 cases of intestinal metaplasia and 104 of atypical hyperplasia of the gastric mucosa.

In vivo studies have found licorice to be potently antioxidant, to stimulant immune activity, to be anticonvulsant, to be potently anti-inflammatory on skin eruptions, to be hepatoprotective, to be cerebroprotective, to heal aspirin-induced ulcers, to be antispasmodic to the lower intestine, to be strongly antitussive, and to protect the mitochondria from damage.

SPECIFIC ACTIONS AS A SYNERGIST

Licorice is a fairly potent synergist through a number of avenues. Importantly, it is directly active against the efflux mechanism AcrAB-TolC in the Enterobacteriaceae family of bacteria, which are Gram-negative organisms. This efflux mechanism can extrude many diverse antibacterials including tetracyclines, fluoroquinolones, and chloramphenicol. Licorice, then, can effectively be added to formulations treating infections from that Gram-negative family, including, among others, *Yersinia, Shigella, Serratia, Salmonella, Morganella, Klebsiella, Enterobacter,* and *Escherichia.*

Licorice increases the potency of both herbs and pharmaceuticals when used with them. It has been found, for example, to enhance the action of antituberculosis drugs, increasing positive outcomes in treatment; to increase the action of hydrocortisone; and to potentiate oseltamivir against resistant influenza strains. Chinese trials have shown that it increases the potency of other herbs in the treatment of rheumatoid arthritis and increases the antioxidant actions of other herbs such as astragalus and the isolated compound lycopene. Licorice enhances the anticancer activity of various herbs against prostate cancer cell lines; increases the effect of the neuromuscular blocking agent paeoniflorin; and significantly increases the immune-stimulating action of herbs such as *Echinacea purpurea* and *Astragalus*.

Licorice increases the strength of tincture formulations if added to the herbs prior to tincturing. For example, it enhances the solubility of compounds from other plants (e.g., the sapogenin isoliquiritigenin, the saikosaponins from ginseng) by a factor of up to 570.

Licorice also reduces toxicity in other plants; it prevents toxicity from aconite alkaloids and reduces the toxicity from a number of herbs used to treat rheumatoid arthritis in Chinese clinical trials.

Ginger

Family: Zingiberaceae. There are about 1,400 members of the family, of which the genus *Zingiber* is usually referred to as the *true* gingers. The species in the *Alpinia* genus are probably the other most commonly used medicinals in the family.

Species Used: There are 85 or maybe 100 species of plants in the genus *Zingiber*. (Why have taxonomy anyway?) *Z. officinale*, the common food ginger, is the most famous and the one generally used for medicine. Many of the species in this family contain similar constituents and can be used medicinally, but their actions do differ. This short monograph looks only at the culinary ginger, *Z. officinale*.

Part Used

The root. The root of ginger is really a rhizome, but nobody cares about the distinction but phytogrammarians, so I will just call it a root, as nearly all people who use language do.

Preparation and Dosage

The best form of the herb is the fresh juice of the root taken as a hot tea; it is most potent like this. Large quantities of the juice can be stabilized with alcohol (in an 80:20 juice-to-alcohol ratio) and then added to herbal combinations to blend the juice's synergistic actions into the formula. *If you are using the plant to treat resistant infections, this is the way to do it in tincture combinations.* Fresh tincture of the root is nearly as good. Dried root is relatively useless.

If you are using ginger as an antiviral, the hot tea from the fresh juice is exceptionally potent. It takes about 30 minutes after drinking the fresh juice hot tea for ginger's compounds to enter the bloodstream; they reach peak concentration in about 60 minutes and then begin to decline. The fresh juice tea should be consumed every 2 to 3 hours in acute conditions to keep the constituents at high levels in the blood.

FRESH GINGER JUICE TEA

Juice one or more pieces of ginger, in total about the size of a medium to large carrot, or four pieces the size of your thumb. *Save the plant matter that is left over* (for making an infusion; see below).

Combine 1/4 cup fresh ginger juice with 12 ounces hot water, 1 tbl wildflower honey, the juice from 1/4 lime (squeeze the juice into the cup, then drop in the rind), and 1/8 tsp cayenne.

Drink 4–6 cups per day. (If you don't own a juicer, use infusion method two, below.)

In acute conditions: Drink 6 cups per day minimum.

INFUSION

Method One: The leftover plant matter from juicing ginger can be put into 1–2 cups hot water, depending on how much you have left, and allowed to steep for 4 to 8 hours, covered. Strain, and use the infused liquid as you would fresh ginger juice in making fresh ginger juice tea (above). It will be almost as useful as the fresh juice but not quite.

Method Two: Grate or chop gingerroot (a piece about the size of

Finding Ginger

Grocery stores everywhere (get organic if you can; if not, use what you can find).

your thumb) as finely as you can. Steep in 8–12 ounces hot water for 2 to 3 hours, *covered* in order to preserve the essential oils in the tea. Drink 4–6 cups daily.

TOPICALLY

Ginger juice is exceptionally good (sometimes) in relieving the pain of burns and speeding up healing. Apply the fresh juice topically to the affected area with a cotton ball. It is also a good antibacterial and antifungal when applied to skin infections.

TINCTURE

Fresh root, 1:2, 95 percent alcohol, 10–20 drops, up to 4x daily. (I do not prefer this approach, as the fresh juice is much, much better—nevertheless it is a million . . . well, okay, a billion . . . times better than using the dried root.)

AS FOOD

In everything and anything, often.

Side Effects and Contraindications

Large doses should be avoided in pregnancy due to the plant's emmenagogue effect, though the dried root can be used to help morning sickness in moderate doses. May aggravate gallstones, so caution is advised. Rarely: bloating, gas, heartburn, nausea—usually when using the dried, powdered root.

Herb/Drug Interactions

The root is synergistic with a number of antibiotics, especially the aminoglycosides, increasing their potency, especially against resistant organisms.

Alternatives: *Alpinia galanga*, also known as galangal, is a close relative of culinary ginger and is also used in cooking, primarily in Asia (it is common in Thai food, for example). It has a similar range

(continued on page 442)

Properties of Ginger

Actions

As an antiviral, ginger inhibits the attachment of viruses to the cell, inhibits hemagglutinin, inhibits viral proteases, inhibits neuraminidase, stimulates antiviral macrophage activity, and is virucidal. It is also:

Analgesic
Anthelmintic
Antiarthritic
Antibacterial
Antidiarrheal
Antiemetic
Antifungal
Anti-inflammatory
Antispasmodic
Antitussive
Carminative
Circulatory stimulant
Diaphoretic
Elastase inhibitor
Hypotensive
Immune stimulant
Synergist

Active Against

Ginger is a synergist, increasing the actions of other herbs and boosting their effectiveness by relaxing blood vessels and increasing circulation, thus carrying the active constituents of the other herbs throughout the body. It has also been used across the world for treating a large range of viral infections including colds, influenza, hepatitis, herpes, yellow fever, measles, chicken pox, and enterovirus. Note: The list that follows contains *only* those viruses (and other microbes) that it has been found effective for in medical research studies; it has been used against a wider range in historical practice.

Given the test range, ginger should be thought of as a narrow-spectrum antiviral—primarily specific for respiratory viral infections, though its range of actions makes it a very good supportive herb for most viral infections. It is active against influenza A, rhinovirus (especially 1B), human cytomegalovirus, hepatitis C, HIV-1, Epstein-Barr, HSV-1 and HSV-2 (resistant or otherwise), Newcastle virus (Ranikhet strain), vaccinia virus, tobacco mosaic virus, and poliovirus (type 3—mildly so).

The herb has a decent range of antimicrobial actions as well, against:

Acinetobacter baumanii
Angiostrongylus cantonensis
Anisakis simplex
Aspergillus niger
Bacillus subtilis
Campylobacter jejuni
Candida albicans
Candida glabrata
Coliform bacilli
Dirofilaria immitis
Escherichia coli
Fusarium moniliforme
Haemonchus contortus

Haemophilus influenzae
Helicobacter pylori (cagA+ strains)
Klebsiella pneumoniae
Listeria spp.
Porphyromonas endodontalis
Porphyromonas gingivalis
Prevotella intermedia
Proteus vulgaris
Pseudomonas aeruginosa
Salmonella typhimurium
Shigella dysenteriae
Shigella flexneri
Staphylococcus aureus
Staphylococcus epidermidis
Streptococcus viridans
Toxoplasma gondii
Trypanosoma evansi

Use to Treat

Ginger is best thought of in the following way: as a respiratory antiviral circulatory stimulant that will calm nausea, reduce diarrhea and stomach cramping, reduce fever (by stimulating sweating), reduce cold chills, reduce inflammation in bronchial passageways, thin mucus and help it move out of the system, reduce coughing (as much as codeine cough syrups), ameliorate anxiety, and provide analgesic relief equal to or better than ibuprofen. It is a synergist, increasing the actions of other herbs and boosting their effectiveness by relaxing blood vessels and increasing circulation, thus carrying the active constituents of the other herbs more efficiently throughout the body.

If used at the onset of a cold or flu, i.e., *the very day you sense it coming on*, it can cut down sick time to 3 days or less and the episode will often be mild. If used once the flu or cold is fully blown, it will help ameliorate the symptoms considerably and shorten the illness. How much depends on your general immune health. If you've been burning the candle at both ends and putting off resting for too long . . . well, get some soup and settle in for some time off.

The herb can also be used in some bacterial diarrheal conditions, especially where there is cramping (cholera, dysentery, *E. coli*, etc.), for reduced circulation with coldness in the extremities, for migraine headache if accompanied by cold hands or feet, and for a sluggish constitution.

of antiviral action. Again, the fresh juice and the ethanol extract of the fresh root are the strongest antiviral forms of the medicine to use. Other edible gingers, such as *Zingiber zerumbet,* another Southeast Asian culinary ginger, are also very high in antiviral activity.

Habitat and Appearance

The exact geographical location of the original ginger plant is unknown—most likely someplace in Asia. It has been cultivated for 4,000 or more years in China and India and reached the West around 2,000 years ago. The genus name *Zingiber* is of ancient Hindu extraction; it means "horn-shaped." ("They" say it's from the shape of the root, but I don't believe it; I've seen gingerroot roots.) The roots form dense clumps as they grow, and that is what everyone harvests.

The plant is a perennial and likes warm, humid climates from sea level up to about 5,000 feet in altitude. It is rarely found wild; it's a cultivated medicinal.

The plant grows 2 to 3 feet in height and looks like sort of a shortish bamboo with a thin central stalk. *Zingiber* plants look much alike and are often confused with the alpinias, another genus in the family.

Cultivation and Collection

Ginger is almost always cultivated from pieces of the living root, like potatoes. Simply allowing some gingerroot to begin budding, then cutting it into pieces, each with a bud, and planting them is usually how it is done. Most ginger plants on Earth are rootstock clones. And it is one of the most heavily cultivated plants on Earth. *Everybody* loves it. The plant is considered a perennial, but it generally depletes the soil in which it is grown so it's usually rotated every other year. Unless it is in the exact right location it won't last once the soil is depleted.

Ginger is a tropical plant. It likes sheltered locations, filtered sunlight, warmth, humidity, rich soil. It hates direct sun and so on; basically it wants to be pampered and protected from the elements. It can't take freezing.

The root cuttings should be planted in late fall or early spring. No direct sun locations. Plant the cuttings 2 to 3 inches deep with the bud upward.

The plants need a lot of water, so don't let the soil dry out. Mulch them thickly. They hate dry air. The leaves die back in 8 to 10 months, and that is when the roots should be harvested. The roots will last a long time before they dry out; they should be used fresh if you are using them as antivirals.

Plant Chemistry

Several hundred constituents, including gingerols, zingiberol, zingiberene, shogaols, 3-dihydroshogaols, gingerdiols, mono- and diacetyl derivatives of gingerdiols, dihydrogingerdiones, labdadiene, and so on. The volatile oils such as the gingerols are very potent but much reduced in the dried roots. They are present at levels 6 to 15 times higher in fresh roots. Many constituents convert to shogaols as the root dries. The volatile constituents are the most antiviral.

Traditional Uses of Ginger

It has been used every place it is grown as a medicine. *Everyone* not trapped in a technological culture uses it as a synergist for healing for colds and flu, nausea, poor circulation, and so on.

In Burma, fresh gingerroot is boiled in water (with palm sap as a sweetener) to get a hot infusion for treating colds and flu. In Congo, ginger is crushed and mixed with mango tree sap for colds and flu. In the Philippines, fresh chopped ginger is boiled with water, and sugar added, to treat sore throat. It is used similarly in China and India. (There is a reason it is done this way.)

Ginger has a long historical tradition in warm climates as a food additive. Like many culinary spices it possesses strong antibacterial activity against a number of foodborne pathogens—especially against three of those now plaguing commercial foods: *Shigella, E. coli,* and *Salmonella.*

Two of the best ways to take ginger as food are the pickled ginger often served along with sushi in Japanese restaurants or candied gingerroot slices. Both make great snacks, can be eaten in large quantities, and are a healthy stimulant for the system.

AYURVEDA

Ginger has a very long history in Ayurveda, which calls it *srangavera* and about 50 other names depending on where you go. It is used for dyspepsia, flatulence, colic, vomiting, spasms of the stomach and bowels attended by fever, cold, cough, asthma, indigestion, lack of appetite, diarrhea, fever. The fresh juice (aha!), mixed with sugar and water, is a common form of preparation.

TRADITIONAL CHINESE MEDICINE

Fresh root: *sheng jiang*. (Dried root: *gan jiang*—a very different medicine.) Considered pungent and warm in traditional Chinese medicine (TCM), it is used as a diaphoretic, antiemetic, mucolytic, antitussive, detoxicant, anti-inflammatory. It is considered specific to warm the lungs, for pathogenic wind-cold conditions (i.e., severe intolerance to cold), slight fever, headache, general ache, nasal congestion, runny nose, cough, vomiting. It is usually prepared by decoction in water or pounded and the juice added to warm water. Ginger is generally combined with other herbs in TCM as it is considered to be a "guide" drug that carries the other herbs where they need to go. Ginger is also considered to be specific for ameliorating the toxic effects of other drugs or herbs. Estimates are that up to half of all Chinese herbal formulas contain it.

WESTERN BOTANIC PRACTICE

Everyone in the West has used ginger in much the same ways, though, historically, most of them tended to focus on its use for stomach and bowel complaints.

Scientific Research

The research on ginger has been problematic in that distinctions haven't been made (or looked for) between the actions of the fresh root and the dried root. (Common among scientists.) Nor has there been clarity about *how* the herb is prepared or what effect that might make on outcomes. (Common among scientists.) It is very rare that fresh preparations have been tested. (Ridiculous since that is the *primary* form of the medicine the world over.) Water extracts of the dried roots show very little antimicrobial activity—though they remain potently anti-inflammatory. If you don't understand the problems inherent in the journal papers, the outcomes found—which vary all over the place—are hard to understand. Sigh. Plants possess very different medicinal actions depending on: when they are harvested, how they are harvested, if they are dried or fresh, how they are prepared as medicines, how often they are taken, how much is taken, and if they are taken in isolation or in combination. Scientists coming from a reductionist orientation have a hard time understanding all that; they don't understand that herbal medicine really *is* rocket surgery.

As an overview: There have been some 30 clinical trials with 2,300 people using gingerroot. Following is just a sampling of a few of those and of a few in vivo and in vitro studies.

Anti-inflammatory action: Gingerol and its related compounds are potent inhibitors of lipopolysaccharide-induced PGE2 production in vitro. Inhibit both COX-1 and COX-2 in vitro through inhibiting several genes involved in the inflammatory response (acting on cytokines, chemokines, 5-lipoxygenase, and COX-2). Of 56 people (28 with rheumatoid arthritis, 18 with osteoarthritis, 10 with muscular discomfort) who took dried ginger, 75 percent reported relief from pain and swelling. In a double-blind, randomized, placebo-controlled clinical trial with 102 people with osteoarthritis, ginger was found to be as effective as ibuprofen in relieving pain and swelling. Numerous other in vivo studies have shown that gingerroot has both anti-inflammatory and analgesic actions; some used the essential oil massaged into the affected area—it works really well.

Antiemetic/antinausea: Various clinical studies have found that gingerroot is especially effective for treating severe morning sickness in pregnant women. The dried root was used, of course, and was found more effective in severe cases. (The fresh root is better for nausea.)

Antiadhesion: In vivo, gingerroot interferes with the adhesion of enterobacterial disease organisms to the intestinal wall. This, in essence, reduces entero-infection of the GI tract, short-circuiting the disease process. Ginger is also an elastase inhibitor. Many bacteria use elastase to break down cellular tissue, helping their penetration of the body. (Ginger also reduces spasms in the intestinal tract, relaxing the intestinal wall at the same time.)

Antidiarrheal: Gingerroot interferes with the colonization of cells by enterogenic bacteria, thus reducing diarrhea, and reducing bacterial load. The root alters bacterial and host cell metabolism through a unique-to-ginger mechanism.

Cerebroprotective: In vivo studies found that gingerroot protects rats from brain damage and memory impairment.

Immunostimulant: In vivo studies with gingerroot have found that it increases immune markers across the board, pre- and post-infection.

Detoxification: In vivo rat studies

found that ginger reduces cadmium levels and toxicity in rats, acting as a heavy metal detoxifier. And gingerroot in vivo reduces the effects of organophosphate insecticides.

Anthelmintic: Ginger was found to be effective in the treatment of endoparasites and stomach problems in ethnoveterinary practice in Pakistan, killing all red stomach worms (*Haemonchus contortus*) in test animals. It has been found active against a number of other endoparasites in other trials.

Other studies have found antiulcerative, antitumor, gastric antisecretory, antifungal, antispasmodic, anticonvulsant, and antiallergenic actions in the plant.

SPECIFIC ACTIONS AS A SYNERGIST

Ginger increases the potency of herbs and pharmaceuticals if added to a protocol, inhibits bacterial resistance mechanisms in pathogens, stimulates circulation, and reduces the toxicity of endotoxins and pollutants. It dilates blood vessels and increases circulation, helping the blood, and the constituents in the blood from other herbs, to achieve faster and more effective distribution in the body.

Ginger is highly effective in reducing the ability of bacteria to extrude antibacterials out of their cells. (In consequence it increases the potency of a number of pharmaceuticals.)

Ginger potentiates the activity of aminoglycoside antibiotics (arbekacin, gentamicin, tobramycin, streptomycin) and other antibiotics such as bacitracin and polymyxin B, against vancomycin-resistant enterococci (which are Gram-positive)—essentially by increasing the permeability of the cell membrane; ginger is a strong p-glycoprotein inhibitor, as strong as the pharmaceutical verapamil. It also increases the effectiveness of daunomycin (used in the treatment of cancer), increasing the accumulation of the pharmaceutical three-fold and significantly reducing the P-gp-mediated efflux of the drug. This is common in P-gp inhibitors since cancer cells tend to use P-gp efflux mechanisms to get rid of pharmaceuticals.

Sublethal levels of tetracycline become lethal against staph organisms when ginger is added; compounds from ginger modify bacterial resistance in *Acinetobacter baumanii;* ginger potentiates the action of nifedipine on antiplatelet aggregation in normal human volunteers and the hypertensive; ginger potentiates the effectiveness of clarithromycin against *Helicobacter pylori* independent of whether the bacterial strain was susceptible to the pharmaceutical or not prior to the addition of ginger.

Ginger also has direct synergistic actions with other herbs. It potentiates their activity, increasing it substantially. For example, constituents in magnolia, but not in ginger, enhance sucrose intake in rats and reduce immobility time in swimming tests. But when ginger volatile oils are added to the mix, sucrose intake is increased exponentially; reduction time for immobility was also increased.

In other studies, when ginger oils are added to magnolia, they combine to produce a tremendously synergistic outcome in the treatment of depression. Serotonin in the brain and noradrenaline levels in the prefrontal cortex increase substantially after ginger is added to subclinical (inactive) doses of magnolia.

Ginger is also considered to be specific for ameliorating the toxic effects of other drugs or herbs used in TCM. In vivo studies found that ginger reduces cadmium levels and toxicity in rats, acting as a heavy metal detoxifier. It also reduces the effects of organophosphate insecticides in vivo.

Black Pepper/Piperine

Species Used: Piperine is a potent alkaloid found in two different peppers, black pepper (*Piper nigrum*) and long pepper (*Piper longum*). It is the primary constituent responsible (along with an isomer of piperine—chavicine) for the spicy pungency of pepper.

Piperine is the most common constituent in black pepper, running from 5 percent to 9 percent. Long pepper has much less, from 1 percent to 2 percent.

The pepper plant itself *can* be used as a synergist if you are so inclined; for a number of reasons I prefer the isolated constituent as a synergist, however. I will talk about both approaches in this section and the reasons why I am suggesting the constituent in this case.

Preparation and Dosage

Because this book is concentrating on the treatment of resistant bacterial organisms, many of which can have severe impacts if not treated effectively, it makes sense to me to use the isolated constituent piperine rather than the whole herb in this instance. The herb itself *can* be used; it is, however, about one-fifteenth as strong as piperine. Since piperine is, at this point, relatively easy to find, I would suggest having some on hand, just in case. If you don't have it or it becomes no longer available (see Finding Black Pepper and Piperine on page 449), you can indeed use the pepper itself.

BLACK PEPPER TINCTURE

Both *Piper nigrum* and *Piper longum* are prepared as tinctures, 1:5, 65 percent alcohol. Dosage: 5–15 drops as needed. Piperine is not very water soluble; you need an alcohol tincture to extract it from the peppercorns. I would highly recommend using whole peppercorns, freshly ground, for making the tinctures. Previously ground pepper is much weaker.

TRIKATU

You can also, if you wish, make trikatu, the traditional Ayurvedic combination that is added to herbs as a formulation synergist. It is prepared using *Piper nigrum* and *P. longum* and gingerroot in a ratio of 1:1:1; that is, equal parts of each herb or their tinctures. I prefer the tinctures. Use a tincture of fresh gingerroot, or, more preferably, the alcohol-stabilized fresh juice (as described in the ginger monograph on page 437) and tinctures of the two peppers as outlined above. Combine them in equal parts and then add that combined tincture to whatever formulation you are making. If you are making 4 ounces of an influenza formulation, then add an extra ounce of trikatu to make a total of 5 ounces. In other words, add 25 percent to any formulation you are making. It is going to be spicy.

PIPERINE

If you wish to use pure piperine, you will need to buy it, as it is a manufactured product. It is relatively inexpensive. Normal dosing, for instance to enhance the uptake of nutrients from food, is 20 mg daily.

Note: I would *not* use piperine as a regular supplement; in my opinion, it is indicated *only* for medical conditions that necessitate its use. If you have a systemic infection, especially if it is Gram-negative, piperine is a highly effective synergist for the herbs you will use to treat it and should be considered as a part of the treatment approach.

Dosage in acute conditions: Piperine should be taken prior to the herbal formulation you are using so that the intestinal wall has already been altered by the time your herbs get to the GI tract. Take 20

Properties of Black Pepper/Piperine

Actions

Analgesic
Antibacterial
Anticonvulsant
Antidiarrheal
Antidysphagic (essential oil)
Antihyperlipidemic (reduces lipid levels in the blood)
Anti-inflammatory
Antimutagenic
Antioxidant
Antispasmodic
Antitumor inhibitor
CYP3A4 inhibitor
Free radical scavenger (potent)
Hepatoprotector
Immunostimulant
Increases oxygen uptake by red blood cells
Intestinal mucosa modulator
Melanocyte stimulant
Modulates thyroid hormone levels in the blood
Neural protector/ stimulant
P-glycoprotein inhibitor
Reduces blood glucose levels
Reduces erythrocyte fragility
Stimulates production and release of pancreatic enzymes, bile acids, and gastric acids
Stimulates the pituitary/adrenal axis
Synergist
Testosterone antagonist
Vasodilator

Finding Black Pepper and Piperine

Both black pepper and piperine are widely available. BioPerine by Source Naturals is a pretty good piperine product.

Potential future problems: Once again, the weight loss, muscle builder, and "herbal high" manufacturers are creating problems. All three are using piperine for their particular neuroses, to enhance either "fat burning" or bloodstream uptake of their particular products. This will, inevitably, be problematical down the road.

mg piperine 15 to 30 minutes prior to your herbs and then again 4 to 6 hours later, 30 minutes before taking your herbs again. Piperine will stay strongly present in the body for about 6 hours.

So . . . take piperine twice daily, 20 mg each time, in acute conditions to a max of 40 mg daily. Generally, not to exceed 7 days. If you are taking your herbs six times daily, you still only need to take piperine twice, once before the first dose, and then again 4 to 6 hours later.

Side Effects and Contraindications

Black pepper can exacerbate gastric reflux problems, but its major side effects occur on the reproductive system. In traditional medicine it is considered a mild contraceptive. The whole herb, however, is generally pretty safe along these lines unless taken in huge doses for extended periods of time. Studies on piperine, on the other hand, have found that it does interfere with egg implantation if taken long term in high doses.

However, the impacts on the male reproductive system are more severe. When taken as a supplement, continued oral intake of piperine decreases the weight of the testes, lowers sperm production, decreases intracellular testosterone, and decreases the fertilizing capacity of sperm. Constant piperine intake has deleterious effects on the Leydig cells, epididymis, and seminiferous tubes even at doses of 1 mg/kg of body weight (that is, roughly, 70–80 mg daily for an adult male).

Piperine should primarily be used for short-term treatment of acute conditions. Women who are trying to become pregnant should not use it. Men with low testosterone levels should be very cautious in its use and not use it for longer than 2 weeks.

Herb/Drug Interactions

Piperine will increase the bioavailability of scores of drugs. (It will decrease the bioavailability of a few others such as diclofenac sodium.) If you are taking pharmaceuticals, you should check for synergy (the list is too long for this book) or simply not take them together. It is highly likely that the supplement *will* increase bioavailability and thus the impacts of the pharmaceutical.

Plant Chemistry

Piper nigrum contains at least 200 identified constituents with more being discovered all the time. The most important is considered to be the alkaloid piperine, which is present at levels of up to 9 percent of the dried peppercorns in black pepper. It is the primary substance responsible for the peppery taste of the spice.

Other major compounds are chavicine, coumaperine, piperidine, numerous piperidine amides, piperettine, piperanine, piperolein A, B, and C, piperonal, and so on.

Traditional Uses of Black Pepper

Piper nigrum is native to southern India, where it is extensively cultivated. The plant is a flowering vine that produces grape-like clusters of dark red berries, at the center of which is a large white seed. The seed, as is sometimes the case, comprises most of the berry; the pulp surrounding it is fairly thin, with the usual thinnish outer rind of the fruit covering that. Basically, it is not a very exciting berry.

The black peppercorns that we use for a spice, however, are produced from the green, unripe berries. The berries are harvested and briefly immersed in hot water, thus slightly cooking them. This ruptures the cell walls in the berry and activates a number of enzymes that will cause the outer pulp and rind that surround the white seed to blacken during drying. The fruits are then spread in the sun to dry for several days. The outer pulp and rind wrinkle and turn black. Once dried the fruits are usually sold whole to preserve the strength of the corns, then ground into the powder that we call black pepper just before use.

White pepper is simply the pepper seeds themselves absent the pulp and rind. In this case the ripe berries are soaked in water for a week until the outer rind and pulp soften and slough off the inner seed. The seed is then dried, sold, and ground into a fine powder.

Black pepper has been used in India for at least 4,000 years as both spice and medicine. It is probably the most common spice in the world after salt.

AYURVEDA

Black pepper has a primary place in Ayurveda, often combined with long pepper (*Piper longum*) and ginger to form a compound called *trikatu* or the three acrids. This combination has been a primary element of Ayurvedic compounding since at least 600 BCE; most Ayurvedic formulations contain it.

Trikatu is considered specific for correcting imbalances in the three *doshas*, psychospiritual aspects of the human body that when out of balance lead to disease expressing itself physically. This formulation is (as are the three herbs individually) considered specific for "activating" the potency of the plants with which it is combined. This has been its main use for millennia.

As a single herb, black pepper (and long pepper) has been used for a variety of conditions (constipation, diarrhea, earache, gangrene, heart disease, hernia, hoarseness, indigestion, insect bites, insomnia, joint pain, liver problems, lung disease, oral abscesses, sunburn, tooth decay, and toothaches), but its main uses have been, internally, for disease conditions accompanied by fever and/or diarrhea, dysentery, GI tract disorders, and urinary problems, and externally for rheumatism and neuralgia.

TRADITIONAL CHINESE MEDICINE

Black pepper was incorporated into the Chinese materia medica during the Middle Ages. It is considered specific for warming the middle, dispersing cold, dispelling phlegm, for wind-cold, and for diarrhea, usually for conditions accompanied by vomiting, diarrhea, and abdominal pain. It is also considered specific for epilepsy. The synergistic actions of the plant are apparently unknown in this system.

Scientific Research

I am splitting this section into two parts: 1) nonsynergist actions and 2) synergist actions. Most of the studies have been on the isolated constituent piperine. (There are several hundred studies on piperine; this is just a sampling; most of the studies have been in these areas.)

NONSYNERGIST ACTIVITY OF BLACK PEPPER AND PIPERINE

Black pepper does have some antibacterial activity itself. In vitro studies of a number of its constituents (not piperine) found them active against *Bacillus subtilis*, *Bacillus sphaericus*, *Staphylococcus aureus*, *Klebsiella aerogenes*, and *Chromobacterium violaceum*. The essential oil of black pepper is effective against *Bacillus subtilis*, *Pseudomonas aeruginosa*, *Candida albicans, Trichoderma* spp., and *Aspergillus niger.* An aqueous solution of black pepper was tested against 12 genera of oral bacteria isolated from 200 individuals and was found to be effective against 75 percent of them (unfortunately the abstract does not list the bacteria; the full paper is regrettably elusive). Piperine itself is active against *Leishmania* spp. and *Trypanosoma cruzi.*

Here is a look at some of the studies.

In vitro: Black pepper is a strong antioxidant, more potent than alpha-tocopherol when used at similar concentrations. One of pepper's constituents is as potent as the synthetic antioxidants BHA and BHT.

In vitro: Black pepper inhibits cholesterol esterification in HepG2 cells; it potently inhibits binding between slCAM-1 and LFA-1 of THP-1 cells, dose dependently.

In vivo, guinea pig and rabbits: Crude extracts of black pepper, at low doses, have a mild laxative effect in constipation. However, in larger doses they are antispasmodic, reducing contractions in the intestine, and are antisecretory and antidiarrheal. Piperine, at lower doses than the pepper extract, acts identically.

In vivo, diarrhea, mice: Piperine inhibits castor oil and arachidonic acid–induced diarrhea.

In vivo, inflammation, mice: 1) Piperine reduces inflammation in both chronic and acute models; 2) inhibits monosodium urate crystal–induced inflammation (specific for gouty arthritis); 3) significantly reduces inflammation around joints in arthritic mice studies. It produces anti-inflammatory, antinociceptive, and antiarthritic actions. It inhibits expression of IL6 and MMP13 and production of PGE2.

In vivo, cancer, animal models: Numerous studies have found that piperine protects animals from induced cancer, reduces tumor incidence in others, and increases life span in terminal cases.

In vivo, neuroprotection, mice/rats: 1) Piperine significantly improves memory and protects the hippocampus from neurodegeneration; 2) blocks convulsions induced by intracerebroventricular injection of kainate; 3) inhibits synchronized oscillation of intracellular calcium in rat hippocampal networks, represses spontaneous synaptic activities, and protects hippocampal neurons from apoptosis.

Human clinical trial, epilepsy in children: Clinical trials (randomized, crossover, placebo-controlled, double-blind) with a piperine derivative in China in the treatment of epilepsy found that it reduced the number of seizures in a majority of the children who used it.

Human clinical trial, dysphagia in elderly: Inhalation of black pepper essential oil by elderly persons suffering from difficulty or inability to swallow (dysphagia) showed remarkable effects in restoring swallowing ability.

SYNERGISTIC ACTIVITY OF BLACK PEPPER AND PIPERINE

The synergistic actions of black pepper and piperine are primarily generated by three things: 1) the circulatory actions of the plant or its isolated constituent; 2) their effects on P-gp and CYP3A4; 3) their impacts on efflux pumps in bacteria.

Pepper and piperine expand blood vessel diameter and increase circulation. Piperine is strongly present in the blood (it binds to albumin for transport) and easily crosses internal organism barriers (organs and systems both: blood-brain barrier and so on). It reaches every part of the body.

Piperine and pepper have specific effects on blood constituents. In my opinion the actions of the plant and its constituent on red blood cells (reducing their fragility and increasing their oxygen uptake) play an important part in their synergistic actions. Pepper and piperine also seem to have specific actions on white blood cells. They do have some immune-stimulating actions, but more importantly they seem to be highly protective of white blood cells, being active against leishmanial and tryposomal parasites of the macrophages. They seem to produce the same effects on white blood cells as they do on red, that is, reducing their fragility and enhancing their normal actions. Although no one has tested for this, it seems as if piperine may play a particular role as a hematoprotector and hematoregenerator not only of red blood cells but also white, though differently than the other plants I have discussed so far.

A smaller role in the plant's synergism is played by the general medicinal actions of the plant—that is, it is to some extent antibacterial, which will give additive effects (at the least) to the antibacterial actions of the other herbs used with it; it is analgesic, helping with pain; it is anti-inflammatory; if you are treating inflammatory infections, its specific actions there will help immensely; and if you are treating CNS problems, it will, in addition to helping other herbs get to the affected area, add its own neuroprotective actions to the mix.

Black pepper and piperine also possess a number of efflux inhibition actions. Piperine inhibits the NorA efflux pump in *Staphylococcus aureus*. It also inhibits ethidium bromide efflux. Ethidium bromide is a substrate for all the efflux pumps in *Staphylococcus aureus* (except NorC). Ethidium bromide is also a substrate in a number of efflux pumps in some Gram-negative bacteria—those that possess the SMR efflux pumps, and in *Mycobacterium* spp. Specifically, piperine has been found to be an inhibitor of the RV1258c efflux pump in *Mycobacterium tuberculosis*.

But perhaps the major strength of the plant and its constituent piperine is the effects they have on permeability glycoprotein (P-glycoprotein or P-gp) and CYP3A4. Black pepper and piperine are potent inhibitors of both.

P-GP AND CYP3A4

All living organisms have to deal with one primary survival reality: determining what is me and not me and then identifying whether or not the "not-me" is going to be harmful to the "me." There are a great many mechanisms that all organisms have to do this, and they have a lot of options available for dealing with unsafe substances that "not-mes" can generate. Basically, they control access to their cells. In general, they all have four mechanisms for this: 1) assisted exclusion; 2) metabolic conversion;

3) solubilizer attachment; 4) reduction in assisted absorption.

In practical terms, this means: When a substance is taken into the body and touches the GI tract membrane, an immediate identification process occurs. What is this thing? And is it safe? If the intestinal wall identifies it as harmful, then it can:

Exclude it; that is, use what is called an efflux pump or an efflux transporter to move the thing out, making sure it does not affect the cell/organism.

Metabolize it; that is, chemically turn it into something else that is not harmful, which is then either used or excreted from the cell/organism. The chemical substances that are thus created are called metabolites.

Attach it; that is, link the substance chemically to a highly water-soluble substance, often glucuronic acid. This creates a new compound that is unable to diffuse through cell membranes. It is then excreted in either urine or feces.

Reduce assisted absorption; that is, inhibit influx transporters. Assisted absorption involves the use of transporter proteins, a.k.a. influx transporters, in the lining of the intestinal wall. These proteins transfer useful substances into the cells of the intestinal wall and from there they are transported to the blood. Influx transporters are strongly active in moving such things as amino acids across the intestinal membrane. One of the most potent is gamma-glutamyltransferase (GGT). It is present in the cell membranes of the intestines, kidneys, bile duct, liver, spleen, heart, brain, and seminal vesicles.

All these responses make it harder for substances to get into the body and affect it. Many pharmaceuticals are considered to be foreign substances and, when these actions take place, up to 85 percent of a pharmaceutical may be inactivated, which is part of the reason doses are so high with some drugs.

Piperine affects all four of those mechanisms that control access to cells. It has particularly strong effects on efflux pumping, metabolization, glucuronic acid attachment, and GGT.

There are a number of efflux transporters. P-gp, or permeability glycoprotein, is one of the more prominent. P-gp is found mainly in the intestinal wall, kidneys, liver, brain, testes, adrenal gland, and uterus. It is also common in cancer cells and a few bacteria. You can visualize P-gp as a barrier lining the intestinal wall and choosing which substances to let into the body and, if so, how much (it also does this at the blood-brain barrier). Piperine significantly reduces the ability of P-gp to block incoming substances. As a result, if you take piperine or black pepper (or the traditional Ayurvedic blend trikatu), more of the medicinal will pass through the intestinal wall and into the bloodstream. Sometimes, the amount getting into the blood is substantially higher, up to 32 times its levels without piperine. This is why particular care needs to be taken if you are using piperine and are also taking pharmaceuticals. It is also why you should never take piperine with severe infections of the intestinal wall such as *E. coli* and cholera. Piperine would allow the bacteria to more easily infiltrate the intestinal wall and get deeper into your system.

CYP3A4 is one of the more important metabolizers in the human body. It affects the broadest range of substances (or substrates as they are called) of any of the CYP family of enzymes, affecting thousands if not hundreds of thousands of substances. It is a main metabolizer in the intestinal wall and liver. Generally, it does one of two things: converts a substance to another that has lower biological activity or makes substances more water soluble, which reduces their ability to move into cells. Inhibition of CYP3A4 means that the substance is left in its original, highly bioactive form when it gets into the body. Piperine strongly inhibits CYP3A4. (It has also been found to inhibit CYP1A2, CYP1A1, and CYP2D6.)

Piperine/black pepper also inhibits AHH or aryl hydrocarbon hydroxylase, which metabolizes aromatic hydrocarbons. (This makes piperine useful for enhancing the impact of herbs like juniper berry, which is high in aromatic hydrocarbons, in the treatment of UTI.)

Piperine/black pepper also strongly inhibits UDP-glucuronyltransferase (a.k.a. UGT). UGT is the enzyme that attaches glucuronic acid to xenobiotics to facilitate their removal from the body. This action by piperine increases the time that foreign substances, e.g., herbs or pharmaceuticals, remain in the body/bloodstream prior to elimination, from 2 to 4 hours longer.

Piperine/black pepper also significantly stimulates the activity of the influx transporter GGT, increasing the movement of substances across the intestinal membrane.

Piperine, and black pepper, thus increase the amount of any substance going into the body, keep it in its most potent form (unmetabolized), and keep it in the body longer. Piperine/black pepper also, for similar reasons, facilitates the movement of substances into the brain and CNS, uterus, testes, adrenals, kidneys, and liver. If any of those systems are being treated for disease, for example, bacterial meningitis or hepatitis C, piperine will increase the amount of herb getting to the meninges or the liver.

At the same time piperine/black pepper stimulates circulation and increases blood vessel size so that the substances are widely circulated throughout the body very rapidly.

A number of studies have looked at the actions of black pepper and piperine along these lines. Most studies have occurred with piperine. However, there has been some work with trikatu, the traditional Ayurvedic blend of the two peppers and gingerroot.

In vivo, goats, pharmaceuticals: If trikatu was preadministered to mountain goats before their treatment with pefloxacin (a fluoroquinolone antibiotic used in India in veterinary practice), the drug levels in the body and its penetration into various parts of the body were substantially increased. Other studies have found that trikatu increases the bioavailability of vasicine and indomethacin.

Human clinical study, pharmaceuticals: Trikatu increased the concentrations of vasicine by over 200 percent and sparteine by over 100 percent in the blood plasma of human volunteers.

In vivo, mice/rats, pharmaceuticals: Piperine increased the effects of pentobarbital-induced hypnosis in mice. Blood and brain pentobarbital levels were higher in treated animals; piperine also prolonged hexobarbital sleeping time and zoxazolamine paralysis; enhanced the bioavailability of aflatoxin B1; enhanced the bioavailability of etoposide; increased the bioavailability of nimesulide, thus allowing the use of reduced, and safer, doses; and delayed elimination of phenytoin.

In vivo, mice/rats, herbs: Piperine increases the movement of radio-labeled L-leucine, L-isoleucine, and L-valine across the intestinal wall, enhancing uptake; increases the uptake of curcumin and its presence in serum; and increases plasma levels of epigallocatechin gallate from green tea.

Human clinical study/trial, pharmaceuticals: A single oral dose of propranolol (40 mg) or theophylline (150 mg) alone or in combination with piperine (20 mg) was given each day for 7 days. Increased oral bioavailability was found in the piperine group. A single dose of piperine (20 mg) administered with phenytoin significantly increased the mean plasma concentration of phenytoin; a crossover, placebo-controlled study found that piperine increased the bioavailability of nevirapine, increased its mean plasma concentrations, and reduced its elimination from the body; another study found it increased the bioavailability of vasicine and sparteine.

Human clinical trial/study, herbs: A crossover study with volunteers given 2 grams curcumin found that its serum levels were either undetectable or very low. When piperine was administered with the curcumin, serum levels were 2,000 percent higher. Piperine enhanced bioavailability, serum concentration, and extent of absorption; a double-blind study found that piperine (5 mg) increased plasma concentrations of CoQ10 by 30 percent.

7

THE FIRST LINE OF DEFENSE: STRENGTHENING THE IMMUNE SYSTEM

The man is not sick because he has an illness; he has an illness because he is sick.

—Chinese proverb

It is the body which ultimately controls infections, not chemicals. Without underlying immunity, drugs are meaningless.

—Marc Lappé

No matter the virulence of a disease, and this includes fierce diseases such as Ebola, some people remain healthy in spite of being exposed. In fact, medical studies have consistently shown the presence of virulent bacteria in most peoples' systems though they never become ill.

Countless studies have found that the healthier your immune system, the less likely you are to get a disease and the more likely you are, if you do get sick, to have a milder episode. This is especially true in diseases such as Lyme. Researchers have consistently noted that the higher certain immune markers are, the less likely that infection will occur and, if it does, the disease will be less severe than if the immune markers are low.

Our immune system is in fact our first line of defense. Its job is to protect us from disease and, if disease occurs, to cure it. A healthy immune system is therefore the first and most important part of health and healing.

The Basic Elements of the Immune System

Some of the specific elements of our immune system are the thymus, spleen, liver, lymph system, lymph nodes, tonsils, appendix (basically a large lymph node), and bone marrow. The thymus coordinates immune activity, the spleen processes worn-out red blood cells and platelets and provides a location to engulf and destroy invaders. The liver cleans toxins from the blood and produces most of the body's lymph. Lymph is the liquid that flows in the lymph system, somewhat similar to a city's sewer system. The lymph system runs parallel to the blood vessels and stores, filters, and circulates waste, especially dead bacteria and the massive numbers of white blood cells produced during active infections. Lymph nodes are large intersections of lymph channels and store or warehouse the waste products being processed through the lymph system. When the lymph nodes are processing a lot of waste, they tend to swell, clog up, and become painful to the touch. When they do, the processing of waste slows down. Keeping the nodes clear helps the body process infections much more quickly. The lymph nodes also produce unique white blood cells called lymphocytes (as does the thymus gland) that are particularly strong elements of the immune system.

The bone marrow, and to some extent the thymus, manufactures other types of white blood cells that fight infections. Two of the most important are phagocytes and neutrophils. Phagocytes exist in three forms (monocytes, macrophages, and granulocytes). As macrophages, they rove the body looking for foreign bodies and help clean up residues of white blood cells and bacteria during and after infections. They also alert the neutrophils, which attack and destroy bacteria and viruses, of the presence of disease organisms.

All these various parts of the immune complex can be supported and kept healthy. A strong immune system means that infections are less frequent and healing is quicker.

Foods for the Immune System

There are things you can do to keep the immune system healthy. Regular touching is one of them, such as receiving Swedish massage on a weekly or monthly basis. Certain foods do help immune health as well. Some of the best foods that support immune health are:

- **Yogurt.** Regular intake does result in fewer sick days. The body's white blood cell count increases substantially, and the GI tract bacterial community remains very healthy, which also helps. Kefir can also be used.
- **Oats and barley.** Farm animals given a mix of the two have many fewer infections, including those from influenza. (And yes, in spite of rumors to the contrary, we actually are animals, too.)
- **Garlic.** Although not as strong an antibiotic as I had formerly thought, regular garlic intake does boost immune function—in one study, those taking garlic were much less likely to catch colds and flu.
- **Selenium-rich foods** have been found to help clear influenza infections from the body. Selenium is found highest (in descending order) in Brazil nuts, fish (tuna, cod, halibut, sardines, flounder, salmon), poultry (chicken and turkey), sunflower seeds, shellfish (oysters, mussels, shrimp, clams, scallops), meat (liver, beef, lamb, pork), eggs, mushrooms, whole grains, wheat germ, onions, garlic, asparagus, broccoli, tomatoes. One ounce of Brazil nuts (usually just called "nuts" in Brazil) will supply 544 mcg of selenium—you don't need many; one Brazil nut can supply a whole day's supply of selenium. To give a comparison, tuna fish contains 68 mcg per

ounce; cod, 32 mcg per ounce; turkey, 27 mcg; sunflower seeds, 23; oysters, 22; and so on.

- **Chicken soup**. Yes, it does work.
- **Black tea.** It significantly increases the immune system's interferon levels. Green tea will also be of benefit.
- **Zinc-containing foods.** Zinc is an essential mineral, especially in immune function. It enhances the actions of many of the immune system's actors, including T cells. Zinc is highest in oysters, wheat germ, liver, seeds (highest in sesame, tahini, pumpkin, squash, and watermelon seeds), roast beef, dark chocolate and cocoa, lamb, peanuts, garlic, chickpeas. To give you an idea of levels: Oysters concentrate zinc (and copper as well). One medium oyster contains about 13 mg of zinc, 3 ounces of wheat germ contains 17 mg, calf liver has about 12 mg per 3 ounces, sesame seeds contain about 8 mg per 3 ounces, and so on.
- **Mushrooms.** But not the usual store-bought variety. Shiitake and maitake can both be used in cooking, and they are both very good for raising immune function, primarily due to their high levels of polysaccharides. Their polysaccharides raise immune function considerably when taken as a regular part of the diet.
- **And of course:** ginger in the diet, broccoli and other members of that family (all have some of the same properties as isatis), red bell peppers (which are, gram for gram, higher in vitamin C than anything else on the planet), and oregano.

And then there are the herbs.

Herbs for the Immune System

A number of herbs stand out when it comes to strengthening, rehabilitating, or enhancing the immune system. All of them can be used long term; few have any side effects. Though some of these herbs are active against specific disease organisms, their strength lies in enhancing various aspects of the immune system, offering protective activity against toxins or disease for specific organs in the body, antitumor activity, and/or tonic and restorative activity for general debility in the body or immune system. Many of these plant medicines are also considered to be antistressors and adaptogens. They protect the body from the effects of stress and stimulate the body, and especially the immune system, to more effectively deal with adverse events—internal or external.

Nine Herbs for the Immune System

Ashwagandha
Astragalus
Boneset
Cordyceps
Echinacea
Eleuthero
Red root
Reishi
Rhodiola

Ashwagandha

Family: Solanaceae

Common Names: *Ashwagandha • Indian ginseng • winter cherry*

Species Used: After intense fisticuffs it was decided that there are six species in this genus. *Withania somnifera* is the species most commonly known as an immune herb. However, two other *Withania* species, *Withania obtusifolia* and *W. coagulans*, are used in much the same manner. *W. obtusifolia* has a long history of use in the Sudan while *W. coagulans* (especially the fruit) has long been used in Pakistan and India. *W. coagulans* is so termed because it is a powerful coagulating agent and is used in place of rennet by Indians to make cheese. (*Obtusifolia* is so named because its leaves are obtuse, that is, "lacking in insight or discernment," and is used in place of aware perception by taxonomists.)

Parts Used

The root is almost exclusively used in Western practice (a few people are starting to use the berry), the whole plant in the rest of the world.

Preparation and Dosage

TINCTURE

Dry root: 1:5, 70 percent alcohol, 30–40 drops up to 3x daily.

Fresh leaf: 1:2, 95 percent alcohol, 10–30 drops up to 3x daily.

Dry seed: 1:5, 65 percent alcohol, 15–30 drops up to 3x daily.

Fresh fruit: 1:2 (grind the whole mess well), 95 percent alcohol, 15–30 drops up to 3x daily.

CAPSULES

Take 500–1,000 mg daily, though in Ayurvedic practice 3–6 grams are used daily.

Some people, sigh, are standardizing the root capsules to 1.5 percent withanolides. Others are producing both 1:4 and 1:2 tinctures. All may be stronger than the whole, not-altered root and root tinctures . . . but maybe not.

Side Effects and Contraindications

Avoid high doses in pregnancy, as it may be abortifacient in large doses. May cause drowsiness. Take the herb after dinner to find out just how sleepy it makes you before using it during the day. In rare instances: diarrhea, GI tract upset, vomiting at large doses.

Herb/Drug Interactions

May potentiate barbiturates (anecdotal); don't use with sedatives and anxiolytics.

Habitat and Appearance

Ashwagandha is native to the dry regions of India and is now fairly prolific throughout northern Africa and the Mediterranean, essentially your warm, semi-arid climates that get some good rain during the rainy season. It's a small, perennial, bushy, woody shrub to about 2 feet tall, though with a lot of care, water, and fertilizer it can grow to 6 feet. The plant produces orange-red fruits looking much like cherries

Properties of Ashwagandha

Actions

Root
Alterative
Amphoteric
Antibacterial
Antifatigue
Anti-inflammatory
Antioxidant
Antipyretic
Antistressor
Antitumor
Anxiolytic
Astringent
Chondroprotective
Collagenase inhibitor
Diuretic
Hematopoietic
Immune tonic
Immunomodulant
Insomnia reliever (especially stress- or disease-induced)
Nervine
Neuroprotective

Leaf and stem
Antibacterial
Antimicrobial
Antipyretic
Antitumor
Astringent
Bitter
Diuretic
Febrifuge
Nervine

Seed
Coagulant
Diuretic
Hypnotic

Fruit
Alterative
Antibacterial
Astringent
Immune tonic

Finding Ashwagandha

Herb stores everywhere, the Internet. Excellent seed stock can be purchased from Horizon Herbs. The plant is very easy to grow.

(hence that common name) that are enclosed in a papery husk. Ashwagandha is similar in appearance to both ground cherry and Chinese lantern. The roots are long, tuberous, and brown.

Cultivation and Collection

The plant is little grown (or known) in the United States but is a rather common agricultural plant in its region. It does well in warm, semiarid to arid climates as long as it gets some water now and then. Perfect for parts of Arizona and Southern California—good in zones 8 and warmer. It is a hardy evergreen perennial to temperatures to just above freezing (and can survive occasional drops to as low as 15°F) but does well as an annual pretty much anyplace it is warm enough. It needs at least a 200-day growing season to reach maturity but will produce a decent root system in 100 days if that's all you've got.

Ashwagandha is propagated by seed and it grows easily. Sow in early spring indoors. Germination is in about 15 days. Plants really like full sun and fast-draining soil with some limestone in it (alkaline soil lover). The plants are intolerant of wet soils. Harvest the roots just after the cherries become ripe. Dry the cherries for use the next year as new seed stock. Cut the roots into smallish pieces, and dry out of the sun. Store in plastic bags when well dried, in plastic tubs in a cool, dark location. The leaves can be harvested at any time.

Plant Chemistry

The major constituents are steroidal alkaloids and steroidal lactones: withanine, somniferine, somnine, somniferinine, withaninine, pseudo-withanine, tropine, pseudo-tropine, ashwagandhanolide, cuscohygrine, anferine, anhydryine, sitoindoside 7 and 8, a lot of other stuff, and a bunch of steroidal lactones in the leaves called withanolides. Withaferin A in the leaves has tremendous antitumor activity.

Traditional Uses of Ashwagandha

The primary traditional uses of the herb have all been in the Ayurveda system in India.

AYURVEDA

A major plant in India for at least 3,000 years, ashwagandha is considered to be tonic, alterative, astringent, aphrodisiac, and a nervine sedative. It has been used for TB, emaciation in children, senile debility, rheumatism, general debility, nervous exhaustion, brain fog, loss of memory, loss of muscular energy, and spermatorrhea. Its primary use is to restore vigor and energy in a body worn out by long-term constitutional disease or old age.

TRADITIONAL CHINESE MEDICINE

Unknown as far as I can determine.

WESTERN BOTANIC PRACTICE

A recent plant to the West, almost an herb-of-the-day.

Scientific Research

There have been an increasing number of studies on ashwagandha since 2000; there are about 400 of them on PubMed as of 2011. Here's a sampling:

Clinical trial, antistressor activity: 100 men and women in a double-blind, placebo-controlled, randomized trial. The herb significantly reduced stress in all who took the herb.

Clinical trial, hemoglobin effects: A double-blind study with 60 healthy children age 8 to 12 years. There was a marked increase in level of hemoglobin at the end of 30 days and in packed cell volume, mean corpuscular volume, serum iron, and hand grip at the end of 60 days.

Clinical trial, hemoglobin effects: A double-blind study with 101 healthy men age 50 to 59 years. Each took 3 grams per day of ashwagandha for 1 year. All showed significantly increased hemoglobin and RBC count, improvement in melanin, and decreased SED rate, and three-quarters of them reported increased sexual performance.

In vitro, antibacterial action: Ashwagandha does have some antibacterial actions; whole-plant extracts have been found active against *Staphylococcus aureus, Pseudomonas aeruginosa, Salmonella* spp., *E. coli,* and *Bacillus subtilis.*

In vitro/in vivo, rats/mice, antineoplastic activity: There have been over 50 studies on the antineoplastic actions of the plant, primarily using the leaves. Tumor growth is retarded, tumor cell proliferation is reduced, side effects of radiation and chemotherapy are reduced, and life expectancy is increased.

In vivo, mice, pain relief: Withaferin A, a constituent of ashwagandha, has been shown to be analgesic and antipyretic.

In vitro studies, cartilage effects: Found the root extract to be highly chondroprotective of damaged human osteoarthritis cartilage matrix. It also was significantly inhibitive of the gelatinase activity of collagenase type 2 enzyme.

In vivo, rats, central nervous system effects: Showed the herb to have anxiolytic and antidepressant actions. Strong antioxidant.

In vivo, mice, central nervous

system effects: Showed the herb to correct scopolamine-induced memory loss in mice.

In vitro, central nervous system effects: Root extracts induce neurite extension and outgrowth in human neuroblastoma SH-SY5Y. Stimulate neuritic regeneration and synaptic reconstruction in damaged cortical neurons. Completely inhibit dendritic atrophy.

In vivo, rats, central nervous system effects: Treatment for 14 days significantly improved nitropropionic-acid-induced cognitive dysfunction and oxidative damage in rats. (Note: There have been at least 30 studies finding cognitive improvements in various animal species from the use of the root.)

In vivo, rats, anti-inflammatory: Strongly anti-inflammatory in various rheumatological conditions.

In vivo, dogs, cardiac effects: Hypotensive, bradycardic, respiratory stimulant actions.

In vivo, mice, white blood cells: Ashwagandha significantly reduced induced leukopenia in mice. White blood cell count significantly increased.

In vivo, mice, thyroid enhancement: Significantly increased thyroid production of T3 and T4.

Astragalus

Family: Leguminosae

Common Names: *Astragalus (English) • huang-qi (Chinese)*

Species Used: This is a huge genus of some 3,000 species, prevalent throughout the world. The primary species used is *Astragalus membranaceus*, a.k.a. *A. membranaceus* var. *mongholicus*, a.k.a. *A. mongholicus*. Sigh . . . now that the number of species in this genus has been, almost, settled, the number of variants is in question. (*Yes*, this one is *Astragalus membranaceus,* but it looks funny. I found it in Mongolia; therefore . . .)

There is not much information on whether any of the other species in the genus can be used similarly.

Note: *Astragalus propinquus* is, in some circles, a synonym for *A. membranaceus*. However, a number of sources now insist (cue shocked expression) that *this* is the correct name for the plant. And of course, *Astragalus mongholicus* is just a rose by any other name.

Parts Used

The plant is a perennial with a long fibrous rootstock. The root, which is the part used for medicine, is often found thinly sliced and dried (a traditional preparation in Chinese medicine) and most closely resembles a yellow (medical) tongue depressor. Bulk quantities of the powdered or coarsely ground organic root are commonly available through herbal suppliers to Western botanic practitioners.

Properties of Astragalus

Actions

- Adaptogen
- Antibacterial
- Antihepatotoxic
- Antiviral
- Cardioprotective
- Diuretic
- Enhances function in lungs, spleen, and GI tract
- Hypotensive
- Immune enhancer
- Immune modulator
- Immune restorative
- Immune stimulant
- Tonic

Astragalus is an immune potentiator and modulator. It strongly regulates interferon-gamma and interleukin-2 levels. If interferon-gamma levels are high, it is strongly active in lowering them. Enhances CD4+ counts and balances the CD4:CD8 ratio. Astragalus is specific for immune atrophy and enhances function in the spleen and thymus.

Active Against

While not specifically an antimicrobial herb, astragalus does possess some antimicrobial actions. Most important for this book, it does have antiviral activity. It is active against influenza A (H1N1, FM1), human

Preparation and Dosage

Many astragalus formulations are standardized, though I'm not sure that the literature really supports standardization with this herb.

The root is usually standardized for either 0.4 percent or 0.5 percent 4′-hydroxy-3′-methoxyisoflavone 7-sug, but the reasons are not entirely clear for doing so. No literature exists that I can find that lays out why in fact this particular constituent was singled out and not the

adenovirus type 3, herpes simplex 1, Coxsackie virus B3, infectious bursal disease virus, cytomegalovirus, Punta Toro virus, Japanese encephalitis virus, porcine parvovirus, hepatitis B and significantly reduces the effects of canine distemper virus in vivo. The herb is strongly protective against infection with Japanese encephalitis virus and bunyavirus if taken prophylactically. Most of its actions come from antivirus stimulation of the immune system.

The herb does have some other antimicrobial effects. It is active against *E. coli*, *Arbiter aerogenes*, *Proteus vulgaris*, *Staphylococcus aureus*, *Salmonella enteritidis*, *Shigella dysenteriae*, *Campylobacter*, *Streptococcus hemolyticus*, *Diplococcus pneumoniae* (a.k.a. *Streptococcus pneumoniae*), *Aeromonas hydrophila*, and *Candida albicans*.

Use to Treat

All viral infections as an immune adjuvant. Many people are beginning to view the herb as a primary immunomodulator to prevent viral infection and illness. It is specific for that purpose.

It is also specific for treating myocarditis from Coxsackie B3 infection. It is specific for reducing the impacts of Japanese encephalitis virus. It is specific as a preventive for reducing the likelihood of infection from Lyme bacteria and reducing the severity of the disease.

Finding Astragalus

Herb stores everywhere and the Internet.

astragalosides. (Astragaloside IV, for instance, is one of the primary active ingredients of the plant in heart disease. It increases exercise tolerance and reduces chest distress and dyspnea and optimizes left ventricular function.) The methoxyisoflavone constituent for which the plant is standardized is an anabolic-type compound that enhances strength and muscle formation and may have some protective actions in upper respiratory infections and on digestive function. Data on its functions are somewhat unclear and hard to come by; I have been unable to locate any clinical or laboratory studies on the constituent—though they must exist somewhere. Their rarity stimulates speculation.

The whole root contains constituents that are essential for carditis and enhanced immune function. And, indeed, the majority of the Chinese studies—clinical and laboratory—were with the whole herb.

The herb may be taken as tea, powder, capsules, or tincture or in food.

TEA

Use 2–3 ounces of herb per pot of tea; drink throughout the day.

TINCTURE

1:5, 60 percent alcohol, 30–60 drops up to 4x daily

POWDER

In chronic conditions: Take up to 3 tbl per day.
In acute conditions: Take up to 6 tbl per day.

FOOD

Astragalus has been used for centuries as an additive to meal preparation. The sliced root is placed in soups and removed before eating, or a strong infusion of the root is made and used to cook rice and as a stock for soups.

Side Effects and Contraindications

No toxicity has ever been shown from the regular, daily use of the herb nor from the use of large doses. The Chinese report consistent use for millennia in the treatment of colds and flu and suppressed immune function without side effects.

Astragalus is contraindicated, however, in late-stage Lyme disease because it can exacerbate autoimmune responses in that particular disease.

Herb/Drug Interactions

Synergistic actions: Use of the herb with interferon and acyclovir may increase their effects. The herb has been used in clinical trials with interferon in the treatment of hepatitis B; outcomes were better than with interferon alone. It has also shown synergistic effects when used with interferon in the treatment of cervical erosion; antiviral activity is enhanced.

Drug inhibition: Use of the herb with cyclophosphamide may decrease the effectiveness of the drug. Not for use in people with transplanted organs.

Herb/Herb Interactions

Synergistic with echinacea and licorice in the stimulation of immune function.

Habitat and Appearance

Of the more than 3,000 species of astragalus in the world, 16 grow in the United States. The leaf structure looks like a typical member of the pea family. It is a short-lived, sprawling perennial and grows up to 4 feet in size.

The medicinal astragalus is native to northeast China, though it has been planted a great many other places, including the United

States. Wild populations are still rare in the West, though it is under wide cultivation as a medicinal in the United States and escape to the wild is imminent.

Cultivation and Collection

Astragalus is started from seeds in the early spring indoors. The seed coat needs to be scored with something like sandpaper prior to planting. Growers (e.g., Elixir Farm in Missouri) have found that it prefers a sunny location with, as the Elixir Farm website notes, "deep, sandy, well-drained, somewhat alkaline soil. It does not like mulch or deep cultivation. The crowns of the emerging plants are very sensitive to compost and respond well after they have gained some momentum in the spring." Not surprisingly, given the plant's medicinal actions, it is highly resistant to insect damage, crown rot, mildew, and drought.

The plant grows larger and more woody each year, with the roots harvested beginning the fall of the third year or spring of the fourth. Spring and fall harvests occur in China.

Plant Chemistry

Astragalosides 1-7, astraisoflavan, astramembranagenin, astrapterocarpan, beta-sitosterol, betaine, formononetin, GABA, isoastragaloside 1, 2, and 4, isoliquiritigenin, linoleic acid, linolenic acid, soyasaponin I, kumatakenin, choline, glucuronic acid, 4′-hydroxy-3′-methoxyisoflavone 7-sug, a couple of dihydroxy-7, 4-dimethylisoflavones, 3′-hydroxyformonontin, calcium, folic acid, choline, copper, iron, magnesium, manganese, potassium, sodium, zinc.

Traditional Uses of Astragalus

Astragalus, first mentioned in the 2,000-year-old Chinese text *Shen Nong Cao Jing*, is one of the 50 fundamental herbs in Chinese medicine and is considered to be one of the superior tonic herbs. The plant has developed into one of the primary immune herbs used worldwide over the past four decades.

AYURVEDA

Five species of astragalus are used in the materia medica of India, none of them this species. They are minor herbs, used primarily as emollients.

TRADITIONAL CHINESE MEDICINE

Astragalus has been a major herb in Chinese medicine for between 2,000 and 4,000 years. Its traditional uses are for spleen deficiency with lack of appetite, fatigue, and diarrhea. It is specific for disease conditions accompanied by weakness and sweating, stabilizes and protects the vital energy (qi), and is used for wasting diseases, numbness of the limbs, and paralysis. Other uses are: for tonifying the lungs, for shortness of breath, for frequent colds and flus; as a diuretic and for reduction of edema; for tonifying the blood and for blood loss, especially postpartum; for diabetes; for promoting the discharge of pus, for chronic ulcerations, including of the stomach, and sores that have not drained or healed well.

WESTERN BOTANIC PRACTICE

The herb was not used in Western botanic practice until the tremendous East/West herbal blending that began during the 1960s. It is now one of the primary immune tonic herbs in the Western pharmacopeia.

Scientific Research

A considerable amount of scientific testing has occurred with astragalus, including clinical trials and both in vivo and in vitro studies. Medline lists 799 citations for studies with astragalus, and this does not include the many Chinese studies that have never been indexed for Medline. Two U.S. patents have been granted for the use of astragalus for immunostimulation. What follows is merely a sampling.

IMMUNE FUNCTION

Most of the clinical studies and trials regarding immunostimulation have been focused on the use of astragalus in the treatment of cancer and/or as an adjunct to chemotherapy to help stimulate chemo-depressed immune function. A number of other studies have examined its immune effects with a range of different conditions.

The herb has been used with children suffering tetralogy of Fallot after a radical operation to correct the condition. Tetralogy of Fallot is a complex of four heart abnormalities that occur together, generally at birth. Surgery is used to correct it. Astragalus was found to decrease abnormal levels of IgG, Igm, C3, C4, CD8+, and CD19+ while increasing levels of CD4+ and CD56+. The ratios of CD4:CD8, CD3:HLA-DR, and CD3:CD16 normalized between the second and third week of use. IL-6 and TNF-alpha both began decreasing in the first week and by week 4 were in the normal range.

When astragalus was used in the treatment of herpes simplex keratitis, levels of Th1, including IL-2 and IFN-gamma, increased and Th2 levels, including IL-4 ad IL-10, decreased, showing that the herb modulated Th1 and Th2 levels. This same kind of effect has been found in the treatment of numerous cancers. For example, in a study of 37 lung cancer patients astragalus was found to reverse the Th2 status normally present in that condition. Th1 cytokines (IFN-gamma and IL-2) and its transcript factor (T-bet) were enhanced and Th2 cytokines were decreased.

A clinical study with 63 people suffering serious abdominal traumatic injury found that the addition of astragalus to the treatment regimen significantly increased cellular immunity.

In clinical trials with a number of different cancers and congestive heart conditions, astragalus has been found to increase CD4+ levels, reduce CD8+ levels, and significantly increase the CD4:CD8 ratio. The plant has been found to have a broad immunostimulatory effect. Use of the herb with cancer patients undergoing chemotherapy found that white blood cell counts improved significantly (normalizing). The herb has been found to be specifically useful in preventing or reversing immunosuppression from any source: age-related, bacterial, viral, or chemical. It enhances phagocytosis and increases superoxide dismutase production from macrophages.

HEART DISEASE

There have been numerous clinical trials with the herb for treating heart disease. The herb has been found specific for inhibiting Coxsackie B infections, both as an antiviral and as a heart protector. It will reverse damage to the heart in a number of conditions. With respect to Lyme carditis probably the most important are its impacts on left ventricular function, angina, and shortness of breath. While it is not completely protective for atrioventricular (AV) block, it does improve electrophysiological parameters and ameliorates AV block to some extent.

In a trial of astragalus for 2 weeks with 19 people with congestive heart failure, 15 people experienced alleviation of symptoms of chest distress and dyspnea, and their exercise tolerance increased substantially. Radionuclide ventriculography showed that left ventricular modeling and ejection function improved, and heart rate slowed from 88.21 to 54.66 beats/minute.

In another trial, 43 people suffering from myocardial infarction were tested with astragalus. Left ventricular function strengthened. Superoxide dismutase activity or red blood cell levels increased, and lipid peroxidation of plasma was reduced.

In a study with 366 cardiac patients astragalus was found to be effective when compared to lidocaine and mexiletine (which were not found effective). With astragalus the duration of ventricular late potentials shortened significantly.

In the treatment of 92 patients suffering ischemic heart disease, astragalus was more successful than nifedipine. Patients were "markedly relieved" from angina pectoris. EKG test results improved 82.6 percent.

ANTI-INFLAMMATORY ACTIVITY

Astragalus has been found to possess anti-inflammatory activity by inhibiting the NF-kB pathway and blocking the effect of interleukin-1 beta in leukotriene C production in human amnions. The constituent astragaloside IV inhibits increases in microvascular permeability induced by histamine. The whole-herb decoction has been found to reduce capillary hyperpermeability.

NEUROLOGICAL ACTIONS

Astragalus has been found to improve anisodine-induced impairment of memory acquisition and alcohol-elicited deficit of memory retrieval. After use of the herb the number of errors was reduced. The plant has been found to exert potent antioxidant effects on the brain, helping to prevent senility.

FATIGUE

Astragalus has been found effective in alleviating fatigue in heart patients and in athletes. In one trial, 12 athletes were randomly separated into two groups, and six were given astragalus. Astragalus was found to positively influence anaerobic threshold, enhance recovery from fatigue, and increase fatigue threshold.

A double-blind, randomized, controlled trial with 36 adults with chronic fatigue found that a mixture of astragalus and Salviae Radix significantly decreased fatigue scores.

HEPATITIS

A number of trials have found the herb effective in the clinical treatment of hepatitis B and liver disease. Liver function is improved, the liver is protected from damage, and regeneration is stimulated.

IMMUNE-ENHANCING BROTH

Robyn Landis and K. P. S. Khalsa share a tasty recipe for an immune-enhancing astragalus broth in their book, *Herbal Defense* (Warner Books, 1997).

Immune-Enhancing Broth

INGREDIENTS

- 3 cups water or vegetable broth
- 1 ounce astragalus (five "tongue depressor" lengths of the sliced root)
- 1 bulb (5 to 10 cloves) fresh garlic, sliced or whole
- Salt and pepper to taste

Combine the water, astragalus, and garlic and simmer for several hours, until the garlic is soft. Season with salt and pepper to taste. Consume all the broth if you feel an infection coming on, or take a cup or two several times during the week to prevent infection. Consume the garlic separately, leave in the broth, or use as a spread on toast.

Immune-Enhancing Rice

INGREDIENTS

- 1½ ounces sliced astragalus root
- 4 cups water, plus more as needed
- 2 cups (uncooked) brown rice

Add the astragalus to the water, bring to boil, and simmer, covered, for 2 hours. Remove from the heat and let stand overnight. Remove the astragalus, and add enough water to bring the broth volume back up to 4 cups. Add the rice, bring to a boil, then reduce the heat and simmer, covered, until the rice is done, approximately 1 hour. Use this rice as you would any rice, as a base for meals throughout the week.

Boneset

In addition to its antiviral properties, boneset is a potent immunostimulant. In fact, clinical trials have shown that boneset works better than echinacea for this purpose, is analgesic (at least as effective as aspirin), and reduces cold and flu symptoms. In mice it has shown strong immunostimulant activity and cytotoxic action against cancer cells. To learn more about boneset, turn to page 400.

Cordyceps

Family: Ophiocordyceps

Species used: *Cordyceps sinensis* almost always, though *C. militaris* is considered interchangeable (and by some, stronger), and many of the others in the genus are usable as well.

In total, there are 140 or 480 or 670 members of the *Cordyceps* genus or the *Ophiocordyceps* genus or the *Metacordyceps* genus, or the *Elaphocordyceps* genus, or all of them together . . . or something. (I read the whole 55-page peer-reviewed journal article—three times—but despite having opposable thumbs and a degree in advanced basket weaving, I still can't follow it. Let's see, the seraphim are the ones that hang from the top of the cave . . . ?).

All of these (prefix) cordyceps mushrooms are endoparasitoids (as distinct from elastoparanoids, i.e., taxonomists). This 10-dollar word simply means that they are parasitic on other living organisms, mostly insects, though a few parasitize other fungi (*turning* on their own kind). The fungus invades and takes over the host's body, replacing its tissues with its own. The main medicinal species that most people use, *Prefix-or-not-cordyceps sinensis,* is a parasite on caterpillars, specifically the larvae of the ghost moth (which is why it is sometimes called the caterpillar fungus). The fungal spores invade the caterpillar (which lives underground), and they sprout into active mycelia (which spread throughout the caterpillar body via the circulatory system), eventually killing the caterpillar (which then mummifies). The mycelia ultimately fill the corpse, leaving the exoskeleton intact, and the mushroom sprouts from the body (via the head) the next summer, and, hey, we got medicine. (Yum!)

Cordyceps species of one sort or another are common throughout the world. Each species is a parasite of either a different arthropod or the one particular mushroom species it likes to parasitize. The range of insect hosts is large: beetles, moth and butterfly pupae and larvae, ants, spiders, grasshoppers, locusts, cicadas, centipedes, bees, and cockroaches, and probably more that no one has found out about yet. Each species of cordyceps has somewhat different medicinal actions, no doubt coming, in part, from what kind of host species it infects (and no, no one has studied this as yet either).

This particular species of *I-guess-it's-a-cordyceps* that we are talking about, the primary one used in medicine, is specific to the Tibetan plateau and the Himalayas in India, Nepal, and Bhutan. It is generally hand-harvested by the local people and is, at this point in time, tremendously expensive (a recent estimate I was given—in 2012—was US $1,600 to $2,000 per pound; prices are increasing about 20 percent per year). Cordyceps mushrooms provide a major source of income for people in those regions. Several hundred tons are harvested each year, making up about half the yearly income of the local peoples and about 10 percent of Tibet's GDP.

To lower the cost and to make the herb more widely available, the mycelia, in China, are now grown (fermented) in vats much like is done with penicillin and other pharmaceuticals. Those manufactured in the West are usually grown on grains (*vegan* cordyceps?). All of the commercial varieties of cordyceps you are likely to find are grown, not wild.

Synonyms: *Sphaeria sinensis, Cordyceps sinensis, Ophiocordyceps sinensis.*

Common names: Cordyceps, caterpillar fungus, yartsa (or yatsa) gunbu (Tibetan), keera jhar (India), dong chong xia cao (Chinese, and it translates as "worm in winter, herb in summer"), chong cao (Chinese again, but this term usually refers to species other than *C. sinensis*), tochukaso (Japanese), aweto (Maori, New Zealand), club mushroom (United States—we are a poetic people but we walk really softly).

Part Used

Grown varieties: the mycelium. Wild-harvested: the whole damn thing—caterpillar body, fruiting mushroom, and all.

Preparation and Dosage

Cordyceps needs to be viewed as a medicinal *food*, not a raw drug to be taken in minute doses. The Chinese tonic dosages are normally rather large, 3–9 grams per day, and during acute disease conditions they can go as high as 50 grams, nearly 2 ounces, per day.

If you think of the herb as a food, then eating 2 ounces, say, as you do of asparagus or potatoes, doesn't seem like all that much. In China, cordyceps is often added to soups and stews (just as astragalus is) as a food ingredient for chronic illness. Sometimes the Chinese decoct it in water and drink it as a tea; however traditional healers for millennia in Tibet and India (and in parts of China) used the herb only after soaking it in an alcohol/water combination, usually the local alcoholic drink. And in fact a number of the constituents are only extractable in alcohol.

The best way to use the herb is either as a powder preparation, taken directly by mouth (allowing the stomach acids and bile, etc., to extract for you), or as a tincture.

For acute viral infections, especially in the brain and CNS, and systemic mycoplasma, especially with brain/CNS involvement, I would recommend you buy the powder in bulk from someone such as 1stChineseHerbs.com and then take 3–4 tbl of the powder blended in water or juice three times daily.

The tepid U.S. dosages, 500–1,000 mg daily, are useless for any active disease condition.

CAPSULES

The Chinese brands, if you buy capsules, run around 900–1,000 mg per capsule, and the suggested dose is 6,000 mg (6 grams) per day—just for a tonic dose. If you want to use the capsules for active viral infections in the brain and CNS, I would double that.

TINCTURES

As a tonic: $^1/_4$–$^1/_2$ tsp 3x daily.

For active infections: $^1/_2$–1 tsp 3–6x daily.

Note: If you are going to make your own tincture from cordyceps powder, then use a 50 percent alcohol solution in a 1:5 herb:liquid ratio. Add the cordyceps powder to the water *only*. Starting with cold water, bring the mixture to a boil, then cover and let steep overnight. *Then* add the alcohol and let it steep for a few weeks. This will more efficiently extract the polysaccharides from the root.

Some sources recommend taking cordyceps with vitamin C to help assimilation. There isn't anything in the scientific literature on this and the Asians used the herb (and noted its beneficial effects) for thousands of years before vitamin C was discovered, so . . . not sure where that urban legend came from.

Side Effects and Contraindications

There are no side effects noted in the literature. Up to 5 grams per kilogram of body weight per day have been used in rats long term with no side effects. That would be 350 grams—i.e., about 12 ounces or $^3/_4$ pound—in a person weighing 150 pounds. Double that dose was used with rabbits for 3 months with no side effects.

The only reported side effects I can find are occasional reports of dry mouth, nausea, diarrhea. One case of an allergic reaction that subsided when the herb was discontinued.

Herb/Drug and Herb/Herb Interactions

Cordyceps sinensis is synergistic with cyclosporine A, and the amount of the drug needed is lessened if cordyceps is taken. The hypoglycemic actions of the herb also reduce the dosage needs for those on antidiabetic medications. There is some concern as well that cordyceps might be synergistic or additive with antiretroviral drugs, thus affecting dosage requirements, but nothing has yet been reported in the literature.

Habitat and Appearance

The most common cordyceps medicinal species are what are called club mushrooms by all the mushroom hunters I know, though some mycofanatics are given to Latinizing, often rolling the consonants trippingly across their tongues. They are generally brownish-to-orangish in color (the mushrooms, not the tongues, though if the tongues *were* brownish-to-orangish this medicine would help clear them up). They look somewhat like a tiny club, narrowing at the bottom, widening at the top, up to 5 inches or so tall (the mushrooms, not the mycologists, though there was this one guy . . .). Basically a very tiny version of something Fred Flintstone might use. Normally they are a bit wrinkled along the sides. There are some other species that have a cap, like other mushrooms, but I have never seen one in person; they tend to be a bit rare in my part of the woods. *Cordyceps militaris* is the one most often found in the United States; it's the only one I have met, and collected, personally, in the Rocky Mountains at 8,000 to 10,000 feet. (*C. sinensis* develops at high altitudes between 10,000 and 16,000 feet, on and in prairies rather than in forests, and tends to be more brownish; *C. militaris* tends more toward orange.)

Most of the cordyceps species specialize in their preferred hosts, but *Cordyceps militaris* (go figure) parasitizes the pupae and larvae of numerous moth species and, I have heard, beetles as well. All of the cordyceps tend to sprout from the head of whatever insect they infect. (What *is* this about anyway? Doctrine of signatures? Good for treating mental disorders?) *Cordyceps*, by the way, means "club head," *cord* being club, *ceps* head, while *y* is a query referent, e.g., why.

Most of the species that have been found exist in Asia (about 100 in China alone), but there are somewhere between 5 and 20 in the United States depending on how many digits the taxonomists are using to count them. The U.S. species commonly parasitize cicadas, beetles, and moth larvae and pupae. *Cordyceps cardinalis* for example is moderately common in the southern Appalachian mountains of the eastern United States (and also in southeastern Japan). It is closely related to *C. militaris* (or *C. pseudomilitaris*, which only pretends to be violent), the species that has the largest geographical distribution, having been found on all continents except Antarctica. (Antarctica means "no bears," another useless fact I can't get out of my brain.)

C. militaris grows throughout the United States and is especially common in the Rocky Mountains, the Carolinas, and along the East Coast, often in mountainous regions. It is the primary medicinal species that is easy to find wild in this country. It is used similarly to *C. sinensis* and there have been some decent studies on its effects (150 or so on PubMed, versus 300 on *C. sinensis*).

Cultivation and Collection

I have seen photos of *Cordyceps militaris* being intentionally grown on grain. In fact, the main method to develop fruiting bodies of cordyceps, rather than just the mycelium, is to use grains as a substrate—the first used, and still most common, is rice. There is also a company in Texas, called Unicorn Bags, that sells *C. militaris* spores with detailed inoculation information on how to use live pupae (that is the stage between caterpillar and butterfly). Not my thing really but if you are excited about it look them up (unicornbags.com). (First, grasp the pupa firmly, then take your hypodermic needle and . . .)

There is some speculation, but there is little research on it as yet, that the fruiting mushrooms grown on grain have different medicinal actions and chemistry than those found wild and this is true of the vat-grown mycelium as well.

Studies of the gross constituents show a high similarity between the grown and wild species and, when tested, the grown varieties do have very similar impacts in the body. The one in-depth study I have seen does show a variation in chemistry—the same compounds are in both but in differing quantities, the grown having much more of some, less of a few others. One other analysis found that there were some particular compounds in the insect-host-grown cordyceps that were not in the vat-grown. Those compounds tend to be named after the insect host itself, e.g., cicadapeptins. And those compounds do have medicinal actions themselves. Nevertheless, most studies have been with the grown varieties, not the wild, and they have been shown to have a range of action very close to that of the wild species.

If you wish to harvest wild cordyceps, especially in the United States, you will most likely find *C. militaris.* I, personally, don't know any of the others in their wild state, though some mycofanatics do know of them, find them, and utilize them with supposedly good results. *C. militaris* does have the best research outside of *C. sinensis*; I don't think there is any doubt that the two can be considered interchangeable in action. The Chinese, in practice, apparently agree, and some even think *C. militaris* is better. So, if you want to hunt the wild cordyceps, look for *C. militaris*. (Easiest way? Join the local mycological society and go hunting with them.)

The best time to harvest the mushroom is in the summer after a good wet winter or spring—depending on the local climate they can be found from April to August. I have found them only in the mountains, in pine forests, usually in July/August. Once you've located one, carefully dig the entire mushroom, including the host insect, which will be belowground or embedded in rotted wood (or something). Bag it separately from all the other mushroom species you have collected, take it home, and dry it on an open-air tray in the dark. Watch it carefully to make sure it does not decay as mushrooms are wont to do (though these generally are not as wet as most of the other types and so are less prone to decay once picked). When dry, store in whole form in plastic bags in plastic tubs, out of the sun.

(continued on page 486)

Properties of Cordyceps

Actions

Adrenogenic	Antitumor	Immunomodulator
Antiasthmatic	Antitussive	Insecticidal
Antibacterial	Bronchial regulator	Mitochondrial adaptogen
Anticonvulsant	Cardiotonic	Nerve sedative
Anti-inflammatory	Expectorant	Neuroprotective
Antimetastic	Hepatoprotective	Renoprotective
Antimicrobial	Hypoglycemic	Sleep regulator
Antioxidant	Hypolipidemic	Steroidogenic
Antipyretic	Immunoadaptogen	

Cordyceps is a rather potent immunoadaptogen. If immune activity is high, it reduces it; if low, it enhances it. When taken regularly, if the immune system is stressed by, say, a bacterial organism, the herb will stimulate the immune system in just the right way to respond to the stressor while lowering the levels of or inhibiting entirely the bacterial-induced cytokines that are generated.

As a mitochondrial adaptogen, it increases oxygen utilization in the mitochondria, stimulates ATP production by the mitochondria, and protects mitochondria from adverse events. As a hepatoprotective, it offers autoimmune protection, reduces fibrosis, reduces and inhibits cirrhosis, and protects against hepatitis B. As a renoprotective, it protects from toxicity, inhibits renal failure, and reverses glomerulonephritis. And as a cardiotonic, it is hypotensive, strengthens heartbeat, is antiarrhythmic, and improves myocardial ischemia.

Active Against

Cordyceps is not primarily an antibacterial but is rather a systemic tonic and adaptogen. Still it does have some antimicrobial actions. It is active against some viruses, a few strongly so—influenza virus (H1N1, H9N2), herpes simplex virus 1, HIV-1 protease, hepatitis B, Newcastle virus—and a number of other microbes such as *Mycobacterium tuberculosis*, *Plasmodium* spp., *Clostridium* spp., *Staphylococcus aureus* (resistant and nonresistant), *Enterococcus faecalis*, *Bacillus subtilis*, *Candida albicans*, and various cancers (breast, thyroid, kidney, bladder, prostate, lung, Leydig cell tumor, melanoma). Its antiviral actions make it a perfect immune adjunct for use in treating most major viral infections.

The herb, while not generally active against bacteria, is, however, highly protective of the human body when bacterial infections occur. For example, in one study, mice were fed either phosphate buffered saline (PBS) or *Cordyceps sinensis* mycelium for 3 days and then infected with *Streptococcus pyogenes*. The PBS group showed bacterial dissemination throughout their bodies, while those in the cordyceps group did not. Only 40 percent of the PBS group survived until day 8, while at day 10 70 percent of the cordyceps group were still alive. In addition the PBS group showed extensive skin necrosis, none in the cordyceps group did.

Survival was significantly increased if the cordyceps group received more cordyceps every other day. In fact, *all* of the cordyceps-treated group then survived while ALT and AST levels remained normal. Use of the extract, in vitro, against the same bacterial strain showed *no* direct antibacterial activity at all.

Use to Treat

Any respiratory viral infection, any inflammation in the brain or CNS—especially encephalitis and meningitis, fatigue and weakness, especially after long illness or in chronic infections, poor mitochondrial function, chronic wasting, unproductive cough from no known cause, joint inflammation, mental fog and confusion, low libido, lung infections, kidney infections, thick mucus in the lungs that will not move, immune dysregulation, dizziness, tinnitus, nocturia, and cancer. It is especially effective for mycoplasma infections.

Finding Cordyceps

You can get bulk powder and capsules from 1stChineseHerbs.com as well as many other places on the Internet. If you want to spend enormous amounts of money, you can also buy the wild-crafted mushroom itself. Or . . . you can join the local mycological society (find a fun one, usually it *won't* include guys with mathematically shaven beards) and learn to find it in the wild.

Plant Chemistry

Three constituents are, at present, considered to be the major active chemicals in cordyceps: cordycepin (a.k.a. 3′-deoxyadenosine, a purine alkaloid and a derivative of adenosine), cordycepic acid (a.k.a. D-mannitol), and cordyceps polysaccharide. Some commercial formulations are standardized for cordycepic acid (usually 10 percent), others for 7 percent cordycepin or 0.1 percent adenosine (sort of the same thing). Most are made from cordyceps mycelium and will state as much on the label.

Vat-fermented cordyceps mycelium contains a lot more cordycepin than the wild mushrooms, 40 mcg per gram versus 5 mcg/g. Cordycepic acid varies in wild populations, comprising anywhere from 7 percent to 29 percent by weight depending on time of year, location, and so on. The fruiting bodies contain from 30–85 mg per gram of cordycepic acid; the mycelial content is much higher (which is part of the reason the whole caterpillar is harvested for medicine, not just the club mushroom itself).

Cordyceps, like most mushrooms, has a very high polysaccharide content. The main one is considered to be cordyceps polysaccharide and is primarily composed of D-mannose and D-galactose in a ratio of 3:5. It runs from 3 percent to 8 percent by weight of the harvested fungus. Most of the rest of the polysaccharides in the herb are simply labeled by identifiers such as P70-1, CPS-1, and so on. As with many mushrooms, there are a lot of them, 36 so far.

The fungus is very high in nucleotides, the molecular components of the nucleic acids RNA and DNA. The main ones are guanosine, adenosine, and uridine in that order. The nucleotides tend to be higher, often much more so, in vat-grown cordyceps mycelium than in the wild fungus.

There are various sterols. Ergosterol is a primary one, a precursor of vitamin D_2. It is much higher in the fruiting body itself (10 mg/g) than in the grown mycelium (1.5 mg/g). Others are sitosterol, daucosterol, and campesterol.

Cordyceps has very high levels of 18 different amino acids. The mycelial powders have the highest content. Glutamate, arginine, and aspartic acid are the highest.

The mushroom also has very high levels of fatty acids, in this order: linoleic acid, oleic acid, palmitic acid.

It also contains substantial quantities of 13 different minerals (and traces of 7 more), in this order: potassium, phosphorus, magnesium, calcium, sodium, iron, aluminum, zinc, manganese, silicon, boron, copper, selenium.

And, of course, vitamins: E, K, B_1, B_2, B_{12}.

There are a few other compounds in the fungus including cordymin, various aminophenols, some unusual cyclic dipeptides, various dihydroisocoumarins, cordypyridones A and B, various diphenyl ethers, myriocin, and various polyamines (cadaverine, spermidine, spermine, putrescine, and so on).

The constituents of *C. militaris* are very similar.

Note: Research is showing that some of the active compounds in the various cordyceps species are specific to the insect host upon which they form, e.g., cicadapeptins 1 and 2 that *Cordyceps heteropoda* creates from the chemicals in the cicadas upon which it develops. Again, this type of research is very new and very uncommon.

Traditional Uses of Cordyceps

Cordyceps was first recorded in Tibet in the fifteenth century in the medical text *Mennag chewa rinsel* by Zurkhar Namnyi Dorje. Oddly enough, in spite of the fact that cordyceps first appeared in Tibetan healing texts, and continued to do so through the nineteenth century, it is rarely used as a medicine there. Those who do use it do so primarily as a liquid tonic that they take throughout the day for increasing vigor and strength and as an aphrodisiac. Generally, the liquid is prepared by placing four or five cordyceps mushrooms in arak (a rice or barley liquor) and leaving it to steep in a cool, dark place for 2 to 3 months (sometimes up to a year).

While rarely mentioned in Tibetan texts, and not considered all that important an herb in that tradition, its range of actions in that system are increasing the energy of the body, increasing and restoring semen, and increasing kidney strength. It is considered specific for altitude sickness.

Though the Tibetans didn't find cordyceps to be a major medicine, the Chinese did. It has, since its discovery, been a major trade item with China, sometimes worth more than gold.

The herb came to Western prominence in 1994 when a Chinese track coach insisted that his team won so handily in the 1994 Asian Games in Hiroshima, Japan, beating the world records in the 1,500-, 3,000-, and 10,000-meter events, because he had them use the herb regularly as part of their training regimen.

AYURVEDA

In spite of cordyceps being indigenous in India, there is little, if any, mention of the herb in traditional Ayurvedic texts. There is some speculation that the herb "sanjivani" mentioned in the older texts is cordyceps, but it's a guess.

In India, the use of cordyceps primarily occurs in community herbal practice, not in formal Ayurvedic healing. It is commonly used among traditional healers in Sikkim, a landlocked Indian state in the Himalayan mountains that borders both Nepal and Tibet. It is recommended as a tonic for all illnesses, improving energy, appetite, stamina, libido, and endurance and normalizing sleep. It is considered to be a longevity herb and specific for colds and flu, coughs, asthma, cancer, tuberculosis, diabetes, erectile dysfunction, BHP, jaundice, and hepatitis. Although occasionally prepared as a water extraction, it is generally infused in an alcoholic liquor, as in Tibet.

TRADITIONAL CHINESE MEDICINE

Cordyceps is described variously as having a neutral property and sweet taste or as being sweet/acrid with a warm property. It acts on the lung and kidney channels, is lung nourishing, kidney vital essence and vital energy tonifying, hemostatic, and phlegm resolvent, that is, a mucolytic. It is generally prescribed for overall debility after sickness and for the aged. It is considered to be one of the three primary invigorating medicinals in Chinese medicine along with Asian ginseng and deer antler.

It is specific for tonifying the lungs, arresting bronchial bleeding, dispelling phlegm, chronic cough, asthma, wasting, and tonifying the kidneys. It is also used for impotence, low libido, poor seminal emissions, aching of loins and knees, and as a tonic for spontaneous sweating, aversion to cold, tinnitus, chronic nephritis, general weakness, and sexual hypofunction.

WESTERN BOTANIC USE

Until 1994, none. Now, lots of interest, primarily based on the Chinese and Japanese research and cordyceps's reputation as a longevity herb and aphrodisiac. (We seek our youth and we will not be denied.)

Scientific Research

Most of the scientific studies have occurred since 1995, after the Asian Games, and the numbers of published articles are increasing every year. There were four studies published in 1995, by 2011 there were 80. And those are just the ones accessible through PubMed; there are scores more in the Chinese, Japanese, and Korean databases, most not translated into English. Of those 80, only 13 were not Korean, Japanese, or Chinese and about half of those 13 were not studying the medicinal actions of the plant. The Western world is still betting that those buggy whip orders will pick up again . . . any day now.

The majority of the studies I am citing were with *C. sinensis* or *C. militaris* herbs or their isolated compounds.

IN VITRO STUDIES

Cordyceps downregulates a number of inflammatory cytokines and upregulates others such as IL-10, TGF-ß, and IL-1ra that are specific for controlling overactive inflammation responses in the body. In underactive immune systems, it will upregulate cytokines to help the body deal with disease. In overactive immune circumstances it will downregulate them.

It downregulates or inhibits NF-κB, TNF-α, IL-1ß, IL-12, NO, iNOS, SOD, elastase, luceriferase, ERK, JAK-2 (Janus kinase-2), JNK, p38, PGE2, spleen tyrosine kinase (Syk), STAT-1, AP-1, MMP-3, MMP-9, and H_2O_2 hemolysis, and it scavenges hydroxyl radicals.

When cells are challenged by lipoproteins from the bacterial cytoplasmic membrane, cordyceps strongly downregulates TNF-α, IL-12, and NO. In lipopolysaccharide-activated macrophages it inhibits NF-κB, NO,

TNF-α, IL-1ß, IL-6, IL-12, IFN-γ, AP-1, COX-2, the phosphorylation of p38 MAPK and Akt, as well as inhibiting PGE2 levels and suppressing Syk/NF-κB, IKKε/IRF-3, and p38/AP-1 pathways.

Treatment with cordyceps or the cordyceps constituent cordycepin, or adenosine, causes lipopolysaccharide-stimulated macrophages to return to their original inactivated shape. This dynamic is dose dependent and needs relatively high levels of the herb.

Cordycepin suppresses TNF-α and MMP-9 expression in human bladder cancer cells, inactivates the phosphoinositide 3-kinase (PI3K) pathway in LNCaP cells, and increases levels of TIMP (tissue inhibitor of metalloproteinase) 1 and 2, and thus downregulates MMP-3 and MMP-9 in prostate cancer cells.

Cordyceps possesses a potent sphingomyelinase inhibitor that inhibits the breakdown of sphingomyelin in the body, especially in the brain, making it specific for mycoplasma. It strongly inhibits hydrogen peroxide oxidation and activity against cells and actively protects the mitochrondria (reducing oxidative stress and mitochondrial depolarization). It acts as an intracellular antioxidant and is a strong hydroxyl radical scavenger. All these actions are dose dependent.

Cordycepin strongly inhibits lipopolysaccharide-activated inflammation in microglia cells. It significantly inhibits the production of NO, PGE2, and proinflammatory cytokines in the microglia. It suppresses NF-κB translocation by blocking IkappaBalpha degradation and inhibits phosphorylation of Akt, ERK-1 and ERK-2, JNK, and p38 kinase. A compound of cordyceps, coptidis rhizoma, and Chinese skullcap was shown to have powerful neuroprotective effects on lipopolysaccharide-activated microglial cells. It inhibited NO, iNOS, COX-2, PGE2, gp91 phox, iROS (intracellular reactive oxygen species), TNF-α, IL-1ß, and IkappaBalpha degradation. It upregulated heme oxygenase-1 and increased cell viability and mitochondrial membrane potential. The three-herb compound was found to strongly protect neural cells from toxicity.

Cordyceps is strongly modulatory on immune cells. In vitro it acts as an activator and maturation stimulant to monocytes and immature dendritic cells by stimulating the expression of costimulatory molecules and proinflammatory cytokines, enhancing dendritic-cell-induced allogeneic T cell proliferation and reducing the endocytic ability of dendritic cells. *However*, during lipopolysaccharide stimulation cordyceps suppresses the proinflammatory cytokines involved. It suppresses the lipopolysaccharide-induced, dendritic-cell-elicited allogeneic T cell proliferation and shifts the immune response from a potent Th1 to a Th2 dynamic. In the absence of infection, it potentiates Th1 immune activity. During active infection, it actively modulates the extreme upregulation of lipopolysaccharide cytokines and balances the overreactivity of the Th1 response.

Cordyceps has a lot of effects on airway epithelial cells. It acts to normalize cellular function in airway epithelia by normalizing ion transport. It blocks airway inflammation by blocking NF-κB production in airway epithelial cells. It significantly reduces epidermal-growth-factor-stimulated mucous hypersecretion in lung mucoepidermoid cells by downregulating COX-2, MMP-9, and MUC5AC gene expression through blocking NF-κB and the p38/ERK MAPK pathways. It strongly regulates the inflammation that occurs in the bronchii and regulates bronchoalveolar lavage fluids by doing do. It downregulates IL-1ß, IL-6, IL-8, and TNF-α. It is highly protective of epithelia and normalizes the function of the surface epithelium.

In rheumatoid arthritis synovial fibroblasts it inhibits IL-1ß-induced MMP-1 and MMP-3 expression. MMP-1 degrades fibrillar collagens, MMP-3 the extracellular matrix. It also inhibits MAPK activation, specifically p38 and JNK. It is a fairly potent inhibitor of p38 phosphorylation.

Cordyceps is highly protective of renal tubular epithelial cells in vitro. It is antiadipogenic. It is antiatherogenic by blocking MAPK, specifically ERK, JNK, and p38. It suppresses the expression of diabetes-regulating genes. It reduces platelet aggregation.

Cordyceps stimulates ATP generation by mitochondria and also antioxidant activity, and it modulates immune responses intracellularly. It protects mitochondria from ROS and enhances the mitochondrial antioxidant defenses. The effects are dose dependent.

IN VIVO STUDIES

Cordyceps militaris, grown on soybeans, was used to prepare a hot water extract that was then given to mice infected with influenza A virus. Significantly reduced virus titers in lung tissue were observed after 3 days when compared with mice not given cordyceps. A polysaccharide, presumed to be the most active antiviral agent, was extracted and given intranasally to mice infected with lethal strains of influenza A. Mortality dropped from 70 to 18 percent. The polysaccharide was determined to be a type of arabinogalactan, similar to those extracted from larch and juniper.

In rats, cordycepin attenuated neointima formation (a thickened layer of arterial tissue) in vascular smooth-tissue muscle cells by inhibiting ROS. Cordymin, a constituent of cordyceps, was found to be strongly anti-inflammatory in induced gastric inflammation in mice by inhibiting IL-1ß, TNF-α, and total oxidant levels. It was also found to be strongly analgesic. Cordyceps (*militaris*) extract suppressed induced acute colitis in mice and significantly reduced the production of inflammatory cytokines from macrophages and mast cells. NO, iNOS, and TNF-α were all strongly inhibited. Cordyceps extract inhibited airway inflammation in rats by blocking NF-κB. It significantly inhibited ovalbumin-induced airway inflammation in sensitized guinea pigs and rats that mimics the human condition of asthma. Likewise, *Cordyceps militaris* reduced airway inflammation in a mouse asthma model.

Lipopolysaccharide-injected mice, experiencing induced inflammation, showed a remarkable reduction of IL-1ß, TNF-α, iNOS, COX-2, and PGE2 when given an extract of *Cordyceps pruinosa*.

Cordyceps extract increased CD4+ and CD8+, IL-4, and IL-10 in mice, especially in mesenteric lymph node lymphocytes. Regular daily doses of cordyceps extract prevented disuse-induced osteoporosis in rats. And an extract increased glutathione levels, reduced oxidants, and lowered blood glucose levels in rats with streptozotocin-induced diabetes.

Cordyceps extract significantly improved learning and reduced memory impairment in mice. *Cordyceps militaris* extract (and cordycepin) protected hippocampal neurons in gerbils from ischemic injury. Cordycepin was found to be strongly protective of neurons against cerebral ischemia/reperfusion. It considerably lowered levels of MMP-3 in the brain, increased SOD, and decreased malondialdehyde, significantly reducing oxidation. In one study *Cordyceps sinensis* mycelium strongly protected rat neurons from ischemic injury by inhibiting NF-κB, PMNs (polymorphonuclear neutrophils), IL-1ß, iNOS, TNF-α, ICAM-1, and COX-2. A cordymin extract pretty much did the same thing in another study. In still another study cordyceps extract protected the brain from injury after middle cerebral artery occlusion-induced cerebral ischemia in rats. And in yet another study cordycepin prevented postischemic neuronal degeneration in mice.

Cordyceps sinensis extract significantly reduced renal ischemia/reperfusion injury in rats. Various forms of renal injury in rats were ameliorated by the use of several types of *Cordyceps cicadae* extracts.

Mice exposed to ionizing radiation experienced restored immune function from a polysaccharide of *C. sinensis* through modulation of the secretion of IL-4, IL-5, and IL-17. A butanol extract of *Cordyceps bassiana* was shown to inhibit induced atopic dermatitis in mice. And in hamsters, cordycepin was shown to prevent hyperlipidemia.

Other studies have shown cordycepin to be strongly steroidogenic. It stimulated testosterone production in mouse Leydig cells. And serum testosterone and sperm count and motility were strongly increased in rats after supplementation with *Cordyceps militaris*.

HUMAN CLINICAL STUDIES AND TRIALS

Cordyceps extract inhibits the proliferation and differentiation of Th2 cells and reduces the expression of related cytokines by downregulating GST-3 mRNA and upregulating FOXP3 mRNA and relieves chronic allergic inflammation by increasing IL-10 in the blood of children with chronic asthma.

In one study, 60 asthmatic patients were split into two groups. Thirty used an inhaler, the rest used *Cordyceps sinensis* (CS) capsules. IgE, solubal ICAM-1, IL-4, and MMP-9 were all lowered in the cordyceps group (though not as much as in those using an inhaler). Another study at the Beijing Medical University with 50 asthma patients found that the symptoms in the group treated with CS were reduced by 81 percent in 5 days versus 61 percent over 9 days in the pharmaceutical group.

There have been a number of other trials of the herb in the treatment of chronic obstructive pulmonary disease (COPD), asthma, and bronchitis that have not been translated into English. The herb was effective for all these conditions; it is especially indicated for COPD.

One trial split 65 renal dialysis patients into two groups. The 33 in the second group took cordyceps (330 mg) and ginkgo (230 mg) three times daily for 3 months. At the end of that period microinflammation, a problem in renal hemodialysis, was significantly lowered in the herb group. Levels of hs-CRP (high-sensitivity C-reactive protein), IL-6, and TNF-α were all much lower.

In one study with 51 patients suffering chronic renal failure, the use of 3–5 grams/day of CS significantly improved renal function and increased immune function. Another study with 57 people suffering gentamicin-induced renal damage split the subjects into two groups; one received CS, the other conventional pharmaceuticals. After 6 days those in the CS group had recovered 89 percent of their kidney function versus 45 percent in the other group.

Sixty-one people with lupus nephritis were split into two groups. One received 2–4 grams of cordyceps (before meals) and 600 mg of artemisinin (after meals) three times daily for 3 years. They were observed for an additional 5 years after treatment. Twenty-six had no recurrence, four had mild, and for one the herbs did not work.

A randomized trial of cordyceps in the treatment of 21 aged patients (divided into two groups) found that cordyceps ameliorated aminoglycoside nephrotoxicity.

Cordyceps sinensis (CS) was used in the long-term treatment of renal transplant patients. Long-term survival was no different in the treated and untreated groups, however the incidence of complication was significantly lower in the CS group. The CS group needed much lower doses of cyclosporine A, and serum levels of IL-10 in the CS group were much higher. Another renal transplant study with 200 transplant patients showed the same outcomes.

Three separate studies with a combined patient population of 756 men and women who were experiencing reduced sex drive found that after 40 days 65 percent of those taking cordyceps reported improved libido and performance versus 24 percent of those taking placebo. In another study with elderly patients complaining of decreased libido, impotence, and other sexual malfunctions 3 grams/day of cordyceps was administered for 40 days. Increased sperm survival time, increased sperm count, and decreased numbers of malformed sperm were all found in the majority of males. Improvements in hypoleukorrhagia, menoxenia, and sex drive were reported in a majority of the women.

There have been a number of clinical studies of the herb in cancer treatment, along with chemo and radiation. In one study of 50 patients taking cordyceps, tumors reduced in 23. In another, after 2 months, most patients taking cordyceps reported improved subjective symptoms. White blood counts stayed at 3000/mm^3 or higher. The use of cordyceps during radiation and chemo has been found to counteract the negative immune effects of those procedures.

There have been a number of Chinese studies on using the herb for treating heart conditions, liver problems, hypercholesterolemia, and male/female sexual dysfunction, but few of them have been translated into English. There have also been a few studying exercise tolerance and improvement, e.g., 20 adults aged 50 to 75, in a double-blind, placebo-controlled trial showed improved exercise performance while taking cordyceps. However, the main studies in the United States have been on exercise tolerance with young athletes, and they all showed no improvement. The dosages were extremely low.

The best overall look at the herb, its history, and its medical uses is probably John Holliday and Matt Cleaver, *On the Trail of the Yak: Ancient Cordyceps in the Modern World* (June 2004). You can find it online and download it for free by searching online, or at websites such as Natural Healthcare Products (natural-healthcare-products.eu).

Note: To be effective for anything, cordyceps *must* be dosed appropriately. That means a minimum dose of 3 grams daily, but the best results occur with 6 grams daily as the baseline, especially in acute conditions. The renal studies usually used from 3–4.5 grams. This dose range can also work for lung problems, except in truly acute conditions when it should be 6–9 grams (in mycoplasma treatment as well).

Echinacea

Family: Compositae

Common Names: *These days "echinacea" pretty much is the name, though "purple coneflower" is exceptionally common among gardeners who don't know about the medicinal actions of plants.*

Species Used: All nine members of the genus can be used; however, the most common are *Echinacea angustifolia* and *E. purpurea.* I don't particularly think that *purpurea* is all that strong in comparison to *angustifolia.* I really haven't found it all that effective, in spite of what everyone says, and I avoid it if possible. I would strongly suggest the use of *angustifolia* if you can get it. (There is some evidence that *Echinacea pallida* is more potent than *angustifolia,* but I haven't worked with it personally.)

Parts Used

Root primarily, but the flower heads in seed are also potent. The Germans, however, use the *juice* of *purpurea* as their primary medicinal.

Preparation and Dosage

The most potent medicinal forms of the plant are tincture of the root and the fresh juice of the aerial plant.

Note: Echinacea extracts standardized for phenolic acid or echinocaside content have been found to be inactive as immunostimulants but do still retain their anti-inflammatory actions.

FRESH JUICE

Juice the aerial parts of the plant, when in flower if possible. Take immediately or stabilize with 20 percent to 25 percent alcohol (see page 437). Take 1–3 tsp per day, or up to 6x daily in acute episodes.

TINCTURE

E. angustifolia dry root, 1:5, 70 percent alcohol. (Or fresh flower heads of *purpurea* if you must, 1:2, 95 percent alcohol.)

Note: *The tincture's effectiveness is much reduced if taken in water* (unless you are taking large doses for septicemia or collagen support) and I would strongly recommend against doing so, especially in the treatment of strep infections of the throat.

For strep throat/tonsillitis: Direct contact with the tissue at the back of the throat with a tincture of echinacea (30 drops each hour minimum) liberally mixed with saliva is certain in these kinds of conditions. Echinacea actively stimulates saliva and numbs the tissue it comes into contact with, making it perfect for this (or any sore, swollen throat infections). I have found this reliably effective, again if treatment is assertive and consistent. In a number of cases (including a doubting physician who was ill himself) the throat had been positively cultured for strep; healing generally occurs within 24 hours.

As a mouth/gum wash for sores and ulcers: The tincture, 30 drops, hold in mouth until saliva is well stimulated, swish it around to cover all surfaces well, hold for 30 seconds, swallow. Repeat 3x or 4x daily.

For onset of colds and flus: Not less than 1 dropperful (30 drops) of

Properties of Echinacea

Actions

Analgesic	Antiviral	Immune stimulant
Antibacterial	Hyaluronidase inhibitor	Sialagogue
Anti-inflammatory	Immune modulator	Stimulates antibody production

Finding Echinacea

E. purpurea is everywhere. I strongly advise against using it, ever, unless you are juicing the fresh plant yourself—which you should if it is growing in the garden; there's no need to kill the plant by digging it up. *Angustifolia* is harder to find; few herb shops carry it in tincture form. You can, however, find *angustifolia* tinctures here and there on the Internet. Try SageWomanHerbs.com. Pacific Botanicals carries *angustifolia* root in bulk. Excellent quality. See Sources of Supply on page 599.

tincture each hour until symptoms cease. (Note: Echinacea is more effective for cold and flu onset in combination with licorice root and red root.)

For septicemia, typhoid, diphtheria, and so on: 1 tsp *E. angustifolia* root tincture in very little water every half hour until the situation normalizes. If the tincture is held in the mouth for a minute or so, it will enter the bloodstream quite rapidly. Better outcomes will be achieved this way. If taken 30 minutes after piperine, its movement into the bloodstream will be very rapid.

For collagen tissue protection and repair: ¼–1 tsp tincture, 3x daily for extended periods (weeks).

For external wounds: Because of its capacity to correct tissue abnormality, echinacea is perfect for this application. Its anti-inflammatory, antibacterial, and cell-normalizing actions all come into powerful play for any external wounds. In the case of infected wounds, take the tincture, frequently, diluted in a bit of water. In severe cases take ½–1 tsp of *angustifolia* root tincture each half hour to hour.

For venomous stings and bites: Mix the tincture with an equal amount of water and wash the affected area liberally every 30 minutes, and take 30 drops to 1 tsp of the tincture each half hour to hour depending on the type of bite/sting. For infected bites or stings, more; for venomous bites/stings, more; for simple bee or wasp stings, less. (You can also use a wash for this purpose: Boil 2 ounces ground flower heads or root in 8 ounces water for 15 minutes, let steep 1 hour, strain, and use to wash wounds and venomous bites and stings liberally, as often as needed.)

POWDER

As a wound powder: Powder the dried root (or seed heads) as finely as possible and sprinkle liberally over new or infected wounds. Best in combination with other herbs such as goldenseal, usnea, oak, and wormwood.

Poultice: Mix powder with water until thick and place on the affected area.

For abnormal Pap smear: Echinacea can easily correct even stage three dysplasia. Whenever echinacea is placed directly on cells that are displaying abnormal properties, the cells tend to return to normal relatively quickly as long as the treatment is assertive and consistent. I have seen no other herb that comes even close to echinacea's reliability in this regard. Use as a suppository; see page 575 for details.

Side Effects and Contraindications

Rarely: Joint pain may occur with large doses taken for extended periods of time. Increased shoe size may occur from large doses for extended periods. Current collagenosis? Don't take a lot for a long time.

Echinacea is not an immune tonic; it is an immune stimulant. Continued immune stimulation in instances of immune depletion to avoid necessary rest or more healthy lifestyle choices will always result in a more severe illness than if the original colds and flus were allowed to progress. Echinacea should not be used if you are getting sick a lot and are only using echinacea to stave off illness without using the time gained to heal the immune system itself through deep healing and recuperation.

Herb/Drug Interactions

None have been noted; however, echinacea decreases the action of the influx transporter OATP-B by 50 percent. It may decrease the absorption of OATP-B substrates. Phenobarbital, chloral hydrate, and meprobamate can inhibit the anti-inflammatory actions of echinacea.

Herb/Herb Interactions

Synergistic with astragalus and licorice in the stimulation of immune function.

Habitat and Appearance

The echinaceas are perennials, indigenous to eastern and central North America, usually in moist or dry prairies and open woodlands. *E. purpurea* is a major garden plant pretty much everyplace that has gardens. It is also a major agricultural crop everywhere on Earth, including China, so this member of the genus, even if no others, has colonized numerous countries around the globe.

The plants are unbranched, erect, with wide-bladed leaves and grow 3 to 5 feet tall. Writers often describe the plant leaves as hairy with a rough texture. To me the experience is more like touching Velcro; the plant doesn't mess around. The stems are strong, the plants vigorous, intense. They are not *oooooh* love/mushy plants and have no resemblance to puppies or kittens.

All the species except *purpurea* have strong taproots, brown, vigorous, intense. *Purpurea*'s roots are some sort of strange, glumpy, fibrous sort of paleish-tannish thing. I never have been attracted to that species and besides I don't think it is all that good medicinally so I am prejudiced; the rootish things it produces just look wimpy to me, sort of like a bag of earthworms curled around an irregular sort of tannish lump. But, you know, go ahead and use *purpurea* if you want.

Cultivation and Collection

The reason why so many people use *purpurea* for medicine rather than *angustifolia* (which I think much stronger) is that it is easier to grow. (Ah hah!) Throw the seeds in the ground in the fall and up they come in the spring. Like all the echinaceas they prefer a period of cold before germinating, but I have talked to people who just planted seeds in the spring and found them to be decent if not spectacular germinators. You can also separate the *purpurea* root thingies into chunks and propagate them that way. From personal experience, and from everyone I have talked to, the other species of echinacea are decidedly cranky; you have to work at it to get them to grow. *Angustifolia* is a poor germinator until you figure out just what it likes; stratification is essential for the plant—however, soaking the seeds in ethephon for 10 minutes will help germination tremendously, much more than stratification.

At one time it was almost impossible to get anything other than *purpurea* to put in a garden, but that has changed—many people now have seedlings available of most of the echinacea species. Horizon Herbs (see Sources of Supply on page 599) has one of the best selections. The plants self-seed once established, so beginning with seedlings and tending them carefully until they take is a good route to go if you want this medicinal as a permanent member of your herb garden.

Fall-harvest the roots—after 3 years or so in the ground—after the leaves turn brown. Harvest the seed heads just after the seeds mature. I prefer my root tincture to be from dried roots rather than fresh, but then I use *angustifolia* and am in a minority in this; most people use the fresh *purpurea* roots. In any event, let the (*angustifolia*) roots dry whole, then store them in plastic bags in the dark in a cool location. They will last for years if properly stored. (Studies on years-old dried roots found them just as effective as the fresh roots in their actions.)

You can harvest the fresh plants for juicing anytime, the German approach, and that won't kill the plant as taking the roots does. The plants are most potent if you take them in full flower, then run them through a juicer, and stabilize the juice with 20 percent alcohol by volume (see page 437).

Plant Chemistry

Echinacoside, echinacin, echinoline, echinacein, polyacetylenes, hydrocinnamic acid, betaine, alkylamides, caffeic acid glycosides, inulin, isobutyl amides, isobutylalkamines, sesquiterpene esters, and so on.

Traditional Uses of Echinacea

AYURVEDA

Nope.

TRADITIONAL CHINESE MEDICINE

Nein.

WESTERN BOTANIC PRACTICE

The various echinacea species were used for a very long time by the indigenous cultures of North America, who then passed on the knowledge to the nascent American medical movements (who really went with it). The native cultures used the plants, most often the roots, for wounds and sores; as a poultice for swellings; for septic wounds, sores in the mouth or gums, respiratory infections, sore throat, tonsillitis, enlarged glands, fevers, mumps and measles; as a wash for the pain of burns; for toothache and cavities; for snakebites and poisonous bites from insects and spiders; stomach cramps, GI tract distress, arthritis, and rheumatism. They took large frequent doses.

The Eclectics were first alerted to the plant by its usefulness for snakebite treatment but went on to use it as one of their primary medicines. Generally, they used it much like the native cultures. They, however, felt the herb specific for septicemia, infected blood, severely infected wounds (with blood infection), generally infected mucous membrane systems of the throat, tongue, mouth, lungs, and stomach, tonsillitis, respiratory infections with foul smell, diphtheria, infected insect bites, and on and on and on. They used large frequent doses—every half hour to hour. The Eclectics *only* used *angustifolia*; they did not consider *purpurea* a legitimate substitute for it nor a very good herb in and of itself.

The use of *Echinacea purpurea* came about not only because of ease of growth but due to intense German interest in the plant; it is part of their standard-practice medicine. (They used *purpurea* because it was easy to grow and was already present in the country.) Most, if not all, of the German studies and use, however, have been with the expressed juice of the plant—which they often use parenterally (by injection) rather than taken by mouth; they don't use the root of *purpurea*. *Hello*—they don't use the root of *purpurea*. They do use the root of *E. pallida* as an ethanolic extract taken by mouth. *Purpurea* root came into vogue in the United States during the herbal renaissance of the late twentieth century *because* of the German use of the expressed juice of the aerial parts of the plant in flower (an invalid generalization to the root from the actions of the fresh juice) *and* because it was easily available in the eastern United States. It is native to the eastern United States and is widely grown there in gardens.

E. purpurea is used in Germany as a *supportive* therapy for colds, for chronic infections of the respiratory and lower urinary tract, or externally for poorly healing wounds and chronic ulceration. The tincture of *E. pallida* root is used as supportive therapy for influenza-like infections. Supportive, not primary.

(continued on page 504)

Time for a Rant

Like goldenseal, echinacea is a North American plant and, as such, most of the studies in the United States are still arguing about whether it works or not (just as with goldenseal). The Germans are under no such illusions; it is part of their standard-practice medicine. Most of the early research occurred in Germany; the rest of the world is just starting to catch up. Unfortunately a great deal of the research has devoted itself to deciding whether the herb works or not (generally not), and way too many of the studies look at the use of the herb as a preventive for colds—in adults and children. Very few of them have looked at the traditional uses and dosages of the herb and oriented their studies around that, so that they are discovering it useless for what they are testing it for. What a shock. Basically, they are giving capsules of *purpurea* in small doses a few times a day to help prevent colds—some good double-blind studies, too. (That's where they poke out *both* of the researcher's eyes and . . .)

If I had a nickel for every person who has told me they had a cold and had taken some echinacea—usually *purpurea*—(dropperful 3x daily) and didn't notice any difference, I would be rich.

To be clear: The herb is very good, *if you are using it properly for the right things*. It is relatively useless for preventing colds. The overuse of the herb for that (especially combined with goldenseal—what a waste) is due entirely to marketing ploys by the larger herb companies. Echinacea *can* help at the onset of a cold or flu *if used in large doses every half hour or hour exactly at the onset of the cold or flu*. If the infection gets established, use lomatium, because echinacea just ain't gonna cut it. I have also found that echinacea is much less effective as a flu and cold treatment for people past the middle age shift. It is, however, very good for younger people *if used properly*.

Nevertheless, I don't consider that the main strength of the plant. In general, it is very good for exactly what the native peoples and Eclectics used it for: *severe* infections of the throat, infected wounds that stink, insect bites, snakebites, nastily infected mucous membranes especially if accompanied by foul smell, septicemia, wounds and sores, sores in the mouth and gums, and so on. If your condition is similar and you treat it aggressively, the plant can save your life.

The herb does enhance immune function, but most people think of it as an immune tonic. It isn't. Rhodiola and ashwagandha are tonics but not echinacea. Echinacea is an immune *stimulant*.

I have found the herb to be excellent for raising immune function in *active* infections if taken internally in the right doses and to be very specific for correcting problems in the skin or mucous membranes if used topically—basically anyplace the herb can touch the affected part. But the doses have to be high and frequent or else forget it. And again, if you have any kind of circulating infection, especially if there is bacteria in the blood (septicemia), the herb is very potent if taken properly.

The herb also has some good specific actions on the mucous membranes and collagen tissues of the body, but you really have to know what you are doing to get good outcomes. And again, I just haven't found *purpurea* to be as reliable as *angustifolia* for serious conditions. Some of the herbalists I know in Europe insist that they have, but I have personally tried really large doses of *purpurea*, for myself and others, and it just isn't up to snuff. The native cultures almost always used *angustifolia* for serious conditions (so did the Eclectics); *purpurea* had a very small profile in indigenous medicine in the United States. I tend to think they were on to something, as I have, as they apparently did, found *purpurea* weak.

If I had a nickel for every person who has told me they had a cold and had taken some echinacea and didn't notice any difference, I would be rich.

Does *purpurea* work at all? Well, yes, but we are talking pretty good doses of the fresh plant juice here (6 to 15 ml, i.e., 1 to 3 teaspoons daily) and using it in specific ways for specific conditions and still—for colds and influenza even the Germans consider it to be only *supportive*. Its real strength in their system is as a topical treatment for wounds and sores.

There are very few if any commercial products in the United States that use the fresh juice or suggest the right dosing strategies and amounts. The main thing is . . . *angustifolia* (and the others) are just better. Much better.

Scientific Research

Most of the usable studies on echinacea have used the fresh juice of *Echinacea purpurea*. Unless otherwise noted, that is what these studies are referring to. There have been hundreds of papers published on the plant; this is just a sampling.

But first . . . echinacea (all species) really has two primary actions: it stimulates the immune system and it is a very potent hyaluronidase inhibitor. Many of its most potent medicinal actions come from these two things.

Hyaluronidase (HYL) is an enzyme that breaks down hyaluronic acid (HA), a glycosaminoglycan that is widely distributed throughout connective, epithelial, and neural tissues. It is, as well, a major part of the extracellular matrix. Inhibition of hyaluronidase has a number of beneficial actions: 1) In inflammatory diseases such as various forms of arthritis, the use of a hyaluronidase inhibitor stops the normal (and abnormal) breakdown of cartilage (and synovial fluid), which increases the amount of cartilage (and fluid) in and around the joints, helping counteract, even reverse, the condition. Combined with the anti-inflammatory actions of the herb, this means that large doses can be highly useful for reversing various forms of arthritis and rheumatism. 2) Hyaluronic acid is a major component of the skin and is highly involved in skin repair. HA contributes to tissue dynamics, cell movement and proliferation, and the generation of new cellular tissues. HA is strongly present in new wounds and enhances cellular filtration. It is an essential element of granulation; that is, the new cellular tissue that slowly takes the place of the clotted blood (scab) that first forms over a wound. This tissue forms from the bottom of the wound upward. The more HA, the faster and better it forms. Hyaluronidase inhibition means that more HA is present in the skin/wound area and skin repair is significantly enhanced. 3) With many types of cancer, hyaluronidase plays a major role in metastasis. It degrades the extracellular matrix and allows cancer cells to escape the main tumor mass. HYL also degrades other cellular structures, allowing the cancer cells to penetrate them as well. It also plays a role in the formation of the new blood vessels that cancerous tumors need to survive. HYL inhibition, then, produces a particular kind of anticancer, or antitumor, action. 4) Some bacteria (*Staphylococcus aureus*, *Streptococcus* spp., *Clostridium* spp., *Enterococcus* spp., *Mycobacterium* spp., etc.) create and release hyaluronidase in order to loosen the connective tissue matrix and facilitate their penetration into new areas of the body. Part of what echinacea does is to strengthen the structure of the mucous and skin membranes of the body by stopping their structural breakdown through HYL inhibition while at the same time counteracting the HYL release by bacteria. This stops the bacterial movement into the body. A number of viruses also use HYL to help them penetrate the body; this is especially true of cancer viruses. 5) Hyaluronidase is also found in some snake venoms. It increases the lethality of the venom, in part by allowing it to penetrate more easily into the body.

ANTIVIRAL ACTIVITY

Echinacea is antiviral; it's been found active against HIV and influenza H5N1, H7N7, and H1N1 (swine origin). However, in order to inactivate the influenza strains, it needs *direct contact* just prior to or right at the moment of infection. Echinacea inhibits receptor cell binding activity of the virus, interfering with its entry into the cells while at the same time strengthening the protective power of the mucous membranes through HYL inhibition.

ANTIBACTERIAL ACTIVITY

Echinacea is antibacterial; it inactivates *Streptococcus pyogenes*, *Haemophilus influenzae*, *Propionbacterium acnes*, and *Legionella pneumophila*. It also completely reverses the inflammatory processes that are initiated by those organisms. Echinacea is less active against *Staphylococcus aureus* and *Mycobacterium smegmatis* but also completely reverses the inflamation that they cause. Again, *direct contact* is necessary.

Echinacea is also active against *Leishmania major* promastigotes and *Leishmania enrietti*. *E. angustifolia* is active against *Pseudomonas aeruginosa*.

Echinacea is also active against numerous species of *Candida*. In vitro research found that a hexane extract of echinacea inhibited *Candida shehata*, *C. kefyr*, *C. albicans*, *C. steatulytica*, and *C. tropicalis*. In other studies echinacea increased the proliferation of phagocytes in spleen and bone marrow and the migration of granulocytes to peripheral blood. These studies found that echinacea was specifically active against systemic candida in the blood. In fact, mice were then protected from lethal injections of the yeast directly into the blood. In mice whose levels of leukocytes in the peripheral blood had been reduced through injection of cyclophosphamide, echinacea initiated an influx of neutrophil granulocytes that protected the mice from candida infection.

In a study of recurrent candida vaginal yeast infections, half the women were treated with econazole nitrate (EN) alone, the other half were treated with EN and echinacea. Those using EN alone had a 60 percent recurrence rate, while those using EN and echinacea had only a 17 percent recurrence rate.

WOUND-HEALING ACTIVITY

The alcoholic extract of *E. pallida* reverses stress-delayed wound healing in mice. *E. purpurea* enhances wound healing in vocal fold wounds in pigs. Echinacea (type not stated but probably *purpurea*) enhances fibrin formation in skin grafts, decreases wound healing time, stimulates the formation of new connective tissue, and reduces leukocytic infiltration.

ANTI-INFLAMMATORY ACTIONS

Angustifolia, *purpurea*, and *pallida* are all potent inhibitors of nitric oxide. *Pallida* is the strongest. Arginase activity is significantly increased by all three, but only *pallida* inhibits inducible nitric oxide synthase.

Most echinacea species strongly inhibit PGE production; *sanguinea* is strongest, followed by *angustifolia* and *pallida*.

Constituents of echinacea (echinacoside, etc.) protect collagen from free-radical-induced degradation.

PAIN RELIEF

Angustifolia is 10 times more potent a pain reliever than capsaicin. It acts by desensitizing the TRPV1 channel.

ANTICANCER/RADIATION PROTECTION

Echinacea reversed the system effects of gamma-irradiated mice: Red blood cell parameters, white blood cell parameters, and bone marrow cell parameters were all ameliorated. Echinacea (type not stated) was found to significantly abate leukemia and extend the life span of leukemic mice.

IMMUNE ACTIVITY

Echinacea increases the expression of CD69 and CD25 immune cells in vitro.

In vitro studies on the effects of seven species of echinacea on peripheral blood mononuclear cells (PBMC) found that tinctures from four (*angustifolia, pallida, paradoxa,* and *tennesseensis*) stimulated proliferation of PBMCs and increased interleukin-2 (IL-2). Two tinctures (*sanguinea* and *simulata*) stimulated proliferation only. *E. purpurea* stimulated IL-2 only. None of the extracts affected IL-4 or tumor necrosis factor-alpha (TNF-alpha). However, if volunteers were first immunized against influenza and *that* blood tested, tinctures from four (*pallida, paradoxa, sanguinea,* and *simulata*) diminished influenza-specific IL-2. None affected influenza-specific IL-10 or interferon-gamma (IFN-gamma). With blood drawn 6 months postvaccination, four tinctures (50 percent alcohol, *angustifolia, purpurea, simulata,* and *tennesseensis*) augmented IL-10 production and diminished IL-2, with no effect on IFN-gamma. Two (*paradoxa* and *sanguinea*) were similar though weaker. *E. pallida* suppressed all cytokines. The authors note that the various species have different immune-modulating actions.

Three echinacea species were tested for in vivo (mice) enhancement of innate and adaptive immune functions. All three (*angustifolia, purpurea,* and *pallida*) significantly increased antibody response, altered cytokine expression by splenic cells, significantly increased interferon-alpha production, and inhibited the release of TNF-alpha and IL-1 beta. Only two (*angustifolia* and *pallida*) strongly enhanced T cell proliferation, significantly stimulated IL-4 production, and decreased IL-10.

Alkamides from echinacea (type not stated) were found to potently inhibit inflammation in human blood and to exert modulatory effects on various cytokine expression (up-regulating IL-6 and inhibiting TNF-alpha, IL-1 beta, IL-12p70).

A butanol fraction from *purpurea* stems and leaves significantly up-regulated specific genes for IL-8, IL-1 beta, IL-18, and the chemokines CXCL2, CCL5, and CCL2 within

4 hours after treatment of immature dendritic cells.

In vivo studies on mice vaccinated with killed *Salmonella typhimurium* vaccine or an inactivated pertussis vaccine consisting of diphtheria/tetanus toxoids and inactivated virulence factors of *Bordetella pertussis* found that *E. angustifolia* and *purpurea* significantly increased antibody production and proliferation as well as IL-12 levels.

A rather large number of studies found that echinacea activates cellular immunity and stimulates phagocytosis of neutrophils in vitro, in vivo, and, in one case, after rinsing of the mouth cavity. In numerous studies echinacea increases interferon-gamma production, stimulates T helper cell production and proliferation, and strongly enhances CD4 and CD8 subsets.

Echinacea has a wide range of actions on the immune system and is both highly stimulatory and modulatory. It is an effective modulator of macrophage immune responses. It enhances antibody responses to infection. It is 30 percent more effective, for example, than sodium alginate in the stimulation of antivenom (snake) antibodies. It stimulates the production of neutrophils, macrophages, and T and B cells.

Eleuthero

Family: Araliaceae

Common Names: *(English) eleuthero • Siberian ginseng • touch-me-not • devil's shrub*

Species Used: There are 25 or maybe 38 species (thanks, guys) in the genus, and while the primary one used is *Eleutherococcus senticosus,* there is emerging evidence that a number of the species are also medicinally active in similar ways. *Eleutherococcus sessiflorus* is used in Korea, identically to eleuthero. *Eleutherococcus cissifolius* is used in Tibet, fresh juice for eczema.

Eleutherococcus spinosus (a.k.a. *E. pentaphyllus*, fiveleaf aralia) is an invasive in the United States in Connecticut, Indiana, Kentucky, Massachusetts, Utah, and West Virginia, and, as well, Ontario, Canada. It is used similarly to eleuthero as a tonic adaptogen for general debility, rheumatic pains, and weakness. Its use should be explored as a now locally established, important immune plant and adaptogen.

Note: *Acanthopanax senticosus* is sometimes given as a synonym for *E. senticosus.*

Parts Used

The root is the most commonly used part of the plant, but the bark from the woody stems is actually higher in what is considered to be the most active constituent of the plant (eleutheroside B). The fruits are also usable and the leaves have some activity as well. The Chinese use every part of the plant in various ways for this and that.

Preparation and Dosage

There are, in general, three primary forms of eleuthero that are used:
1) the Russian high-concentration formulations, generally 2:1, 1:1, or 1:2;
2) lower-strength 1:5 tincture formulations; and, finally,
3) capsules, usually standardized in some way or another (though I prefer the powdered herb myself).

If you are growing the plant and making your own extracts, the eleutheroside B content in the bark of woody stems is about four times that of the roots, so use that rather than kill the plant to get the roots.

RUSSIAN/HIGH-STRENGTH FORMULATIONS

Most of the Russian studies were conducted using a 1:1 tincture in 30 percent to 33 percent alcohol. The dosage ranged from 2 to 20 ml per day (the smaller dose is a smidgeon under ½ teaspoon). This means people were taking from 1/16 to ⅔ ounce (and in some instances up to 1½ ounces) of tincture per day. At an average cost of $7 to $12 per ounce of tincture (in the United States) this can be prohibitively expensive at the upper dosage ranges.

The Russians generally dosed 2–16 ml, one to three times daily for 60 days with a 2- to 3-week rest period in between. Russian researchers, at these kinds of dosages, saw responses within a few days or even hours of administration.

In this concentration, and at those doses, eleuthero is an immune *stimulant*, not a tonic. Using it at those doses in this concentrated a form is, in my opinion, specific for debilitating diseases accompanied by severe fatigue, brain fog, depression, muscle weakness, tendency to start getting better with inevitable relapse, and chronically depressed immune function.

You can, of course, take lower doses of the concentrated extracts, which would indeed make the tincture more tonic in nature.

Dosage of the Russian formulation in treating chronic, debilitating disease: *Please read carefully.* In chronic, highly debilitated conditions, the stronger Russian formulation is the only type of tincture that should be used—at least initially. I suggest the product sold by Herb Pharm, which is the only company I know of that actually exceeds the Russian specifications. Their formula is a 2:1 rather than a 1:1 (i.e., 2 parts herb to 1 part liquid rather than 1 and 1).

For the first 30 to 60 days: 1 tsp, 3x daily, the last dose occurring no later than 4 P.M. This dose can be increased if necessary.

After 60 days: Discontinue the herb for 2 weeks.

Then: Repeat if necessary.

If symptoms decrease after using the Russian formulation for a while and immune function seems better, you can change to either an encapsulated form or a 1:5 alcohol/water tincture (see below). Both of these are weaker, but more tonic, in their actions.

If symptoms and overall health are better on the stronger extract but worsen once you stop it, or if the presenting symptoms are severe, then the extract may be a better choice for continual use instead. Continue the dosage of the stronger extract: 30 to 60 days on, 2 to 3 weeks off, 30 to 60 days on, and so on.

TONIC FORMULATIONS AND DOSAGES

I have generally used, and prefer in conditions other than persistent chronic disease (e.g., Lyme disease) or severe chronic fatigue, a weaker tincture, as do many American herbalists and herbal companies: 1:5, 60 percent alcohol, 1 dropperful (1/3 tsp) of the tincture, 1–3x daily for up to a year.

In my experience this dosage and pattern of use is less stimulating

Properties of Eleuthero

Actions

- Adaptogen (a substance that increases non-specific resistance to adverse influences)
- Adrenal tonic
- Antidepressant
- Antifatigue
- Antistressor
- Helps restore task endurance
- Immune potentiator
- Immune tonic
- Immunoadjuvant
- MAO inhibitor
- Mental clarity stimulant

Finding Eleuthero

Herb stores everywhere; the Internet. But really, if you are in a region in which the plant will grow easily, buy a few seedlings and plant them. Once established, the plant will spread and provide medicine for you forever.

to the system and the long-term effects are better. The body gradually uses the herb to build itself up over time, the herb acting more as a long-term tonic and rejuvenative than an active stimulant. With this type of tincture it is not necessary to stop every 1 to 2 months, nor have I seen any of the side effects that can occur with the stronger Russian formula. The Chinese, much less given to tincturing anyway, use 4.5–27 grams, often as a decoction or powder.

This weaker American tincture in my clinical experience takes 6 months to become really effective and should be used at least that long; a year is better. It is great for long-term, mild chronic conditions that won't resolve and that present, in Caucasians, with a pallid face, poor elasticity in the skin, mild skin eruptions, weak energy, monotonic voice, and general passivity.

ENCAPSULATED HERB

For the encapsulated form I suggest 1,200 mg minimum daily. In acute conditions 3x that amount. Some manufacturers used to standardize the herb to 0.8 percent eleutherosides B&E, but that is becoming less common as the herb is understood better. I am not sure it is necessary.

POWDERED HERB

I like this form of the root and, in conditions such as severe, long-term chronic fatigue, blend it with some other powdered herbs that I buy by the pound (Pacific Botanicals—see Sources of Supply on page 599—is good for this): 2 parts each eleuthero, astragalus, milk thistle seed, and spirulina, and 1 part each licorice, chlorella, turmeric, and ashwagandha. Take it for a year, 1/4 cup of the blend, every night just before bed, mixed in 8–12 ounces juice or water in a blender. It will turn the condition around.

I also use it by itself sometimes, a tablespoon in a bit of water or juice.

Side Effects and Contraindications

Insomnia and hyperactivity can occur with use of the stronger Russian formulation, especially when taken in large doses. *Do not take after 4 P.M.*, just an FYI on that one.

Eleutherococcus is, in general, completely nontoxic and the Russians have reported the use of exceptionally large doses for up to 20 years with no adverse reactions. It is especially indicated for people with pale unhealthy skin, lassitude, and depression.

For almost all people no side effects have been noted. A very small number of people have experienced transient diarrhea. It may temporarily increase blood pressure in some people. This tends to drop to normal within a few weeks. Caution should be exercised for people with very high blood pressure (180/90) especially if eleuthero is combined with other hypertensives such as licorice.

With extreme overuse: tension and insomnia.

Herb/Drug Interactions

Increases the effects of hexobarbital, monomycin, kanamycin.

Habitat and Appearance

Siberian ginseng, a persistent, aggressive shrub from 3 to 15 feet in height, grows throughout parts of China, Russia, Korea, and even a bit in the northern islands of Japan. The plant is native to, as Richo Cech at Horizon Herbs puts it, "cold northern lakeshores and woods of China and Siberia." Essentially, it likes mixed and coniferous mountain forests that have good soils and get a bit cold. I have found related aralias growing to 9,500 feet in the Colorado mountains in similar terrain. The American ginseng grows in similar, though wetter, and not nearly so high, terrain in the Midwest and northeastern United States, often among oaks or oak/pine mixed forest. Eleuthero will apparently grow wherever other aralias have established themselves—similar-terrain sort of thing.

Eleuthero's stem is covered with spines and the plant, when mature, presents an aggressive, intimidating presence that has given rise to some of its common Russian names: touch-me-not and devil's shrub. After flowering, it produces clusters of blue-black berries a bit similar to blueberries in appearance. Typical aralia/ginseng family leaves.

Due to its popularity as a medicinal, it is undergoing heavy planting in the United States and has begun to escape captivity. Soon it will be, like a number of important medicinals (among them Japanese knotweed and about half of the plants discussed in this book), a naturalized, aggressive weed with qualities unknown to those it irritates. (It is currently considered invasive in Ohio and Tennessee.)

Cultivation and Collection

The plant is generally cultivated from seeds, but it will, so they say, apparently sprout easily from stem and root cuttings as well—strip or prune off the lower leaves from the stems, stick into moist potting soil or well-drained garden soil—in autumn. Keep moist until well rooted.

Eleuthero, according to gardeners whom I trust, likes rich soil, lots of water, and deep woods. However, some other sources indicate the plant is hardy to zone 3 and can grow in sandy, loamy, or clay soils, even if they are nutritionally poor, even in full or partial sun. I don't know, I haven't seen an aralia or ginseng grow in those kind of soils or conditions. Nice, though, if true.

Horizon Herbs (see Sources of Supply on page 599) sells stratified seeds in hydrated coir, pretty much guaranteed to germinate. Once established, the plant never goes away. It takes about 4 years before the plant is mature enough to produce flowers and seeds. The eleutheroside content is much higher by the fourth year. Don't harvest before then.

The roots and stem bark are harvested in the fall. Cut the larger roots into smaller pieces, peel the stem bark off in strips. Leave in a drying tray until antihydration is completed. Store as usual—plastic bags, in plastic bins, out of the light in a cool location. I would strongly suggest harvesting the fruit and drying it for later use in syrups.

Commercially purchased root in bulk will already be cut and sifted or powdered to industry standards.

Plant Chemistry

Eleutherosides A through M, ciwujianosides, eleutherans, isofraxidin, friedelin, beta-sitosterol, daucosterol, ethylgalactoside, chlorogenic acid, rosmarinic acid, and so on. A lot of people think the eleutherosides are the important adaptogenic and immune constituents, especially eleutheroside B and perhaps E.

Chlorogenic acid is a fairly strong antioxidant and antihyperglycemic with antiviral, antibacterial, and antifungal actions. It slows the movement of glucose into the blood. Rosmarinic acid is also potently antioxidant and anti-inflammatory, with antiviral and antibacterial actions as well.

Eleutheroside B content in the bark of the woody stems (400 mg/100 gm) is nearly four times that of the roots; eleutheroside E content, however (30 mg/100 gm), is only about one-third that of the roots. The fruits have about the same eleutheroside E content as the stem bark but only about one-tenth the eleutheroside B content. The stem bark (850 mg/100 gm) has 50 percent more chlorogenic acid than the roots but half the rosmarinic acid (11 mg/100 gm). The fruits have half as much chlorogenic acid but eight times the rosmarinic acid as the stem bark. The fruits are high in rutoside (150 mg/100 gm), the stem bark not so much (66 mg/100 gm).

Traditional Uses of Eleuthero

Though used in China for several thousand years, *Eleutherococcus* was brought to prominence by intensive Russian research in the latter half of the twentieth century. Then the emerging herbal renaissance in the United States caught wind of it, retitled the plant Siberian ginseng, and the boom was born. It became a major herb-of-the-day for a while, then was supplanted by rhodiola—the new kid on the block.

AYURVEDA

No record of it in my library or anyplace else I can find.

TRADITIONAL CHINESE MEDICINE

Acanthopanax gracilistylus and *A. senticosus* (a.k.a. *Eleutherococcus senticosus*) are both used in Chinese medicine. The former plant goes by *wu jia pi* and is used for relieving rheumatic conditions, for strengthening the tendons and bones, and for rheumatic arthralgia, weakness in the legs, retarded walking in children (striking image), and general weakness and debility. It does have some of the same eleutherosides in it.

Eleutherococcus senticosus goes by *ciwujia* in the Chinese system and does have a fairly strong presence in Chinese medicine. The Chinese use the root but also consider the stems, leaves, and fruit to be effective medicinals. Eleuthero is, in their system, vital-energy tonifying, spleen invigorating, kidney tonifying, and tranquilizing. It is used primarily for asthenia of the spleen and kidney, weakness and soreness of the lower back and knees, physical weakness, insomnia, frequent dreaming, and anorexia.

The Chinese have done some pretty good research on it as well.

WESTERN BOTANIC PRACTICE

Unknown in the West (unless you count Russia) until the herbal boom in the latter half of the twentieth century.

Scientific Research

Eleutherococcus has a number of complex effects on the body; there are four important ones: 1) on the hypothalamus/pituitary/adrenal system; 2) on the immune system; 3) on the liver and pancreas; and 4) on the heart and circulatory system. All these actions combine to produce the plant's unique adaptogenic actions.

The hypothalamus/pituitary/adrenal system: *Eleutherococcus* maintains the functioning of the hypothalamus/pituitary/adrenal system at optimum levels, altering its function in response to external factors. (As well, the herb appears to act as an adrenal tonic, helping restore function and health in both overworked and damaged adrenals.) If a person is under severe stress, the system ramps up; if the stress is less, the system activity lowers—in essence, the definition of an adaptogen. It helps the body adapt to external stressors, no matter what they are. The result of this is more energy, greater endurance, and enhanced response capacity to demands on the system.

The immune system: The herb has the same effects on the immune system; in other words, it maintains its functioning at optimum levels in response to outside stressors. In this instance, the stressors are disease organisms entering the body. Studies have found that *how* the immune system responds depends on what kind of disease stressor is affecting it. The different parts of the immune system are activated to match the particular type of stressor affecting the organism. Eleuthero has particularly strong effects on the spleen and spleen functioning.

The liver and pancreas: *Eleutherococcus* strongly affects the way the body deals with glucose in both the liver and pancreas, essentially optimizing how both organs affect glucose and then optimizing the actions of glucose in the body. This substantially increases energy levels. Essentially, it is fuel optimization.

The heart and circulatory system: The herb affects heart and vessel function, optimizing oxygen uptake, availability, and use in the body, thus increasing energy and endurance. Tendency toward hypoxia is reduced, no matter the cause.

Pharmacokinetic studies have found that the constituents from *Eleutherococcus* are first concentrated in the liver, kidneys, spleen, and pancreas. Within 2 to 4 hours they concentrate in the pituitary, heart, and adrenals. There are lesser concentrations in the thymus, testes, and brain. The concentration in the adrenals is three times that of the other organs. The constituents, once they reach the organs, begin exerting specific effects.

In the pancreas, the constituents concentrate in the islets of Langerhans, which are responsible for insulin synthesis. *Eleutherococcus* stimulates more efficient functioning of the islets, protects them from damage, and can both reverse and prevent alloxan-induced injury to them. This is part of the way the plant exerts effects on glucose metabolism. The resynthesis of glycogen is enhanced in the liver and throughout the body. Thus, as glycogen levels fall during exertion, they are resynthesized very rapidly so that energy levels remain high.

In the spleen, eleuthero stimulates the production of antibodies and facilitates the removal of antibody-coated bacteria. The production of monocytes is increased and their movement to injured tissues is facilitated, as is their transformation into macrophages. This increases phagocytosis, macrophage activity, and both innate and adaptive immune responses. Dendritic cell numbers and function are also increased. Dendritic cells are highly present in tissues that contact the external environment—skin, nose, lungs, stomach, intestines—as well as in the blood. They interact with T and B cells to initiate and shape adaptive immune responses. They are a crucial and major part of the immune system, and they are highly activated by *Eleutherococcus*; in essence, they become more potently adaptable in their immune responses.

Again, *Eleutherococcus*'s effects on the immune system are both stimulatory and modulatory; that is, the potency and sensitivity of the system is increased but how it behaves after that depends on the stressors the body is experiencing. Numerous studies, in vivo, show that *Eleutherococcus* significantly increases the survival time and number of survivors of mice injected with lethal microbes, irrespective of the disease organism used. It is highly stimulatory of the adaptive immune response to disease. The plant also helps the body more effectively deal with pollutants and toxic overload.

Additionally, *Eleutherococcus* does have some antiviral action. It inhibits human rhinovirus, respiratory syncytial virus, and influenza A virus in vitro. This, combined with its immune actions, makes it a perfect herb in helping prevent viral infections. One Russian study on young men using the herb found a significantly reduced incidence of influenza infection compared to those who did not use the herb. Another Russian study of 13,000 auto workers found that those who took the herb developed 40 percent fewer respiratory infections than was normal for their group. And in yet another one, conducted from 1973–1975, 1,200 auto workers were given the herb with tea annually for 2 months each time; disease incidence decreased by 20 percent to 30 percent, depending on the year.

A number of clinical trials have shown significant immune-enhancing activity, including significant increases in immunocompetent cells, specifically T lymphocytes (helper/

inducers, cytotoxic, and natural killer cells). Tests of the herb have repeatedly shown that it increases the ability of human beings to withstand adverse conditions, increases mental alertness, and improves performance. People taking the herb consistently report fewer illnesses than those who do not take the herb. Part of its power is its ability to act as a tonic stimulant on the adrenal glands. It normalizes adrenal activity and moves adrenal action away from a cortisol/catabolic dynamic to a DHEA/anabolic orientation. Basically, this reduces stress and normalizes physiological functioning throughout the body.

In another Russian clinical trial, 2,100 healthy adults were given the herb and were found to better handle stressful conditions. They showed increased ability to perform physical labor, withstand motion sickness, and work with speed and precision despite loud surroundings. Their ability to accurately proofread documents increased, and they more readily adapted to diverse physical stresses: high altitudes, heat, and low-oxygen environments.

Other studies have found that the herb heightens mental alertness, improves concentration, and boosts the transmission of nerve impulses in the brain.

There are scores of Russian studies; this just touches on them. A number of other studies have been conducted in the United States and Europe, most often on athlete endurance—which the herb helps.

The Chinese have done a number of studies on the plant. In vivo studies have found the plant to have significant calming actions in the CNS, to be highly regulatory of the body's response to nonspecific stimuli, to increase tolerance to hypoxia, to be protective from radiation exposure, to be actively detoxicant, to be a potent antistressor, to rectify endocrine disorders, to modulate both red and white blood cell levels and blood pressure levels, to have a wide range of immune modulation actions, to be antineoplastic and anti-inflammatory, to optimize heart function, to be gonadotrophic, and to stimulate tissue regeneration.

Chinese clinical studies found the herb useful in treating physical symptoms due to anxiety (insomnia, palpitations, anxiety, dizziness, and so on), to reverse leukopenia due to radiation, to be highly effective in treating coronary diseases of various etiology, and to be effective in acute obstructive cerebral thrombosis, chronic bronchitis in elderly patients, altitude sickness, arthritis, and chronic fatigue.

Eleutherococcus senticosus is strongly antihepatotoxic and hepatoprotective in vivo against CCL4-induced hepatotoxicity and is a hepatoregenerator, significantly stimulating liver regeneration in animals with portions of their liver surgically removed. Other studies have found the plant to have anticancer, antioxidant, and anti-inflammatory activity, to be of value in ischemic stroke, and to be fairly neuroprotective, while at the same time increasing mental alertness and acuity.

Red Root

In addition to its antiviral properties, red root is known as a lymph system stimulant and an anti-inflammatory for both the liver and spleen. It's a strong coagulant and low doses can markedly reduce blood clotting time. Historically it has been used to treat asthma, dysentery, syphilis, and more. To learn more about red root, turn to page 408.

Reishi

Family: Ganodermataceae

Common Names: *Reishi, which is the Japanese name for the plant, has become the most common name for the herb in the West.*

Species Used: There are 80 or maybe 250 species of ganoderma (taxonomy is a science?). A number of them are used medicinally. The primary medicinal is considered to be *Ganoderma lucidum* but *G. luteum, G. tsugae, G. applanatum, G. australe, G. capense, G. tropicum, G. tenue,* and *G. sinense* are also used.

In the Chinese system all are considered to possess slightly different effects. The mushrooms are grouped, medicinally, by their color. Blue (sour) is considered to improve eyesight and liver function and calm the nerves; red (bitter) is considered the most medicinally potent, and aids internal organs, improves memory, enhances vitality; yellow (sweet) strengthens spleen function, calms the spirit; white (hot) improves lung function, gives courage and strong will; black (salty) protects the kidneys; and purple (sweet) enhances function of the ears, joints, muscles, and helps the complexion.

Part Used

Generally the fruiting body, i.e., the mushroom itself, and sometimes the mycelium.

Preparation and Dosage

May be taken as tablets, tincture, syrup decoction, or powder, or even used as a soup base.

TABLETS

Take three 1-gram tablets (bought retail) up to 3x daily.

TINCTURE

1:5, 20 percent alcohol, 10–20 ml (2–4 tsp), up to 3x daily.

The tincture is best made by first making a decoction of the herb; this will extract the polysaccharides most efficiently. If you have 16 ounces of powdered reishi, you would then use 80 ounces of liquid, 64 ounces of which would be water, and 16 alcohol. Add the powdered or chopped-up reishi to the water, bring to a boil, cover, and slow-boil for 30 minutes. Allow to cool with the lid on. When cool, pour into a large jar, add 16 ounces pure grain alcohol, cover, and allow to steep for 2 weeks. Decant, press, and store.

SYRUP DECOCTION

Use 2–5 grams of reishi per quart of water depending on strength desired. Slowly bring to boil and simmer at lowest boil obtainable for 2 hours, uncovered, until the volume of water is reduced by two-thirds. Cool and strain. Consume in the evening before bed or in three equal amounts over the course of the day. In acute conditions the amount consumed can be increased as much as desired.

POWDER

Take 3–6 grams a day in chronic disease, 9–15 grams a day in acute conditions, equally divided in three doses. Stir into water and drink or encapsulate (6–12 "00" capsules in chronic disease, 18–30 in acute conditions).

For mushroom poisoning: Take 120–200 grams of dried powdered reishi in water, 3–5x daily.

Side Effects and Contraindications

Contraindicated in cases of obstructed bile duct. Occasionally, skin rash, loose stool, dry mouth, sleepiness, bloating, frequent urination, sweating, nausea may occur. Adverse reactions cease upon discontinuance of the herb. In the case of nausea take with meals.

Herb/Drug Interactions

Reishi is synergistic with cefazolin, interferon-alpha, and to some extent interferon-gamma, and potently so with acyclovir. Caution should be exercised if you are on immunosuppressive drugs. There may be an additive effect with blood-thinning medications such as aspirin or warfarin.

Habitat and Appearance

Reishi is a hard, tough, woody mushroom that has a shiny or varnished appearance to the cap. The Latin word for the primary medicinal species, *lucidum*, means "shiny" or "brilliant." Essentially, so does the genus name *Ganoderma*, from the Greek, *gano* meaning "sheen" or "brightness," *derma* meaning "skin." So . . . the Latinate term for the plant, created by botanists, means "shiny skin shiny." (Latin terminology is not all that philosophically deep. The sonorous sound of the words just makes us think so.)

The various species range in cap color from yellow to black, but the most common one found wild in the United States, *G. lucidum*, is red.

Reishi mushrooms grow on a wide variety of trees, often dead or dying, especially deciduous trees such as oak, elm, maple, willow, sweet gum, magnolia, plum, and locust. They will sometimes grow on coniferous trees such as pine, larch, and spruce. They tend to grow in temperate regions.

Cultivation and Collection

The fruiting mushroom bodies can be harvested at any time. They don't need any special treatment. Just let them sit out and dry thoroughly, then store in plastic bags in plastic tubs out of the light. They will last for years.

Properties of Reishi

Actions

Analgesic
Antiallergenic
Antibacterial
Antihepatotoxic
Antihyperbilirubinemic
Antihyperlipemic
Antihypertriglyceridemic
Anti-inflammatory
Antinephrotoxic
Antitumor
Antiviral
Cholagogue
Choleretic
Coronary vasodilator
Cytotoxic
Hepatoregenerator
Hypocholesterolemic
Hypotensive
Immunomodulator
Immunostimulant
Spleen and thymus tonic

As an immune stimulant, reishi stimulates interleukin 1 and 2, phagocytosis, and lymphocyte proliferation, enhances natural killer cells, activates macrophages, enhances polymorphonuclear leukocytes, protects and enhances T cells, enhances thymus weight and functioning, and stimulates gamma-interferon production. As an antitumor agent, it also reduces the proliferation of tumor cells and inhibits tumor necrosis factor. And as an antiviral, it's been shown to be active against numerous viruses, including HBV and HIV.

Finding Reishi

Herb shops everywhere, the Internet, or you can grow your own fairly easily—try Fungi Perfecti (fungi.com), which sells easy-to-use starter kits.

Reishi can be easily cultivated through the use of inoculated wooden dowels or plugs. It does best in nonaromatic hardwoods. Cut a log into sections, let it sit out for a few months, then drill and insert the plugs, generally in early spring after the last frost. The mycelium will spread through the log the first year and begin producing mushrooms the second year. Try Fungi Perfecti (fungi.com) for inoculated plugs and much more information.

Plant Chemistry

Over 400 different bioactive constituents have been identified in reishi so far. One hundred forty of them are triterpenes, primarily ganodermic acids, though there are 10 specific groups. Over 100 additional compounds are polysaccharides, which produce many of the plant's immune actions. There are numerous other compounds, one of which—the LZ-8 protein—has fairly strong immune-stimulating actions in the spleen and on peripheral lymphocytes.

Traditional Uses of Reishi

AYURVEDA

Apparently unknown, though there is a similar mushroom recorded in Indian lore, a mysterious *chih* fungus considered to be an herb of immortality. Versions of the Indian legends of the fungus are rife in ancient Chinese literature and are considered, by many historical figures, to be *ling chih*, or reishi. I can't find any reference to reishi in Ayurvedic practice in my library, however.

TRADITIONAL CHINESE MEDICINE

Ganoderma is known as *ling chih* or *ling zhi* (mushroom of immortality) in China and *reishi* (ten-thousand-year mushroom) in Japan, under which name it is now commonly known in the West. The reputation of the herb is as a longevity and vitality-enhancing tonic.

Reishi has been used in China and Japan for at least 4,000 years in the treatment of debility from prolonged illness, for "deficiency" fatigue, as an antiaging herb, and for coronary heart disease, hepatitis, kidney disease, arthritis, hypertension, sleep disorders, asthma and bronchitis, ulcer, and nerve pain.

In TCM it is considered warming, tonic, nourishing, antitoxic, astringent, and dispersing of accumulations. At least five species of *Ganoderma* are used in traditional medicine in China and Japan, each for different disorders. *Ganoderma lucidum,* in many respects, is considered to be the most potent.

WESTERN BOTANIC PRACTICE

Apparently unknown until its introduction by traditional Chinese practitioners in the mid-to-late twentieth century. Western use has been stimulated by the extensive studies carried out in Japan (for the most part).

Scientific Research

The best overviews of *Ganoderma,* I think, are S. Bhagwan et al., "*Ganoderma lucidum:* A Potent Pharmacological Macrofungus," and R. Russel and M. Paterson, "*Ganoderma*: A Therapeutic Fungal Biofactory."[1] They cover about everything, however . . . a brief look:

In vivo and in vitro studies have found reishi to be liver regenerative, liver protective, choleretic, liver enzyme normalizing, analgesic, antiallergenic, anti-inflammatory, antibacterial, antiviral, antioxidant, antitumor (inhibiting or regressing tumors), hypotensive, a bronchial relaxant, immunostimulant, immunomodulating, cardiotonic, expectorant, and antitussive.

Human trials have found effectiveness for neurasthenia, insomnia, dizziness, duodenal ulcers, liver pain, rhinitis, muscular dystrophy, stress, Alzheimer's disease, hyperlipidemia, liver failure, diabetes, cancer, immune enhancement, and hepatitis.

Although not primarily thought of as such, reishi is antibacterial, antifungal, and a fairly potent antiviral against a number of pathogens.

Reishi is antibacterial against *Helicobacter pylori, Pseudomonas syringae, P. aeruginosa, E. coli, Bacillus subtilis, Staphylococcus aureus, Klebsiella pneumoniae, Salmonella typhi, Micrococcus flavus,* and *Micrococcus luteus.*

Reishi is a strong antiviral, especially against hepatitis viruses. It is active against influenza A viruses, potently so against herpes simplex virus 1 and 2 (it also inhibits their attachment and penetration into cells), and strongly so against vesicular stomatitis virus, Epstein-Barr virus, and HIV.

Reishi is active against *Candida* spp., *Microsporum canis, Trichophyton mentagrophytes.* It is also active against plasmodial parasites.

Like eleuthero, reishi has profound effects on the immune system, especially the spleen, stimulating its immune responses considerably. Reishi is strongly mitogenic, especially on splenocytes, stimulating the generation of highly active immune cells. It activates immune effector cells such as T cells, macrophages, and natural killer cells and increases the production of cytokines, including interleukins, tumor necrosis factor-alpha, and interferons. Reishi potently stimulates macrophages and their activity in the body against pathogens. The primary clinical studies on the enhancement of immune function have occurred with cancer patients; most immune studies have been in vivo or in vitro.

Reishi has a number of fairly potent anticancer actions, which are generating a lot of interest. It reduces angiogenesis, the formation of new blood cells by tumors, is antiproliferative, has direct anticancer effects on a number of cancer cell lines, including prostate, colon, leukemia, lymphoma, and myeloma cells, strongly inhibits intracellular signaling and invasive behavior of cancer cells, protects the body from radiation damage during cancer treatment, and mediates cancer cell growth through enhancement of host immune defenses.

Here is a sampling of a few clinical trials: In one human trial of 355 people with hepatitis B, with a combination formula containing reishi, 92.4 percent of patients showed improvement. Another trial found that patients with hepatitis B experienced the alleviation of hepatitis symptoms and lowering of SGOT and SGPT levels. Other trials showed reduction in blood pressure in all patients with hypertension who took reishi over a 6-month period. In trials with over 2,000 patients with chronic bronchitis, 60 percent to 90 percent experienced alleviation of symptoms, marked improvement, and weight gain. Studies with people with high blood pressure have consistently showed improvement in blood pressure levels and people with impaired memory or thinking have shown increased mental clarity and memory.

Reishi has a long history of folk and historical clinical use in protecting the liver against *Amanita phalloides* poisoning, though I could locate no specific trials.

Rhodiola

Family: Crassulaceae

Common Names: *Rhodiola • golden root • roseroot • stonecrop • arctic root. The fresh roots smell a bit like roses, hence the origin of that name. They are golden in color, thus golden root.*

Species Used: There is, as usual, confusion among those with advanced degrees in plant science as to just how many species of rhodiola there are: 36, or maybe 60, or probably 90. It's like stamp collectors ("No, look at that tiny ink spot on the edge"); I just want to scream.

The primary medicinal that most people use is *Rhodiola rosea,* but many of the related species are used medicinally in the regions in which they grow. Because of the interest in *R. rosea*, the genus is being intensively studied for activity: I have found medicinal studies of one sort or another on *R. crenulata*, *R. quadrifida*, *R. heterodonta*, *R. semenovii*, *R. sachalinensis*, *R. sacra*, *R. fastigiata*, *R. kirilowii*, *R. bupleuroides*, *R. imbricata*, *R. rhodantha*, and *R. integrifolia*.

There have been some extravagant claims (easily found on the Internet) that *only* Russian *Rhodiola rosea*, harvested near the Arctic Circle (presumably by fasting virgins as the northern lights first emerge over the rim of Earth), contains the necessary active constituents for the herb to be useful. However, *all* the *Rhodiola rosea* plants, irrespective of where they grow or in what country, have nearly identical chemistry. They are all perfectly usable as medicine.

But please note: The exact chemical profile of the *R. rosea* plants themselves differs depending on time of year, time of day, and geographical location (this valley in Russia or *that* one) irrespective of whether they are harvested at the Arctic Circle in Russia by fasting virgins or not. In other words, you can pick *R. rosea* from this location in May and again in September and the chemical profile of the plant *won't* be the same. The same is true of every species in the genus—and of every medicinal plant on Earth. Part of the art of herbalism is being able to determine medicinal potency of the plants you are harvesting by using the most sophisticated scientific instrument ever discovered—the focused power of human awareness. Machines just aren't a reliable substitute for the capacity to reason *and* feel simultaneously. Furthermore . . . oops! Sorry. Got carried away again.

Studies on 14 other species in the genus have found the same constituents in them as in *R. rosea*. They can all be used medicinally, they all do pretty much the same things, and they all work identically to the usual commercial-variety *R. rosea*—see Scientific Research (page 531) for more. *Rhodiola integrifolia*, by the way, is considered to be a natural hybrid between *Rhodiola rhodantha* and *R. rosea*; you can consider it pretty much identical to *R. rosea*.

Properties of Rhodiola

Actions

Adaptogen	Cardiotonic (potent)	Immune tonic
Adrenal protectant	Endocrine tonic	Mental stimulant
Anticancer	Ergogenic	Mitochondrial tonic and protectant
Antidepressant	Hippocampal protectant and tonic	Muscular stimulant
Antifatigue	Hypoxia antagonist (potent)	Nervous system tonic
Antioxidant (strong)		Neural protectant
Antistressor		

Possibly a synergist, the plant is a strong inhibitor of P-glycoprotein and CYP3A4. See the piperine monograph (page 447) for specifics.

Active Against

Again, this herb is not primarily an antimicrobial but it does have some antiviral actions. It is active against influenza viruses due to its neuraminidase inhibitory activity. It has been found active against H1N1 and H9N2 viral strains. It is also active against the hepatitis C and Coxsackie B3 viruses. One of its constituents, kaempferol, is specific against Japanese encephalitis virus and enterovirus 71. It has some antibacterial activity as well, against *Staphylococcus aureus* (strong), *Bacillus subtilis* and *Mycobacterium tuberculosis* (moderate), *E. coli* (weak).

Use to Treat

Brain fog	Chronic fatigue syndrome	Low immune function
Chronic disease conditions with depression	Chronic, long-term fatigue	Nervous exhaustion
		Recurrent infections

Rhodiola can also be used to accelerate recovery from debilitating conditions and long-term illness and infections.

Other Uses

The leaves of most species can be eaten, chopped finely and added to salads, or cooked as a pot herb. The plants are very high in vitamin C, with 33 mg per gram of fresh plant.

Finding Rhodiola

You can buy it pretty much everywhere. If you live in the right climate you can probably find it wild or grow it yourself.

Note: The rhodiolas look much like sedums and were once included in that genus, so you will see rosea sometimes listed as *Sedum rosea* and so on.

Parts Used

The root.

Preparation and Dosage

Generally used as capsules or tincture.

TINCTURE

Dried root, 1:5, 50 percent alcohol. Some people use a 1:3 formulation. I am not sure it is necessary.

Tonic dose: 30–40 drops, 3x or 4x daily, usually in water.

In acute conditions: ½–1 tsp, 3x daily for 20 to 30 days, then back to the tonic dose.

CAPSULES

The root is most often used in capsule form, 100 mg each. Usual dose is 1 or 2 capsules per day. In acute conditions up to 1,000 mg a day can be taken. The capsules are often standardized to contain 2 percent to 3 percent rosavins and 0.8 percent to 1 percent salidroside. They are usually taken just before meals.

Side Effects and Contraindications

Some people experience jitteriness from the herb; you should not take it at night until you know if you are one of them.

Herb/Drug Interactions

None noted.

Habitat and Appearance

Rhodiolas are plants that like high altitude and cold, either will do. They are a circumpolar genus of the subarctic and cool, mountainous regions of the northern hemisphere and are common in eastern Russia, parts of China, Tibet (which has many species), the mountains and northern climes of Europe, Canada, and the mountainous and colder regions of the United States. The United States, Europe, and Tibet appear to have the largest populations, with Tibet having the most species.

The rhodiolas are typical succulents with fleshy, moisture-filled, grayish-green leaves. The plants grow to about 12 inches, and they will have, depending on the species, a cluster of yellow, pink, red, or orange flowers at the top of the stalk. *R. rosea*'s flowers are yellow.

The root system is fairly large if the plants grow in a nutrient-rich environment. The farther north they grow, and the poorer the soils, the smaller the root.

There are three species of rhodiola in North America: *Rhodiola rosea* grows in the mountains of North Carolina, and in Pennsylvania through New England, into Canada, and all the way to the Arctic Circle. *R. rhodantha* grows in the Rocky Mountain states from New Mexico and Arizona up to the Canadian border. *R. integrifolia* has the widest distribution in North America. It ranges from the Rocky Mountain spine (New Mexico, et cetera, westward) up into Canada and into the Arctic. There are populations as well in Minnesota and New York State. Most of the eastern rhodiolas are considered to be endangered.

If you are in the western United States and wanting to wild-harvest your own roots, look for *R. integrifolia*; it is just as useful as *R. rosea* medicinally *and* it is not endangered as many of the eastern United States *R. rosea* populations are.

Cultivation and Collection

Due to the popularizing of the plant as an antiaging and chronic fatigue medicinal, wild populations of *R. rosea* are becoming endangered; the Russians have put them on their red list of threatened plants. The largest populations of the plant were formerly in the Altai region of southern Siberia. However, over 45 companies have been harvesting the plant for export ("*Real* Russian rhodiola") and those plant populations have been severely reduced.

If you live in a region in which rhodiola grows, you can harvest your own roots; you won't need to harvest much for yourself and your family. Commercial harvesting, except for very limited amounts in abundant areas, is highly discouraged.

If you find the plant in your area, harvest the roots in the fall after seeding or in the spring just as it is coming up. The roots will be bigger and, in my opinion, more potent in the spring. Slice the bigger roots; the interior of the root will change from white to a brown or reddish color as it begins to dry.

Due to the heavy worldwide demand for the plant, there are increasing efforts to make the plant an agricultural staple in regions where it will grow; Bulgaria, Canada, and Finland are early innovators in growing the crop. The yields are low, only about 3 tons per hectare, and they are labor intensive. Since the roots are taken, and only after 5 years, agricultural growing of the plant demands a minimum of five fields, planted in rotation so they can be harvested in successive years in order to keep up continual production.

The seeds are tiny; a thousand of them weigh only 0.2 gram. The germination rates are low, 2 percent to 36 percent; they are happier with a little stratification. Thirty days at 23°F will increase germination rates to 50 percent to 75 percent. Soak the seeds in water overnight, mix into moist soil, store for 1 month at a temperature of 36° to 39°F. You will then get about a 75 percent germination rate.

In Finland they get 95 percent to 100 percent germination if they sow the seeds on the surface of a sand/peat mix and keep the trays outside all winter under the snow. In April/May the boxes are brought into a greenhouse at a temperature of 64° to 72°F. Germination begins in 3 days to a week.

If you keep the seedlings inside for a year before transplanting, yields are significantly higher. They like sandy, loamy soil that is neutral or slightly acidic. NPK: 50/50/70. They don't need additional fertilizer after the first year. The easiest method, however, is to divide the roots of an established plant and plant the root cuttings, much like potatoes.

The plant takes a minimum of 3 years to mature, but the roots should not be harvested for 5 years. Dig in the fall, slice, let dry out of the sun. Store in plastic bags, inside plastic containers, in the dark.

Plant Chemistry

Most people think that salidroside (a.k.a. rhodioloside) is the most important compound in the root, others insist it is the rosavin. Others say, yeah, those and . . . rosin, rosarin, and tyrosol. Studies have found, as usual, that salidroside is much more effective when combined with rosavin, rosin, and rosarin. So I'm guessing, just a wild shot here, that it's the whole root that is most active.

There are, of course, a great many other compounds in the root, at least 85 essential oils and another 50 water-soluble nonvolatiles. Many of the usual plant compounds are present.

Traditional Uses of Rhodiola

Rhodiola, as far as I can tell, and in spite of assertions that it is a long-standing medicinal in traditional Chinese medicine (TCM), was a contribution to the medicinal plant world by the Russians due to their interest in adaptogens. This is pretty much a Russian-introduced category of medicinal herb—a plant that enhances general overall functioning, somewhat like a tonic but one that increases the ability of the organism to respond to outside stressors of whatever sort, diseases included. It enhances an organism's general resistance to multiple adverse influences or conditions. Rhodiola, like the stronger preparations of *Eleutherococcus*, is considered to be not just adaptogenic but an adaptogenic stimulant—part of the reason it can cause jitteriness and wakefulness in some.

AYURVEDA AND TCM

Rhodiolas have been used in TCM, Tibetan medicine, and Ayurveda for a very long time—according to many reports. But my library, extensive, doesn't list the genus in any of my source books for those systems of healing.

However, a few other, obscure sources reveal that the plants were used in traditional Russian folk medicine to increase physical endurance, work productivity, longevity, resistance to altitude sickness and for fatigue, depression, anemia, impotence, GI tract ailments, infections, and nervous afflictions.

In central Asia the tea has been used for a long time as the most effective local treatment for colds and flu. Mongolian physicians use it for TB and cancer. The plant is a part of traditional Tibetan medicine for promoting blood circulation and relieving cough.

WESTERN BOTANIC PRACTICE

The plant never was a huge medicinal even though there are traces of its use as far back as the seventeenth century in the Scandinavian countries. *Rhodiola rosea* and *R. integrifolia* were used by the indigenous tribes of Alaska as a food, the root eaten for sores in the mouth, for TB, stomachache, and GI tract troubles. A couple of the sedums were recognized by the Eclectics but none of the rhodiolas before their name change.

Scientific Research

There is a lot of research on this plant right now, and more studies are occurring daily. There have been, unlike the case for many other newish medicinal plants, a lot of human clinical trials with this herb. I am primarily going to look at the neuroprotective/neuroregenerative, immune, and antistress/antifatigue actions of the plant—they are strongly interrelated. The potent antioxidant actions of the plant are deeply interrelated with those as well.

ANTIVIRAL/ANTIBACTERIAL

A number of the rhodiolas have been found to have antiviral and antibacterial actions. *Rhodiola kirilowii* is active against the hepatitis C virus and *Mycobacterium tuberculosis*; *Rhodiola rosea* is active against H1N1 and H9N2 viral influenza strains as well as Coxsackie virus B3.

NEUROPROTECTIVE/NEUROREGENERATIVE

Numerous rhodiola species have been found to be highly neuroprotective.

In vitro: Compounds in both *Rhodiola sacra* and *R. sachalinensis* protect neurons against beta-amyloid-induced, stauroporine-induced, and H2O2-induced death. Salidroside, a common compound in many rhodiolas, protects cultured neurons from injury from hypoxia and hypoglycemia; protects neuronal PC12 cells and SH-SY5Y neuroblastoma cells against cytotoxicity from beta-amyloid and against hypoglycemia and serum limitation; and protects neurons against H2O2-induced death. It does so by inducing the antioxidant enzymes thioredoxin, heme oxygenase-1, and peroxiredoxin-1, down-regulating the pro-apoptotic gene Bax, and up-regulating the anti-apoptotic genes Bcl-2 and Bcl-X(L). It also restores mitochondrial membrane potential negatively affected by H2O2 and restores intracellular calcium levels.

In vivo: *Rhodiola rosea* enhances the level of 5-hydroxytryptamine in the hippocampus, promotes the proliferation and differentiation of neural stem cells in the hippocampus, and protects hippocampal neurons from injury. *R. rosea* protects against cognitive deficits, neuronal injury, and oxidative stress induced by intracerebroventricular injection of streptozotocin. Salidroside protects rat hippocampal neurons against H2O2-induced apoptosis. A combination of rhodiola/astragalus protects rats against simulated plateau hypoxia (26,000 feet). It inhibits the accumulation of lactic acid in brain tissue and serum.

Human clinical trial: A double-blind, placebo-controlled, randomized study with 40 women, ages 20 to 68, who were highly stressed, found that a *Rhodiola rosea* extract increased attention, speed, and accuracy during stressful cognitive tasks. *Rhodiola rosea* was used with 120 adults with both physical and cognitive deficiencies: exhaustion, decreased motivation, daytime sleepiness, decreased libido, sleep disturbances, concentration deficiencies, forgetfulness, decreased memory, susceptibility to stress, irritability; after 12 weeks, 80 percent of patients showed improvements. A combination formula (Xinnaoxin capsule) of *Rhodiola rosea*, *Lycium chinense* berry, and fresh *Hippophae rhomnoides* fruit juice was given to 30 patients with chronic cerebral circulatory insufficiency; after 4 weeks the condition was significantly improved. A double-blind, crossover 3-week study on stress-induced fatigue on the mental performance of healthy physicians during night duty found that *Rhodiola rosea* extract decreased mental fatigue and increased cognitive functions such as associative thinking, short-term memory, calculation and concentration, and speed of audio-visual perception.

ANTIFATIGUE/ANTISTRESS

In vitro: Salidroside stimulates glucose uptake by rat muscle cells; *Rhodiola rosea* extract stimulates the synthesis or resynthesis of ATP and stimulates reparative processes in mitochondria.

In vivo: *Rhodiola rosea* extracts increased the life span of *Drosophila melanogaster*, lowered mitochondrial superoxide levels, and increased protection against the superoxide generator paraquat. Four weeks' supplementation with *R. rosea* extract significantly increased swimming time in exhausted mice—it significantly increased liver glycogen levels;

SREBP-1, FAS, and heat shock protein 70 expression; Bcl-2/Bax ratios; and oxygen content in blood. Salidroside protected the hypothalamic/pituitary/gonad axis of male rats under intense stress—testosterone levels remained normal rather than dropping, secretary granules of the pituitary gland increased, and mitochondrial cells were strongly protected. *R. rosea* extract completely reversed the effects of chronic mild stress in female rats—that is, decreased sucrose intake, decreased movement, weight loss, and dysregulation of menstrual cycle. Rhodiola suppressed increased enzyme activity in rats subjected to noise stress—glutamic pyruvic transaminase, alkaline phosphatase, and creatine kinase levels all returned to normal, and glycogen, lactic acid, and cholesterol levels in the liver also returned to normal. *R. rosea* reduced stress and CRF-induced anorexia in rats. And so on.

Human clinical trial: Twenty-four men who had lived at high altitude for a year were tested to see the effects of rhodiola on blood oxygen saturation and sleep disorders. Rhodiola increased blood oxygen saturation significantly and increased both sleeping time and quality. In a double-blind, placebo-controlled study of the effects of *R. rosea* on fatigue in students caused by stress, physical fitness, mental fatigue, and neuro-motoric indices all increased (other studies found similar outcomes). *R. rosea* intake in a group of healthy volunteers reduced inflammatory C-reactive protein and creatinine kinase levels in the blood and protected muscle tissue during exercise. *Rhodiola rosea* in a placebo-controlled, double-blind, randomized study was found to increase physical capacity, muscle strength, speed of limb movement, reaction time, and attention—in other words it improved exercise endurance performance. A similarly structured study found that 1 week of rhodiola supplementation decreased fatigue and stress levels but more interestingly decreased photon emissions on the dorsal side of the hand. In another study *Rhodiola rosea* increased the efficiency of the cardiovascular and respiratory systems and prevented fatigue during an hour of continuous physical exercise. A phase three clinical trial found that rhodiola exerts an antifatigue effect that increases mental performance and concentration and decreases cortisol response in burnout patients with fatigue syndrome; other studies have found similar outcomes, including the amelioration of depression and anxiety.

IMMUNE ACTIONS

In vitro: *Rhodiola imbricata* protects macrophages against tert-butyl hydroperoxide injury and up-regulates the immune response. Additionally it potently stimulates the innate immune pathway and initiates strong immunostimulatory actions, increasing Toll-like receptor 4, granzyme B, and Th1 cytokines. *Rhodiola sachalinensis* extract enhances the expression of inducible nitric oxide synthase in macrophages. *Rhodiola quadrifida* stimulates granulocyte activity and increases lymphocyte response to mitogens. *Rhodiola algida* stimulates human peripheral blood lymphocytes and up-regulates IL-2 in Th1 cells and IL-4, 6, and 10 in Th2 cells.

In vivo: *Rhodiola kirolowii* enhances cellular immunity—stimulating the activity of lymphocytes, increasing phagocytosis in response to microbial organisms. *Rhodiola imbricata* enhances specific immunoglobulin levels in response to tetanus toxoid and ovalbumin in rats—the plant has adjuvant/immunopotentiating activity in both humoral and cell-mediated immune response.

Human clinical use: *Rhodiola rosea* (in combination with schizandra, eleuthero, and leuzea) significantly increased both cell-mediated and humoral immune response in ovarian cancer patients. Rhodiola significantly reduced problems and infection after the treatment of acute lung injury caused by massive trauma/infection and thoracic-cardio operations. A combination formula of rhodiola, eleuthero, and schizandra significantly enhanced positive outcomes in the treatment of acute nonspecific pneumonia. *Rhodiola rosea* increased the parameters of leukocyte integrins and T-cell immunity in bladder cancer patients.

OTHER ACTIONS

Rhodiola, various species, has been found effective in the treatment of breast cancer. It inhibits the tumorigenic properties of invasive mammary epithelial cells, inhibits superficial bladder cancer, suppresses T241 fibrosarcoma tumor cell proliferation, and reduces angiogenesis in various tumor lines. *Rhodiola imbricata* is highly protective in mice against whole-body lethal radiation.

The plant has also been found highly antioxidant in numerous studies, to be liver protective, and to be highly protective of the cardiovascular system.

The plant is adaptogenic; that is, it increases the function of the organism to meet whatever adverse influences are affecting it, whether stress or illness. Most of the attention has been paid to its ability to increase endurance and mental acuity, but its effects on the immune system, though less studied than eleuthero's, are similar.

8

A HANDBOOK OF HERBAL MEDICINE MAKING

[Our bodies] are not distinct from the bodies of plants and animals, with which we are involved in the cycles of feeding and the intricate companionships of ecological systems and of the spirit. They are not distinct from the earth, the sun and moon, and the other heavenly bodies. It is therefore absurd to approach the subject of health piecemeal with a departmentalized band of specialists. A medical doctor uninterested in nutrition, in agriculture, in the wholesomeness of mind and spirit is as absurd as a farmer who is uninterested in health. Our fragmentation of this subject cannot be our cure, because it is our disease.

—Wendell Berry, *The Unsettling of America*

Tremendous empowerment comes from learning to recognize the medicinal plants that surround us, even more in learning how to make them into medicines for healing. And though it takes time, as your knowledge increases, as you learn how to tend to your illnesses and those of your family, the sense of helplessness that so many of us have experienced when we become ill, often ingrained since birth, begins to dissipate.

We have been trained to place our health in the hands of outside specialists who, very often, know neither ourselves nor our families, not the fabric of our lives, nor the communities in which we live. They have no understanding of, and often no interest in, the complexity in which we live and from which our illnesses emerge. But for most of us, those specialists are the *only* place we know to go when we are ill, uncertain, and afraid, to seek help—for ourselves or our loved ones.

The world, however, is a great deal more complex than that frame allows, and there are many more options to healing than that system acknowledges. All of us live, all the time, in the midst of a living pharmacy that covers the surface of this planet. And that living pharmacy is there for you, or anyone, to use—anytime you wish. Once you *know* that, once you have been healed by the plants in that living pharmacy, often of something that physicians said could not be healed, things are never the same again. You begin to break the cycle of dependence on which the health care system depends.

Taking back control over personal health and healing is one of the greatest forms of personal empowerment that I know. It does take time and effort, this kind of learning, but the learning goes quickly. Harder, perhaps, is learning to trust the plants with your life. It is a truly frightening moment, that moment of decision, when trust is extended in that way, for, before it occurs, there is no way to experientially *know* what the outcome will be. Most people on this planet, though, people who do not live in the Western, industrialized nations, make that decision every day of their lives. It is a trust they extend every moment of every day. Trusting the healing capacities of the plants is not a new experience to the human species.

The next step in the journey is learning how to turn the plants you are learning about into medicines for yourself and your family. It isn't that hard—people all over the globe have been doing it for 100,000 years. At least.

To Begin With . . .

The first thing to understand is that there are no mistakes. You are learning a new skill and *everyone* learns what works by learning what doesn't. That is how human beings do it; we all learn to cook well by first cooking badly. So . . . enjoy the process and give yourself permission to make mistakes, to learn as you go.

If you are wildcrafting your medicines, the first step, of course, is getting to know the plants themselves, learning to recognize them in the wild, getting to know them where they live. I prefer finding a local plant person to help me with this; I like to be introduced to plants by someone who already knows them. It just seems more polite than learning about them from a book. An important part of this is increasing the acuteness of your *seeing*; you have to learn to see what is right in front of you. That is often hard with plants, as most of us have relegated them to the background as a sort of insentient and colorful backdrop to our city life.

One of the most common experiences herbalists have is going into the wild, looking diligently for a plant, not finding it, then giving up and sitting on a rock to rest and discovering they are in a field full of the very plant they are looking for.

As you increase your noticing, you will begin to see the plants sharply defined, as individuals, and you will find the ones you know everywhere. And as your experience of this new world opens up, you will find that plants are living beings and just like people they have their quirks, oddities, differences—plants of the same species don't always look the same. Where they live changes them (just as it does us).

If you learn them in the high mountains of Colorado and then seek them in eastern Washington State, they will look entirely different. Plants such as red root hug the ground at 9,000 feet above sea level but will stand 6 feet tall at lower elevations. Plants that are pulled into themselves, conserving water resources, in semi-arid and arid regions will plump out in the humid tropics, grow fat and big with all the abundance of an easy life. They will often change so much from eco-range to eco-range that they don't appear to be the same plants—and, of course, their medicinal actions will change as well. They don't need to make the same chemicals in the Olympic Peninsula as they do in the south of Spain.

Plants, just like people, live in neighborhoods, in certain regions and habitats. Part of the journey is learning those neighborhoods and habitats, learning where they like to grow, learning how they appear in different regions, different continents, altitudes, climates, and how their medicine changes in each of those climates as well. It also means learning how they appear at different times of the year.

Plants go through cycles, and these cycles are more pronounced if there is a cold winter where they live. Once you make the acquaintance of a plant, learn where it lives, you can visit it in all seasons of the year, learn how it looks as the seasons progress, learn the differences in its medicine in each of those seasons. Illness comes at any time; if you wildcraft you will need to know your medicines no matter the time of year. If you live in a climate that is very cold with deep snow, then it becomes important to learn the trees, for they can be found and made into medicines in any season. It is important, too, to make enough medicine of the plants that sleep through the winter so that you have them on hand if you need them. All of the *vegetalistas*—plant people—that I know have an herb room, a place where they keep their medicines and store the plants they have harvested but not yet made into medicines.

Trusting the healing capacities of the plants is not a new experience to the human species.

As you learn the plants, you will come to know how they *look* but also how they feel to the hand, how they smell, how they taste, even how they *sound*. Aspens make a sound completely unlike any other tree as the wind moves among them. You also learn, over time, how a plant subtly changes your body the moment you take it inside you. *All* plants have different effects and this becomes part of the knowledge as well.

Learn, also, to pay attention to how the plant *feels* to your non-physical sensing. You have learned to pay attention to how a restaurant or someone's home *feels* to you when you first walk in the door, to notice whether it feels welcoming or not, emotionally warm or not, safe or not. This kind of sensing can be extended to the plants you use for your medicines. Pay attention to whether or not the plant you are harvesting feels healthy and vital to you. Your medicines will only be as good as the plants you use to make them.

And . . . thank the plants as you harvest them. This is a form of saying grace for food, only now you are doing it for your medicines. This may not be a regular part of your life, this kind of thankfulness, but after 25 years of this work, I can tell you, it does make a difference to the quality of the medicines you make and of the relationship you will ultimately have with the plants you use for healing.

Harvesting

Making plant medicines is a full-immersion, full-sensory experience; it's very physical. Harvesting plants often means walking miles to find the ones you are looking for. If you are working with roots, you will be digging, of course, and some plants are very difficult to dig. You will need a shovel, sometimes a pick. Other plants, such as nettles or devil's club, have stinging hairs or thorns; you will need gloves. And despite their use, you will get bitten by the plant—*everybody* does. It's part of the journey.

Take an easy-to-carry bag, with a fold-up shovel, plant cutters, a knife, and plastic bags to put the plants in. Big plastic bags. Paper is relatively useless; it won't hold up to walking miles in the field and it is much bulkier than plastic. You can use a woven basket instead of a bag, but it's better to keep the herbs you are harvesting in their own bags, not roughly mixed together in a basket. Take Band-Aids and tweezers and comfortable walking shoes and a staff, a hat and water and a lunch to eat. Also: Don't walk any farther than half the distance you have the energy for. (Just an FYI on that one.)

Preparing Medicinal Plants

Once you have harvested the plants, take them home and begin preparing them as medicine right away; they will rot if you leave them in the plastic bags, or dry badly if you just dump them in a pile on the table and leave them too long. Never, never, never leave them in the truck overnight. (*Everyone* puts plant preparation off sooner or later and then has to throw the plants away. It *only* takes once . . . usually.)

Roots should be shaken and brushed to get the dirt off. Washing them is generally a bad idea unless, due to the nature of the root (e.g., coral root), they have to be washed. (Washing removes essential oils and the outer bark—things you don't want to lose.) Some roots are as tough as steel once they dry (e.g., red root), so cut them into small pieces while they are fresh. (*Everyone* fails to do this once.)

DRYING TRAYS

Get a good drying tray for seeds, roots, bark, and so on. Flattish trays that are fairly shallow are best. I like woven ones that let the air circulate or high-impact plastic trays. You will always drop and break a glass one. (Eventually.) Metal has too many reactions with plant chemicals and moisture and can contaminate the herb.

Leafy plants can be tied together—you will need some good twine—and hung from the rafters to dry unless you are making medicine from the fresh leaves. They dry well that way.

Storing Supplies and Medicines

Label *everything*. Everyone, and I mean *everyone*, thinks they will never forget the plant they just harvested, but everyone, and I mean *everyone*, does if it is not labeled. Then you will find yourself with a lot of unidentifiable plant matter on your hands that you can't use (and no, using them for illnesses you can't identify either won't work). And . . . label *all* your medicines once you've made them as well. You *will* forget what is in that bottle.

You will need bottles, of course, to store your finished medicines in. Tiny ones are nice for salves. Brown ones are nice for tinctures; they keep the light out and minimize degradation. Everything is best if kept in the dark; light has a strongly negative impact on the life of your medicines. (You will need droppers too—they are ridiculously expensive compared to the bottles they go with.)

If you are making tinctures, you will need Ball jars or something

The Different Kinds of Herbal Medicines

Herbal medicines, in general, fall into two groups: 1) those for internal use, and 2) those for external use.

The main forms of herbal medicines for internal use are:

- Water extracts (infusions and decoctions)
- Alcohol extracts (tinctures)
- Percolations (water or alcohol)
- Fluid extracts
- Syrups/oxymels/electuaries
- Glycerites
- Fermentations
- Vinegars
- Fresh juice (stabilized or not)
- Powders (plain or encapsulated)
- Food
- Suppositories/boluses
- Douches
- Essential oils
- Steams
- Smokes

The main forms of herbal medicines for external use are:

- Oil infusions
- Salves
- Evaporative concentrates
- Washes
- Liniments
- Lotions
- Compresses/poultices
- Essential oils
- Smudges

Most of these you can make yourself. Essential oils need special distilling equipment and I won't spend much time on them in this chapter—just a bit about using them as medicine.

similar for the herbs to macerate in. I often get old olive or pickle jars, the *big* ones, from restaurants to use for larger batches. Make sure they are clean—the smell does get into the tincture if you don't. There are other things you will find you need as you go along. I will mention a number of them when I talk about the particular kinds of medicines you can make.

In general, there are only a few kinds of herbal medicines: salves, infusions, tinctures, and powders. The list on the opposite page appears more complicated than that, but that is pretty much all it comes down to. There are just a number of different *forms* to those four types of medicines. Most of them you will never need; still, I'm going to tell you about them. You never know what might come in handy.

Remember: Have fun. This is an art as much as a science, and art always, *always*, has a depth of feeling and intuition to it that can never be captured and quantified. Trust your *feelings* and understand that your heart is as important to listen to as your head. Life without heart, you know, is not much of a life at all.

A Comment on Solvents

Unless you are using the plant itself in some form—as powder, food, juice, or so on—what you will be doing when you make your medicines is extracting the chemical constituents of the plant in some kind of liquid solvent. (When you take the whole herb internally, the stomach acids, bile salts, and so on *are* the solvent media. They leach out the active constituents of the plants for you.)

Every solvent has its own properties and people use different ones for many different reasons, some of which I will go into in this chapter. Generally, a solvent is referred to as a *menstruum*. It comes from *menstruus*, a Latin word meaning "month." It was felt, in the old days, that the moon and its cycle of 28 days had an influence on liquids, just as it does on the tides. So, herbs were placed in liquids—on particular days by the fanatical—and left in there for one cycle of the moon.

Hence *menstruum*. Though derided as superstition by scientists, there is some legitimacy to this kind of thinking. Plants really are stronger when harvested on certain days, the moon does affect the underground aquifers of the earth, just as it does the oceans (causing the ground to breathe out moisture-laden air), leeches really are useful (surgeons use them regularly now), maggots really do clean gangrenous wounds better than anything else, and . . . oops, sorry, got carried away again.

Anyway, the solvent is called the *menstruum*, herbs are placed in the menstruum, and once there they begin to *macerate*. Maceration is the soaking of something—usually a plant of some sort—in a solvent until the cell walls begin to break down so the compounds in the herb will leach into the solvent, where they are held in suspension. When you later separate the liquid (now containing the medicinal compounds) from the solids, the solids that are left are called the *marc*. The liquid is called whatever kind of medicine you were making: tincture, infusion, or so on.

Water is considered to be *the* universal solvent; it works for most things to some extent. For most of human history, it has been the primary solvent people have used. Alcohol is the next most effective solvent. Combining them will give you the most comprehensive solvent medium that exists.

Just as with the plants you harvest, use the best-quality solvents you can get. Your water, especially, should be well, spring, or rain water—if you can get it. If you use tap water, have a filter on the water line if you are at all able to do so. Or else buy a good-quality water. The better the water, the better the medicine. (Tap water is, as well, filled with minute quantities of pharmaceuticals—you really don't want to ingest them. They are highly bioactive.)

Another thing to understand is that the more finely powdered your herb, the more surface area that is exposed to the solvent. This allows more of the chemical constituents to leach into the solvent.

When you are making extracts, part of what you learn, and develop in your practice, is knowledge of just what kinds of solvents are right for which herbs and in what combinations. The goal is to get as many of the medicinal compounds as possible into the extractive medium. Each herb is different and needs different combinations of water and alcohol—that is, a different formula for preparation. Some do better in pure alcohol, some in pure water. Some need oils to extract the active constituents (*Artemisia annua* is an example of this; artemisinin is more easily soluble in fats than in either alcohol or water). Some need boiling, some prefer cold liquids.

Pharmacists, prior to World War II (before pharmaceuticals began to dominate medicine), were extensively trained in very sophisticated forms of herbal medicine making—many of which are beyond the scope of this book (and of most pharmacists these days). This is why pharmacists are still called "chemists" in England and the drugstores there the "chemist's" shops. Distressingly, that kind of training no longer occurs; it is now a lost art. I doubt there is a medicinal pharmacist in practice anywhere in the Western world who can prepare a tincture of *Colchicum officinale* and determine, exactly, the amount of colchicine in it—as all pharmacists could do in 1920.

In becoming an herbal medicine maker, you are learning how to be a practical dispensing pharmacist. Part of what that means is discovering how to best prepare the herbs and with which solvents. Chapter 9 is an herbal formulary that will give you the ratio of alcohol and water for several hundred plant tinctures.

Water Extractions

The two most common forms of water extractions are infusions and decoctions. Two lesser-known forms are evaporative concentrates and percolations.

Infusions

Teas are, at heart, weak infusions. When making medicine, however, you are usually working with what would formally be called an infusion. Infusions are stronger than teas since the herbs sit, *infuse*, in the water for a much longer period.

An infusion is made by immersing an herb in either cold or hot, not boiling, water for an extended time. Again, the water you use should be the purest you can find, *not* tap water. Water from rain, a healthy well, or a spring is best.

The weakness of infusions, cold or hot, is that they do not keep well; they tend to spoil very quickly. Refrigeration will only slow the process a little. Infusions, unless you stabilize them with something like alcohol, need to be used shortly after you make them. Their strength is that nearly everyone has access to enough water to make them without resorting to the expense of buying alcohol.

HOT INFUSIONS

Although the guidelines below call for short timelines for hot infusions, I often make my infusions at night just before bed and let them infuse overnight. I usually make enough for one day, then drink the infusions throughout the next day.

Most *hot* infusions are consumed, confusingly, not hot but warm or at room temperature; the infusion periods are too long for the water to stay hot. *Hot* infusion, in this sense, is a description of the extraction process, not of its temperature when used.

Some herbs, however, are best consumed while still hot, such as diaphoretics that stimulate sweating. For example, yarrow, if being used to help break a fever, is best consumed hot (steeped 15 minutes, covered). If being used for GI tract distress or to stimulate menstruation, though, it is best prepared as a hot infusion but consumed hours later at room temperature.

To prepare a hot infusion, bring water to a boil, then combine it with the herb in the following manner:

- **For leaves:** 1 ounce per quart of hot water, let steep 4 hours, tightly covered. Tougher leaves require longer steeping. The more powdered the leaves (if dried), the stronger the infusion. If you are using fresh leaves, cut them finely with scissors or chop them as finely as possible with a sharp knife.

- **For flowers:** 1 ounce per quart of hot water, let steep 2 hours, tightly covered. More fragile flowers require less time. Most flowers can be infused whole.
- **For seeds:** 1 ounce per pint of hot water, let steep 30 minutes, tightly covered. More fragrant seeds such as fennel need less time (15 minutes), rose hips longer (3 to 4 hours). Most seeds possess very strong seed coats to protect them from the world until they sprout. You will need to break the seed coat in order for the solvent to work; the seeds should be powdered as finely as possible.
- **For barks and roots:** 1 ounce per pint of hot water, let steep 8 hours, tightly covered. Some barks, such as slippery elm, need less time (1 to 2 hours). Most barks and roots are infused after being dried; powder them as finely as possible. If you are using fresh roots, mince them as finely as possible.

If you keep the containers tightly covered, the volatile components in the herb will remain in the liquid rather than evaporating into the air. The heat will vaporize the volatiles and they will rise up in the steam, then collect on the underside of the lid. As the mixture cools, the volatiles will condense and drip from the lid back into the infusion. This ensures that the essential oils, which are very volatile, will remain. You can easily identify an herb that has a high volatiles content; it will have a strong essential oil or perfumey smell to it. These must always be covered when making a hot infusion.

When you are ready to use the infusion, pour off the water and squeeze out the marc as much as possible. The liquid in the saturated herbs is often much stronger than the infused liquid, so keep it if you can.

COLD INFUSIONS

Cold infusions are preferable for some herbs. The bitter components of herbs tend to be less soluble in cold water. Yarrow, for instance, is much less bitter when prepared in cold water. Usually cold infusions need to steep for much longer periods of time; each herb is different.

The necessity for a cold infusion rarely arises; nevertheless, it may. If so, place the herb in room-temperature water, cover, and let steep overnight.

Infusion Equipment

There are many kinds of infusion pitchers and mugs that are available to buy; they are pretty common. Most of them have some form of basket in which to place the herbs (and a lid to cover them). The basket is suspended at the top of the mug or pitcher so that the herbs and the liquid do not mix together. It does make it a bit easier. (Avoid plastic if

Measuring Herbal Medicines

It seems nearly everyone uses a different way to describe how much to take; some say milliliters (ml), some say drops, some say dropperful, some say teaspoon or tablespoon, so here is a conversion table for you. It may help.

A drop: A drop is not always a drop (see why there's confusion?). A drop of water and a drop of alcohol are about the same, but a drop of glycerine is bigger—about five times bigger than a drop of water—because it is so viscous. Nevertheless, pretty much everyone treats a drop as a drop. Now, is that clear or what?

Dropperful: A 1-ounce glass tincture bottle has a standard glass dropper that fits in it, and when it's full of tincture that is what I call a dropperful. It generally holds around 30 drops, so I consider a dropperful to be 30 drops, or 1.5 ml. Normally, a glass dropper will fill only halfway with one squeeze, so it takes two to get a full dropper.

A milliliter is, for water or alcohol, 20 drops, or two-thirds of a dropperful.

A teaspoon is 5 ml or 100 drops or three and one-third dropperfuls.

A tablespoon is 1/2 ounce, 15 ml, 3 teaspoons, 300 drops.

An ounce is in the neighborhood of 600 drops.

you can; use stainless steel, glass, or pottery infusers.) You can also buy (or make) small cloth bags to hold the herbs, which you then suspend in whatever container you are using. A tea ball will also work, but I don't find them as effective; they don't usually hold enough herb.

The best infusers work by holding the herb in the upper part of the pot, so that only the upper portion of the liquid is in contact with the herb. As the water at the top of the infuser becomes saturated with the herbal constituents, it gets heavier and sinks to the bottom. This creates a circulating current in the water that brings the unsaturated water to the top of the jar where it can then infuse as well. This will make the strongest infusion. You can just put the herb in a jar with hot water and cover it; it will work fine, but it won't be quite as strong as this method. (See Percolations on page 555 for more on the dynamics of this.)

A Hot Infusion for Parasites

INGREDIENTS:

- 2 ounces dried alchornea leaf
- 2 ounces fresh gingerroot, chopped finely
- 2 ounces dried sida leaf
- 2 ounces dried wormwood leaf (*Artemisia absinthium*)
- 2 quarts water

Place herbs in container, pour near-boiling water on top, cover tightly, and let sit overnight. Strain and press the marc to extract as much liquid as possible. Drink 1 cup four times per day. This amount will last 2 days. Make it again every 2 days until you have been using it for 8 days. This is a good infusion for treating intestinal worms (you can just use the wormwood and ginger if you wish). It will be very bitter, though the ginger will help that a bit.

Decoctions

Decoctions are much stronger than infusions. Basically, they are boiled infusions. There are two forms of decoctions: 1) simple decoctions, and 2) concentrated decoctions. A simple decoction is any water extract that is boiled for a short length of time. Concentrated decoctions are boiled until the water is reduced to some extent. Normally, herbs that are highly resinous or filled with volatile oils are not decocted. Only herbs whose constituents are not damaged by heat are boiled.

It is important to begin with cold water, not warm or hot, add the herbs, and bring to a boil. The extraction will be more efficient if you begin with cold water as different constituents extract better at different temperatures.

Some herbs, such as isatis, are stronger if they are boiled for a few minutes simply because the higher heat is a better extractant. Herbs high in polysaccharides such as reishi are also often helped by boiling; polysaccharides tend to extract more efficiently when decocted. In essence, anytime an herb is boiled, no matter how short a time, it is considered to be a decoction. If you are just boiling the herb to better extract the constituents, you are making a simple decoction.

Simple Decoction

INGREDIENTS:

- 1 ounce herb
- 1 pint cold water

Combine herb and water. Bring to boil. Boil at least 15 minutes (some herbs will need longer). Let cool enough that you can handle it. Strain the decoction to remove the herb. Press the herb to extract all liquid. Add enough water to bring the liquid back to 1 pint. Take as directed.

In a concentrated decoction, which is more common than simple decoctions, the herb is boiled in water long enough that the amount of water you began with is reduced to some extent, often by half, sometimes more. This acts to concentrate the constituents in less liquid, making the medicine stronger. Concentrated decoctions are not often drunk as a tea (reishi is an exception). However, they are sometimes used in smaller doses similarly to a tincture. Once the decoction is made, it is allowed to cool, the liquid strained, then dispensed a tablespoon at a time—usually three or four times a day depending on the herb and the disease. The usual dosage range for concentrated decoctions, depending on the herb, is 1–4 fluid ounces a day.

The most common form of medicine made from concentrated decoctions is a cough syrup. They are also used to make a fomentation—that is, a very condensed water extract that is soaked into a cloth and applied to the surface of the body (to treat pain and inflammation in a joint, for example). Decoctions are also used as enemas—should the need arise, which everyone hopes it won't. This gets a very strong concentrate into the bowel where it will, usually, rather easily move across the membranes of the colon into the bloodstream.

When you are making your concentrated decoctions, use porcelain, glass, or stainless steel pots if you can; iron and aluminum will often contaminate the mix. When the decoction is cool, prepare it as needed for whatever you are going to use it for. Concentrated decoctions will last longer than infusions, especially if kept cold. Syrups will often last a year in a refrigerator just fine.

As an Aside

Oxymels, which I won't discuss more than this, have been used for thousands of years. The basic form is 40 ounces of honey to which is added 5 fluid ounces of water and 5 fluid ounces of vinegar. Oxymels were often used for colds, flu, and sore throats. However, a more medicinal form of an oxymel is made using a concentrated decoction for the water part of the recipe. Electuaries, on the other hand, are medicinal pastes (the core of which can be a concentrated decoction to which powdered herbs are added) that are made palatable by the addition of sweeteners such as honey or syrups. Marsh mallows, originally, were not candy but a particular kind of electuary that made the medicine more palatable. This is still a good way to take powdered herbs: mix the powdered herbs you wish to take very well, then add enough honey to make a ball only slightly sticky to the hand, then eat it.

A Concentrated Decoction for Colds and Flu

INGREDIENTS:

- 1 ounce dried white or culinary sage leaf
- Pinch of cayenne
- 3 cups cold water
- Wildflower honey
- Juice of 1 lemon

Combine sage and cayenne with water. Bring to boil, then reduce heat and simmer, uncovered, until liquid is reduced by half. Let cool enough that you can work with it. Strain the liquid and press sage to extract as much liquid as possible. Add wildflower honey to taste. Add juice of 1 lemon. Store in refrigerator. Take 1 tablespoon or more as often as needed at the onset of throat or upper respiratory infection.

Cough Syrup Recipe

INGREDIENTS:

- 3 ounces horehound leaves/stems
- 2 ounces cherry bark
- 2 ounces elder berries
- 2 ounces elecampane root
- 2 ounces licorice root
- 2 ounces mallow root
- 1 ounce slippery elm bark
- 1 ounce vervain leaf
- 1 ounce lomatium (or osha) root
- 7 pints water
- 3 ounces glycerine
- Wildflower honey
- 2 ounces mullein tincture
- 1 ounce grindelia tincture

Combine the horehound, cherry bark, elder berries, elecampane, licorice, mallow, slippery elm bark, and vervain, along with half the lomatium, in the water in a large pot. Bring to a boil. Stir frequently as it heats to prevent sticking. Once it boils, reduce heat a bit and, stirring constantly, cook until the liquid is reduced by half. Let cool. (You can put the pot in a bath of cold water to cool it faster. Don't let it tip over.) Strain the liquid, and press the marc in a cloth to extract as much liquid as you can.

(The mucilaginous herbs—the licorice and mallow—can make it hard for the liquid to pass through the weave of the cloth you are using to press the marc. So, conversely, you can keep the licorice and mallow out of the mix and, once the marc is pressed, reheat the liquid, adding the licorice and mallow to the pot in a muslin bag. Bring to a boil and let simmer, stirring constantly, for 30 minutes. Remove the bag, let it cool, then squeeze it out as best you can.)

Warm the liquid again, just enough that it will dissolve the honey and glycerine. Add the glycerine, then the honey to taste. Powder the remaining lomatium to a fine powder—a nut or coffee grinder or mortar and pestle is good for this—then add it to the liquid. Let the mix cool, then add the mullein and grindelia tinctures.

The honey, glycerine, and two tinctures help stabilize the syrup, keeping it from going bad. I do keep the whole thing in the refrigerator, though. It will last a year very easily. Generally, it is best to make this kind of a syrup in the fall, after the berries are ripe and ready for harvest, and just before flu season. (You can substitute similar herbs for any used in this recipe.) Use as needed—I just drink it from the bottle—it is very effective.

Washes

Washes are simply infusions or decoctions that are used directly on the skin. If you have hurt your skin, an abrasion or sunburn for example, any wash that contains a tannin herb such as oak or acacia or older pine needles and soothing herbs such as mallow or chamomile will facilitate healing immensely—prickly pear (a soothing mucilaginous herb) is immensely good for this.

If you have a skin infection or a wound that you want to keep from becoming infected, use a wash of the applicable herbs from this book. If you don't know what kind of infection it is, use the antibacterial wash described below.

General Antibacterial Wash

INGREDIENTS:

- 2 ounces antibacterial herbs, such as artemisia (the *absinthium* species is very good), cryptolepis, or sida
- 2 ounces echinacea
- 2 ounces evergreen needles (any kind)
- 1 quart water

Combine the herbs with the water. Cover, bring to boil, and simmer uncovered for 30 minutes. Let cool and strain. Then wash the affected skin liberally with the decoction four times daily.

Steams

Steams are excellent for upper respiratory infections. They can be used as often as desired or needed. Wonderful steams can be made from most of the artemisias, any of the evergreens, any of the sages, and many other aromatic plants. You can also make them with essential oils.

The process involves putting a highly aromatic, antibacterial herb in water, boiling it, and breathing the steam.

A Steam for Upper Respiratory Infections

Though this steam recipe calls for dried herbs, it can be prepared with fresh herbs if desired.

INGREDIENTS:

- 2 ounces young eucalyptus leaves, dried
- 1 ounce sage leaf, dried
- 1 ounce juniper leaf or berry, dried
- 1 gallon water

Place herbs in water (in glass, stainless steel, or ceramic-coated pot) and bring to roiling boil. Remove from heat, hold head over steam, and cover head and steaming pot with large towel. Breathe steam deep into lungs. Bring herbs to boil and repeat as often as necessary. Replace herbs when their strong smell begins to noticeably diminish.

Essential oil steam: This steam method can also be undertaken with essential oils. Use 30 drops each of the essential oil of rosemary, sage, juniper, eucalyptus, and bergamot in 1 quart of water.

Wound wash: This recipe can also be prepared as a wash for infected or weeping wounds. Rather than boiling, bring the mixture to the edge of boiling, remove from heat, and let steep until lukewarm. Strain, use it to wash the wound thoroughly, then apply a wound powder.

Evaporative Concentrates

Evaporative concentrates are remarkable medicines but are rarely used in herbal practice and are poorly understood. The most common evaporative concentrate in the United States is made from chaparral leaf and is used for treating mastitis in women. However, the primary reason to use evaporative concentrates—in my opinion—is that this is the one process I know of to create a topical corticosteroid cream as potent as those made by pharmaceutical companies.

An evaporative concentrate is made by making a very, *very* slow-cooking decoction. A slow cooker (or Crock-Pot) is necessary; I don't know of another way to do it. You need a cooking pot where you can keep the heat at the slowest simmer possible, very slightly below boiling or very slightly over it.

To make a corticosteroid herbal cream, you need to begin with an anti-inflammatory herb. There are many of these and it is worth exploring different plants to find which ones work best for you. I tend to use the ones that contain a lot of salicylates, like aspen or willow, and are water soluble. When the decoction is finished, it will be very thick—the consistency of a hand cream. When used on the skin, for rashes, varicose veins, skin eruptions, and inflammations, it is as potent as pharmaceutical corticosteroids. The only drawback—not solvable—is that the concentrates are nearly black in color. It's very visible on the skin. Difficult if it is your face you are treating.

I usually refrigerate these concentrates, but when I haven't, even after months, they have never gone bad. The chemical concentration is apparently too high for bacteria to deal with. Needless to say, these concentrates are *not* for internal use.

Herbal Corticosteroid Evaporative Concentrate

INGREDIENTS:

32 ounces water

6 ounces powdered willow (or aspen) bark

Put the water in a slow cooker, and add the herb. Cover and turn the cooker on high. As the water warms, stir the mix well. When the water has come to a boil, reduce the heat to just under or just slightly over a simmer. Leave the cooker on that setting, covered, for 2 days.

Turn off the cooker, let the mix cool, and strain out the herb, squeezing the marc in a cloth to extract as much as possible. Clean the slow cooker and then put the liquid back in it. Turn on high and bring to a boil. Reduce immediately to just under or just slightly over a simmer. Keep it covered. Cook until the liquid is reduced to nearly nothing, essentially 1–2 ounces. This will take up to a week.

As the liquid begins to approach 1–2 ounces, watch it carefully. At this point it can lose the remaining water very quickly and it will burn once it does. *Once the liquid is this low, the remainder will go very fast.* It helps to stir it regularly at this point to get an idea of how much liquid is left. Once it has reduced enough, turn off the cooker, let it cool, and then place the concentrate in a jar. Label well. *Not* for internal use.

Percolations

Percolations are just the same as drip-grind coffee. You are letting liquid drip slowly through the herb—which is held in filter paper—into a container.

Percolations are handy to know about in case you run short of a tincture and need some in a hurry. They take a few hours rather than a few weeks. They are also the best way to make a cold-process water extract, much better than letting the herb steep in cold water. The main strength of a percolation, however, is its potency. This is due to the nature of solvents.

In essence, a solvent is a pure liquid; it doesn't have anything in it but itself. As a solvent leaches chemical constituents into itself, it begins filling up, or getting saturated as they say. Once it is saturated, it can't take any more into itself. A good way to visualize this is to see, in your imagination, the liquid on one side, the herb on the other. The herb is full, the liquid is empty. As the two combine, the constituents in the herb begin to flow into the liquid. However, once the amount of constituents in the liquid are in equilibrium with those in the herb—like a weight scale where equal weights are on each side of the scale—it is very difficult for the constituents to keep flowing into the liquid. A saturation point is being reached.

The way a percolator works, however, means that the liquid never becomes saturated; the liquid that is touching the herb is always pure. So, the extract becomes very strong. You will see how this works when I describe how the percolator works in practice.

To make a percolation, however, you will need a percolator—this is why so few people make them. It is a bit more complex than using a jar to make a tincture or a coffee cone to make coffee. Some people do make their own percolators (it can be done fairly simply), or you can buy one from a scientific glass supplier.

Most scientific percolators are several feet long and look somewhat like a giant glass ice cream cone, wider at the top (big enough to easily put your hand and arm into) and narrowing to a point at the bottom. There is a narrow opening at the bottom that flows into an integral glass tube with a control knob on it, a spigot essentially, that you turn to control the flow of liquid out of the percolator.

(You can make your own percolator by cutting the bottom off a glass water bottle—don't use plastic—such as a mid-sized Perrier container. *Sand the edges well.* Until they are smooth. Keep the cap; you will need it.)

To use a percolator, you first determine what kind of percolation you are going to make, water or an alcohol and water mix. Make up the liquid mixture you are going to need and keep it close. Then take the dried herb and grind it as finely as possible. Percolation will not work with fresh herbs; they have to be dried. For a percolation to work well, the herb really does need to be as close to a powder as possible. You need as much plant surface area exposed to the liquid as possible. Once the herb is powdered, and before you start percolating, put the herb in a large bowl and add enough alcohol to the herb to moisten it—not wet, just moist. This will begin breaking down the cell walls of the plant and make the extraction more efficient.

Let the moist herb sit a couple of hours, but if you are impatient, at least 30 minutes. Then take some filter paper—I use the same coffee filters as are used for drip-grind coffee cones—and place it in the bottom of the percolator. It helps if the inside of the percolator is slightly dampened first so that the paper will adhere to the glass and fit snugly. Press the paper into place, being sure to not punch a hole in it with your fingers. Once that is done, carefully put the moistened herb in the cone, making sure you don't get any between the filter paper and the glass. Press it lightly into place—you don't want it compacted though, since liquid has to flow through it.

Depending on the amount of herb you use, the percolator can be filled nearly to the top with plant matter. When all the plant material is in the percolator, put a circular piece of filter paper on top of the herb and put something heavy on that to keep the paper, and the herb, from floating up—a small stone works well. (Not scientific, I know, but very aesthetic.)

Then, slowly, begin pouring the liquid into the percolator. Do it slowly so that you don't stir up the powdered herb. The liquid will slowly percolate down into the plant matter, and air bubbles will come up. (You may not be able to get all the liquid into the percolator in one go. If so you will have to add the rest as the liquid level drops.) When the herb is fully saturated, put a container under the spigot and very slowly open the spigot. (Some people run a plastic hose from the spigot into a container—needless to say, the percolator has to be held in the air on a stand of some sort in order to work.) You want to get one drop per second coming out of the spigot, so adjust the spigot until you get just that rate of drip.

The reason this makes such a good tincture (or cold water infusion) is that *only* clean liquid is flowing over the herb. This means that the liquid is completely unsaturated; its extraction capacity remains very high. So as the liquid flows over the herb, it pulls chemical compounds out of the plant, then more clean liquid comes behind and pulls more out. It's very elegant.

If you are using a homemade percolator, prepare it the same way, but when you are ready to percolate, very slightly open the bottle cap—just enough that a very slow drip comes out. Again, one drip per second is very effective.

Alcohol Extractions

Because alcohol extractions, i.e., tinctures, keep so well over time and because they are so easily dispensed, many herbalists prefer them over infusions. They are made by immersing a fresh plant in full-strength alcohol or a dried plant in an alcohol and water mixture.

I am a fan of using pure grain alcohol for tinctures. What that means in practice, however, is using an alcohol that is 190 proof, or 95 percent alcohol. (There is such a thing as 100 percent or 200-proof alcohol, but the only people who generally use it are scientists or large commercial enterprises; you will probably never see it.) Most people buy their 190-proof alcohol at their local liquor store; the most common brand in the United States is called Everclear.

Some states—some countries—will not allow their citizens to buy 190-proof alcohol (for their own good, of course). If you live in such a place, you will have to cross state (or country) lines and buy your alcohol from a more enlightened place or else make do with what they allow you to buy. In such places, most people use a 40 percent to 50 percent alcohol-content vodka; that is, 80 to 100 proof. Get the highest proof you can—you will see why this is important as we go on.

In the United States, the amount you pay for liquor, regardless of what you are buying, is directly proportional to its alcohol content. The actual cost of a gallon of 190-proof alcohol is about $1.00. The rest of the cost is federal and state taxes—which are then taxed again by sales tax when you buy the thing. So you may be tempted to buy a lower-proof vodka because it is cheaper. That is a bad idea. Your tinctures will be weak.

The Origin of "Proof"

As an aside: In the eighteenth century the English navy paid sailors partly in rum. The watering of drinks has always been a problem. So to test their rum before accepting it as pay, the sailors would soak gunpowder with it. If the gunpowder would still burn, the rum was "proved." Hence 100 proof. The rum had to be a minimum of 57.5 percent alcohol for the gunpowder to burn, but that has been watered down to a simple rule of thumb: 50 percent alcohol = 100 proof.

Fresh Plant Tinctures

Fresh herb tinctures, again, are made by putting the fresh herb in pure grain alcohol. These tinctures are nearly always made in a one-to-two ratio, which is written 1:2. (There are a few exceptions.) This ratio means you are using 1 part herb (dry weight measurement) to 2 parts liquid (liquid measurement). The amount of herb in such ratios is always indicated by the first number, the amount of liquid by the second number.

So, for example, if you have 3 ounces (dry weight measure) of fresh echinacea flower heads, you would place them in a jar with 6 ounces (liquid measure) of 190-proof alcohol. I generally use well-sealed Mason or Ball jars, stored out of the sun and shaken daily. At the end of 2 weeks the herb is decanted and squeezed through a cloth until as dry as possible (an herb or wine press is good for this), and the resulting liquid is then stored in labeled, amber bottles.

Fresh plants naturally contain a certain percentage of water, and alcohol is a very good extractor of water. (One of the main symptoms of a hangover comes from the alcohol extracting the water from your body—you get the same kind of headache from too much alcohol as you do from dehydration.) Alcohol will pull not only the medicinal constituents out of the plant but the plant's water as well.

The water in the fresh plant dilutes the alcohol, how much depends on the kind of plant it is. Peppermint has a lot of water in it, 50 percent or more by weight. So what you get when you tincture fresh peppermint leaves is a tincture that is about 50 percent alcohol and 50 percent water. Myrrh gum has virtually no water in it, so you end up with a tincture that is 95 percent alcohol and 5 percent water—and all that water was already in the alcohol, assuming you began with 95 percent alcohol.

Fresh leafy plants may be chopped or left whole before placing them into the alcohol or pureed with the alcohol in a blender. Fresh roots should be ground with the alcohol in a blender into a pulpy mush. (I generally think it better to make root tinctures from dried roots, but there are a few exceptions; coral root is one.)

Dried Plant Tinctures

Plants, as they dry, lose their natural moisture content (the amount of water you combine with alcohol to make a tincture is the amount of water that the plant loses when it dries). Tables detailing the moisture content of many medicinal plants are available. When making a tincture of a dried plant, you always add back the amount of water that was present in the plant when it was fresh. This enables the extraction of the water-soluble constituents to occur.

Dried plants are usually tinctured at a one-to-five ratio, which is written 1:5. (There are, as always, exceptions.) That means 1 part dried herb to 5 parts liquid. Fresh *Echinacea angustifolia* root, for example, contains 30 percent water by weight. If you have 10 ounces of powdered root (dry weight) you would then add to it 50 ounces of liquid (liquid measurement). This gives you your 1:5 ratio. The tricky part for many people comes in figuring out how much of that liquid should be water and how much alcohol. In this instance you are wanting your liquid to be 30 percent water (fresh echinacea root's water content); that is, 30 percent of 50 ounces, which would be 15 ounces water. The rest of the liquid will be alcohol; that is, 35 ounces.

Pressing Herbal Tinctures

When your tinctures are done, and you pour off the liquid, the marc will still have some, often a great deal of, liquid in it. The marc needs to be pressed to remove the remaining tincture. Most people do this by hand. The best thing to use is a good-quality cloth with a close weave to it—I use the same surgical cloths hospitals do; they hold up really well. An herb press facilitates this immensely, though a cider press, depending on the style, will work very well, too. You will get a lot more out of a press than when doing it by hand, but they do tend to be expensive.

With fresh plants you can generally get out about as much liquid as you put in; with dried material, especially roots, you get out as much as you can. Sometimes this isn't much.

A formula for this particular plant tincture would look something like this:

> *Echinacea angustifolia:* fresh root tincture 1:2; dried root tincture 1:5, 70 percent alcohol. Dosage: 30–60 drops as needed. In acute conditions: 30 drops minimum each hour.

It is just *assumed* that you already know that all fresh plant tinctures at 1:2 will be using 95 percent alcohol. (Note: Everyone I know just assumes that the 95 percent alcohol they are using is 100 percent; no one I know takes that 5 percent into account in figuring this stuff out. Life is too short.)

Again, don't use tap water if you can avoid it. Powder the herbs you are tincturing as finely as possible—many people in the United States use a Vitamix for this. It is a pretty indestructible mixer/grinder, especially if you get a commercial-grade unit. (The demo video shows them grinding 2×4s into sawdust.) I have had mine for 25 years and have replaced the blades only twice in spite of the heavy use I've subjected it to.

Unless the herbs become tremendously hard when dried (as red root does), it is best to store herbs as whole as possible until they are needed. This reduces the cell surface area that is exposed to air. Oxygen degrades plant matter fairly quickly.

Dry plant tinctures, like fresh, are left to macerate for 2 weeks, out of the light, before decanting.

Combination Tincture Formulas

In spite of our aversion in the United States toward the metric system, all scientific glassware in the United States is metric. Most herbalists use a *graduated cylinder* to measure the amount of tincture they are pouring out (available from any scientific glassware company). Most herbal bottles, of course, are in ounces, while the measuring cylinders are in milliliters. Roughly, 30 milliliters is equal to 1 ounce.

As an example, if you were going to make a combination tincture formula for the early onset of colds and flu, a good mix would be

How Long Will Tinctures Last?

Tinctures should be kept out of the sun—a dark, cool room is good. Keeping them in dark or amber-colored glass jars is even better—though if they are in the dark, you can leave them in clear jars as many of us do with our larger quantities of tinctures. Tinctures will, in general, last many years. However, you should know about precipitation, a very neglected area of herbal medicine.

The constituents that you have extracted from the herbs are held in suspension in a liquid medium. Over time, some of these constituents will precipitate out and settle on the bottom of the tincture bottle. Some herbs such as *Echinacea angustifolia* root are heavy precipitators, while others, like elder flower, are such light precipitators that you will almost never see a precipitate in the bottle. Unfortunately, there has been little study on this, nor has a chart of herbal precipitation rates ever been prepared (as far as I know; intent searching has never turned one up). Technically, we need one that shows both the rate of precipitation and the amount of precipitation for each plant.

Some herbalists will add 1–2 ounces of glycerine to every 16 ounces of tincture (10 percent to 15 percent of the total liquid) to help slow down or eliminate precipitation. It does help retard the precipitation of tannins; I am not sure how well it works for other constituents or over time but you might try it and see how it works if precipitation becomes a concern for you.

You will find that some herbs will produce an ever larger precipitate on the bottom of your storage bottles as time goes by. It is not possible to get that precipitate back into solution. Most herbalists simply shake the bottle prior to dispensing and suggest the user do the same before ingesting it. I do it this way and it seems to work fine, medicinally speaking.

There is, as yet, no data on whether the efficacy of a tincture is affected by precipitation. Certainly the ones that do not precipitate are good for decades if kept in a dark, cool location in well-sealed bottles.

10 milliliters each of echinacea, red root, and licorice tinctures mixed together. This would give you 1 fluid ounce total.

You can mix something like this in the graduated cylinder, as long as your hand is steady, then pour the mixture into a 1-ounce amber bottle with a dropper lid. Dosage would be one full dropper at least each hour during the onset of upper respiratory infections. This will usually prevent the onset of colds and flu if your immune system is relatively healthy.

Glycerites

Glycerine can also be used for making extracts; it has become a popular alternative for children's tinctures and for people who don't like alcohol.

Glycerine is technically a kind of alcohol, though most people don't know it (and when told they don't seem to think it evil). It is formed through the hydrolysis of oils or fats, usually animal or vegetable. It is a common by-product of the industrial production of soap. Glycerine is a relatively new substance (to people), discovered in 1789 and used medicinally only since the mid-1800s.

Glycerine is fairly viscous and very sweet; I've never had any undiluted glycerine go bad, even after years of being unrefrigerated. It is very stable, like alcohol, and possesses its own antimicrobial properties. It is not as efficient an extractive as water or alcohol; it won't extract gums, resins, or volatile or fixed oils, so its range of use is limited.

If you do dilute the glycerine, as you will have to do in making an extract, it won't hold up as well as an alcohol tincture. Most people add 10 percent to 15 percent alcohol to glycerites to ensure stability.

One of the very good things about glycerine is that it is moisturizing, demulcent, emollient, and soothing to the skin. I have found it to be exceptional for making extractions to be used for ear infections. Unlike alcohol, it won't irritate the inside of the ear but will soothe it instead while still carrying antimicrobial constituents to the place they need to go.

Glycerine is only about 60 percent as extractive as water or alcohol; glycerites will be 40 percent less strong than those other extractions. Glycerites should be dosed at one and a half to two times the dosage for tinctures. If you would normally dose with ½ dropperful (15 drops) of tincture, you would, with a glycerite, give ¾ dropperful (22 drops) to 1 full dropper (30 drops).

MAKING GLYCERITES FROM DRIED HERBS

The ratio is the same as for alcohol tinctures, 1:5. The liquid, however, to better preserve the glycerine and to help the extraction be more effective, should contain at least 10 percent 190-proof alcohol, then 60 percent glycerine, and finally 30 percent water.

As an example: If you are starting with 5 ounces of powdered echinacea root, then you would need 25 ounces of liquid, of which 2.5 ounces would be alcohol, 15 ounces would be glycerine, and 7.5 ounces would be water.

It is more effective if you add the alcohol to the powdered herbs first and let it sit for 24 hours, then add the glycerine and water, mix well, and leave in a jar with the lid on for 2 weeks. Decant and store as with alcohol tinctures.

Ear Infection Glycerite

INGREDIENTS:

- 1 ounce berberine plant
- 1 ounce cryptolepis (or sida or alchornea)
- 1 ounce echinacea
- 1 ounce juniper (or other evergreen needles)
- 1 ounce usnea lichen
- 2.5 ounces grain alcohol
- 15 ounces glycerine
- 7.5 ounces water

Powder herbs well, place in jar, add alcohol, mix thoroughly, and let sit for 24 hours. Mix glycerine and water together, and add to powdered herbs in jar. Let macerate 2 weeks, then decant and strain. Store in amber jar. Use 1–3 drops in the ear up to six times daily for ear infections.

A Comment on Alcohol

There has been a tremendous resurgence of puritanitis in the United States and a few other parts of the globe (notably the United Kingdom) over the past 20 years or so. One object of attention of this spasming of the puritan reflex has been the evils of alcohol. Many on the right and on the left seem to think it is some sort of inherently evil substance that is going to destroy Western civilization or at least make God really, really mad.

Alcohol existed long before human beings emerged out of the ecological matrix of this planet. It is a highly natural substance, both inside and outside of our bodies. *All* living beings partake of it, including trees, bees, and elephants. (Not kidding.) All of them enjoy it. It facilitates the functioning of the body, enhances organ function in many respects, and reduces the incidence of many diseases. It is not an evil substance.

One of the continual queries about tinctures concerns the alcohol content. Many people are afraid to take tinctures because of the evil alcohol in them.

To be really specific: The amount of alcohol in tinctures is incredibly tiny. Less than you will get from eating a few pieces of bread (yes, bread does have alcohol in it, enough to produce a breathalyzer reading of 0.05 just by itself). If you are taking 20 drops of a 60 percent alcohol tincture *every* hour for an acute condition, you will get about 1/17 of an ounce of alcohol over the course of a day (less than 2 milliliters). If you are taking a general dose (20 drops three times daily), you will be getting about 1/30 of an ounce over a day. Again, this is less than you will get from eating two slices of bread.

If this truly is a problem for you, you can make infusions or use glycerites—though the glycerites really aren't as effective and the water extractions won't extract some of the more important alcohol-soluble constituents. Some people heat their tinctures to remove the alcohol; it doesn't work very well and I suspect the heat alters the quality of the tincture. I don't recommend it.

MAKING GLYCERITES FROM FRESH HERBS

This is made with the usual 1:2 ratio for fresh herbs. In this instance, however, use 15 percent pure alcohol and 85 percent glycerine. So if you have 5 ounces fresh herb, you would want 10 ounces of liquid, of which 1.5 ounces would be 95 percent alcohol and 8.5 ounces would be glycerine.

Herbal Honeys

Honey can be used just like glycerine, following the same directions for making a glycerite. Make sure to use a good wildflower honey.

Nasal Sprays

Nasal sprays are excellent for helping with the onset of upper respiratory or sinus infections. Simply take an herbal tincture and place up to 10 drops or so in a 1-ounce nasal spray bottle (available from pharmacies). Add pure water and spray up nostrils as often as needed.

Nasal Spray Formula for Sinus Infections

INGREDIENTS:

- 5 drops cryptolepis tincture
- 5 drops bidens tincture
- 5 drops juniper berry tincture
- 5 drops usnea tincture

Combine the tinctures in a 1-ounce nasal spray bottle, add enough pure water to make 1 ounce, replace cap, and spray into nostrils as often as desired. (You could substitute 2 drops each of the essential oils of eucalyptus, sage, rosemary, and juniper for the tinctures if you wish.)

Vinegar Tinctures

I don't use these much, but they have a long history of use in many different cultures. One of their strengths is that vinegar itself is a highly medicinal substance; another is that they don't go bad, no matter how long you keep them. Natural vinegars should be used; most people use an unpasteurized, organic apple cider vinegar. Make your tinctures at a 1:2 ratio if using fresh herbs, or 1:5 if using dried. You don't need to add any water to vinegar tinctures.

Fluid Extracts

Not many people make their own fluid extracts any more, though a few herbal companies sell them. Herb Pharm's *Eleutherococcus* tincture is one of the better known. Essentially, 1 gram of fluid extract is supposed to be equivalent to 1 gram of the herb. They are very concentrated alcohol tinctures. In the nineteenth century they generally contained other substances such as vinegar or sugar. *All* trained pharmacists could make fluid extracts in the nineteenth and early twentieth centuries. They would make them in their pharmacies, in the lab in back, and keep them on hand for when needed. Most companies that make fluid extracts these days use specialized equipment to do so.

Here are the directions for a fluid extract of ipecac, from an early U.S. pharmacopeia.

> Moisten 16 Troy ounces ipecacuanha in fine powder with 6 fluid ounces alcohol; press it firmly into a conical percolator, and displace 3 pints of tincture, or until the ipecacuanha is exhausted. Distill the tincture over a water-bath until the residue is of a syrupy consistence. Mix with 1 fluid ounce acetic acid and 10 fluid ounces water; boil until reduced to ½ pint, and the resinous matter has separated. Filter when cold, and add water through the filter to make the filtrate up to ½ pint. Mix with ½ pint alcohol.

An alternate form of a fluid extract would be an evaporative concentrate. For example, make up a willow bark concentrate as described earlier but save the marc. Add to the marc 5 ounces of 190-proof alcohol and let it macerate as you reduce your decoction in the slow cooker. Once the decoction is reduced to 1 ounce of a very thick liquid, press out the alcohol from the marc and combine it with the concentrate. This will give you approximately 6 ounces of a fluid extract, essentially a 1:1 ratio. The dosage for internal use would be tiny, 1 to 3 drops. It is much stronger than a regular tincture.

This form of a fluid extract will work only with plants that have primarily water-soluble constituents. A percolator really is necessary for those that need alcohol extraction.

Here is Michael Moore's recipe for a fluid extract using a percolator:

> Briefly, take 8 ounces of Tabebuia (Pau D'Arco), grind it, make up an arbitrary amount of menstruum (let's say four times as much, or 32 ounces). The tincture lists a 50% strength; make your fluidextract menstruum 20 percent higher in alcohol content (i.e. 70%). Mix 22.4 ounces of alcohol with 9.6 ounces of water to get a quart of 70 percent alcohol menstruum. Take the Tabebuia, moisten it, digest it for TWO days, pack a larger [percolator] cone with it, and drip (very slowly) a first batch of tincture that is only 75% of the volume as the original dried herb weighed. This means after you have dripped 6 fluid ounces, take it away, and continue dripping everything else into a second jar. As the rest of the menstruum finally starts to sink below the top of the herb column, start adding water into the cone. This second drip can be any amount you wish . . . a quart, 2 quarts, whatever. You will need to evaporate it all in a double boiler until it is reduced to 25% in volume of the herb weight . . . 2 ounces in this case. Add the vile remnant of the second percolation to the 6 ounces from the first percolation, and you now have 8 ounces of fluidextract, made from 8 ounces of Tabebuia Bark. A fluidextract is by definition 1:1 in strength.[1]

Douches

The easiest way to make a douche is to add ½ ounce of tincture to 1 pint of water. This is especially effective in the treatment of vaginal infections. Usnea is particularly valuable as a douche, as are the berberines. In general, douching twice a day for 3 days is sufficient.

You can also make a strong infusion or decoction and, when cooled, douche with that. Sida and cryptolepis would be good as either an infusion or a decoction.

Liniments

Liniments are generally made with rubbing alcohol. Use a 1:2 ratio with fresh plants, 1:5 with dried. You don't need to add any additional water. I use these for topical use, generally for arthritis and sore muscles. Cayenne is a very good liniment herb for both: 3 ounces powdered cayenne in 15 ounces rubbing alcohol, macerate for 2 weeks, decant, and press. I just pour a bit in my hand and rub the affected area as often as needed. **Caution:** Wash your hands afterward and *never, ever, ever* touch *any* mucous membranes before you do. Cuts are nearly as bad. And for sure, never, never go to the bathroom and then wipe yourself after using one of these unless you have washed your hands really, really well first. Just an FYI on that one.

Oil Infusions

Oil infusions are exceptionally useful for burns, sunburn, chapped and dry skin, skin infections; as ear drops; and for use on wounds as salves. With oil infusions the medicinal properties of the plant are transferred to an oil base rather than water or alcohol. A salve is just an oil infusion thickened by the addition of beeswax.

Oil Infusions with Dried Herbs

To make an oil infusion of *dried* herbs, grind the herbs you wish to use into as fine a powder as possible. Place the herbs in a glass baking dish, and pour enough oil on top of them to soak them well. Stir the powdered herbs to make sure they are well saturated with oil; add just enough extra oil to cover them by 1/4 inch or so. I generally use olive oil because it is very stable; it doesn't go rancid easily and is, itself, strongly antimicrobial.

Some people just leave the mix, covered, in a sunny location for a few weeks. That will work fine as long as they do get sun and are warmed well every day. I prefer using the oven. I cover the container, put it in the oven on low heat just before bed, and leave it overnight. Some herbalists prefer to cook the herbs for as many as 10 days at 100°F in a slow cooker. (Most of us are too impatient for that.) However you do it, when the mix is done, let it cool, then strain the oil out of the herbs by pressing through a strong cloth with a good weave.

Herbal Oil for Skin Infections

INGREDIENTS:

- 1 ounce dried artemisia leaf (any species)
- 1 ounce dried berberine plant (any species; root, bark, or leaf as the case may be)
- 1 ounce dried cryptolepis (or sida or bidens or alchornea leaf)
- 1 ounce dried echinacea root or seed
- 1 ounce dried evergreen needles (any species)
- 1 ounce dried usnea
- 1 quart olive oil

- Grind all the herbs as finely as you can, then place them in a glass or ceramic pot—do not use metal. Pour in enough oil to saturate the herbs, stir the mix well, then add enough extra oil to cover the herbs by ¼ inch. Heat the mixture, covered, overnight in the oven with the setting on low (150° to 200°F) or on low in a slow cooker for 7 days. Let the mixture cool. Press the oily herb mixture through a cloth to extract the oil. Store the oil in a sealed glass container out of the sun. It does not need to be refrigerated.

Oil Infusions with Fresh Herbs

To make an oil infusion from *fresh* herbs, place the herbs in a clear glass jar and cover them with just enough oil to make sure no part of the plant is exposed to air. Let the jar sit in the sun for 2 weeks (or cook in a slow cooker for 5 days at low setting). Then press the herbs through a cloth. Let the decanted oil sit. After a day the water that is naturally present in fresh herbs will settle to the bottom; carefully pour off the oil and discard the water. Note: You may have to do this two or three times to get all the water out. If any water remains in the oil, it will spoil.

Some herbalists prefer to start the oil infusion by pouring just a bit of alcohol over the herb and letting it sit in the alcohol for 24 hours. This begins breaking down the cell walls of the plant, making the oil extraction stronger.

Salves

To make a salve, all you do is take the oil you have made (the recipe at the top of the preceding page is a good one) and add beeswax to it. *Only* beeswax should be used, not petroleum waxes. For a variety of reasons beeswax is better, among them: beeswax itself has antimicrobial properties.

So . . . after pressing out the oil from your cooled oil infusion, put it in a glass, ceramic, or stainless steel pot and slowly reheat it. It needs to be reheated just enough to melt the beeswax.

It usually takes somewhere around 2 ounces of beeswax per cup of infused oil to make a salve. It goes a lot faster if the beeswax is in the form of beads or is as finely chopped as you can get it.

When the beeswax is melted and stirred in, place a few drops from the pot on a small plate and let it cool. Touch it; if it is too soft add more wax, if too hard add a bit more oil. A perfect salve should stay hard for a few seconds as you press your fingertip on it and then suddenly soften from your body heat. If you do make up your salve and it is too soft, you can just reheat it slowly and add a bit more beeswax. If too hard, you can add a bit more oil.

I used to make my salves and put them into scores of tiny salve jars. Now, I just put them into a larger container such as a Ball or Mason jar, slowly reheat it if I need some to use, and then pour that into a smaller container to carry with me.

Lotions

Contrary to popular belief, oil and water do mix. It's called a lotion. You can make water infusions of herbs, then blend them with oil (and an emulsifier) to make a lotion for the skin. Many herbs that are good for the skin can be blended into these kinds of lotions. Some of the best information on this (not my thing really) can be found online.

Using Whole Herbs

Herbs don't have to be made into tinctures or infusions; they can be taken directly in various forms: as powders, as food, as juice. They are very effective in these forms for a variety of ailments.

Wound Powders

Some wounds do not respond well to a wet dressing like a salve. However, dried herbs placed directly on the wound are exceptional in such cases. Herbal combinations, when powdered well, will stop bleeding and facilitate rapid healing while preventing infection. After the wound has begun healing, you can switch to a salve or even honey directly on the wound.

(As an aside, I once accidently shot a 16d nail through the first joint of the index finger on my left hand—a complicated misfire by a compressed air nail gun. After I used a hammer to remove my finger from the board it was nailed to, I poured some cryptolepis tincture on the nail, then pulled it out of the finger. I used a wound powder, much like the one in this book, on the wound for 2 days, then switched to pure honey dressings for a week. It worked fine; full function restored.)

There is probably no more powerful way to treat wound infections than with powdered herbs. I have yet to find an infection that will not respond to one.

The herbs need to be powdered as fine as possible. I usually begin with a Vitamix, which will give me a semi-small grind, then switch to a nut or coffee grinder for further powdering. This will get the herbs about as fine as you can get them. A mortar and pestle will do very well, but they are time consuming.

After the herbs are powdered, they should be sifted through a fine-mesh sieve, so make sure you are getting only the finest powder possible. (Discard any pieces that refuse to reduce to a powder or save them for use in an oil infusion later.) Once it has been sieved, put the powder in a tightly sealed container and keep it in a freezer or in a cool location away from sunlight. Powdered herbs lose their potency fairly quickly unless protected. Replace the powder every 6 months, unless you are keeping it frozen, which will allow it to last several years.

When needed, sprinkle the powder liberally on wet wounds. It will stop the bleeding, prevent infection, and stimulate cell wall binding. Infected, oozing, pus-filled wounds should be opened up, cleaned with an antibacterial herbal wash, then liberally sprinkled with the powder as often as needed. Once the wound is healing cleanly it should not be disturbed (i.e., by scrubbing or trying to open it up again)—just add more wound powder, or switch to honey, as needed.

A Good Wound Powder

INGREDIENTS:

- 1 ounce berberine plant (root or bark, as the case may be)
- 1 ounce cryptolepis root or sida, bidens, or alchornea leaf
- 1 ounce echinacea root or seed
- 1 ounce juniper leaf
- 1 ounce lomatium root
- 1 ounce usnea lichen

Powder all herbs as finely as possible, and strain through a sieve. Use as needed. This same formula can be sprinkled onto feet or into shoes and socks for athlete's foot fungal infections. It may also be used on babies for diaper rash.

Herbal Powders for Internal Use

Herbs are often powdered and then pressed into tablets or put into capsules for internal use, generally by commercial companies. You can get a simple herbal capsule machine if you wish. Packing a lot of capsules by hand is tremendously tedious. These days, I usually just take the herbs internally in their powdered form. Many people don't like to do it this way because of the flavor of the herbs—they are often bitter. (I just use juice or honey; I am very lazy.)

Although many herbs are available as capsules or tablets, for some conditions the herbs really do need to be taken as powders; they shouldn't be encapsulated. This is especially true in cases of severe stomach ulceration. The herbs should be powdered, then mixed with liquid and consumed. This allows the herb to make contact with the entire affected area.

If the ulceration is in the duodenum, which lies just below the stomach, then capsules *should* be used. The capsules tend to sit at the bottom of the stomach and then drop through into the duodenum where they are needed. Duodenal ulcers are often accompanied by painful cramping or spasming. This can be alleviated by the addition of a few drops of peppermint essential oil to the herbal mixture before encapsulating it.

Herbal Regimen for an Ulcerated Stomach

INGREDIENTS:

- 4 ounces dried licorice root
- 4 ounces dried marsh mallow root
- 4 ounces dried comfrey root
- 2 ounces berberine plant tincture
- 1 quart wildflower honey

Powder licorice, marsh mallow, and comfrey roots (as finely as possible) and mix together in equal parts. Take 2 tablespoons, twice a day (morning and evening), mixed in any liquid (e.g., apple juice), for 30 days. For the next 60 days use just powdered licorice and marsh mallow roots (omitting the comfrey), again mixed in equal parts; take 1 tablespoon in the morning only. The herbs should not be in capsules in order to allow them to fully coat the stomach lining. (For duodenal ulcers, you would take them in capsules.)

At the same time, as you first begin the treatment with the powder, take 1 teaspoon of the berberine plant tincture three times daily for 15 days. And . . . take 1 tablespoon honey six times daily for 30 days.

Suppositories

Suppositories can be made from powdered herbs to treat things such as vaginal infections and hemorrhoids. I have recommended the use of echinacea suppositories for abnormal Pap smears for many years; they work very well. The powdered herbs are combined with enough liquid to make them hold together, be shaped properly, and be inserted.

Suppository for an Abnormal Pap Smear

INGREDIENTS:

Echinacea angustifolia root
Vegetable glycerine
Flour
Usnea tincture
Calendula tincture

Powder the echinacea root as finely as you can, then mix it with enough vegetable glycerine to bring it to the consistency of cookie dough. At this point it will still be a bit sticky, so mix it with enough flour (any kind—chlorella or spirulina can also be used) to bring it to the consistency of bread dough. Once you have, take a bit of the mix and press it into the shape of a suppository, about the size of your thumb. Repeat until you've used up all the mixture. Place the suppositories on a tray and put them in the freezer. They won't freeze; they will remain pliable but manageable.

Each evening, after you are in bed, place one suppository up against the cervix. The next morning, use a douche made from a mix of equal parts usnea and calendula tinctures, ½ ounce in 1 pint water (otherwise the remains of the suppository will drip out throughout the day—messy). Repeat every day for 14 days.

Using Fresh Herbs

Some herbs are particularly potent if used fresh and taken internally. The most obvious form of this is food. Our ancestors ate several hundred plants over the course of the year, most of them wildcrafted. Our bodies are used to it and in many respects a number of our diseases come from the lack of wild plants in our diets. Nearly all plants can be eaten for food and their medicinal constituents then become a part of the regular diet. I won't go into that in any depth here but do want to mention a few herbs that really are best if used fresh, primarily when juiced.

Medicinal Plant Juices

Ginger, of course, is only strongly effective if used fresh, and the best way to do that is to juice the plant. (See the ginger monograph on page 437 for more.) The fresh leaf juices from bidens and *Artemisia annua* are also much more potent than using the plants in their dried form. And, of course, the fresh juice of *Echinacea purpurea* is part of standard-practice medicine in Germany. Some of the other plants that possess particularly potent medicinal juices are cabbage and plantain.

Cabbage is particularly high in S-methylmethionine (SMM)—it used to be called vitamin U. (This substance is also strongly present in malted barley.) SMM is exceptionally effective in healing and protecting the GI tract from ulceration and inflammation. It is present in its most active form, and at the highest concentrations, in fresh cabbage juice. One of the best combinations for treating irritable bowel syndrome, Crohn's disease, or ulceration in the GI tract is the juice from one piece of cabbage about the size of a carrot and six leaves of plantain. (I prefer to also add the juice of two carrots, one beet, and four stalks of celery.)

Although the juicing of fruits and vegetables has a long history, there are few people exploring the use of medicinal plant juices in any depth. It is a very open field with a lot of potential for development. Many of the plants are much stronger if their fresh juice is used.

You can juice the plants, then stabilize the juice with the addition of 20 percent alcohol by volume. That is, if you have 5 ounces of juice, you would add 1 ounce of pure grain alcohol to keep the juice from spoiling. The juice can then be dispensed much like a tincture, though in somewhat larger doses.

Essential Oils

Essential oils are made by distilling volatile oils from plants. From 0.5 percent to 5 percent of a plant's weight is composed of volatiles, or what we call essential oils. Most plants tend toward the lower end of that scale. To get an idea of how much plant it takes to make an essential oil: If a plant has 1 percent essential oil, it will take 100 ounces of the plant (a little over 6 pounds) to get 1 ounce of essential oil.

To make essential oils, distillation is necessary. In recent years a number of herbalists have begun to reclaim home distilling in order to make their own essential oils, but most of us just buy them already made.

Essential oils are used as medicine, mainly, in three ways: 1) placed directly on the skin, sometimes diluted, sometimes not; 2) inhaled (i.e., aromatherapy); and 3) in minute doses internally.

Essential oils move through the skin fairly easily. Lateral epicondylitis (a.k.a., tennis elbow) is a very painful and often debilitating inflammation of the nerve in the elbow, usually from repeated stress on the joint. Birch essential oil, rubbed on the area and about 5 inches around it, will usually reduce both the inflammation and the pain within 15 minutes. (It takes months for it to heal, but this does help immensely.)

Essential oils can be added to hot water and inhaled as steams or added to water and used as nasal sprays, for instance.

It *is* possible to take essential oils internally, but great caution should be exercised. Because so much plant matter is used to make an essential oil, these oils are incredibly potent. If you were foolish enough to take a whole ounce of essential oil by mouth—a very, very bad idea—you would be consuming 6 pounds of a medicinal plant in a form that would go into the bloodstream almost instantly. This is why essential oils are greatly diluted when put into formulations, used in diffusers, or taken internally in tiny, tiny doses (from 1–5 drops at a time). Generally, for internal use, I stick to things like peppermint oil, 1 drop at a time, for severe indigestion.

Treatment of Children

Children's bodies are much smaller than adults' and if you are using herbal medicines with them, you need to adjust the dosages. You can determine the dosages for children through one of three approaches:

Clark's Rule: Divide the weight in pounds by 150 to give an approximate fraction of an adult's dose. For a 75-pound child the dose would be 75 divided by 150, or half the adult dose. (This is the one I find most useful.)

Cowling's Rule: The age of a child at his or her next birthday divided by 24. For a child coming 8 years of age, the dose would be 8 divided by 24, or one-third the adult dose.

Young's Rule: The child's age divided by (12 + age of child). For a 3-year-old it would be 3 divided by (12 + 3; that is, 15) for a dose of one-fifth the adult dose.

Childhood Ear Infections

Most childhood ear infections can be treated successfully with herbs. Tinctures, glycerites, honeys, teas, and herbal steams are all effective approaches.

Children are most susceptible to ear infections from antibiotic-resistant strains of *Haemophilus influenzae, Staphylococcus aureus, Streptococcus pneumoniae,* and *Branhamella catarrhalis*. These kinds of treatment plans have been found highly effective for treating them, individually or together.

Children's Ear Oil

INGREDIENTS:

- 5 cloves garlic
- 4 ounces olive oil
- 20 drops eucalyptus essential oil

Chop garlic finely, place in small baking dish with olive oil, cook over low heat overnight, and strain, pressing cloves well. Add essential oil of eucalyptus to garlic oil and mix well. Place in amber bottle for storage. To use: Hold glass eyedropper under hot water for 1 minute, dry well (quickly), and suction up ear oil from bottle. Place 2 drops in both ears every half hour or as often as needed for 2 to 7 days.

Brigitte Mars's Herbal Tea for Ear Infections

INGREDIENTS:

- 1 ounce elder flower (*Sambucus* spp.)
- 1 ounce licorice root
- 1 ounce Mormon tea (*Ephedra viridis*)
- 1 ounce peppermint leaf
- 1 ounce rose hips
- 1 quart water
- Wildflower honey (optional)

Roughly crush all herbs. Bring water to a near boil, then pour over the herbs and allow to steep until cooled enough to drink. Consume as hot as is comfortable for drinking. Sweeten with honey if desired. As much as is wanted can be consumed. The Mormon tea is a decongestant, the rose hips are slightly astringent and anti-inflammatory and high in vitamin C, the elder flowers are slightly sedative and reduce fevers, the licorice root is anti-inflammatory and tastes good and is antiviral and antibacterial, and the peppermint helps reduce fevers and decongests and is calming. Catnip can be added to help lower fever.

Ear Infection Tincture Combination

INGREDIENTS:

- 1 ounce echinacea tincture
- 1 ounce ginger tincture
- 1 ounce licorice tincture
- 1 ounce red root tincture

- Mix together the tinctures. Give one full dropper (30 drops) of the mixture each hour per 150 pounds of body weight until symptoms cease. Best administered in juice. Dosage should be altered for the child's weight. Eucalyptus and sage tinctures can also be used. You can also prepare this as a glycerite or a medicinal honey.

Children's Diarrheal Diseases

Children are also susceptible to diarrheal infections from *E. coli* O157:H7 bacteria and antibiotic-resistant strains of *Shigella dysentariae*. When they get extremely ill with these bacteria, they may also experience high fever and diarrhea. The berberine plants are the best for this.

To Lower a Fever in a Child

The best herb for lowering seriously high fevers is coral root (*Corallorhiza maculata*), as either a tea or tincture. Dosage is one teaspoon of the root steeped in 8 ounces hot water for 30 minutes and drunk or up to 30 drops tincture for a child of 60 pounds. Brigitte Mars's herbal tea for ear infections (page 578), with the addition of catnip, is also exceptionally effective in lowering fevers. Finally, bathing with cool water will also work very well.

Treating Diarrhea in Children

The use of a tea and tincture combination together is usually effective.

Rosemary Gladstar's Tea for Diarrhea

INGREDIENTS:

- 3 parts blackberry root
- 2 parts slippery elm bark

Mix the herbs together (for example, 3 ounces blackberry root and 2 ounces slippery elm bark). Simmer 1 teaspoon of the herb mixture in 1 cup water for 20 minutes. Strain and cool. Take 2 to 4 tablespoons every hour or as often as needed.

Tincture Combination for Diarrhea

INGREDIENTS:

- 1 ounce acacia tincture
- 1 ounce berberine plant tincture
- 1 ounce cryptolepis tincture
- 1 ounce evergreen needle tincture

Combine the tinctures, and shake well. Give 1 full dropper (30 drops) for every 150 pounds of body weight every 1 to 2 hours in water or orange juice until symptoms cease.

A Final Note

You, more than anyone else ever will, know how you are feeling in your body. Pay close attention to how you respond to any medicines you take. If you don't feel right when you take an herbal medicine, stop taking it.

9

AN HERBAL FORMULARY

All the technical information has been stolen from reliable sources and I am happy to stand behind it.
—Edward Abbey

When making herbal tinctures, you need to know the proportion of water to alcohol—among other things. *Everyone* needs a handy list of medicinal plants and their tincture requirements. This list won't have every plant you will ever need on it, but it does have many of them.

By the way, this list was compiled from a number of sources: Michael Moore, King's Eclectic Dispensatory, several Chinese materia medicas, various lists I have received over the years, and my own work with a number of plants that either were on no lists at all or whose formulations in the literature I found to be ineffective. Michael Moore's work is the most comprehensive and valuable, and you can access it on the website for his school, the Southwest School of Botanical Medicine (swsbm.com). **Note:** Plants are listed here by botanical name. If you're searching by common name, check the index to cross-reference.

***Abies* (the firs).** Tincture, fresh needles (must include spring growth), 1:2; dried needles, 1:5, 50 percent alcohol. Dosage: 5–20 drops. Infusion: internal, 1–3 fluid ounces; external, as needed.

***Acacia greggii* (catclaw acacia).** Standard infusion, pod/leaf: 2–4 fluid ounces.

***Achillea* (yarrow).** Tincture, fresh plant in flower, 1:2; dried plant, 1:5, 50 percent alcohol (note: not preferred, as the volatiles are lost). Dosage: 10–30 drops up to 4x daily. Infusion: 3–6 cups daily as needed.

***Acorus calamus* (calamus, sweet flag).** Tincture, fresh root, 1:2; dried root, 1:5, 60 percent alcohol. Dosage: 15–45 drops up to 4x daily.

***Actaea rubra* (baneberry, red cohosh).** Tincture, fresh root, 1:2; dried root, 1:5, 80 percent alcohol. Dosage: 10–20 drops up to 3x daily.

***Adiantum* (maidenhair fern).** Infusion, dried herb: 1–3 fluid ounces.

***Aesculus hippocastanum* (horse chestnut).** Tincture, dried bark or nut, 1:5, 50 percent alcohol. Dosage: 3–10 drops daily.

***Agave* (century plant).** Tincture, fresh leaf, 1:2; dried root, 1:5, 50 percent alcohol. Dosage: 30–60 drops up to 4x daily.

***Agrimonia* (agrimony).** Tincture, fresh leaf, 1:2; dried leaf, 1:5, 50 percent alcohol. Dosage: 1/4–1 tsp up to 4x daily.

***Agropyron repens* (couchgrass).** Tincture, dried root, 1:5, 50 percent alcohol. Dosage: 30–60 drops up to 6x daily. Cold infusion: 2–4 fluid ounces.

***Ailanthus altissima* (tree of heaven).** Tincture, dried inner bark, 1:5, 50 percent alcohol. Dosage: 1/2–1 tsp up to 6x daily for acute diarrheal conditions, 1/2–1 tsp up to 3x daily for giardia, 30–90 drops up to 3x daily for everything else. Cold infusion: 1–2 ounces up to 5x daily.

***Alchemilla* (lady's mantle).** Tincture, fresh plant, 1:2. Dosage: 30–90 drops up to 3x daily. Infusion: as needed.

***Alchornea* (alchornea).** Tincture, dried leaf or bark, 1:5, 50 percent alcohol. Dosage: 1/4 tsp every 4 hours.

***Allium sativum* (garlic).** Fresh juice of the bulb: 1/4–1 tsp. Tincture, fresh bulb, 1:2. Dosage: 15–40 drops. Caution: Fresh juice is emetic in larger doses.

***Alnus serrulata* (tag alder).** Decoction, bark (fresh or recently harvested only): internal use, 1/2–2 tbl up to 3x daily; external use (as a wash), as needed.

***Alpinia* (galangal).** Tincture, dried root, 1:5, 65 percent alcohol. Dosage: 30–90 drops as needed.

***Althaea* (marsh mallow or hollyhock).** Tincture, fresh root, 1:2; dried root (the fresher the better), 1:5, 50 percent alcohol. Dosage: as needed.

***Ambrosia* (ragweed).** Tincture, fresh or recently dried plant only, 1:2. Dosage: 20–40 drops up to 4x daily.

***Ammi visnaga* (khella, bishop's weed).** Tincture, seed, 1:5, 60 percent alcohol. Dosage: 60–120 drops up to 4x daily.

***Anemone hirsutissima* (pulsatilla ludoviciana, pulsatilla patens, anemone patens, pulsatilla hirsutissima, pasque flower, eastern pasque flower).** Tincture, fresh plant in flower, 1:2. Dosage: 10–15 drops, as needed, not more often than each hour. May cause vomiting in large doses.

***Anemone tuberosa* (desert anemone, desert pasque flower).** Same as for *A. hirsutissima.*

***Anemopsis* (yerba mansa).** Tincture, fresh root, 1:2; dried root, 1:5, 60 percent alcohol. Dosage: 20–60 drops up to 5x daily. Cold water percolation: 2–4 fluid ounces up to 5x daily—if you can stand it.

***Angelica* (angelica).** Tincture, fresh root, 1:2; dried root, 1:5, 65 percent alcohol. Dosage: 30–60 drops up to 4x daily. Tincture, seed, 1:2. Dosage: 10–30 drops up to 4x daily.

***Angelica sinensis* (dong quai).** Tincture, cured Asian root, 1:5, 70 percent alcohol. Dosage: 15–30 drops up to 3x daily.

***Anisum* (anise).** Tincture, seed, 1:5, 60 percent alcohol. Dosage: 3–15 drops on the tongue as needed. Infusion: 2–4 fluid ounces as needed.

***Antennaria* (cat's paw, pussy toes, mountain everlasting).** Standard infusion, whole plant: 3–6 fluid ounces up to 4x a day.

***Anthemis nobilis* (Roman chamomile).** Tincture, fresh flowering herb, 1:2, 50 percent alcohol. Dosage: 30 drops in water as needed. Infusion: 2–4 fluid ounces.

***Apium* (celery).** Tincture, fresh seed, 1:2. Dosage: 15–80 drops in water up to 3x daily. Infusion, dried seed: ½–1 tsp seeds in 1 cup hot water up to 4x daily.

***Aralia californica* (California spikenard, elk clover).** Tincture, fresh root, 1:2; dried root 1:5, 50 percent alcohol. Dosage: 10–30 drops up to 3x daily.

***Aralia hispida* (bristly sarsaparilla).** Tincture, dried root or bark, 1:5, 50 percent alcohol. Dosage: 5–25 drops up to 3x daily.

***Aralia nudicaulis* (sarsaparilla).** Tincture, dried root, 1:5, 60 percent alcohol. Dosage: 15–30 drops up to 6x daily.

***Aralia racemosa* (spikenard).** Tincture, fresh root, 1:2; dried root, 1:5, 50 percent alcohol. Dosage: 10–30 drops up to 3x daily.

***Aralia spinosa* (devil's walking stick).** Tincture, dried root or bark, 1:5, 50 percent alcohol. Dosage: 5–25 drops up to 3x daily.

***Arctium* (burdock).** Tincture, dried root, 1:5, 60 percent alcohol. Dosage: 30–90 drops up to 3x daily. Tincture, seed, 1:5, 60 percent alcohol. Dosage: 10–25 drops up to 3x daily.

***Arctostaphylos* (uva ursi, bearberry).** Tincture, dried leaf, 1:5, 50 percent alcohol. Dosage: 30–60 drops in 8 ounces water up to 3x a day.

***Argemone corymbosa* (prickly poppy, Mojave prickly poppy).** Tincture, fresh herb in seed, 1:2. Dosage: 5–15 drops as needed.

***Argemone mexicana* (prickly poppy, Mojave prickly poppy).** Same as for *A. corymbosa.*

***Arnica* (arnica).** Tincture for external use, fresh plant in flower, 1:2, 70 percent rubbing alcohol; apply as needed to affected area. Tincture for internal use, fresh plant in flower or fresh root, 1:2. Dosage: 1–5 drops up to 3x daily. Do not exceed recommended dosage.

***Artemisia absinthium* (wormwood).** Tincture, fresh plant in flower, 1:2; dried plant, 1:5, 60 percent alcohol. Dosage: 30–90 drops up to 6x daily. Cold infusion, fresh plant in flower: 1–3 fluid ounces up to 3x daily.

***Artemisia annua* (sweet Annie).** Tincture, fresh plant in flower, 1:2. Dosage: 30–90 drops up to 6x daily.

***Artemisia tridentata* (sagebrush).** Same as for *A. absinthium.*

***Artemisia vulgaris* (mugwort, California mugwort).** Tincture, fresh plant, 1:2; dried plant, 1:5, 50 percent alcohol. Dosage: 15–30 drops up to 3x daily.

***Asarum* (wild ginger).** Tincture, fresh root, 1:2; dried root, 1:5, 60 percent alcohol. Dosage: 20–50 drops in water up to 3x daily.

***Asclepias asperula* (immortal root).** Tincture, dried root, 1:5, 50 percent alcohol. Dosage: 5–30 drops up to 3x daily. Best if used in combination tinctures.

***Asclepias cornuta* (common milkweed).** Same as for *A. asperula.*

***Asclepias incarnata* (swamp milkweed).** Same as for *A. asperula.*

***Asclepias subulata* (desert milkweed).** Tincture, dried root, 1:5, 50 percent alcohol. Dosage: 10–20 drops in water up to 3x daily.

***Asclepias tuberosa* (pleurisy root).** Tincture, fresh root, 1:2; dried root, 1:5, 50 percent alcohol. Dosage: 30–90 drops up to 3x daily.

***Asparagus officinale* (asparagus).** Tincture, fresh root, 1:2; dried root, 1:5, 50 percent alcohol. Dosage: 30–60 drops up to 3x daily.

***Aspidosperma* (quebrache bark).** Tincture, dried bark, 1:5, 50 percent alcohol. Dosage: 15–30 drops up to 3x daily.

***Astragalus membranaceus* (astragalus).** Tincture, dried sliced root, 1:5, 60 percent alcohol. Dosage: 30–60 drops up to 4x daily. Cold water percolation: 2–3 fluid ounces up to 3x daily.

***Avena* (wild oats).** Tincture, fresh milky seed top, 1:2. Dosage: 10–30 drops up to 4x daily. Infusion, dried plant: 4–8 fluid ounces daily.

***Balsamorhiza* (balsam root).** Tincture, fresh root, 1:2; dried root, 1:5, 65 percent alcohol. Dosage: 25–45 drops up to 4x daily. Note: Cut the root well before grinding it as it contains tough threads that will wrap around your blender blades and freeze them up.

***Baptisia tinctoria* (wild indigo root).** Tincture, dried root, 1:5, 65 percent alcohol. Dosage: 10–25 drops up to 3x daily.

***Berberis vulgaris* (common barberry).** Tincture, dried root, 1:5, 50 percent alcohol. Dosage: 10–60 drops up to 3x daily. Infusion or cold water percolation: 1–3 fluid ounces to 3x daily. More in acute GI tract conditions.

***Bidens* (same insulting names as for *B. pilosa*).** Same as for *B. pilosa* except most species will be weaker. *B. pinnata* dosage should be 50 percent more than that of *pilosa.*

***Bidens pilosa* (beggar's ticks, Spanish needles).** Best if fresh. Tincture, fresh herb, 1:2. Dosage: 45–90 drops in water up to 2x daily, or in acute conditions ¼–1 tsp on up to 1 tbl in water up to 6x daily. Fresh juice: dosage is same as for tincture; stabilize with 20 percent to 25 percent alcohol if you intend on storing it.

Brickellia grandiflora **(brickellia).** Tincture, dried herb, 1:5, 50 percent alcohol. Dosage: 30–60 drops up to 3x daily. Infusion: 2–4 fluid ounces, to 2x daily.

Bursera microphylla **(elephant tree).** Tincture, small twigs and dried leaves (such as they are), 1:5, 70 percent alcohol. Dosage: 10–30 drops daily. Best if used in combination formulas. Tincture, gum, 1:5, 80 percent alcohol. Dosage: 5–20 drops daily.

Calendula officinalis **(marigold).** Tincture, fresh flower, 1:2; dried flower (must be brilliant orange/yellow), 1:5, 70 percent alcohol. Dosage: 5–30 drops up to 4x daily.

Capsella bursa-pastoris **(shepherd's purse).** Tincture, fresh whole plant, 1:2; very recently dried plant (would not recommend unless desperate), 1:5, 50 percent alcohol. Dosage: 10–30 drops up to 2x daily.

Capsicum **(cayenne).** Tincture, dried seed pod, 1:5, 95 percent alcohol. Dosage: 5–15 drops, normally in hot tea of some sort.

Cardamomum **(cardamom).** Tincture, seed, 1:5, 50 percent alcohol. Dosage: 5–10 drops.

Carum **(caraway seed).** Tincture, seed, 1:5, 50 percent alcohol. Dosage: 10–20 drops in liquid of one sort or another.

Castela emoryi **(holacantha emoryi, chaparro amargosa).** Tincture, dried plant, 1:5, 50 percent alcohol. Dosage: 20–50 drops up to 2x daily.

Caulophyllum **(blue cohosh).** Tincture, dried root, 1:5, 60 percent alcohol. Dosage: 5–20 drops. Rarely used alone; best in combination formulas.

Ceanothus **(red root).** Tincture, dried root, 1:5, 50 percent alcohol. Dosage: 30–90 drops up to 4x daily. Best if used in combination unless you are using it specifically for lymph problems. Cold water percolation: 2–4 fluid ounces daily.

Centaurium **(centaury).** Tincture, fresh plant, 1:2. Dosage: 10–20 drops before meals.

Centella asiatica **(gotu kola).** Tincture, fresh plant, 1:2. Dosage: 15–30 drops up to 3x daily. Tincture, dried plant, 1:5, 50 percent alcohol. Dosage: 20–40 drops up to 4x daily.

Cercocarpus **(mountain mahogany).** Tincture, twigs/stems, 1:5, 50 percent alcohol. Dosage: 15–45 drops in water up to 3x daily. Decoction: 2–3 fluid ounces to 3x daily.

Cereus grandiflorus **(night-blooming cereus).** Tincture, fresh plant, 1:2. Dosage: 5–25 drops up to 4x daily.

Chamaecyparis lawsoniana **(Lawson's cypress).** Tincture, fresh needles/stems, 1:2, 5 percent glycerine. Tincture, recently dried needles, 1:5, 60 percent alcohol, 5 percent glycerine. Dosage: for diarrhea, 20 drops as necessary, usually not for more than 3 days; for gum infections, 5 drops in water, used to wash mouth. Not for long-term use internally. Infusion, dried needles/twigs: 2–4 fluid ounces, generally for GI tract problems.

***Chamaecyparis nootkatensis* (yellow cedar).** Same as for *C. lawsoniana.*

***Chamaelirium* (helonias, unicorn root).** Tincture, dried root, 1:5, 50 percent alcohol. Dosage: 10–40 drops daily. Best if used in combination formulas.

***Chelidonium* (greater celandine).** Tincture, fresh plant, 1:2. Dosage: 10–25 drops. Short-term use.

***Chelone* (balmony).** Tincture, fresh herb, 1:2. Dosage: 10–20 drops up to 3x daily.

***Chilopsis linearis* (desert willow).** Tincture, dried bark and twigs, 1:5, 50 percent alcohol. Dosage: ¼–1 tsp up to 3x daily for systemic candida. Decoction or cold water percolation: 3–6 fluid ounces up to 3x daily.

***Chimaphila* (pipsissewa).** Tincture, fresh herb, 1:2; dried herb, 1:5, 50 percent alcohol. Dosage: 20–50 drops up to 4x daily.

***Chionanthus* (fringetree).** Tincture, fresh bark, 1:2; dried bark, 1:5, 65 percent alcohol. Dosage: 30 drops up to 2x daily. Cold water percolation, bark or leaf: 2–4 fluid ounces.

***Cimicifuga racemosa* (black cohosh).** Tincture, dried root, 1:5, 80 percent alcohol. Dosage: 10–25 drops up to 3x daily.

***Cinchona* (quinine bark).** Tincture, dried bark, 1:3, 45 percent alcohol. Dosage: 15–30 drops up to 3x daily; for malaria, ¼–1 tsp up to 3x daily, not to exceed 7 days, and repeat in 2 days. Cold water percolation: 2–3 fluid ounces up to 3x a day, not to exceed 7 days.

***Cinnamomum* (cinnamon).** Tincture, dried powdered bark, 1:5, 60 percent alcohol, 5 percent glycerine. Dosage: 20–60 drops up to 4x daily.

***Clematis* (virgin's bower).** Tincture, freshly dried herb, 1:5, 50 percent alcohol. Dosage: 10–40 drops up to 3x daily.

***Cnicus benedictus* (blessed thistle).** Tincture, fresh herb in flower, 1:2; dried herb, 1:5, 60 percent alcohol. Dosage: 20–40 drops in hot water up to 3x daily.

***Collinsonia* (stone root).** Tincture, dried root, 1:5, 60 percent alcohol. Dosage: 45–60 drops up to 4x daily. Michael Moore considers the tincture of the fresh plant to be far superior to that of the dried root. Tincture, fresh plant, 1:2, 20–40 drops up to 4x daily.

***Commiphora* (myrrh).** Tincture, dried resin, 1:5, 95 percent alcohol. Dosage: 5–20 drops up to 3x daily.

***Conyza canadensis* (Canadian fleabane).** Tincture, fresh flowering herb, 1:2. Dosage: 15–20 drops up to 3x daily. Infusion, dried flowering herb: 2–4 fluid ounces up to 4x daily.

***Coptis* (goldthread).** Tincture, dried root, 1:5, 50 percent alcohol. Dosage: 30–60 drops up to 3x daily.

***Corallorhiza* (coral root).** Tincture, fresh root, 1:2. Dosage: for acute conditions, 15–30 drops no more than each hour, as needed; as a tonic, 30–90 drops up to 3x daily. I don't think the dried root is a good choice for this herb, however—tincture, dried root, 1:5, 60 percent alcohol.

***Coriandrum* (coriander).** Tincture, dried seed, 1:5, 65 percent alcohol. Dosage: 10–20 drops as needed.

***Cornus sericea* (red osier dogwood).** Cold water percolation or infusion, dried root or bark: 3–6 fluid ounces up to 3x daily.

***Corydalis aurea* (goldensmoke).** Tincture, dried herb, 1:5, 50 percent alcohol. Dosage: 10–15 drops up to 4x daily.

***Crataegus* (hawthorn).** Tincture, dried berries, 1:5, 60 percent alcohol; fresh flowering branches, 1:2. Dosage: 10–30 drops up to 3x a day.

***Crocus* (saffron).** Tincture, dried stigmas (expensive), 1:5, 95 percent alcohol. Dosage: 5–20 drops.

***Cubeba* (cubeb berries).** Tincture, unripe fruit, 1:5, 80 percent alcohol. Dosage: 10–30 drops up to 3x daily. Not for long-term use.

***Cupressus* (true cypress).** Tincture, fresh needles/stems, 1:2, 5 percent glycerine; recently dried needles, 1:5, 60 percent alcohol, 5 percent glycerine. Dosage: for diarrhea, 20 drops as necessary, usually not for more than 3 days; for gum infections, 5 drops in water, used to wash mouth. Not for long-term use internally. Infusion, dried needles/twigs: 2–4 fluid ounces, generally for GI tract problems.

***Curcuma* (turmeric).** Tincture, dried root, 1:5, 50 percent alcohol. Dosage: 10–30 drops up to 2x daily.

***Datura* (jimsonweed).** Tincture, fresh or dried leaf, 1:3, 70 percent rubbing alcohol. For external use.

***Daucus carota* (wild carrot).** Tincture, dried seed, 1:5, 60 percent alcohol. Dosage: 20–60 drops up to 2x daily.

***Dicentra formosa* (bleeding heart).** Tincture, fresh root, 1:2. Dosage: 10–20 drops up to 3x daily. Tincture, dried root, 1:5, 50 percent alcohol. Dosage: 15–30 drops up to 3x daily.

***Dioscorea villosa* (wild yam).** Tincture, dried root: 1:5, 60 percent alcohol. Dosage: 30–100 drops up to 4x daily.

***Dipsacus* (teasel).** Tincture, freshly dried autumn first-year root or spring second-year root, 1:3, 45 percent alcohol. Dosage: 1–30 drops up to 3x daily depending on whether you are a homeopathic herbalist or a regular one.

***Dracontium* (symplocarpus, skunk cabbage).** Tincture, freshly dried root, 1:5, 50 percent alcohol. Dosage: 20–60 drops up to 3x daily.

***Echinacea angustifolia* (purple coneflower).** Tincture, fresh flower heads in seed, 1:2; dried root, 1:5, 70 percent alcohol. Dosage: acute, 30 drops each hour; tonic, 30–100 drops up to 3x daily.

***Echinacea pallida* (purple coneflower).** Same as for *E. angustifolia*.

***Echinacea purpurea* (purple coneflower).** Same as for *E. angustifolia*, except I consider the plant to be much less effective, so dosage needs to be much higher, 1–2 tsp up to 5x daily.

***Eleutherococcus* (eleuthero, Siberian ginseng).** Tincture, dried root, 1:5, 60 percent alcohol. Dosage: as long-term tonic, 20–60 drops daily.

Fluid extract: dried root, 1:1, 60 percent alcohol. Dosage: as a tonic, 10–15 drops up to 3x daily; for acute conditions with severe fatigue, ½–1 tsp 2x daily, 20 days on, 10 days off, then repeat.

***Ephedra viridis* (Mormon tea, American ephedra).** Tincture, dried herb, 1:5, 50 percent alcohol. Dosage: 15–30 drops. Best if used in combination formulas.

***Ephedra vulgaris* (ma huang).** Tincture, dried herb, 1:5, 50 percent alcohol. Dosage: 10–15 drops. In my opinion, should only be used in combination formulas. Note: now illegal in the United States.

***Epipactis gigantea* (stream orchid).** Tincture, fresh plant, 1:2; dried root, 1:5, 60 percent alcohol. Dosage: 30–90 drops. A very nice nervine.

***Equisetum arvense* (horsetail).** Tincture, fresh spring plant, 1:2. Dosage: 15 drops to ½ tsp up to 5x daily. Infusion, dried spring or early summer herb: 2–4 fluid ounces daily.

***Equisetum hyemale* (scouring rush).** Same as for *E. arvense.*

***Eriodictyon* (yerba santa).** Tincture, fresh leaf, 1:2; dried, 1:5, 75 percent alcohol. Dosage: 15–30 drops up to 5x daily. I prefer this tincture in combination formulas. Infusion: 2–4 fluid ounces as needed.

***Eschscholtzia californica* (California poppy).** Tincture, fresh flowering plant, 1:2. Dosage: 15–25 drops up to 3x daily.

***Eucalyptus* (eucalyptus).** Tincture, dried leaf, 1:5, 65 percent alcohol. Dosage: 5–15 drops in hot water up to 5x daily. Infusion: 2–4 fluid ounces up to 4x daily.

***Eupatorium perfoliatum* (boneset).** Tincture, fresh flowering herb, 1:2. Dosage: 20–40 drops in hot water up to 3x daily. Infusion, dried herb: 6–8 fluid ounces up to 3x daily.

***Eupatorium purpureum* (gravel root, queen of the meadow, joe-pye weed).** Tincture, fresh root, 1:2; dried root, 1:5, 60 percent alcohol. Dosage: 30–90 drops in hot water up to 3x daily. Decoction, dried root: 2–4 fluid ounces up to 4x daily.

***Euphrasia* (eyebright).** Tincture, dried herb, 1:5, 50 percent alcohol. Dosage: 30–90 drops, orally, up to 4x daily. I prefer this tincture in combination formulas. Decoction, dried herb: 2–4 fluid ounces up to 4x daily.

***Filipendula* (meadowsweet).** Tincture, fresh flowering herb, 1:2. Dosage: 60–90 drops up to 4x daily. Tincture, dried flowering herb, 1:5, 50 percent alcohol, 90–120 drops up to 4x daily. Infusion, dried herb in flower: 3–6 fluid ounces up to 4x daily.

***Foeniculum* (fennel seed).** Tincture, dried seed, 1:5, 60 percent alcohol. Dosage: 10–15 drops directly on the tongue or 30–60 drops in warm water as needed. Infusion: as needed.

***Fouquieria splendens* (ocotillo).** Tincture, fresh bark, 1:2. Dosage: 10–30 drops up to 4x daily.

***Fragaria* (strawberry):** Infusion, dried herb: as needed.

***Galium aparine* (cleavers, bedstraw).** Tincture, fresh plant, 1:2.

Dosage: 1–2 tsp up to 4x daily. Fresh plant juice: up to 1/4 ounce daily. Or plant juice stabilized with 25 percent alcohol: same dosage as tincture. Infusion: as needed.

***Ganoderma* (reishi).** Tincture, fruiting body, 1:5, 20 percent alcohol. Dosage: 10–20 ml (2–4 tsp) 3x daily. Note: Prepare a decoction of the herb in the amount of water to be used in tincturing. Add to cold water, bring to boil, cover, slow-boil for 30 minutes. Turn off heat, allow to cool. Pour into jar, add alcohol, put on lid, and let sit 2 weeks. Decant and store. You can also use a slow cooker to slow-cook it, covered, for 24 to 72 hours.

***Garrya* (silk tassel).** Tincture, fresh leaf, 1:2; dried leaf, 1:5, 50 percent alcohol. Dosage: 45–60 drops up to 5x daily. Tincture, root bark, 1:5, 50 percent alcohol. Dosage: 10–20 drops up to 5x daily.

***Gentiana* (gentian).** Tincture, dried root, 1:5, 50 percent alcohol. Dosage: 5–20 drops before meals, if you can take it.

***Geranium* (cranesbill).** Tincture, dried root, 1:5, 50 percent alcohol, 10 percent glycerin. Dosage: 30 drops–1 tsp up to 4x daily. Decoction: 1–4 fluid ounces up to 4x daily.

***Glycyrrhiza glabra* (licorice).** Tincture, dried root, 1:5, 50 percent alcohol. Dosage: 10 drops up to 3x daily. Best if used in formula combinations. I do not recommend this herb singly.

***Glycyrrhiza lepidota* (American licorice):** Same as for *G. glabra*.

***Gossypium* (cotton).** Tincture, fresh root bark, 1:2. Dosage: 30–60 drops up to 3x daily. Tincture, freshly dried root bark, 1:5, 50 percent alcohol. Dosage: 1–2 tsp up to 4x daily. Try to avoid commercial cotton; it's highly chemicalized.

***Grindelia* (gumweed).** Tincture, fresh flowering top, 1:2; freshly dried flowering herb, 1:5, 70 percent alcohol. Dosage: 15–40 drops up to 5x daily.

***Guaiacum officinale* (lignum vitae).** Tincture, dried bark or wood, 1:5, 95 percent alcohol. Dosage: 5–15 drops in water, frequently.

***Hamamelis* (witch hazel).** Tincture, fresh twigs and leaves, 1:2. Dosage: 10–60 drops as needed.

***Harpagophytum procumbens* (devil's claw).** Tincture, dried root, 1:2, 60 percent alcohol. Dosage: up to 1 tsp 2x daily. Cold water percolation: 4–6 fluid ounces daily.

***Heracleum* (cow parsnip).** Tincture, fresh seed, 1:2. Dosage: 5–10 drops as needed for hiatus hernia. Tincture: fresh root, 1:2. Dosage: 5–10 drops as needed as oral antimicrobial for gums.

***Heterotheca* (camphor weed).** Tincture for external use, fresh flowering herb, 1:2, 70 percent rubbing alcohol; recently dried, 1:5, 70 percent rubbing alcohol. Topically as liniment. Powdered dried root as antifungal for athlete's foot.

***Humulus* (hops).** Tincture, fresh strobiles (i.e., flowery things on the vine), 1:2; dried strobules, 1:5, 65 percent alcohol. Dosage: 30–90 drops up to 3x daily.

***Hydrangea arborescens* (seven barks).** Tincture, fresh root, 1:2; dried root, 1:5, 50 percent alcohol. Dosage: ½–1 tsp in water up to 4x daily.

***Hydrastis* (goldenseal).** Tincture, dried root, 1:5, 70 percent alcohol. Dosage: 20–50 drops up to 4x daily. Would highly recommend berberine alternatives.

***Hyoscyamus niger* (henbane).** Tincture, fresh flowering top, 1:2. Dosage: 3–10 drops up to 3x daily. Caution is advised.

***Hypericum* (St. John's wort).** Tincture: fresh flowering top, 1:2. Dosage: 20–30 drops up to 3x daily. Dried plant is useless.

***Illicium* (star anise).** Tincture, dried seed, 1:5, 50 percent alcohol. Dosage: 5–10 drops as needed.

***Impatiens* (jewelweed).** Juice of fresh plant, stabilized with 20 percent alcohol. Topical use for poison ivy and other itchy rashes as needed. (Fresh plant tincture not quite as good.)

***Inula* (elecampane).** Tincture, fresh root, 1:2; dried root, 1:5, 60 percent alcohol. Dosage: 10–30 drops up to 4x daily.

***Iris missouriensis* (blue flag).** Tincture, dried root only, 1:5, 80 percent alcohol. Dosage: 5–20 drops up to 3x daily. Not for long-term use.

***Iris versicolor* (blue flag).** Same as for *I. missouriensis*.

***Isatis* (woad).** Tincture, dried leaf or root, 1:5, 25 percent alcohol. Both leaves and root should be heated in the water to be used for the tincture, to a boil, and left to steep until cool; then add alcohol. Dosage: as a tonic, 30 drops up to 6x day; for acute conditions, 1 tsp up to 10 times day. Decoction, root: 10–30 grams (⅓–1 ounce) of the root boiled for 30 minutes. Dosage: 1 cup 3x daily for a max of 3 weeks. Decoction, leaf: 9–15 grams of the leaf as a tonic, 60–120 grams in acute conditions, boiled for 30 minutes. Dosage: 1 cup 3x daily.

***Juglans major* (black walnut).** Tincture: fresh leaf, 1:2; dried leaf, 1:5, 50 percent alcohol. Dosage: 30–90 drops up to 3x daily. Tincture, dried hull, 1:5, 50 percent alcohol. Dosage: 20–50 drops up to 4x daily.

***Juniperus* (juniper).** Tincture, dryish berries, 1:5, 75 percent alcohol. Dosage: 10–20 drops up to 3x daily. Tincture, fresh needles, 1:2. Dosage: 30–50 drops up to 4x daily.

***Krameria* (rhatany).** Tincture, dried root, 1:5, 50 percent alcohol, 10 percent glycerin (or not; I haven't noticed a problem without glycerin). Dosage: 20–50 drops up to 3x daily. World-class astringent.

***Lactuca* (wild lettuce).** Tincture, fresh herb in seed, 1:2. Dosage: ½–1 tsp up to 3x daily.

***Larrea* (chaparral).** Tincture, leaves and small twigs, 1:5, 75 percent alcohol. Dosage: 20–60 drops up to 3x daily.

***Leonurus cardiaca* (motherwort).** Tincture, fresh flowering herb, 1:2. (Would not suggest using the dried plant at all.) Dosage: 30–60 drops up to 4x daily. Up to ¼ fluid ounce at a time, in water. Exceptional if combined with *Pedicularis*, equal parts.

***Leptandra* (Culver's root).** Tincture, dried root, 1:5, 65 percent alcohol.

Dosage: 10–30 drops up to 3x daily. I prefer this herb in combination formulas. Nice herb but very strong.

***Ligusticum porteri* (osha).** Tincture, dried root, 1:5, 70 percent alcohol. Dosage: 20–60 drops up to 5x daily. Very intense.

***Lobelia inflata* (lobelia).** Tincture, fresh flowering plant, 1:4, pure grain alcohol. Dosage: 5–20 drops up to 4x daily. Skip the dried plant; it's relatively useless. Tincture, fresh seed, 1:5, 65 percent alcohol. Dosage: 3–10 drops.

***Lomatium dissectum* (lomatium).** Tincture, fresh root, 1:2; tincture, dried root, 1:5, 70 percent alcohol. Dosage: 10–30 drops up to 4x daily.

***Lycium pallidum* (wolfberry).** Tincture, fresh herb, 1:2. Dosage: 15–40 drops up to 4x daily.

***Lycopus* (bugleweed, water horehound).** Tincture, fresh herb, 1:2. Dosage: 15–40 drops up to 3x daily.

***Lysichiton americanum* (western skunk cabbage), my favorite.** Tincture, freshly dried root, 1:5, 50 percent alcohol. Dosage: 20–60 drops up to 3x daily.

***Mahonia* (Oregon grape).** Tincture, dried root, 1:5, 50 percent alcohol. Dosage: 10–60 drops up to 3x daily. Infusion or cold water percolation: 1–3 fluid ounces up to 3x daily. More in acute GI tract conditions.

***Malva neglecta* (mallow).** Infusion: 2–6 fluid ounces as needed. Highly useful as part of decoction mix for cough syrups.

***Marrubium* (horehound).** Tincture, fresh flowering herb, 1:2; dried plant, 1:5, 50 percent alcohol. Dosage: 30–90 drops up to 4x daily. (Yuck, talk about bitter.) Exceptionally useful as part of a combination decoction for cough syrups.

***Matricaria* (chamomile).** Tincture, fresh flower, 1:2; dried flower, 1:5, 45 percent alcohol. Dosage: 100–150 drops up to 3x daily.

***Matricaria matricarioides*, a.k.a. *discoidea* (pineapple weed).** Same as for *Matricaria.*

***Medicago sativa* (alfalfa).** Infusion, dried flowering plant: usually in the morning, or as needed. Exceptionally good blended with red clover and wild oat straw, equal parts.

***Melissa officinalis* (lemon balm).** Tincture, fresh flowering herb, 1:2; recently dried flowering herb, 1:5, 50 percent alcohol. Dosage: ½–1 tsp in warm water up to 4x daily. Tincture for external use: 1:3, 25 percent alcohol, 30 percent glycerine, 45 percent water; use topically for itching skin blisters/shingles.

***Mentha arvensis* (poleo mint).** Tincture, fresh herb (in flower if possible just for the added mass), 1:2. Dosage: 1 drop on up.

***Mentha piperita* (peppermint).** Same as for *M. arvensis.*

***Mentha spicata* (spearmint, yerba buena).** Same as for *M. arvensis.*

***Menyanthes* (buckbean, bogbean).** Tincture, whole fresh plant, 1:2; dried plant, 1:5, 50 percent alcohol. Dosage: 10–30 drops up to 3x daily.

***Mitchella repens* (squaw vine).** Tincture, fresh plant, 1:2; dried plant,

1:5, 50 percent alcohol. Dosage: ½–1 tsp up to 3x daily.

***Myrica* (bayberry).** Tincture, fresh root bark, 1:2; dried root bark, 1:5, 60 percent alcohol. Dosage: 20–60 drops up to 3x daily; in acute conditions ½–1 tsp up to 4x daily. Cold water percolation: 2–4 fluid ounces up to 3x daily; in acute conditions up to 6x daily.

***Nepeta cataria* (catnip).** Tincture, fresh flowering herb, 1:2; recently dried herb if you must, 1:5, 50 percent alcohol. Dosage: ½–1 tsp up to 4x daily.

***Nuphar* (yellow pond lily).** Tincture, fresh root, 1:2. Dosage: 10–20 drops up to 3x daily.

***Oenothera* (evening primrose).** Tincture, fresh flowering herb stalk, 1:2. Dosage: 30 drops up to 1 tsp as needed. Tincture, seed, 1:5, 60 percent alcohol, 10 percent glycerine. Dosage: 3–10 drops up to 6x daily.

***Olea europaea* (olive).** Tincture, fresh leaf, 1:2; dried leaf, 1:5, 60 percent alcohol. Dosage: 20–40 drops up to 3x daily.

***Oplopanax horridus* (devil's club).** Tincture, dried root bark, 1:5, 60 percent alcohol. Dosage: 10–40 drops up to 3x daily.

***Opuntia* (prickly pear).** Fresh pad juice, stabilized with 25 percent alcohol: 1–3 fluid ounces up to 2x daily.

***Osmorhiza occidentalis* (western sweet cicely).** Tincture, dried root, 1:5, 65 percent alcohol. Dosage: 45–60 drops up to 3x daily.

***Paeonia* (peony).** Tincture, dried root, 1:5, 60 percent alcohol. Dosage: 10–25 drops up to 4x daily.

***Panax ginseng* (Asian ginseng).** Tincture, cured (red) root, 1:5, 70 percent alcohol. Dosage: 5–30 drops up to 3x daily. Tincture, uncured (white) root, 1:5, 70 percent alcohol. Dosage: 20–40 drops.

***Panax quinquefolium* (American ginseng).** Tincture, all forms of dried roots, 1:5, 70 percent alcohol. Woods-grown dosage: 10–20 drops 3x daily. Field-cultivated dosage: 20–40 drops 3x daily.

***Parietaria* (pellitory-of-the-wall).** Tincture, flowering herb, 1:5, 50 percent alcohol. Dosage: 60–90 drops up to 5x daily.

***Passiflora* (passionflower).** Tincture, fresh flowering herb (if you can get it in flower; otherwise, just the whole herb), 1:2; dried, 1:5, 50 percent alcohol. Dosage: ½–1½ tsp up to 4x daily.

***Paullinia cupana* (guarana).** Take this one as a powder of the seed, 1 tsp in a little water. Makes the mind *clear* and the self energetic. Very unlike caffeine. Tincture the dried seed if you want, 1:5, 65 percent alcohol. Dosage: ¼–1 tsp.

***Pausinystalia* (yohimbe).** Tincture, dried bark, 1:5, 65 percent alcohol. Dosage: 5–30 drops. Careful with this one.

***Pedicularis* and *P. groenlandica* in particular (lousewort, elephant head).** Same as for *P. bracteosa* on page 593. A lot of people use the species interchangeably, but *groenlandica* and fernleaf lousewort (*P. bracteosa*) are the only two I have tried, and I think *groenlandica* tastes dreadful. Michael Moore notes the pediculari are semi-parasitic and pick up stuff from their hosts. I generally harvest the fernleaf lousewort that grows among aspen groves and haven't noticed a problem. Moore suggests that you avoid species growing in close proximity to *Senecio* species or toxic legumes. I think the dried herb is useless.

***Pedicularis bracteosa* (betony, fernleaf lousewort).** Tincture, fresh plant, 1:2. Dosage: 30 drops up to ½ fluid ounce in water as needed. My favorite of the pediculari. Very nice as a general muscle relaxant, especially if combined in equal parts with motherwort tincture.

***Petasites* (western coltsfoot).** Tincture, fresh herb, 1:2. Dosage: 30–60 drops up to 3x daily.

***Petroselinum* (parsley).** Tincture, dried root, 1:5, 60 percent alcohol. Dosage: 30–60 drops up to 3x daily; I'd mix the tincture in water with this one.

***Phytolacca* (poke).** Tincture, dried root, 1:5, 50 percent alcohol. Dosage: 5–15 drops up to 3x daily. Not nearly as unsafe as portrayed; nevertheless, use with awareness and be careful with that dose.

***Picraena* (quassia).** Tincture, dried bark, 1:5, 50 percent alcohol. Dosage: 30–60 drops up to 3x daily.

***Pilocarpus* (jaborandi).** Tincture, dried leaf, 1:5, 60 percent alcohol. Dosage: 15–30 drops in warm water.

***Pinus* (pine).** Tincture, needles, 1:5, 60 percent alcohol. Dosage: 10–30 drops up to 3x daily. Powdered: topically as needed.

***Pinus* pollen (pollen pini).** Tincture, 1:5, 60 percent alcohol. Dosage: as a tonic, 10 drops up to 3x daily; as a treatment for specific conditions, 30 drops 3x daily. Not for men under 45 without a specific medical condition. Not generally for women except in certain medical conditions. Not for muscle builders. Contains high amounts of testosterone. Large doses (½ fluid ounce a day or more) will shrink testes and reduce normal testosterone production.

***Piper methysticum* (kava kava).** Tincture, dried root, 1:5, 60 percent alcohol. Dosage: 30–90 drops up to 4x daily. The fresher the root, the better.

***Piper nigrum* (black pepper).** Tincture, dried fruit (i.e., peppercorns), 1:5, 65 percent alcohol. Dosage: 5–15 drops.

***Plantago major* (plantain).** Fresh leaf juice, really the only good way to use this plant: 1–2 tbl up to 4x daily. Can be frozen or stabilized with 20 percent to 25 percent alcohol. Specific for Crohn's, IBS, intestinal ulceration. Topical poultice of the fresh leaf for splinters, basically, embedded things in the skin. Magic.

***Polygonatum* (Solomon's seal).** Tincture, fresh root, 1:2. Dosage: 10–30 drops up to 3x daily.

***Polygonum bistorta* (bistort root).** Tincture, dried root, 1:5, 50 percent alcohol, 10 percent glycerin. Dosage: 30–90 drops up to 3x daily.

***Polypodium glycyrrhiza* (licorice fern).** Tincture, dried root, 1:5, 50 percent alcohol. Dosage: 10–30 drops up to 3x daily.

***Populus balsamifera* (balsam poplar).** Tincture, fresh early-spring leaf buds, 1:2; very recently dried early-spring leaf buds, 1:5, 75 percent alcohol. Dosage: 15–30 drops up to 3x daily. You can also infuse the early-spring leaf buds in oil for topical use. Yum.

***Populus tremuloides* (quaking aspen).** Tincture, freshly dried bark, 1:5, 50 percent alcohol. Dosage: 10–30 drops up to 3x daily.

***Prinos* (black alder).** Tincture, freshly dried bark, 1:5, 65 percent alcohol. Dosage: 10–30 drops up to 2x daily.

Propolis (from the hive). Tincture, 1:5, 95 percent alcohol. Dosage: 5–15 drops in a little honey or straight if you can take it. Doesn't mix well with others.

***Prunella* (self-heal, heal-all).** Tincture, fresh plant, 1:2. Dosage: as needed. A highly underrated plant.

***Prunus* (choke cherry).** Tincture, late summer or fall bark, 1:5, 60 percent alcohol, 10 percent glycerin. Dosage: 30–90 drops up to 4x daily. I prefer the small, high-mountain varieties, especially in syrups. They really are better. The berries should be dried and added to the syrup decoction as it is cooking.

***Prunus persica* (peach tree).** Tincture, recently dried leaf, 1:5, 50 percent alcohol. Dosage: 10–60 drops up to 3x daily.

***Ptelea* (wafer ash, hop tree).** Tincture, bark, seed, or leaf, 1:5, 65 percent alcohol. Dosage: 10–30 drops up to 3x daily.

***Ptychopetalum* (muira puama, potency wood).** Tincture, dried bark, 1:5, 70 percent alcohol. Dosage: 30–60 drops. Careful, this one does have an effect on the male organs of reproduction.

***Pulmonaria* (lungwort).** Tincture, fresh flowering herb, 1:2. Dosage: 30–90 drops as needed.

***Pygeum africanum* (African prune).** Tincture, dried bark, 1:5, 50 percent alcohol. Dosage: 40–80 drops up to 3x daily.

***Pyrola* (false wintergreen).** Tincture, 1:5, 60 percent alcohol. Dosage: 20–40 drops up to 3x daily.

***Quercus* (oak).** Tincture, dried root, 1:5, 50 percent alcohol, 10 percent glycerin. Dosage: 30 drops to 1 tsp up to 4x daily. Decoction: 1–4 fluid ounces up to 4x daily.

***Rhamnus californica* (California buckthorn, coffeeberry).** Tincture, well-dried bark, 1:5, 50 percent alcohol. Dosage: 1–2 tsp.

***Rheum officinale* (rhubarb).** Tincture, dried root, 1:5, 50 percent alcohol, 10 percent glycerin. Dosage: 15–30 drops up to 4x daily. Note: Vitamin C powder is a much better solution for constipation.

***Rhodiola rosea, R. integrifolia* (rhodiola, golden root, rose root).** Tincture, dried root, 1:5, 50 percent alcohol (some people use a 1:3). Dosage: as a tonic, 30–40 drops 3–4x daily; in acute conditions, ½–1 tsp 3x daily for 20 to 30 days, then back to the tonic dose. The tincture is usually taken in water—the plant is extremely astringent.

***Rhus aromatica* (sweet sumac).** Tincture, dried root bark, 1:5, 50 percent alcohol, 10 percent glycerin. Dosage: 20–40 drops up to 4x daily.

***Rhus glabra* (smooth sumac).** Tincture, dried leaf or fruit, 1:5, 50 percent alcohol, 10 percent glycerin. Dosage: 20–40 drops up to 4x daily.

***Rosmarinus* (rosemary).** Tincture, dryish leaf, 1:5, 60 percent alcohol. Dosage: 30–60 drops up to 3x daily.

***Rubus idaeus* (raspberry).** Infusion, dried leaf: as often as needed. Excellent for diarrhea.

***Rubus villosus* (blackberry).** Infusion or decoction, dried root bark: 2–4 fluid ounces. Really excellent for diarrhea. If it just won't quit, use this. I don't know why more people don't.

***Rumex crispus* (yellow dock).** Tincture, dried root, 1:5, 50 percent alcohol. Dosage: 30–75 drops up to 3x daily.

***Rumex hymenosepalus* (canaigre, red dock).** Decoction, dried root. Dosage: not a lot. World-class astringent; it will suck the moisture out of your body starting at your toes and then go all the way up. Great topically as either powder or cooled decoction for any kind of seeping wounds. Tincture, dried root, 1:5, 50 percent alcohol, 10 percent glycerin. Great in gum toner combinations.

***Ruscus aculeatus* (butcher's broom).** Tincture, fresh root, 1:2. Dosage: 30–60 drops up to 3x daily.

***Salix* (willow).** Decoction, dried bark: 2–4 fluid ounces to 4x daily. Evaporative concentrate for topical use.

***Salvia* (sage).** Tincture, fresh herb (in flower), 1:2; dried herb, 1:5, 50 percent alcohol. Dosage: 30–60 drops as needed. Decoctions and infusions are also useful.

***Sambucus* (elder).** Tincture, fresh flower, 1:2. Dosage: 30–90 drops up to 3x daily. Tincture, fresh leaf, 1:2. Dosage: 10 drops, not more than once per hour (good nervine). Tincture, dried berry, 1:5, 50 percent alcohol. Dosage: 20–40 drops up to 3x daily. If nausea occurs, back off on the dose.

***Scoparius* (broom).** Tincture, dried flowering top, 1:5, 50 percent alcohol. Dosage: 20–40 drops up to 4x daily.

***Scrophularia* (figwort).** Tincture, fresh herb, 1:2. Dosage: 30–60 drops up to 3x daily.

***Scutellaria* (skullcap).** Tincture, fresh plant, 1:2. Dosage: 20–60 drops or more to 3x daily. Some people are highly responsive to it, others—nothing. Would skip the dried herb unless very recently harvested; fairly useless otherwise: 1:5, 50 percent alcohol.

***Serenoa* (saw palmetto).** Tincture, dried berry, 1:5, 80 percent alcohol. Dosage: 30–90 drops up to 3x daily. Yuck. Fetid soap.

***Sida* (sida).** Tincture, fresh leaf, 1:2; dried leaf, 1:5, 60 percent alcohol. Dosage: 20–40 drops up to 4x daily; in acute conditions, ½ tsp–1 tbl, 3–6x daily, generally for less than 60 days.

***Silybum marianum* (milk thistle).** Tincture, dried seed, 1:3, 70 percent alcohol. Dosage: 30–60 drops up to 5x daily minimum; or 1–2 tsp 3x daily in liver disease. For liver disease, though, the standardized capsules are much better, 1,200 mg daily. In tonic liver mixes, the powdered seeds are good in larger doses.

***Smilacina racemosa* (false Solomon's seal).** Tincture, fresh root, 1:2. Dosage: 10–20 drops up to 3x daily. The dried root is very good in syrups.

***Smilax* (sarsaparilla).** Tincture, fresh root, 1:2; dried root, 1:5, 60 percent alcohol. Dosage: 30–90 drops up to 3x daily.

***Solanum dulcamara* (bittersweet).** Tincture, fresh stem, 1:2; dried stem, 1:5, 60 percent alcohol. Dosage: 10–20 drops 1–2x daily. The plant is a lot milder than its reputation.

***Solidago* (goldenrod).** Tincture, fresh plant in flower, 1:2. Dosage: 20–60 drops up to 3x daily.

***Stachys officinalis* (European betony).** Tincture, fresh flowering herb, 1:2; dried herb, 1:5, 50 percent alcohol. Dosage: 3 drops to 1 tsp up to 4x daily.

***Sticta* (lobaria pulmonaria, lungwort moss).** Tincture, lichen, 1:5, 60 percent alcohol. Dosage: 20–30 drops up to 4x daily.

***Stillingia sylvatica* (queen's root).** Tincture, fresh root, 1:2; recently dried root, 1:5, 50 percent alcohol. Dosage: 10–30 drops daily.

***Swertia radiata*, a.k.a. *Frasera speciosa* (green gentian, cebadilla).** Powdered root, recently dried: mix with petroleum jelly and place on skin cancers, cover with bandage, leave 72 hours, remove.

***Symphytum* (comfrey).** Tincture, dried root: 1:5, 50 percent alcohol. Dosage: 30–60 drops up to 3x daily for up to 30 days. Root powder for ulceration in GI tract: 1 tsp 3x daily for 30 days.

***Tabebuia* (pau d'arco).** Tincture, dried bark, 1:5, 50 percent alcohol. Dosage: ½–1 tsp up to 4x daily.

***Tanacetum* (feverfew).** Tincture, fresh plant, 1:2; dried plant, 1:5, 50 percent alcohol. Dosage: 30–60 drops up to 4x daily. Cold infusion, fresh plant in flower: 2–4 fluid ounces.

***Taraxacum* (dandelion).** Tincture, fresh root, 1:2; fresh leaf, 1:2. Dosage: ½–1 tsp up to 4x daily. Don't take the leaf before bed; it's a strong diuretic.

***Thuja* (arborvitæ, red or yellow cedar).** Tincture, fresh herb, needle, or leaf, 1:2. Dosage: 5–15 drops in water up to 4x daily.

***Thymus* (thyme).** Tincture, fresh herb, 1:2; dried herb, 1:5, 45 percent alcohol. Dosage: 20–40 drops up to 3x daily.

***Tribulus* (puncture vine).** Tincture, dried seed (and herb if you must), 1:5, 60 percent alcohol. Dosage: 30–40 drops up to 2x daily.

***Trifolium pratense* (red clover).** Infusion or decoction, flowering herb: 4–6 fluid ounces daily.

***Trillium* (beth root).** Tincture, fresh plant, 1:2. Dosage: 15–25 drops up to 3x daily.

***Turnera diffusa* (damiana).** Tincture, fresh flowering herb, 1:2. Dosage: 20–30 drops up to 3x daily (yum). The dried plant isn't really worth it, but it would be 1:5, 60 percent alcohol. Fresh plant is the way to go.

***Ulmus pumila* (Siberian elm).** Cold infusion, powdered or shredded bark. Dosage: as needed for GI tract problems, debility. Note: *Ulmus fulva*, slippery elm, is endangered. Siberian elm is the primary elm that is an exact substitute for slippery elm. It is an invasive and should be used with abandon. It is really good, plus the fresh seeds are highly edible and tasty, especially if lightly cooked in butter. The dried seeds make a great flour.

***Umbellularia* (California bay, Oregon myrtle).** Tincture, fresh leaf, 1:2; recently dried leaf, 1:5, 65 percent alcohol. Dosage: 10–20 drops up to 3x daily.

***Uncaria tomentosa* (cat's claw).** Tincture, dried root bark or vine inner bark, 1:5, 60 percent alcohol. Dosage: 40–60 drops up to 3x daily.

***Urtica* (nettles).** Infusion, whole herb: as needed.

***Usnea* (old man's beard).** Tincture, dried herb, 1:5, 50 percent alcohol. Dosage: 30–60 drops up to 4x a day. Herb should be well ground, moistened with a little alcohol, then added to the proper amount of water to be used in the tincturing process, brought to a boil, slow-boiled, covered, for 30 minutes, then allowed to cool, still covered. Then the alcohol should be added, the whole mess put in a jar and allowed to macerate for 2 weeks, decanted, and bottled. A slow cooker can also be used instead of the boiling; let cook on the low setting for a couple of days.

***Valeriana* (valerian).** Tincture, dried root, 1:5, 70 percent alcohol. Dosage: 30–90 drops up to 3x daily. Old sock special.

***Verbascum* (mullein).** Tincture, fresh flowering head stalk, 1:2. Dosage: 20–40 drops up to 4x daily.

***Verbena* (blue vervain).** Tincture, fresh flowering herb, 1:2; dried flowering herb, 1:5, 60 percent alcohol. Dosage: 30–90 drops up to 4x daily.

***Viburnum* (cramp bark, black haw).** Tincture, root bark, and bark, 1:5, 50 percent alcohol. Dosage: 30–90 drops up to 4x daily.

***Vinca major* (periwinkle).** Tincture, fresh herb, 1:2; dried herb, 1:5, 50 percent alcohol. Dosage: 20–40 drops up to 2x daily.

***Vinca minor* (periwinkle).** Same as for *V. major*.

***Viola odorata* (violet).** Tincture, fresh plant in flower, 1:2. Dosage: 1–2 tsp up to 2x daily.

***Vitex agnus-castus* (chaste tree).** Tincture, dried berry, 1:5, 65 percent alcohol. Dosage: 30–60 drops in the morning. Michael Moore suggests using the tincture or the tea in the 2-week period before menses as it strengthens the progesterone phase of the cycle.

***Withania somnifera* (ashwagandha).** Tincture, dried root, 1:5, 70 percent alcohol. Dosage: 30–40 drops up to 3x daily. Tincture, fresh leaf, 1:2. Dosage: 10–30 drops up to 3x daily. Tincture, dried seed, 1:5, 65 percent alcohol. Dosage: 15–30 drops up to 3x daily. Tincture, fresh fruit, 1:2

(grind the whole mess well). Dosage: 15–30 drops up to 3x daily.

***Xanthoxylum* (prickly ash).** Tincture, bark/berry, 1:5, 65 percent alcohol. Dosage: 10–30 drops up to 3x daily.

***Zea mays* (corn silk).** Tincture, fresh silk, 1:2. Dosage: ½–1½ tsp in water. Excellent in UTI combinations.

***Zingiber* (ginger).** Fresh juice of the root, stabilized with 20 percent to 25 percent pure grain alcohol. Add ¼ cup fresh juice of gingerroot to 8 ounces hot water, and add 1 tbl wildflower honey, ⅛ tsp cayenne, and a squeeze of ¼ lime (then drop the peel in). Drink up to 6 cups daily. Fresh root tincture, 1:2. Dosage: 10–60 drops in warm to hot water up to 6x daily.

SOURCES OF SUPPLY

A weed is a plant that has mastered every survival skill except for learning how to grow in rows.

—Doug Larson

Many of the herbs I have talked about in this book—and, of course, a great many others—grow wild. Even if you live in a city, you can find many of them cohabitating with you or only a short drive away. Since many of these herbs are invasives, most people will be glad for you to take them away.

If you need to buy your herbs, the Internet is a good way to seek them. I suggest running a web search for the herbs you are looking for to find the cheapest prices; if you are persistent, you can often save half off normal retail.

If you are going to be buying a lot of herbs and you live in the United States, it makes sense to buy a resale license from your state. The price is often minimal and it will allow you to buy wholesale; most wholesalers will want a resale certificate before they will sell to you.

And, of course, you can grow them yourself. Once established most of the herbs in this book will provide medicine for you and your family forever.

Here are some of the best sources I know of for the herbs in this book. All of them are in the United States.

1stChineseHerbs.com
5018 View Ridge Drive
Olympia, WA 98501
888-842-2049
1stchineseherbs.com
Wonderful people with a very large selection of Chinese herbs, including most of those discussed in this book. Most herbs by the pound.

Elk Mountain Herbs
214 South 2nd Street
Laramie, WY 82070
307-742-0404
elkmountainherbs.com
Wonderful tinctures from local wildcrafted Western plants.

Green Dragon Botanicals

48 Elliot Street, Suite D
Brattleboro, VT 05301
877-591-1874
greendragonbotanicals.com

A good source for Japanese knotweed.

Healing Spirits Herb Farm and Education Center

61247 Route 415
Avoca, NY 14809
607-566-2701
healingspiritsherbfarm.com

Matthias and Andrea Reisen have been growing wonderful medicinal plants for years. The plants just jump out of the bag and laugh when you open it up.

Horizon Herbs, LLC

P. O. Box 69
Williams, OR 97544
541-846-6704
horizonherbs.com

Richo Cech has spent much of his life learning how to grow common and rare medicinals. He has seeds or young stock for most of the plants in this book as well as great information on how to grow them.

Mountain Rose Herbs

P. O. Box 50220
Eugene, OR 97405
800-879-3337
mountainroseherbs.com

A nice selection, sustainably produced.

Pacific Botanicals

4840 Fish Hatchery Road
Grants Pass, OR 97527
541-479-7777
pacificbotanicals.com

This is perhaps the best wholesaler (they also sell retail) in the U.S. Their herbs are magnificent. Normally, all are sold by the pound.

Sage Consulting & Apothecary

108 East Cheyenne Road
Colorado Springs, CO 80906
888-350-3911
sagewomanherbs.com

They have some herbs otherwise hard to get, especially isatis tincture (just the root though).

Woodland Essence

392 Teacup Street
Cold Brook, NY 13324
315-845-1515
woodlandessence.com

Kate and Don make wonderful tinctures and medicines and can sell you many of the herbal tinctures that I discuss in this book; if they don't have them, they can probably point you in the right direction.

Zack Woods Herb Farm

278 Mead Road
Hyde Park, VT 05655
802-888-7278
zackwoodsherbs.com

Melanie and Jeff are wonderful people and grow tremendously beautiful medicinal plants. Very, very high-quality herbs. Usually sold by the pound.

ENDNOTES

Prologue

1. Sarah White, "The Empowered Patient," *Medhill Reports*, December 8, 2010.
2. Denis Campbell and Anushka Asthana, "The 'Catalogue of Errors' That Cost This Father His Life," *The Guardian*, November 27, 2010.
3. "'The NHS Failed My Mum,' Says Distraught Daughter," *Grantham Journal*, December 14, 2010.

Chapter 1—The End of Antibiotics

1. W. J. Powell, "Molecular Mechanisms of Antimicrobial Resistance," technical report #14, Feb. 2000. Online at http://foodsafety.ksu.edu/articles/280/molecular_mechanisms_antimic_resist.pdf, page 2.
2. Stuart Levy, *The Antibiotic Paradox* (NY: Plenum Press, 1992), 94.
3. Ibid., 75.
4. Ibid., 3.
5. Ibid.
6. Quoted in Barbara Griggs, *Green Pharmacy* (Rochester, VT: Healing Arts Press, 1991), 261.
7. Brad Spellberg, *Rising Plague* (NY: Prometheus, 2009), 36–37.
8. R. L. Berkelman and J. M. Hughes, "The Conquest of Infectious Diseases: Who Are We Kidding?" *Annals of Internal Medicine* 119, no. 5 (1993): 426–27.
9. Marc Lappé, *When Antibiotics Fail* (Berkeley, CA: North Atlantic Books, 1995), 187.
10. Steven Projan, "Antibacteria Drug Discovery in the 21st Century," in Richard Wax et al., *Bacterial Resistance to Antimicrobials,* second edition (Boca Raton, FL: CRC Press, 2008), 413.
11. David Hooper, "Target Modification as a Mechanism of Antimicrobial Resistance," in Richard Wax et al., *Bacterial Resistance to Antimicrobials,* second edition (Boca Raton, FL: CRC Press, 2008), 134.
12. Harry Taber, "Antibiotic Permeability," in Richard Wax et al., *Bacterial Resistance to Antimicrobials,* second edition (Boca Raton, FL: CRC Press, 2008), 172.
13. Rob Stein, "New 'Superbugs' Raising Concerns Worldwide," *Washington Post,* October 11, 2010.
14. Olga Lomovskaya et al., "Multidrug Efflux Pumps: Structure, Mechanism, and Inhibition," in Richard Wax et al., *Bacterial Resistance to Antimicrobials,* second edition (Boca Raton, FL: CRC Press, 2008), 46.
15. C. Werry, "Contamination of Detergent Cleaning Solutions during Hospital Cleaning," *Journal of Hospital Infection* 11, no. 1 (1988): 44–49.
16. W. J. Powell, "Molecular Mechanisms of Antimicrobial Resistance," technical report #14, Feb. 2000. Online at http://foodsafety.ksu.edu/articles/280/molecular_mechanisms_antimic_resist.pdf.
17. Abigail Salyers et al., "Ecology of Antibiotic Resistant Genes," in Richard Wax et al., *Bacterial Resistance to Antimicrobials,* second edition (Boca Raton, FL: CRC Press, 2008), 11.
18. Stuart Levy, *The Antibiotic Paradox* (NY: Plenum Press, 1992), 101.
19. Ibid., 87.
20. Quoted in Philip Frappaolo, "Risks to Human Health from the Use of Antibiotics in Animal Feeds," in William Moats (ed.), *Agricultural Uses of Antibiotics* (American Chemical Society, 1986), 102.

21. Quoted in W. J. Powell, "Molecular Mechanisms of Antimicrobial Resistance," technical report #14, Feb. 2000. Online at http://foodsafety.ksu.edu/articles/280/molecular_mechanisms_antimic_resist.pdf.
22. W. J. Powell, "Molecular Mechanisms of Antimicrobial Resistance," technical report #14, Feb. 2000. Online at http://foodsafety.ksu.edu/articles/280/molecular_mechanisms_antimic_resist.pdf.
23. "Staph Bacteria: Blood-Sucking Superbug Prefers the Taste of Humans," *Science Daily*, December 22, 2010.
24. Infectious Diseases Society of America, "Facts about Antibiotic Resistance," April 2011, http://idsociety.org/AR_Facts/.
25. Quoted in Philip Hilts, "Gene Jumps to Spread a Toxin in Meat," *New York Times*, April 23, 1996.
26. Maggie Fox, "Modern Life Comes with Disease Price Tag," Reuters, AOL Online, September 20, 2000.
27. Brandon Keim, "Antibiotics Breed Superbugs Faster Than Expected," Wired.com, December 22, 2010.
28. Nicols Fox, *Spoiled: The Dangerous Truth about a Food Chain Gone Haywire* (NY: Penguin, 1998), 122.
29. Marissa Cevallos, "Meat Contaminated with Resistant Bacteria," LATimes.com, April 15, 2011.
30. Stuart Levy, *The Antibiotic Paradox* (NY: Plenum, 1992), 183.
31. Sarah Bosley, "Are You Ready for a World without Antibiotics?" *The Guardian*, August 12, 2010.
32. Jeffrey Fisher, *The Plague Makers* (NY: Simon and Schuster, 1994), 90.
33. C. G. Daughton and T. A. Ternes, "Pharmaceutical and Personal Care Products in the Environment: Agents of Subtle Change?" *Environmental Health Perspectives* 107, suppl. 6 (1999), 907–38; see also Janet Raloff, "Waterways Carry Antibiotic Resistance," *Science News Online* 155, no. 23 (June 5, 1999).
34. C. G. Daughton and T. A. Ternes, "Pharmaceutical and Personal Care Products in the Environment: Agents of Subtle Change?" *Environmental Health Perspectives* 107, suppl. 6 (1999), 907–38.
35. Stuart Levy, *The Antibiotic Paradox* (NY: Plenum Press, 1992), 175.
36. Lynn Margulis, *Symbiotic Planet* (NY: Basic Books, 1998), 75.
37. Marc Lappé, *When Antibiotics Fail* (Berkeley, CA: North Atlantic Books, 1995), xviii.
38. Ibid., 25–26.
39. Sarah Bosley, "Are You Ready for a World without Antibiotics?" *The Guardian*, August 12, 2010.

Chapter 2—The Resistant Organisms, the Diseases They Cause, and How to Treat Them

1. Brad Spellberg, *Rising Plague* (NY: Prometheus, 2009), 84.
2. "Battling Drug-Resistant Superbugs: Can We Win?" The Forum at Harvard School of Public Health, theforum.sph.harvard.edu/events/battling—drug-resistant-superbugs. (accessed February 24, 2014).
3. Brad Spellberg, *Rising Plague* (NY: Prometheus, 2009), 63.
4. Molly Hennessy-Fiske, "Drug-Resistant 'Superbug' Mostly Limited to Southern California Nursing Homes, Health Officials Say," *Los Angeles Times*, L.A. Now blog, March 24, 2010.

5. "Drug-Resistant 'Superbug' Hits LA County Hospitals, Nursing Homes," CBSLosAngeles.com, March 24, 2011, http://losangeles.cbslocal.com/2011/03/24/drug-resistant-super-bug-hits-la-county-hospitals-nursing-homes/.
6. Steve Sternberg, "Superbug Spreading," *USA Today,* September 17, 2010.
7. Sarah Bosley, "Are You Ready for a World without Antibiotics?" *The Guardian,* August 12, 2010.
8. George Eliopoulos, "Antimicrobial Resistance in the Enterococcus," in Richard Wax et al., *Bacterial Resistance to Antimicrobials,* second edition (Boca Raton, FL: CRC Press, 2008), 256.
9. Brad Spellberg, *Rising Plague* (NY: Prometheus, 2009), 79.
10. Sue Fischer, personal communication, March 2011.

Chapter 3—Emerging Viruses: What We Are Facing

1. Although I don't look at treatments for chikungunya fever virus in this book, some herbs have been found effective against it (in vitro): *Trigonostemon cherrieri, Flacourtia ramontchi, Anacolosa pervilleana.*
2. Frank Ryan, *Virus X: Tracking the New Killer Plagues* (Boston: Little, Brown, and Company, 1997), 9.
3. Lynn Margulis and Dorion Sagan, *What Is Life?* (NY: Simon and Schuster, 1995), 88.
4. Richard Lewontin, *The Triple Helix* (Cambridge, Mass.: Harvard University Press, 2000), 102–3.
5. Ryan, *Virus X,* 10.
6. Lewontin, *The Triple Helix,* 125–26.
7. Ryan, *Virus X,* 51.
8. Ryan, 52.

Chapter 4—Common Viral Illnesses and How to Treat Them

1. In contrast, read the description of the Native American use of lomatium while treating the flu epidemic on page 383.

Chapter 5—About Herbal Medicines

1. Z. K. Maskatia and K. Baker, "Hypereosinophilia Associated with Echinacea Use," *Southern Medical Journal* 103, no. 11 (2010): 1173–74.
2. M. A. Ekpo and P. C. Elim, "Antimicrobial Activity of Ethanolic and Aqueous Extracts of *Sida acuta* of Microorganisms from Skin Infections," *Journal of Medicinal Plants Research* 3, no. 9 (2009): 621–24.
3. Erich Fromm, as quoted by GoodReads, goodreads.com/quotes/show/233200 (accessed March 26, 2010).

Chapter 6—The Materia Medica

1. Nii-Ayi Ankrah, "Treatment of Falciparum Malaria with a Tea-Bag Formulation of Cryptolepis sanguinolenta root," *Ghana Medical Journal* 44, no. 1 (2010): 2.
2. Damintoti Karou et al., "Antibacterial Activity of Alkaloids from *Sida acuta,*" *African Journal of Biotechnology* 5, no. 2 (2008): 195–200.
3. Michael Moore, *Medicinal Plants of the Pacific West* (Sante Fe, NM: Red Crane Books, 1993), 69.
4. Ibid., 71.

5. F. H. Jansen, "The Herbal Tea Approach for Artemisinin as a Therapy for Malaria?" *Transactions of the Royal Society of Tropical Medicine and Hygiene* 100, no. 3 (2006): 285–86.
6. J. Falquet et al., "Artemisia annua as a Herbal Tea for Malaria," *African Journal of Traditional, Complementary, and Alternative Medicines* 4, no. 1 (2007): 121–23.
7. L. Iauk et al., "Activity of Berberis aetnensis Root Extracts on Candida Strains," *Fitoterapia* 78, no. 2 (2007): 159–61.
8. L. Slobodníková et al., "Antimicrobial Activity of Mahonia aquifolium Crude Extract and Its Major Isolated Alkaloids," *Phytotherapy Research* 18, no. 8 (2004): 674–76.
9. Ahmed Ali Sanaa et al., "Protective Role of *Juniperus phoenicea* and *Cupressus sempervirens* against CCl4," *World Journal of Gastrointestinal Pharmacology and Therapeutics* 1, no. 6 (2010): 123–31.
10. A. Schneider, "Tests Show Most Store Honey Isn't Honey," Food Safety News (online), November 7, 2011, foodsafetynews.com/2011/11/tests-show-most-store-honey-isnt-honey/.
11. I have a couple of comments about the scientific journal papers I used as sources of information on the plants.

In general, I tend to give highest credence to studies performed in Asia (primarily Japan), South America (of which there are too few), and Africa (the best). For antibacterials, African researchers are doing the best work. For antivirals, researchers in China, Korea, Japan, and India are doing the best work.

Unfortunately, U.S. researchers are too often biased against plant medicines, too influenced by pharmaceutical money, and too biased in favor of technological medicine to be completely reliable. The unreliability of Western science in this respect is a growing problem, one becoming commonly recognized throughout the world. In fact, our scientific tradition in the West risks becoming an unreliable joke throughout the world in the coming decades.

Marcia Angell, M.D., has commented on this in a number of articles. She comments:

> **It is simply no longer possible to believe much of the clinical research that is published, or to rely on the judgment of trusted physicians or authoritative medical guidelines. I take no pleasure in this conclusion, which I reached slowly and reluctantly over my two decades as an editor of** *The New England Journal of Medicine*. **[M. Angell, "Drug companies and doctors: A story of corruption,"** *New York Review of Books*, **January 15, 2009]**

Angell observes, earlier in that same article:

> **In view of this control and the conflicts of interest that permeate the enterprise, it is not surprising that industry-sponsored trials published in medical journals consistently favor sponsor's drugs—largely because negative results are not published, positive results are repeated in slightly different forms, and a positive spin is put on even negative results. A review of seventy-four clinical trials of antidepressants, for example, found that thirty-seven of thirty-eight positive studies were published. But of the thirty-six negative studies, thirty-three were either not published or published in a form that conveyed a positive outcome.**

John Ioannidis, in a rather remarkable article published in *PLoS Medicine*, **noted:**

> **There is increasing concern that in modern research, false findings may be the majority of, even the vast majority of, published research claims. However, this should not be surprising. It can be proven that most claimed research findings are false. [J. P. A. Ioannidis, "Why most published research findings are false,"** *PLoS Medicine* **2, no. 8 (2005): e124]**

And then he goes on to do just that.

The point of all this is to say that modern scientific research, while useful, is not the last word, nor are Western studies the most reliable. If we are to create a modern healing tradition in the West, in the true sense of that word "healing," then a very different paradigm than the one in use at the moment needs to be developed. So, while I do focus in some depth on journal papers and what are normally considered to be "scientific" studies, I take them with a large grain of salt.

It takes some time to really learn to read journal papers, and I don't mean from this developing an understanding of the terminology. While all the journal papers tend to follow the same structural outline and most use the same type of authorial voice, there are huge differences in the papers. With time and experience it is possible to tell which of the papers' authors know what they are doing and which do not, which are truly deep-thinking and which are barely average researchers, which of them are doing it for the money and which are genuinely interested in understanding what they are studying, which allow their humanity to guide their work and which do not. These factors alter the outcomes of the work considerably, though there has been little study of their influences. However, most people *think* that the use of journal papers confers legitimacy—and to be fair, some of them really are very good.

12. Curiously enough, many of the strongest antibacterial and antiviral plants are invasives. The dynamics of this are complex, not nearly so simple as one might think. Yes, invasives are tremendously potent simply by virtue of their capacity to take over ecosystems into which they are introduced. But this ignores the homeodynamis factors and deeply interwoven feedback systems that exist in the Earth ecosystem. Plants move throughout ecosystems in response to multiple complex factors, not simply because a seed hitchhiked on someone's shoe. Their impacts as they move are extremely complex and often highly sophisticated. And the question must always be asked, "What are they *doing* here?"

To give a very simple view outside contemporary perspectives: Amur honeysuckle (*Lonicera maackii*) is a shrub native to Japan, Korea, China, and Russia. It is an escaped cultivar in the United States and is invasive nearly everywhere it gets established. It is labeled invasive/banned in Connecticut, prohibited in Massachusettes, a noxious weed in Vermont, and invasive in Wisconsin and Tennessee. According to contemporary orientations regarding invasive species, the plant is considered to be a serious threat to ecosystem diversity and health and it is to be eradicated with extreme prejudice. However, the plant strongly affects the numbers of eggs laid by the mosquito *Aedes triseriatus*, a primary vector of La Crosse encephalitis virus (named after La Crosse, Wisconsin), reducing egg numbers considerably. The more honeysuckle there is, the fewer mosquitoes, the less the incidence of the viral disease in those areas. The plant also contains compounds that are specific for reducing inflammation, especially in the brain, during infection. They protect neurons and microglial cells from damage. This particular mosquito is also a vector for dengue fever (and other viruses), which is an emerging virus in the southern United States in such states as Texas and Georgia. Amur honeysuckle is also invasive in both those states. After 30 years of this work, I have continually seen that invasives show up in the regions where they are needed for the exact diseases that are emerging there. I can no longer discount it just because the mechanism for that process can't be seen with reductionist eyes.

13. S. H. Song and Z. Z. Wang, "Analysis of essential oils from different organs of Scutellaria baicalensis," *Zhong Yao Cai* 33, no. 8 (2010): 1265–70.

14. American Botanical Council, *The ABC Clinical Guide to Elder Berry* (Austin, Tex.: American Botanical Council, 2004), 8.

15. L. Johnson, "Elderberry for Cold and Flu Relief," *Healthy Living* (blog), CBN.com, http://blogs.cbn.com/healthyliving/archive/2011/10/13/elderberry-for-cold-and-flu-relief.aspx, October 13, 2011.

16. E. Parziale, "Elderberry," part of the Backyard Herbalist site hosted at Tripod.com, http://earthnotes.tripod.com/elderberry.htm, 1999.

17. F. Vandenbussche et al., "Analysis of the in planta antiviral activity of elderberry ribosome-inactivating proteins," *European Journal of Biochemistry* 271 (2004): 1508–15.

18. Thanks, Adam.

19. M. Moore, *Medicinal Plants of the Pacific Northwest* (Santa Fe, N.M.: Red Crane Books, 1993), 167.

20. Ibid., 167–68.

21. P. S. Beauchamp et al., "Essential oil composition of six *Lomatium* species attractive to Indra swallowtail butterfly (*Papilio indra*): Principal component analysis against essential oil composition of *Lomatium dissectum* var. *multifidum*," *Journal of Essential Oil Research* 21 (2009): 535–42.

22. E. Krebs, *Bulletin of the Nevada State Board of Health,* no. 1 (Carson City, Nev., January 1920).

Chapter 7—The First Line of Defense

1. S. Bhagwan et al., "*Ganoderma lucidum:* A Potent Pharmacological Macrofungus," *Current Pharmaceutical Biotechnology* 10 (2009): 717–42, and R. Russel and M. Paterson, "*Ganoderma:* A Therapeutic Fungal Biofactory," *Phytochemistry* 67 (2006): 1985–2001.

Chapter 8—A Handbook of Herbal Medicine Making

1. Michael Moore, *Herbal Materia Medica,* 5th ed. (Bisbee, AZ: Southwest School of Botanical Medicine, 1995).

In addition to the Endnotes, you will find a Bibliography at http://www.rodalenews.com/herbal-medicine-bibliography.

INDEX

Boldface page references indicate recipes. Underscored references indicate boxed text.

A

Abies (firs), 581
Acacia
  for bacterial diseases, 51, 57, 64, 66–67, 73, 75
  tincture, 581
  in washes, 552
Acetylenes, in bidens, 237, 240
Acetylsalicyclic acid, 186
Achillea (yarrow). *See* Yarrow
Acinetobacter, 19, 24, 28, 43–44, 56–58
Acorus calamus (calamus, sweet flag), 581
Actaea rubra (baneberry, red cohosh), 582
Acyclovir, 133, 158, 160–62, 172, 471
Adaptogens, 214, 484
Adenovirus, 128–29
Adiantum (maidenhair fern), 582
Aedes albopictus, 80
Aesculus hippocastanum (horse chestnut), 582
Agave (century plant), 582
Agrimonia (agrimony), 582
Agropyron repens (couchgrass), 582
Ailanthus altissima (tree of heaven), 582
Alchemilla (lady's mantle), 582
Alchornea (*Alchornea* spp.), 221–29, 224–26
  A. castaneifolia, 223
  actions of, 224
  common name, 221
  cultivation and collection, 223, 225
  finding, 225
  habitat and appearance, 223
  herb/drug interactions, 222
  parts used, 221
  plant chemistry, 225
  preparation and dosage, 222
    powder, 222
    tea, 222
    tincture, 222, 582
  properties of, 224
  scientific research, 226–29
    antimicrobial activity, 226–28
    malaria, 228
    sickle cell anemia, 227, 228
  side effects and contraindications, 222
  species used, 221
  traditional uses of, 225–26, 226
  use to treat, 224
    Aspergillus, 78
    candida, 76–77
    gastrointestinal viruses, 177–78
    Gram-negative bacterial diseases, 57, 59, 62, 64, 66–70, 73–74
    Gram-positive bacterial diseases, 51, 53–54
    malaria, 77–78
Alcohol
  content of tinctures, 565
  proof, 558, 558
  as solvent, 543
Alcohol extractions, 557–69
  described, 557–58
  douches, 568
  fluid extracts, 567–68
  glycerites, 563–66, **564**, 565
  herbal honeys, 566
  liniments, 568–69
  nasal sprays, 566
  tinctures, 559–63, 560, 562
  vinegar tinctures, 566–67
Alkaloids
  in alchornea, 225
  in berberine plants, 263, 265, 272–73, 275–77
  in cryptolepsis, 194, 199–200
  extraction, 187–88, 194
  in isatis, 369
  in sida, 207, 214–15, 218–21
  solubility and water pH, 194
Allium sativum. See Garlic
Alnus serrulata (tag alder), 582
Alpha lipoic acid, 176

Alpha-mannosidosis, 206
Alpinia (galangal), 439, 442, 582
Althaea. See Marsh mallow
Amantadine, 114–15
Ambrosia (ragweed), 582
Ammi visnaga (khella, bishop's weed), 582
Ampelopsis brevipedunculata, 167–68, 398
Andrographis, 170
Anemia, alchornea for, 227, 228
Anemone hirsutissima, 582
Anemone tuberosa (desert anemone, desert pasque flower), 582
Anemopsis (yerba mansa), 353, 582
Angelica (angelica), 583
Angelica sinensis (dong quai), 583
  for Gram-negative bacterial diseases, 68, 70, 73
  for HMGB1 inhibition, 113, 145–46
  for influenza, 126–27
Anisum (anise), 583
Antennaria (cat's paw, pussy toes, mountain everlasting), 583
Anthemis nobilis (Roman chamomile), 583
Anthocyanins, in elder, 340, 350
Antibacterials. *See also* Antibiotics
  adding synergists to systemic, 187
  alchornea, 221–29, 224–26
  artemisia, 242–58, 246–48
  ashwagandha, 466
  berberine, 184
  berberines, 259–80, 265–67
  bidens, 229–42, 232–33
  cryptolepsis, 192–204, 196–97, 200
  echinacea, 505
  golden seal, 184–85
  honey, 289–97, 291–92
  juniper, 280–89, 282
  localized, 184, 259–307
  5'-methoxyhydnocarpin (5'-MHC), 185
  rhodiola, 526, 531
  sida, 204–21, 208–10, 215, 220
  systemic, 184, 189–258
  usnea, 297–307, 299–300
Antibiotic age, 9–11
Antibiotic resistance, 85
  bacterial learning and, 20–23, 22
  deaths from, 8, 13
  developing, mechanisms for, 16–18
    altered uptake, 16
    antibiotic modification, 17
    efflux pumps, 17–18
    super adaptability, 18
    target modification, 16–17
  in ecosystem, 31–34
  as exponential growth curve, 41–44
  factory farms and, 28–31
  hospital-acquired infections, 12–13, 27–28
  resistant microorganisms, 45–78
  rise of, 14–23, 15, 22
  sharing, methods of, 18–20
    plasmids, 19
    transposons and integrons, 19–20
    using viruses, 20
  spread of resistant disease, 23–28
Antibiotics. *See also* Antibacterials; Antibiotic resistance
  end of, 7–38
  environmental contamination with, 10–11
  herbal, 4–5
  limits of, 11–13
  use in animals, 9
  in waste stream, 10
Antimicrobials. *See specific herbs*
Antithrombin III, 115
Antivirals, herbal
  Ampelopsis brevipedunculata, 398
  astragalus, 468–69
  Chinese skullcap, 310–28, 312–13, 317–19
  cordyceps, 479, 484–85
  discussed, 5
  echinacea, 505
  elder, 184, 328–52, 342–44
  eleuthero, 516
  Forsythia suspensa, 398–99
  ginger, 352
  houttuynia, 352–67, 359–61
  isatis, 367–82, 374–76
  Isatis tinctoria, 185–86
  licorice, 382
  lomatium, 383–97, 388–90
  overview, 307–10
  range of, 309
  reishi, 521, 523
  rhodiola, 526, 531
  Sophora flavescens, 399
  Strobilanthes cusia, 399–400
  systemics, 144
Antiviral supplements, 406–7
AP-1 (activator protein-1), 152
Apium (celery), 583

Aralia spp., 583
Archangelisia, 262
Arctium (burdock), 583
Arctostaphylos (uva ursi, bearberry), 583
Ardisia squamulosa, for adenovirus, 128
Argemone, 262, 267, 274, 583
L-arginine, 172, 173, 176
Arnica (arnica), 583
Artemisia (*Artemisia*)
- *A. absinthium* (wormwood), 583
- A. *annua* (sweet Annie), 544, 575–\76, 584
- A. *identata* (sagebrush), 584
- *A. princeps* for adenovirus, 128
- A. *vulgaris* (mugwort, California mugwort), 584
- actions of, 246
- active against, 246
- clinical trials, 258
- common names, 242
- cultivation and collection, 250–51
- finding, 248
- habitat and appearance, 249–50
- herb/drug interactions, 249
- parts used, 242–44
- plant chemistry, 251
- preparation and dosage, 244–49
  - dried herb infusion for malaria, 245
  - fresh herb infusion for malaria, 245
  - fresh herb juice for malaria, 245
  - guidelines for preparing whole herb, 245
  - infusion in milk for malaria, 248
  - scientific research on whole herb *versus* artemisinin, 256–58
  - tincture for malaria, 248
  - tincture with sida and cryptolepsis for malaria, 248
- properties of, 246–47
- scientific research, 254–58
  - anticancer properties, 255
  - antiparasitic properties, 254–55
  - artemisinin resistance, 256
  - clinical trials, 258
  - whole herb *versus* artemisinin, 256–58
- side effects and contraindications, 249
- as systemic antibacterial, 242–58, 246–48
- traditional uses of, 252–54
  - Ayurveda, 253
  - traditional Chinese medicine, 253–54
  - Western botanic practice, 254
- use to treat, 247
  - *Aspergillus,* 78
  - candida, 76
  - Epstein-Barr virus, 170
  - Gram-negative bacterial diseases, 59, 64, 66–67, 73–75
  - Gram-positive bacterial diseases, 51–53
  - malaria, 77–78, 186, 242, 244–45, 248–49, 251–54

Artemisinin, 77–78, 186, 242–44, 248, 249, 251, 251–52, 253, 254–58, 415
Asarum (wild ginger), 584
Asclepias asperula (immortal root), 108, 120–22, 584
Asclepias cornuta (common milkweed), 584
Asclepias incarnata (swamp milkweed), 584
Asclepias subulata (desert milkweed), 584
Asclepias tuberosa (pleurisy root), 108, 120–22, 584
Ashwagandha
- actions of, 464
- cultivation and collection, 464–65
- finding, 464
- for Gram-negative bacterial diseases, 59, 67
- for Gram-positive bacterial diseases, 53
- habitat and appearance, 463–64
- herb/drug interactions, 463
- for immune system, 462, 462–67, 464
- parts used, 462
- plant chemistry, 465
- preparation and dosage, 463
  - capsules, 463
  - tincture, 463, 597
- properties of, 464
- scientific research, 466–67
  - antibacterial action, 466
  - anti-inflammatory, 467
  - antineoplastic activity, 466
  - antistressor activity, 466
  - cardiac effects, 467
  - cartilage effects, 466
  - central nervous system effects, 466–67
  - hemoglobin effects, 466
  - pain relief, 466
  - thyroid enhancement, 467
  - white blood cells and, 467
- side effects and contraindications, 463

species used, 462
traditional uses of, 465–66
Ayurveda, 465–66
Western botanic practice, 466
Asparagus officinale (asparagus), 584
Aspergillus spp., 45, 78
Aspidsperma (quebrache bark), 584
Assam indigo. *See Strobilanthes cusia*
Astragalus (*Astragalus*)
actions of, 468
active against, 468–69
cultivation and collection, 472
cytokine inhibition by, 110, 144
finding, 470
habitat and appearance, 471–72
herb/herb interactions, 471
for immune system, 145, 462, 467–76, 468–69
parts used, 468
plant chemistry, 472
preparation and dosage, 469–71
food, 470–71
powder, 470
tea, 470
tincture, 470, 584
properties of, 468–69
recipes
immune enhancing broth, **475–76**
immune enhancing rice, **476**
scientific research, 473–76
anti-inflammatory activity, 475
fatigue, 475
heart disease, 474–75
hepatitis, 475
immune function, 473–74
neurological actions, 475
side effects and contraindications, 471
species used, 467
traditional uses of, 472–73
Ayurveda, 473
traditional Chinese medicine, 473
Western botanic practice, 473
use to treat, 469
adenovirus, 128
Gram-negative bacterial diseases, 57
Gram-positive bacterial diseases, 51
herpes simplex virus, 172
influenza, 123
shingles, 175
West Nile encephalitis, 146
Astrocytes, 136–37
Astroviruses, 163, 177
Avena (wild oats), 584
Ayurveda, herbs used in
artemisia, 253
ashwagandha, 465–66
astragalus, 473
berberines, 274
bidens, 238
black pepper/piperine, 452
Chinese skullcap, 322
cordyceps, 488
cryptolepsis, 200–201
elder, 347
ginger, 444
houttuynia, 363–64
isatis, 379
juniper, 286
licorice, 433–34
reishi, 522
rhodiola, 530
sida, 216–17
usnea, 305

B

Babesia, artemisia for, 254–55
Baccharis teindalensis, 178
Bacteria. *See also specific species*
as foundation of life-forms, 85
learning, 20–23, 22
as partners, 34–38
Baicalein, 320, 321, 324–28
Balsamorhiza (balsam root), 584
Baptisia tinctoria (wild indigo root), 584
Barberry. *See Berberis*
Barks, for hot infusions, 546
Barleria prionitis, 129
Barley, for immune system, 460
Bartonella, houttuynia tincture for, 354
Basil oil, 62–63, 75
Beeswax, in salves, 569, 571
Bell peppers, for immune system, 461
Berberines
actions of, 265
active against, 265–66
Argemone, 262, 267, 274
Berberis, 259–61, 266–67, 269, 272–75, 277–78
Coptis, 259, 261, 266–67, 272–74

Berberines (*cont.*)
Corydalis, 262, 273–74
cultivation and collection, 270–71
Berberis, 271
Mahonia, 271
Phellodendron, 270–71
finding, 267
genera involved in, 259–62
habitat and appearance, 268–70
Berberis, 269
Mahonia, 269–70
Phellodendron, 268–69
herb/drug interactions, 264, 268
Hydrastis, 259–61, 266–67, 272, 273, 275, 277
as localized antibacterials, 259–80, 265–67
Mahonia, 259, 261, 266–67, 269–70, 273–75
Nandina domestica, 262
parts used, 262
Phellodendron, 259–61, 266–67, 268–69, 270–72, 274–78
plant chemistry, 272–73
preparation and dosage, 263–64
capsules, 264
douche, 263
powder, 263
snuff, 264
tincture, 263
wash, 263
properties of, 265–67
scientific research, 275–80
antibacterial activity, 275–79
berberine alkaloids, 278–80
Phellodendron, 277–78
side effects and contraindications, 264
as synergist, 264, 268
Tinospora, 261, 267
traditional uses of, 273–75
Ayurveda, 274
traditional Chinese medicine, 274
Western botanic practice, 275
use to treat, 267
candida, 76–77
cytomegalovirus, 164
diarrheal diseases in children, 579
gastrointestinal viruses, 177–78
Gram-negative bacterial diseases, 58–59, 64–65, 67–70, 73, 75
Gram-positive bacterial diseases, 50, 52–55
herpes simplex virus, 173
influenza, 127
Berberis (barberry), 259–61, 266–67, 272–75, 277–78
cultivation and collection, 271
for cytomegalovirus, 164
habitat and appearance, 269
for herpes simplex virus, 173
tincture, 584
traditional uses of, 273, 274, 275
Berries, antioxidants in, 338
Bidens (*Bidens*)
actions of, 232
active against, 232
common names, 229
cultivation and collection, 235–37
findings, 233
habitat and appearance, 234–35
herb/drug interactions, 234
parts used, 229–30
plant chemistry, 237
plant juice, 575
preparation and dosage, 230–31
cold infusion, 231
decoction, 231
fresh juice, 231
tea, 231
tincture, 231, 584
water extraction, 230, 231
water infusion, 230
properties of, 232–33
scientific research, 240–42
antibacterial activity, 240
antidiabetic properties, 241
antioxidant/anti-inflammatory activity, 241
antiparasitic activity, 240
antipyretic effect, 241
antitumor activity, 241
hepatoprotectant effect, 241
malaria, 240
for snake envenomation, 240
ulcer protection, 241
vascular tissue relaxant, 241
side effects and contraindications, 234
as systemic antibacterial, 229–42, 232–33
traditional uses of, 237–39
Ayurveda, 238
traditional Chinese medicine, 238
Western botanic practice, 238–39

use to treat, 233
candida, 76
cytomegalovirus, 164
gastrointestinal viruses, 177
Gram-negative bacterial diseases, 58–60, 64–71, 73
Gram-positive bacterial diseases, 51–54
herpes simplex virus, 240
influenza, 127
malaria, 77
Birch bark, 174
Birch essential oil, for tennis elbow, 577
Bishop's weed, 582
Blackberry root, 50, 60, 178
Black cohosh (*Cimicifuga racemosa*), 167–68, 586
Black pepper/piperine (*Piper* spp.)
actions of, 449
finding, 449
for Gram-negative bacterial diseases, 63, 67
herb/drug interactions, 450
plant chemistry, 450–51
preparation and dosage, 447–50
piperine, 448–50
tincture, 448, 593
trikatu, 448
properties of, 449
scientific research, 452–57
nonsynergist activity, 452–53
P-gp and CYP3A4, effects on, 454–56
synergistic activity, 453–54
side effects and contraindications, 450
species used, 447
as synergist, 447–57
traditional uses of, 451–52
Ayurveda, 451–52
traditional Chinese medicine, 452
Black tea, for immune system, 461
Blisters, lemon balm for, 168
Blumea laciniata, for respiratory synctial virus, 129
Bone marrow, functions of, 459
Boneset (*Eupatorium perfoliatum*), 400–406
actions of, 404
active against, 404–5
common names, 401
cultivation and collection, 403
cytokine inhibition by, 109, 110, 137
finding, 403
habitat and appearance, 402–3
for immune system, 400–406, 404–5, 462
interleukin-1β inhibition by, 137
parts used, 401
plant chemistry, 403–4
preparation and dosage, 401–2
cold tea, 401
hot tea, 401
tincture, 402, 588
properties of, 404–5
scientific research, 406
side effects and contraindications, 402
species used, 401
traditional uses of, 405–6
use to treat, 405
dengue fever virus, 147, 165–66
enterovirus 71, 169
Gram-negative bacterial diseases, 73–74
influenza, 124
Bottles, 540
Boussingaultia gracilis, 128
Brazil nuts, selenium in, 460–61
Breakbone fever. *See* Dengue fever
Brickellia grandiflora (brickellia), 585
Broccoli, for immune system, 461
Bunyaviruses, 131
Bursera microphylla (elephant tree), 120–22, 585

C

Cabbage, 576
Caesalpinia benthamiana, as synergist, 421
Caesalpinia pulcherrima, for adenovirus, 128
Calendula officinalis (marigold), 585
Campylobacter jejuni, 58
Candida, treating, 76–77, 196, 266505
Capsella bursa-pastoris (shepherd's purse), 585
Capsicum (cayenne), 585
Capsules, herbal powder in, 573–74
Cardamomum (cardamon), 585
Carica papaya, for gastrointestinal viruses, 178

L-carnitine, for postherpetic nerve pain, 176
Carum (caraway seed), 585
Castela emoryi (holacantha emoryi, chaparro amargosa), 76–77, 585
Casticin, 186
Catnip, for fever in children, 579
Cat's claw (*Uncaria tomentosa*), 147, 165–66, 597
Caulophyllum (blue cohosh), 585
Cayenne, in liniments, 569
C-C chemokine ligands (CCLs), 107, 109, 110, 136
CCR1/CCR2/CCR5, 136
CD4+ count enhancement, by astragalus, <u>468</u>, 474
CD4 fusion inhibitor, 345
Ceanothus. *See* Red root
Centaurium (centaury), 585
Centella asiatica (gotu kola), 421, 422, 585
Cercocarpus (mountain mahogany), 585
Cereus grandiflorus (night-blooming cereus), 585
Chamaecyparis lawsoniana (Lawson's cypress), 585, 586
Chamaecyparis nootkatensis (yellow cedar), 586
Chamaelirium (helonias, unicorn root), 586
Chamomile (*Matricaria*), 552, 591
Chaparral, in evaporative concentrate, 553
Chaparro amargosa (*Castela emoryi*), 76–77, 585
Chelidonium. *See* Greater celandine
Chelone (balmony), 586
Chemists, 544
Chemokine cascade, 136–40
Chicken pox, 161–62, 174
Chicken soup, for immune system, 461
Chikungunya fever, 80–81
Children, treating, 577–80
  diarrheal diseases, 579, **580**
  dosages, 577–78
  ear infections, 578, **578–79**
  fever, 579
Chilopsis linearis (desert willow), 76–77, 586
Chimaphila (pipsissewa), 586
Chinese proverbs, 458
Chinese senega root (*Polygala tenuifolia*)
  COX-2 inhibition, 138
  cytokine inhibition by, 109, 110, 137
  for encephalitis viruses, 147–48
  for postherpetic nerve pain, 175
  for regeneration of damaged neural structures, 145
Chinese skullcap (*Scutellaria*)
  actions of, <u>317</u>
  active against, <u>317–19</u>
  as antiviral, 105, 310–28, <u>312–13</u>, <u>317–19</u>
  COX-2 inhibition, 138
  cultivation and collection, 316, 320
  cytokine inhibition by, 109–10, 137, 144
  finding, <u>319</u>
  habitat and appearance, 316
  herb/drug interactions, 314–16
  herb/herb interactions, 314–16
  indoleamine 2,3-dioxygenase (IDO) inhibition, 140
  interferon inhibition, 111
  matrix metallproteinase inhibition, 137
  melatonin and, 139–40, 311, <u>313</u>, 321
  for neural protection, 144
  part used, 310–11
  plant chemistry, 320–21
  p38 MAPK inhibition by, 110, 140
  preparation and dosage, 311–14
    powder, 313–14
    tincture, 311–12
    wash, 314
  properties of, <u>317–19</u>
  scientific research, 324–28
    human studies, 327–28
    in vitro studies, 324–25
    in vivo studies, 325–27
  side effects and contraindications, 314
  species used, 310, <u>312–13</u>
  as synergist, 314
  traditional uses of, 322–24
    Ayurveda, 322
    traditional Chinese medicine, 323
    Western botanic practice, 323
  use to treat, <u>319</u>
    adenovirus, 128
    encephalitis viruses, 144
    enterovirus 71, 168–69
    Epstein-Barr virus, 169, 170
    influenza, 105, 120–22, <u>127</u>, 326–27
    for inhibition of viral infection of neural cells, 145
    parainfluenza virus, 129
    respiratory synctial virus, 129
    seizures, 143
    shingles, 175

Chionanthus (fringetree), 586
Chlamydia, 88, 279
Cholera, 26, 74–75
Chondroitin sulfate, 143
Chrysophlenetin, 186
Chrysospenol-D, 186
Cicer arietinum, for parainfluenza virus, 129
Cilial structures, treatments supporting, 127
Cimicifuga racemosa (black cohosh), 167–68, 586
Cinchona (quinine bark), 586
Cinnamomum (cinnamon), 586
Cissampelos pareira (velvet leaf), 146–47, 165–66
Citrus aurantium (bitter orange), 421
Clark's Rule, 577
Cleaning plants, 540
Cleavers, 411, 588
Clematis (virgin's bower), 586
Clostridium difficile, 4, 25, 45, 50
Cnicus benedictus (blessed thistle), 586
Coconut oil, 407
Coelocline, 262
Colchicum officinale, 544
Cold, common, 129–30
Cold infusions, 546–47
Collecting plants, 539
Collinsonia (stone root), 586
Combinations of plants, 186–87
Commiphora (myrrh), 421, 586
Common cold, 129–30
Conyza canadensis (Canadian fleabane), 586
COPD, cordyceps for, 492–93
Coptis (goldthread), 259, 261, 266–67, 272–74
  for cytomegalovirus, 164
  for Gram-negative bacterial diseases, 70–71
  tincture, 586
Coral root (*Corallorhiza* spp.), 125, 579, 586
Cordyceps
  actions of, 484
  active against, 484–85
  common names, 479
  COX-2 inhibition, 138
  cultivation and collection, 482–83
  cytokine inhibition by, 109–10, 137, 144
  finding, 485
  habitat and appearance, 481–82
  herb/drug interactions, 481
  ICAM-1 inhibition by, 137
  for immune system, 145, 462, 477–94, 484–85
  for inhibition of viral infection of neural cells, 145
  interferon inhibition by, 111
  matrix metallproteinase inhibition by, 137
  monocyte maturation and, 109
  for neural protection, 144
  part used, 479
  plant chemistry, 486–87
  p38 MAPK inhibition by, 110, 140
  preparation and dosage, 479–80
    capsules, 480
    as medicinal food, 479
    tinctures, 480
  properties of, 484–85
  scientific research, 489–94
    human clinical studies and trials, 492–94
    in vitro studies, 489–91
    in vivo studies, 491–92
  side effects and contraindications, 480
  species used, 477–78
  traditional uses of, 487–89
    Ayurveda, 488
    in Tibet, 487–88
    traditional Chinese medicine, 488–89
    Western botanic practice, 489
  use to treat, 485
    enterovirus 71, 169
    Epstein-Barr virus, 169–70
    herpes simplex virus, 172
    influenza, 123, 127, 491
    shingles, 175
Coriandrum (coriander), 587
Cornus sericea (red osier dogwood), 587
Corticosteroid evaporative concentrate, 554, **554–55**
Corticosteroids
  for reduction of inflammation, 115
  for Varicella Zoster virus, 162
Corydalis (goldensmoke), 262, 273–74, 587
Cough, treatment in influenza, 125–26
Cough syrup, 125, **125–26**, 550, **551–52**
Cowling's Rule, 577
COX-2, 136–38, 152, 350, 365
Coxsackie B3, 469, 474, 526

Cranberry juice, for diarrhea, 168
Crataegus (hawthorn), 587
C-reactive protein (CRP), 152
Cream, corticosteroid evaporative concentrate, 554
Crinum latifolium, 140, 146
CRKP (carbapenem-resistant *Klebsiella pneumoniae*), 43, 64
Crocus (saffron), 587
Croton lechleri, 178
Croup, 129
Cryptolepine
  in cryptolepsis, 195, 198, 199–200, 203
  in sida, 207, 214, 218–21
Cryptolepsis
  actions of, 196
  active against, 196
  common names, 192
  cultivation and collection, 198–99
  as douche, 568
  finding, 197
  habitat and appearance, 198
  herb/drug interactions, 198
  parts used, 193
  plant chemistry, 199–200
  preparation and dosage, 194, 194–95
    artemisia tincture with sida and coryptolepsis for malaria, 248
    capsules, 195
    pH of water and, 194
    powder, 194
    tea, 194, 194–95
    tincture, 194
  properties of, 196–97
  scientific research, 202–4
    antibacterial properties, 203–4
    antihyperglycemic properties, 204
    hypotensive property, 204
    hypothermic property, 204
    malaria, 202–3
  side effects and contraindications, 195, 198
  species used, 192–93
  as systemic antibacterial, 192–204
  traditional uses of, 200, 200–202
    Ayurveda, 200–201
    traditional Chinese medicine, 201
  use to treat, 197
    Aspergillus, 78
    Gram-negative bacterial diseases, 57–60, 62, 64–70, 73, 75
    Gram-positive bacterial diseases, 50–55
    malaria, 77–78
Cubeba (cubeb berries), 587
Cupressus (true cypress), 587
Curcuma (turmeric), 587
C-X-C chemokine ligands (CXCLs), 107–11
Cyanide, in elder, 332–34, 336, 346
Cymbopogon citratus, 421
Cynanchum paniculatum, 173
CYP3A4 inhibition, 314–15, 456
Cytokine cascade
  described, 99, 103–10
  infection dynamics and, 103–10
  knotweed as inhibitor of, 148
  natural treatments for reduction of, 144
  supportive formulations to reduce HMGB1 levels during cytokine storms, 126–27
  West Nile encephalitis, 136–40
Cytokines
  inhibitors, 115
  stages of chemokine stimulation, 109–10
Cytokine storm, 99, 111–13, 126–27
Cytomegalovirus (CMV), 154–55, 163–64
Cytotoxicity, of cryptolepine, 195, 198

D

Da-chang-yeh. *See Strobilanthes cusia*
Dalea spp., as synergist, 186, 420
Datura (jimsonweed), 587
Daucus carota (wild carrot), 421, 587
Death, causes of, 84–85
Decoctions, 548–52
  concentrated, 548–50, 550, **551**
    for colds and flu, **551**
    in oxymels and electuaries, 550
  cough syrup, 550, **551–52**
  simple, 548, **549**
Dengue fever, 81, 146–47, 155–57, 164–66
Desert willow (*Chilopsis linearis*), 76–77, 586
Desmethoxyyangonin, 185
Diaphoretic adjunct, yarrow as, 124, 191
Diaphoretic teas, for fever in influenza, 124

Diarrheal diseases
in children, 579–80, **580**
Rosemary Gladstar's tea for, **580**
tincture combination for, **580**
Dicentra formosa (bleeding heart), 587
Dioscorea villosa (wild yam), 587
Dipsacus (teasel), 63, 587
DNA, 19–20, 23, 85–86
DNA virus, 89–91
Dosages. *See specific herbs*
Douches, 568
Dracontium (symplocarpus, skunk cabbage), 587
Dried plant tinctures, 560–61
Drop (measurement), 547
Dropperful (measurement), 547
Droppers, 540
Drying plants, 540
Drying trays, 540
Dye
from alchornea, 224
from cryptolepsis, 197
from isatis, 371, 375
from *Strobilanthes cusia,* 399
Dyer's woad. *See* Isatis

E

E. coli
alchornea for, 226–27
berberines for, 263, 265, 279
factory farms and, 29–30
O157:H7, 26–27, 29, 59, 579
resistant disease, 26–27, 28, 42
treating, 58–60
Ear infections
Brigitte Mars's herbal tea for, **578–79**
causes, 578
children's ear oil, **578**
glycerite for, **564**
tincture combination for, **579**
Earth, as a living system, 88
Ebulin, 341
Ecdysteroids, in sida, 214, 221
Echinacea (echinacea)
actions of, 496
author's rant on, 502–3
bias against, 181
common names, 494
cultivation and collection, 499–500
E. angustifolia, 170, 560–61
finding, 496
fresh juice, 495
habitat and appearance, 498–99
herb/drug interactions, 498
herb/herb interactions, 498
for immune system, 462, 494–507, 496, 502–3
parts used, 494
plant chemistry, 500
powder, 497
for abnormal Pap smear, 497
poultice, 497
as a wound powder, 497
preparation and dosage, 495–97
fresh juice, 495, 576
powder, 497
tincture, 495–97, 560–61, 587
properties of, 496
scientific research, 504–7
antibacterial activity, 505
anticancer/radiation protection, 506
anti-inflammatory activity, 505–6
antiviral activity, 505
hyaluronidase inhibition, 504
immune stimulation, 506–7
pain relief, 506
wound-healing activity, 505
side effects and contraindications, 497–98
species used, 494
tincture
for collagen tissue protection and repair, 496
dried plant, 560–61
for external wounds, 496–97
as mouth/gum wash for sores and ulcers, 495
for onset of colds and flus, 495–96
for septicemia, thyphoid, diptheria, and so on, 496
for strep throat/tonsilitis, 495
for venomous stings and bite, 497
traditional uses of, 500–501
use to treat
candida, 76–77
Gram-negative bacterial diseases, 58, 60, 63–68, 71–72, 74
Gram-positive bacterial diseases, 50–51, 54–55

- *Echinacea* (*cont.*)
  - use to treat (cont.)
    - influenza, 117–18, 505, 508
    - rhinovirus, 129–30
- Eclectics, 412
  - artemisia use, 254
  - bidens use, 238
  - echinacea use, 501
  - isatis use, 380
  - juniper use, 283, 287, 288
  - sida use, 218
- Ecosystem, resistance in, 31–34
- Efflux pump, 17–18, 46, 277, 288, 314
- Efflux pump inhibitors, 185, 277, 288, 418–22, 455
- EGCG, 57, 73, 113, 138, 421
- Elder (*Sambucus*)
  - actions of, 342
  - active against, 342–43
  - alternatives to, 338
  - as antiviral, 184, 328–52, 342–44
  - caution with, 336–37
  - common names, 330
  - COX-2 inhibition, 138
  - cultivation and collection, 340
  - cytokine inhibition by, 109, 137
  - eating fresh berries, 338
  - finding, 344
  - habitat and appearance, 339–40
  - herb/drug interactions, 338
  - herb/herb interactions, 338
  - ICAM-1 inhibition by, 137
  - IL-4 and IL-10 induction, 109
  - parts used, 330–31
  - phytohysteria concerning, 331–33, 346
  - plant chemistry, 340–41, 345–46
  - preparation and dosage, 331–36
    - antiviral elder recipe, **336**
    - elderberry syrup for colds and flu, **335**
    - tincture, 595
  - properties of, 342–44
  - scientific research, 350–52
    - human study, 352
    - in planta, 351
    - in vivo, 351–52
  - side effects and contraindications, 337
  - species used, 328–30
  - synonyms, 330
  - toxicity and, 331–34, 336–37
  - traditional uses of, 346–50
    - Ayurveda, 347
    - traditional Chinese medicine, 347–49
    - Western botanic practice, 347–49
  - use to treat, 343–44
    - adenovirus, 128
    - influenza, 119, 184, 331, 341, 342–43, 346, 351–52
    - parainfluenza virus, 129
    - respiratory synctial virus, 129
    - rhinovirus, 129
  - VCAM-1 inhibition by, 137
- Electuaries, 550
- *Elephantopus scaber*, 129
- Elephant tree (*Bursera microphylla*), 120–22, 585
- Eleuthero (*Eleutherococcus*)
  - actions of, 510
  - common names, 507
  - cultivation and collection, 512–13
  - finding, 510
  - for Gram-positive bacterial diseases, 54
  - habitat and appearance, 512
  - herb/drug interactions, 512
  - for immune system, 462, 507–17, 510
  - for influenza, 516
  - parts used, 508
  - plant chemistry, 513–14
  - preparation and dosage, 508–11
    - capsules, 511
    - powder, 511
    - Russian/high-strength formulations, 508–9
    - tincture, 509–10, 567, 587
    - tonic formulations and dosages, 509–10
  - properties of, 510
  - for respiratory synctial virus, 129
  - for rhinovirus, 129
  - scientific research, 515–17
    - heart and circulatory system effects, 515
    - hypothalamus/pituitary/adrenal system effects, 515
    - immune system effects, 515
    - liver and pancreas effects, 515
  - side effects and contraindications, 511
  - species used, 507
  - traditional uses of, 514–15
    - traditional Chinese medicine, 514–15
    - Western botanic practice, 515

Elm bark, 50
Emblica officinalis, 70
Emmenagogue activity
  of artemisia, 253
  of houttuynia, 356
Emodin, 149
Empowerment, 181, 535–36
Emulsifier, 571
Encephalitis viruses, 130–54
  bunyaviruses, 131
  flaviviruses, 130–31
  infection process, 92
  mechanisms of viral infection, 133–43
    La Crosse encephalitis virus (LCEV), 141–43
    tick-borne encephalitis, 140–41
    West Nile encephalitis, 133–40
  medical treatment, 132–33
  natural treatments for, 143–47
    antiviral systemics, 144
    for dengue encephalitis, 146–47
    immune herbs/adaptogens, 145
    inhibition of HMGB1, 145–46
    inhibition of viral infection of neural cells, 145
    protection of neural cells and neural mitochondria, 144
    protocol overview, 143–44
    reduction of cytokine cascade, 144
    regeneration of damaged neural structures, 145
    stimulation of spleen and lymph node, 144
    for tick-borne encephalitis, 146
    for West Nile encephalitis, 146
  neural herbs for, 147–54
    Chinese senega root (*Polygala tenuifolia*), 147–48
    Japanese knotweed (*Polygonum cuspidatum*), 148–51
    kudzu (*Pueraria lobata*), 152
    lion's mane (*Hericium erinaceus*), 152–53
    pink-striped trumpet lily (*Crinum latifolium*), 153–54
  orbivirus, 131
  phlebovirus, 131
  reovirus, 131
  symptoms, 132
  tick-borne (TBE), 130–32, 140–41, 146
  togaviruses, 130
  vaccines, 130–32
  West Nile, 81, 130–31, 133–40, 146
Endocytosis, 104–5
Endotoxins, 47
Enemas, decoctions as, 550
Entamoeba histolytica, 227, 240
Enterococcus spp., treating, 50–52
Enterovirus 71, 157, 167–69
Ephedra viridis (Mormon tea, American ephedra), 588
Ephedra vulgaris (ma huang), 588
Ephedrine (ephedra), 207, 210, <u>210</u>, <u>214</u>, 588
Epigallocatechin (EGCG), 57, 73, 113, 138, 421
Epipactis gigantea (stream orchid), 588
Epstein-Barr virus, 158, 169–70
Equipment, infusion, 547–48
Equisetum arvense (horsetail), 588
Equisetum hyemale (scouring rush), 588
Eriodictyon (yerba santa), 588
ERK-1/ERK-2, 109, 110, 148–49
Erythromycin, for West Nile encephalitis, 133, 138
ESBL resistance, 42, 64
Eschscholtzia californica (California poppy), 262, 588
E-selectin, 107, 136–37
Essential oils
  described, 576–77
  in hot infusions, 546
  as inhalants for influenza, 128
  steam, 553
Eucalyptus (*Eucalyptus*), 62–63, 73–74, 128, 588
Eupatorium perfoliatum. See Boneset
Eupatorium purpureum (gravel root, queen of the meadow, joe-pye weed), 588
Euphorbia hirta, for gastrointestinal viruses, 178
Euphrasia (eyebright), 588
Evaporative concentrates
  described, 553–54
  herbal corticosteroid, 554, **554–55**
Extracts
  alcohol extractions, 557–69
  plant alkaloids and, 187–88
  solvents, 543–44
  water extractions, 544–57

F

Facilatative herbs, 184
Famciclovir, 160–62
Fanpetals. *See* Sida
Farms, factory, 28–31
Fennel hot infusion, 546
Filipendula (meadowsweet), 588
Firs (*Abies*), 581
Flaviviruses, 130–31
Flavones, of Chinese skullcap, 324
Flavonoids
  in artemisia, 251
  in bidens, 237
  in Chinese skullcap, 324
  in elder, 341
  in sida, 220
Flowers, in hot infusions, 546
Fluid extracts, 567–68
Foeniculum (fennel seed), 588
Folium syringae, 110
Foods
  astragalus added to, 470
  for immune system, 460–61
Forsythia suspensa, 398–99
Fo-ti, for enterovirus 71, 167
Fouquieria splendens (octotillo), 588
Fragaria (strawberry), 588
Frasera speciosa (green gentian, cebadilla), 596
FtsZ inhibitor, berberines as, 265

G

Galangal (*Alpinia*), 439, 442, 582
Galium aparine (cleavers, bedstraw), 588
Ganciclovir, 133, 155, 159
Ganoderma . *See* Reishi
Garlic (*Allium sativum*), 73–74, 129, 460, 582
Garrya (silk tassel), 589
Gastrointestinal viruses, 162–63, 176–78
Genetic rearrangements, 86–87, 91
Gentamicin, 182
Gentiana (gentian), 589
Geranium (cranesbill), 75, 172, 420–21, 589
Germ theory, 84
Giardia, berberine for, 279
Ginger (*Zingiber* spp.), 352
  actions of, 440
  active against, 440–41
  chemistry, 443
  COX-2 inhibition by, 138
  cultivation and collection, 442–43
  cytokine inhibition by, 109–10, 137
  finding, 438
  habitat and appearance, 442
  herb/drug interactions, 439, 442
  parts used, 437
  preparation and dosage, 437–39
    as food, 439
    infusion, 438–39
    plant juice, 118, 437–39, 575
    tea, 438
    tincture, 439, 598
    topical, 439
  properties of, 440–41
  scientific research, 444–47
  side effects and contraindications, 439
  species used, 437
  traditional uses of, 443–44
    Ayurveda, 444
    traditional Chinese medicine, 444
    Western botanic practice, 444
  uses of, 441
    for *Aspergillus,* 78
    for enterovirus 71, 167–68
    for Epstein-Barr virus, 170
    for gastrointestinal viruses, 178
    for Gram-negative bacterial diseases, 57–60, 62–64, 66–71, 73
    for Gram-positive bacterial diseases, 50–51, 53–54
    for immune system, 461
    for influenza, 118–19, 123
    for rhinovirus, 130
    as synergist, 437–47
Ginkgo biloba, 110
Glucobrassicin, in isatis, 378
Glycerine, 562, 563–64
Glycerites, 69, 563–66, **564**, 565
Glycyrrhiza. See Licorice
Glycyrrhizin, 113, 424–28, 433, 436
Goats, sida and, 206
Golden root. *See* Rhodiola
Goldenseal (*Hydrastis*), 259–61, 266–67, 272, 273, 275, 277, 590
  antibacterial activity of, 184–85
  for cytomegalovirus, 164

for herpes simplex virus, 173
for influenza, 118
as synergist, 186
Goldensmoke (*Corydalis*), 262, 273–74, 587
Goldthread. *See Coptis*
Gonorrhea, 25
Gossypium (cotton), 589
Gotu kola (*Centella asiatica*), 421, 422, 585
Graduated cylinder, 561
Gram-negative bacteria, dealing with, 55–75
Gram-positive bacteria, dealing with, 49–55
Gram stain, 45
Greater celandine (*Chelidonium majus*), 146, 168–69, 172–73, 586
Green tea, for HMGB1 inhibition, 113
Grindelia (gumweed), 589
Guaiacum officinale (lignum vitae), 589
Guava, 75

H

Haemophilus influenzae, 24, 61–63
Hamamelis (witch hazel), 589
Hand, foot, and mouth disease. *See* Enterovirus
Harpagophytum procumbens (devil's claw), 589
Harvesting plants, 539
Hawthorn berry, 138
Hemagglutinin, influenza, 104–5
Hemotoxin neutralization, by sida, 219
Hepatitis C virus, mutation rate of, 90
Heracleum (cow parsnip), 589
Herbal corticosteroid evaporative concentrates, 554, **554–55**
Hericium erinaceus. *See* Lion's mane
Herpes simplex virus (HSV)
bidens for, 240
described, 158–61
encephalitis/meningitis, 160, 173
herpes gladiatorum, 160
houttuynia for, 364
ocular, 159–60, 173
treatment of, 160–61
vaginal, 173
Herpes viruses. *See specific viruses*
Herpetic whitlow, 158
Heterotheca (camphor weed), 589
High-mobility group box 1 protein (HMGB1), 111–13, 115, 126–27
Hippophae rhamnoides (sea buckthorn leaf), 146–47, 165–66
HIV
alchornea for, 228
echinacea for, 117
poke root for, 338
Hochu-ekki-to, for rhinovirus, 130
Holistic nonlinear perception, 188
Honey
actions of, 291
active against, 291
content of, 293
in electuaries, 550
finding, 292
herbal, 566
as localized antibacterial, 289–97, 291–92
manuka, 289
in oxymels, 550
preparation and dosage, 290
direct application, 290
internal use, 290
properties of, 291–92
scientific research, 293–97
side effects and contraindications, 290
traditional uses of, 290, 292–93
use to treat, 292
Aspergillus, 78
Gram-negative bacterial diseases, 57, 59, 62–66, 69–71, 73
Gram-positive bacterial diseases, 51, 53–55
Hospital-acquired infections, 12–13
Hot infusions, 545–46
for barks and roots, 546
for flowers, 546
for leaves, 545
for parasites, **548**
for seeds, 546
Houttuynia (*Houttuynia*)
actions of, 360
active against, 360–61
as antiviral, 352–67, 359–61
common names, 353
COX-2 inhibition, 138
cultivation and collection, 357–59
cytokine inhibition by, 109–10, 137, 144

- Houttuynia (*cont.*)
  - for cytomegalovirus, 164
  - for dengue fever virus, 165–66
  - for encephalitis viruses, 144
  - for enterovirus 71, 167–68
  - finding, 359
  - as food, 361
  - habitat and appearance, 356–57
  - for herpes simplex virus, 172–73
  - IL-4 and IL-10 induction by, 109
  - for influenza, 120–22, 360
  - interferon inhibition by, 111
  - parts used, 354
  - plant chemistry, 362
  - p38 MAPK inhibition by, 110, 140
  - preparation and dosage, 354–55
    - capsules, 355
    - docoction, 355
    - fresh plant tincture, 354–55
    - for mycoplasma and bartonella, 354
    - powder, 355
    - for viral infections, 354
  - properties of, 360–61
  - scientific research, 364–67
  - side effects and contraindications, 355–56
  - species used, 352–53
  - synonyms, 353
  - traditional uses of, 362–64
    - Ayurveda, 363
    - traditional Chinese medicine, 363–64
    - Western botanic practice, 364
- Human immunodeficiency virus. *See* HIV
- *Humulus* (hops), 589
- Hyaluronidase inhibitor, echinacea as, 118, 504
- *Hydrangea arborescens* (seven barks), 589
- *Hydrastis. See* Goldenseal
- 3-hydroxykynurenine, 139
- *Hyoscyamus niger* (henbane), 590
- *Hypericum* (St. John's wort), 590

I

- IDO (indoleamine 2,3-dioxygenase), 136–40, 153
- *Illicium* (star anise), 590
- Immortal (*Asclepsias asperula*), 108, 120–22, 584
- Immune system, 458–534
  - basic elements of, 459–60
  - foods for, 460–61
  - herbs for, 458–534, 461–534, 462
    - ashwagandha, 462, 462–67, 464
    - astragalus, 462, 467–76, 468–69
    - boneset, 400–406, 404–5, 462
    - cordyceps, 462, 477–94, 484–85
    - echinacea, 462, 494–507, 496, 502–3
    - eleuthero, 462, 507–17, 510
    - licorice, 435
    - red root, 407–13, 411, 462
    - reishi, 462, 518–24, 521
    - rhodiola, 462, 524–34, 526
  - importance of healthy, 458–59
  - virus protection from, 93
- Immunity, increasing natural, 48–49
- Immunoglobulin A, stimulation by berberines, 276
- *Impatiens* (jewelweed), 590
- Indian pipe (*Monotropa uniflora*), 125
- Industrialized medicine, 180
- Influenza, 96–128. *See also* Influenza treatment
  - avian flu, 102, 103, 111, 113, 116
  - cytokine cascade, 99, 103–10
  - cytokine storm, 99, 111–13
  - deaths from, 100
  - foods for immune system and, 460
  - genetic rearrangements, 91
  - H1N1, 103, 111
  - H3N2, 103, 113
  - H5N1, 111, 113–14
  - infection dynamics, 103–10
  - infection process, 91
  - influenza B and C, 101
  - interferon and, 106–7, 111–12, 114
  - lung and tissue pathology, 113–14
  - medical interventions, 114–16
  - natural treatment protocols, 116–28
  - pandemic, 95, 96–100, 101–2, 111
  - seasonal epidemics, 100
  - swine flu, 81, 102, 103
  - symptoms, 101
  - vaccine, 91, 100
- Influenza treatment
  - complex formulations, 121
  - early-onset treatment, 117–18
    - herbal tincture combination, 117–18
    - oscillococcinum, 117

fever treatment, 124
  boneset tea, 124
  diaphoretic teas, 124
  pasque flower tincture, 124
  wet cloth, 124
headache treatment, 125
  American wood betony, 125
  coral root, 125
  Indian pipe, 125
  motherwort, 125
herbs for
  Angelica sinensis, 126–27
  astragalus, 123
  berberines, 127
  bidens, 127
  boneset, 124
  Chinese skullcap, 105, 120–22, 127, 326–27
  cordyceps, 123, 127, 491
  echinacea, 117–18, 505
  elder, 119, 184, 331, 341, 342–43, 346, 351–52
  elephant tree, 120–22
  eleuthero, 516
  Forsythia suspensa, 399
  ginger, 118–19, 123
  goldenseal, 118
  houttuynia, 120–22, 360
  inmortal, 108, 120–22
  isatis, 120–22
  licorice, 120–22, 127
  list of herbs, 119
  lomatium, 120–22, 127, 385
  osha, 120–22
  peppermint, 124
  pleurisy root, 108, 120–22
  red root, 120–22
  reishi, 523
  rhodiola, 123, 526, 531
  Salvia miltiorrhiza, 126–27
  Sophora flavescens, 399
  Strobilanthes cusia, 400
  yarrow, 124
  yerba santa, 120–22
mild infections, 118–20
  ginger juice tea, 118–19
  herbal tincture combination, 120
moderate and severe infections, 120–23
  antiviral tincture formulation, 120–23
  comments on, 127
  complex formulations, 121
  ginger juice tea, 123
  immune complex tincture formulation, 123
natural treatment protocols, 116–28
supportive additions, 124–28
  for cough, 125, **125–26**
  essential oil inhalants, 128
  for fever, 124
  for headache, 125
  to protect cilial structures and lung mucosa, 127
  to reduce HMGB1 levels during cytokine storms, 126–27
  selenium, 128
  supplements, 128
  zinc, 128
Infusers, 547–48
Infusions, 544–48
  cold, 546–47
  equipment, 547–48
  hot, 545–46
  oil, 569–70, **570**
  strength and weaknesses of, 545
  teas compared to, 544
iNOS, 152, 153
Inositol, for postherpetic nerve pain, 176
Insulin, HMGB1 level reduction with, 115
Integrons, 20
Intercellular adhesion molecule 1 (ICAM-1), 107–8, 136–37, 152
Interferon
  astragalus and, 468, 471
  for encephalitis viruses, 133
  influenza and, 106–7, 111–12, 114
  reishi and, 521
  type 1, 106
  type 2, 107
  type III, 107
  West Nile encephalitis and, 134, 136, 138, 140
Interferon-inducing protein-10 (IP-10), 136
Interleukin-1
  influenza and, 107, 109, 111
  La Crosse encephalitis virus (LCEV) and, 142
  reishi and, 521
  tick-borne encephalitis and, 141
  West Nile encephalitis and, 136–38
Interleukin-2, 138, 468, 521, 534
Interleukin-4, 109, 136

- Interleukin-5, 136
- Interleukin-6, 107, 109–12, 136, 141, 142
- Interleukin-8, 110, 112, 136
- Interleukin-10, 109, 136, 141
- Interleukin-13, 136
- Interleukin-18, 107
- International corporations, 180
- Internet, as information source, 179
- Intestinal parasites, artemisia for, 247
- Intuitive sensing, 188
- *Inula* (elecampane), 590
- Invasive plants, 192
  - *Ampelopsis brevipedunculata,* 398
  - artemisia, 250
  - berberines, 259
  - *Berberis,* 260, 269
  - bidens, 234
  - *Forsythia suspensa,* 398–99
  - houttuynia, 358–59
  - isatis, 371, 373
  - Japanese knotweed, 148
  - *Phellodendron,* 260
  - sida, 209, 211
- Invasivores, 209
- Ipecac, fluid extracts, 567
- *Ipomoea murucoides,* 420
- Iporuru, 223
- *Iris* (blue flag), 590
- Irisolidone, 152
- Isatis (*Isatis*), 185–86
  - actions of, 374
  - active against, 374–75
  - as antiviral, 367–82, 374–76
  - boiled, 549
  - common names, 367
  - COX-2 inhibition, 138
  - cultivation and collection, 376–77
  - cytokine inhibition by, 110, 144
  - finding, 376
  - habitat and appearance, 371–73, 376
  - herb/drug interactions, 371
  - IDO inhibition, 140
  - part used, 368
  - plant chemistry, 378
  - preparation and dosage, 368–70
    - capsules or tablets, 370
    - decoction, 370
    - tincture, 369–70, 590
  - properties of, 374–75
  - scientific research, 380–82
  - side effects and contraindications, 370
  - species used, 367
  - as synergist, 371
  - synonyms, 367
  - traditional uses of, 378–80
    - Ayurveda, 379
    - traditional Chinese medicine, 379–80
    - Western botanic practice, 380
  - use to treat, 375
    - adenovirus, 128
    - *Aspergillus,* 78
    - candida, 76–77
    - cytomegalovirus, 164
    - encephalitis viruses, 144
    - Epstein-Barr virus, 170
    - Gram-negative bacterial diseases, 57, 59, 62–63, 66–68, 72, 74
    - Gram-positive bacterial diseases, 50, 52
    - herpes simplex virus, 172–73
    - influenza, 120–22
    - malaria, 77
    - respiratory synctial virus, 129
    - shingles, 175
- Isothiocyanates, in isatis, 378

J

- Japanese encephalitis virus (JEV), 130–32, 469
- Japanese knotweed (*Polygonum cuspidatum*)
  - COX-2 inhibition by, 138
  - cytokine inhibition by, 109–10, 137, 148
  - for encephalitis viruses, 148–51
  - endothelial cell normalization, 138
  - for enterovirus 71, 167–68
  - E-selectin inhibition, 137
  - for Gram-negative bacterial diseases, 63, 72, 74
  - for Gram-positive bacterial diseases, 52
  - ICAM-1 inhibition by, 137
  - IDO inhibition by, 140
  - interleukin-1β inhibition by, 137
  - for La Crosse encephalitis virus (LCEV), 143
  - matrix metallproteinase inhibition by, 137
  - for neural protection, 144
  - range of actions, 148

VCAM-1 inhibition by, 137
for West Nile encephalitis, 146
Jars, for tinctures, 540, 542
Jatropha curcas, 178
JNK pathway, 109, 110, 148–49
Juglans major (black walnut), 590
Juices, medicinal plant, 575–76
Juniper (*Juniperus*), 280–89
actions of, 282
active against, 282
alternatives, 284
cultivation and collection, 285
finding, 284
habitat and appearance, 283–85
as localized antibiotics, 280–89, 282
plant chemistry, 285
preparation and dosage, 280–81
berries, 281
decoction, 281
essential oil, 281
infusion, 281
powder, 281
steam, 281
tincture, 280, 590
properties of, 282
scientific research, 287–89
side effects and contraindications, 281, 283
species used, 280
traditional uses of, 286–87
Ayurveda, 286
traditional Chinese medicine, 286–87
Western botanic practice, 287
use to treat
Aspergillus, 78
candida, 76
Gram-negative bacterial diseases, 57–60, 64–70, 73
Gram-positive bacterial diseases, 50–55
malaria, 77
Jussiaea suffruticosa, 178

K

Kakkalide, 152
Kavain, 185
Kefir, 460
Kinds of herbal medicines, 541
Klebsiella, 24, 42–43, 64–65
Krameria (rhatany), 590
Kudzu (*Pueraria lobata*), 109–10, 137–38, 144, 152, 167–69, 173
Ku shen. *See Sophora flavescens*
Kynurenic acid, 139

L

Labeling, 540
La Crosse encephalitis virus (LCEV), 141–43
Lactones, 185
Lactuca (wild lettuce), 590
Laggera pterodonta, 129
Larrea (chaparral), 590
Lateral epicondylitis (tennis elbow), 577
Latex, 267
Leaves. *See also specific plants/herbs*
hot infusions, 545
leaf juices, 575–76
Leishmania amazonensis, bidens for, 240
Lemon balm (*Melissa officinalis*)
for blisters, 168
in concentrated sore-relief herbal cream, 174
for shingles, 175
tincture, 591
Leonurus cardiaca (motherwort), 125, 146, 169–70, 590
Leptandra (Culver's root), 590
Lichen. *See* Usnea
Licorice (*Glycyrrhiza* spp.), 382
actions of, 431
active against, 431–32
cultivation and collection, 430, 433
cytokine inhibition by, 109–10, 137
endothelial cell normalization by, 138
finding, 433
habitat and appearance, 429–30
HMGB1 inhibition by, 113, 145
IL-4 and IL-10 induction by, 109
interferon inhibition by, 111
parted used, 424
plant chemistry, 433
preparation and dosage, 424–27
capsules or powder, 426–27
decoction, 426
infusion, 426
tincture, 425–26, 589

- Licorice (*cont.*)
  - properties of, 431–32
  - scientific research, 435–37
  - side effects and contraindications, 427–28
  - species used, 423–24
  - traditional uses of, 433–35
    - Ayurveda, 433–34
    - traditional Chinese medicine, 434
    - Western botanic practice, 434–35
  - uses of, 432
    - for adenovirus, 128
    - for candida, 76–77
    - in concentrated sore-relief herbal cream, 174
    - for cytokine cascade reduction, 144
    - for cytomegalovirus, 164
    - for dengue fever virus, 165–66
    - for encephalitis viruses, 144
    - for enterovirus 71, 167–68
    - for Epstein-Barr virus, 170
    - for E-selectin inhibition, 137
    - for gastrointestinal viruses, 178
    - for Gram-negative bacterial diseases, 59–60, 62–64, 67–71, 73–74
    - for Gram-positive bacterial diseases, 50–54
    - for herpes simplex virus, 172–73
    - for influenza, 120–22, 127
    - for inhibition of viral infection of neural cells, 145
    - for malaria, 77
    - for parainfluenza virus, 129
    - for respiratory synctial virus, 129
    - for rhinovirus, 130
    - scientific research on, 435–37
    - for shingles, 175
    - as synergist, 186, 423–37
  - vascular cell adhesion molecule-1 (VCAM-1) inhibition by, 137
- Life, definition of, 88
- *Ligusticum porteri* (osha), 120–22, 591
- *Ligusticum wallichii*, 143, 146
- Liniments, 568–69
- Lion's mane (*Hericium erinaceus*)
  - for encephalitis viruses, 152–53
  - for enterovirus 71, 168–69
  - JNK pathway inhibition by, 110
  - for postherpetic nerve pain, 175–76
  - for regeneration of damaged neural structures, 145
  - for seizures, 143
- *Listeria*, 29, 30
- Liver, functions of, 459
- Living system
  - Earth as, 88
  - soft boundaries of, 86
- *Lobelia inflata* (lobelia), 591
- Locoweed, 206
- Lomatium (*Lomatium dissectum*), 591
  - actions of, 388
  - active against, 388–89
  - as antiviral, 383–97, 388–90
  - common names, 384
  - cultivation and collection, 390–92
  - finding, 390
  - as food, 390
  - habitat and appearance, 387
  - parts used, 384
  - plant chemistry, 392–95
  - preparation and dosage, 384–85
    - decoction, 385
    - infusion, 385
    - steam inhalant, 385
    - tincture, 384–85, 591
  - properties of, 388–90
  - scientific research, 397
  - side effects and contraindications, 386
  - species used, 383
  - synonyms, 383–84
  - traditional uses of, 395–97
  - use to treat, 389
    - *Aspergillus*, 78
    - cytomegalovirus, 164
    - gastrointestinal viruses, 178
    - Gram-negative bacterial diseases, 57, 59, 62–63, 66–67, 69, 71, 73
    - Gram-positive bacterial diseases, 50, 52–55
    - influenza, 120–22, 127, 385
    - West Nile encephalitis, 144
- *Lonicera japonica*, 110
- Lotions, 571
- *Lycium pallidum* (wolfberry), 591
- *Lycopus* (bugleweed, water horehound), 421, 591
- Lyme disease
  - artemisia for, 251
  - astragalus for, 469, 471, 474
- Lymph nodes
  - functions of, 459
  - in influenza infection, 108

Lymph system, 459
functions of, 459
red root for, 411, 412–13
Lysichiton americanum (western skunk cabbage), 591
L-lysine, 172, 176

M

Maceration, 543
Macrophages, functions of, 459–60
Magnolia officinalis, 110
Mahonia (Oregon grape), 259, 261, 266–67, 269–70, 273–75, 591
Malaria
alchornea for, 228
artemisia for, 186, 242, 244–45, 248–49, 251–54
bidens for, 229, 231, 240
cryptolepsis for, 194, 200, 200, 201, 202–3
sida for, 219
spread of resistant disease, 25–26
Mallow, in washes, 552
Malva neglecta (mallow), 591
Mangifera indica, for gastrointestinal viruses, 178
Marc, 543, 560, 567
Markhamia lutea, for respiratory synctial virus, 129
Marrubium (horehound), 591
Marsh mallow (*Althaea*), 50, 550, 582
Mastitis, chaparral leaf for, 553
Matricaria (chamomile), 552, 591
Matricaria matricarioides a.k.a. *discoidea* (pineapple weed), 591
Matrix metallproteinase inhibitors, 137, 138
Matrix metallproteinases (MMPs), 136, 148–49
MCP-1, 109–12, 136
MCP-3, 111
Measuring herbal medicines, 547
Medicago sativa (alfalfa), 591
Medical model, Western, 180
Medicine making, 535–80
alcohol extractions, 557–69
for children, 577–80
combinations of plants, 186–87
essential oils, 576–77
harvesting plants, 539
importance of preparation methods, 187–88
jars, for tinctures, 540, 542
kinds of herbal medicines, 541
learning process, 536–38
lotions, 571
measuring herbal medicines, 547
oil infusions, 569–70, **570**
preparing medicinal plants, 539–40
salves, 571
solvents, 542–44
storing supplies and medicines, 540, 542
water extractions, 544–57
with whole herbs, 572–76
with fresh herbs, 575
plant juices, 575–76
powders for internal use, 573–74, **574**
suppositories, 574, **575**
wound powders, 572–73, **573**
Medihoney, 289
Melatonin
in Chinese skullcap, 139–40, 311, 313, 321
for West Nile encephalitis, 139–40
Melissa officinalis. See Lemon balm
Menstruum, 542–43
Mentha arvensis (poleo mint), 591
Mentha piperita. See Peppermint
Mentha spicata (spearmint, yerba buena), 591
Menyanthes (buckbean, bogbean), 591
5'-methoxyhydnocarpin (5'-MHC), 185, 277, 418–19
Milk thistle (*Silybum marianum*), 170, 595
Milliliter (measurement), 547
M2 inhibitor, 105, 114–15
Minocycline, 115, 133
MIP-1α, 109, 111
Miracle drugs, 9, 13–14
Mitchella repens (squaw vine), 591
Mitochondria
cordyceps as adaptogen, 484
protection of neural, 144
Mitogen-activated protein kinases (MAPKs), 148
Monolaurin, 407
Mononucleosis, 158
Monotherapy, changes in Western, 416–17
Mosquitoes, chikungunya fever and, 80–81
Motherwort (*Leonurus cardiaca*), 125, 169–70.146, 590
MRSA. *See Staphylococcus aureus*

Multidrug-resistance (MDR) inhibitors, 186, 277, 418–19
Mushrooms. *See also* Lion's mane (*Hericium erinaceus*)
  cordyceps, 462, 477–94, 484–85
  in diet for immune system, 461
  poisoning, reishi for, 519
  reishi, 462, 518–24, 521
Mussaenda pubescens, 129
Mycobacterium tuberculosis. See Tuberculosis
Mycoplasma, houttuynia tincture for, 354
Myocarditis, from Coxsackie B3 infection, 469
Myrica (barberry), 592
Myrrh, 421, 559, 586

N

N-acetylcysteine, for Epstein-Barr virus, 169
Nandina domestica, 262
Narcissus tazetta, 129
Nasal sprays
  described, 566
  for sinus infection, **566**
Neem leaf, for enterovirus 71, 167–68
Neisseria gonorrhoeae, 65
Neospora caninum, artemisia for, 255
Nepeta cataria (catnip), 592
Nerve growth factor, 147–48
Nerve pain, herbs and supplements for, 175–76
Neural cells, 144, 145
Neuraminidase, influenza, 104–5
Neuraminidase inhibitors, 104, 114–15
Neutrophils, functions of, 460
Nigella sativa, 110
Nigrin, 341
NorA efflux pump, 277, 288, 314
Noroviruses, 162–63, 176–78
Norwalk virus, 163, 176
Nuphar (yellow pond lily), 592

O

Oak (*Quercus*), 59–60, 552, 594
Oats, for immune system, 460
Ocimum basilicum, for adenovirus, 128
Oenothera (evening primrose), 592
Oil infusions
  with dried herbs, 569
  with fresh herbs, 570
  salves from, 571
  for skin infections, **570**
  uses, 569
Old man's beard. *See* Usnea
Olea europaea (olive), 592
Oleorupin, 144
Olive oil, 127, 144
Oncovirus, 158
Oplopanax horridus (devil's cub), 592
Opuntia (prickly pear), 592
Orbivirus, 131
Oregano oil, 51, 57–58, 71, 73–74, 461
Oregon grape. *See Mahonia*
Oroxylin A, 315, 320, 325
Orthoreovirus, 163, 177
Oscillococcinum, for influenza, 117
Oseltamivir, 114–15
Osha (*Ligusticum porteri*), 120–22, 591
Osmorhiza occidentalis (western sweet cicely), 592
Ounce (measurement), 547
Oxymels, 550
Oysters, zinc in, 461

P

Paeonia (peony), 110, 592
Palmitic acid, 345
Panax ginseng (Asian ginseng), 592
Panax quinquefolium (American ginseng), 592
Papaver mume, 130
Papaver pseudocanescens, 129
Pap smear, suppository for abnormal, 574, **575**
Parainfluenza virus, 129
Parasites
  artemisia for, 247, 254–55
  cordyceps mushrooms as, 477–78
  hot infusion for, **548**
  houttuynia for, 365
Parietaria (pellitory-of-the-wall), 592
Pasque flower (*Pulsatilla patens*), 124, 169, 173
Passionflower (*Passiflora* spp.), 169–70, 592

Pastes, 550
Paullinia cupana (guarana), 592
Pausinystalia (yohimbe), 592
Pedicularis spp., 125, 592, 593
Penicillin, early use of, 9
Peppermint (*Mentha piperita*)
 for fever in influenza, 124
 in herbal powders, 574
 for indigestion, 577
 for influenza, 124
 tincture, 591
 water content of, 559
Percolations, 555–57
Percolator, 555–57
Perforin, 136
Permeability glycoprotein (P-gp) inhibitors, 186, 264, 276, 315, 454–55
Petasites (western coltsfoot), 593
Petroselinum (parsley), 593
Phagocytes, functions of, 459–60
Pharmaceutical companies, 183
Pharmaceutical/technological model, 180
Pharmacists, 544
Phellodendron, 259–61, 266–67, 268–69, 270–72, 274–78
Phenolics, in sida, 220
Phlebovirus, 131
pH of water, 194
Phyllanthus, for cytomegalovirus, 164
Phytolacca (poke), 593
Phytorationalists, 190
Phytoremediation, bidens and, 234
Picraena (quassia), 593
Pilocarpus (jaborandi), 593
Pine (*Pinus*), 552, 593
Pine pollen cream, for shingles, 175
Pink-striped trumpet lily (*Crinum latifolium*), 153–54
Pinus pollen (pollen pini), 593
Piperine, 48
 dosage, 448–50
 finding, 449
 for Gram-negative bacterial diseases, 66, 68, 70, 74
 for Gram-positive bacterial diseases, 52
 scientific research, 452–57
 as synergist, 447–57
Piper methysticum (kava kava), 185, 593
Piper nigrum. *See* Black pepper/piperine
Plantago major (plantain), 593
Plants
 drying, 540
 harvesting, 539
 learning to recognize in the wild, 537–38
 preparing medicinal, 539–40
 sensing, nonphysical, 538–39
 thanking, 539
Plasmids, 19
Plasmodium, 45, 77–78. *See also* Malaria
Pleurisy root (*Asclepsias tuberosa*), 108, 120–22, 584
Poke root (*Phytolacca americana*), 338, 411
Polio, 82, 308
Polyacetylenes, in bidens, 237, 240
Polygala tenuifolia. *See* Chinese senega root
Polygonatum (Solomon's seal), 593
Polygonum bistorta (bistort root), 593
Polygonum cuspidatum. *See* Japanese knotweed
Polyphenols, in sida, 220, 220
Polypodium glycyrrhiza (licorice fern), 593
Pomegranate (*Punica granatum*), 59, 75, 165–66, 168, 421–22
Populus balsamifera (balsam poplar), 594
Populus tremuloides (quaking aspen), 594
Porcelain berry (*Ampelopsis brevipedunculata*), 167–68, 398
Postherpetic nerve pain, herbs and supplements for, 175–76
Powder
 for internal use, 573–74, **574**
 for percolation, 556
 wound powders, 572–73, **573**
Precipitation, in tinctures, 562
Preparation methods, importance of, 187–88
Prickly pear, in washes, 552
Prinos (black alder), 594
Proof, 558, 558
Propionbacterium acnes, 266
Propolis, 289, 594
Prosopis juliflora, 421
Prostaglandin E2 (PGE2), 136–37, 152
Protein kinase C-delta, 149
Proteus spp., 65–67
Prunella (self-heal, heal-all), 594
Prunus (choke cherry), 594
Prunus persica (peach tree), 594
Pseudomonas aeruginosa, 24, 43–44, 67–69, 196, 226
Ptelea (water ash, hop tree), 594

p38 MAPK, 109, 110, 112, 136, 140, 148
Ptychopetalum (muira puama, potency wood), 594
Pueraria lobata. See Kudzu
Puerarin, 152
Pulmonaria (lungwort), 594
Pulsatilla patens (pasque flower), 124, 169, 173
Punica granatum. See Pomegranate
P2X receptors, 152, 162
Pygeum africanum (African prune), 594
Pyrola (false wintergreen), 594

Q

Qing qiao. *See Forsythia suspensa*
Quercetin, 113, 129, 186
Quercus. See Oak
Quinolinic acid, 139

R

Radiation protection, by echinacea, 506
RANTES, 107, 110, 111, 112, 136
Raoulia australis, for rhinovirus, 130
Rauwolfia spp., as synergist, 421
Reactive oxygen species (ROS), 152, 153
Red peony root, 167–68
Red root (*Ceanothus* spp.)
  actions of, 411
  appearance of, 537
  for candida, 76
  common names, 408
  contraindications, 409
  cultivation and collection, 409–10
  for Epstein-Barr virus, 170
  finding, 411
  for Gram-negative bacterial diseases, 63–64, 66–69, 71
  for Gram-positive bacterial diseases, 53–54
  habitat and appearance, 409
  herb/drug interactions, 409
  for immune system, 407–13, 411, 462
  for influenza, 108, 120–22
  parts used, 408
  plant chemistry, 410–11
  preparation and dosage, 408–9
    capsules, 409
    gargle, 408
    strong decoction, 408
    tea, 408
    tincture, 408, 585
  properties of, 411
  for rhinovirus, 130
  scientific research, 412–13
  species used, 407–8
  for spleen stimulation, 144
  toughness of, 540
  traditional uses of, 412
Reishi (*Ganoderma*)
  actions of, 521
  for candida, 76–77
  common names, 518
  cultivation and collection, 520–22
  finding, 521
  for Gram-negative bacterial diseases, 59–60, 64, 67
  for Gram-positive bacterial diseases, 53–54
  habitat and appearance, 520
  herb/drug interactions, 520
  for herpes simplex virus, 172
  for immune system, 462, 518–24, 521
  for influenza, 523
  parts used, 518
  plant chemistry, 522
  preparation and dosage, 519
    powder, 519
    syrup decoction, 519
    tablets, 519
    tincture, 519, 589
  properties of, 521
  scientific research, 523–24
  side effects and contraindications, 520
  species used, 518
  traditional uses of, 522–23
    Ayurveda, 522
    traditional Chinese medicine, 522–23
    Western botanic practice, 523
Reovirus, 131
Resin, 267
Resistant organisms, 39–78. *See also specific species*
  Gram-negative bacteria, 55–75
  Gram-positive bacteria, 49–55
  herbal remedies, 47
  nonbacterial variants, 75–78

treating
endotoxins and, 47
herbal remedies, 47, 47–49
increasing natural immunity, 48–49
synergists, 47–48
Respiratory syncytial virus, 129
Respiratory viral infections
adenovirus, 128–29
influenza, 96–128
parainfluenza virus, 129
respiratory syncytial virus, 129
rhinovirus, 129–30
Resveratrol, 138, 149–51
Rhamnus californica (California buckthorn, coffeeberry), 594
Rhein, 149
Rheum officinale (rhubarb), 594
Rhinovirus, 129–30
Rhodiola (*Rhodiola*)
actions of, 526
active against, 526
common names, 524
cultivation and collection, 528–30
for cytokine cascade reduction, 144
finding, 526
in food, 526
habitat and appearance, 527–28
for hypoxia, 143
for immune system, 145, 462, 524–34, 526
for neural protection, 144
part used, 527
plant chemistry, 530
preparation and dosage, 527
capsules, 527
tincture, 527, 594
properties of, 526
scientific research, 531–34
antifatigue/antistress, 532–33
antiviral/antibacterial, 531
immune action, 533–34
neuroprotective/neuroregenerative, 531–32
side effects and contraindications, 527
species used, 524–25, 527
traditional uses of, 530–31
Ayurveda, 530
in Tibetan medicine, 530–31
traditional Chinese medicine, 530
Western botanic practice, 531
use to treat, 526
Aspergillus, 78
Epstein-Barr virus, 169–70
Gram-negative bacterial diseases, 57, 66, 70–71
Gram-positive bacterial diseases, 51–52, 54
influenza, 123, 526, 531
shingles, 175
Rhus spp. (sumac), 595
Ribavirin, 114, 133, 134
Ribosome-inactivating proteins (RIPs), 341, 342
Rickettsia, 88
Rimantidine, 114
RNA, 85–86
RNA virus, 89–91
Roots. *See also specific plants/herbs*
cleaning, 540
hot infusions, 546
tinctures from, 559
Rosemary (*Rosmarinus*)
for Gram-negative bacterial diseases, 73–74
leaf in concentrated sore-relief herbal cream, 174
oil in inhalant for influenza, 128
as synergist, 421
tincture, 595
Rotaviruses, 162–63
Royal jelly, 289, 294
Rubbing alochol, in liniments, 568–69
Rubus idaeus (raspberry), 595
Rumex spp. (dock), 595
Ruscus aculeatus (butcher's broom), 595
Rust fungus, 377

S

Sage (*Salvia*)
for dengue fever virus, 165–66
endothelial cell normalization, 138
for Gram-negative bacterial diseases, 68, 70, 73
for HMGB1 inhibition, 113, 145–46
for influenza, 126–27
oil in inhalant for influenza, 128
tincture, 595
Salix (willow), 595

Salk vaccine, 82
Salmonella, 29, 30, 69–70
Salves, 571
Sambucol, 351
Sambucus. See Elder
SARS, 81, 380
Schefflera octophylla, 129
Schisandra, 169
Schistosomiasis, artemisia for, 255
Scoparius (broom), 595
Scrophularia (figwort), 595
Scutellaria. See Chinese skullcap
Sea buckthorn leaf (*Hippophae rhamnoides*), 146–47, 165–66
Sechium edule, 57, 73, 78
Seeds, in hot infusions, 546
Selanginella sinensis, 129
Selenium, for influenza, 128
Selenium-rich foods, for immune system, 460–61
Sensing
intuitive, 188
nonphysical, 538–39
Serenoa (saw palmetto), 595
Serissa japonica, 128
Serratia marcescens, 70–72
Sesquiterpene lactones, 251–52
Shigella spp., 72–73, 579
Shingles, 161–62, 173–76
Sialic acid, 104, 113–14
Sickle cell anemia, alchornea for, 227, 228
Sida (*Sida* spp.), 204–21, 208–10, 215, 220
actions of, 208
active against, 208
antimicrobial activity of, 182, 208, 218–20
broom production from, 209
common names, 204
cultivation and collection, 213
as douche, 568
finding, 210
habitat and appearance, 211–13
North American range, 211–12
worldwide range, 212–13
hemotoxin neutralization, 219
herb/drug interactions, 210
for malaria, 77
parts used, 205
plant chemistry, 214, 214–15
preparation and dosage, 205–7
artemisia tincture with sida and coryptolepsis for malaria, 248
capsules, 206
hot water extraction, 205, 207
powder, 206
tea, 206
tincture, 206, 595
properties of, 208–9
as protein food source, 209
scientific research, 218–19
antimicrobial activity, 218–20
extractions, 218–19
side effects and contraindications, 207
species used, 205
traditional uses of, 215, 215–18
Ayurveda, 216–17
traditional Chinese medicine, 217–18
Western botanic practice, 218
use to treat, 209
Aspergillus, 78
candida, 76–77
Gram-negative bacterial diseases, 57–60, 62–63, 65–67, 69–70, 73
Gram-positive bacterial diseases, 51–54
herpes simplex virus, 172
Sieve, 572
Silybum marianum (milk thistle), 170, 595
Sinus infection, nasal spray for, **566**
Skin infections, oil infusion for, **570**
Sleep, Chinese skullcap for, 311, 321, 324
Slippery elm, in hot infusion, 546
Slow cooker, 554, 569
Smallpox, 83, 308
S-methylmethionine (SMM), 576
Smilacina racemosa (false Solomon's seal), 596
Smilax (sarsaparilla), 596
Snake venom
bidens for, 240
sida for, 219
Solanum dulcamara (bittersweet), 596
Solidago (goldenrod), 596
Solvents, 542–44
percolations and, 555
Sophora flavescens, 129, 399
Sore-relief herbal cream, concentrated, **174**
Spleen, functions of, 459
Stachys officinalis (European betony), 596
Staph infections
alchornea for, 223, 226
bidens for, 231

- cryptolepsis for, 194
- sida for, 206

Staphylococcus aureus
- antibiotic resistance, 13–14, 30
- methicillin-resistant (MRSA), 14, 28, 41–42, 45, 53–54
  - alchornea for, 226
  - 5'-MHC efflux inhibitor and, 185
  - personal stories of, 3
- spread of resistant disease, 23–24, 28
- treating, 53–54

Steams
- described, 553
- essential oil, 553
- for upper respiratory infections, 553, **553**

Stenotrophomonas maltophilia, 73–74
Stephania, 52, 63, 72, 74
Sticta (lobaria pulmonaria, lungwort moss), 596
Stillingia sylvatica (queen's root), 596
Stomach flu, 163
Storing supplies and medicines, 540, 542
Streptococcus spp.
- berberine interference with adherence of, 265
- *S. pyogenes,* 485
- spread of resistant disease, 24
- treating, 54–55

Streptomycin, 9
Strobilanthes cusia, 399–400, 400
Superbugs, 1–6
Superoxide dismutase, 475
Supplies, storing, 540, 542
Suppositories, for abnormal pap smear, 574, **575**
Swainsonine, 206
Swertia radiata (green gentian, cebadilla), 596
Swine flu, 81, 102, 103
Symphytum (comfrey), 596
Synergists, 186, 414–16
- changes in Western monotherapy, 416–17
- defined, 184, 309, 416
- synergistic plants, 420–57
  - berberines, 264, 268
  - black pepper/piperine, 447–57
  - *Caesalpinia benthamiana,* 421
  - *Centella asiatica* (gotu kola), 421, 422
  - Chinese skullcap, 314
  - *Citrus aurantium* (bitter orange), 421
  - *Commiphiora,* 421
  - *Cymbopogon citratus,* 421
  - *Dalea* spp., 420
  - *Daucus,* 421
  - *Geranium caespitosum,* 420–21
  - ginger, 437–47
  - *Ipomoea murucoides,* 420
  - isatis, 371
  - licorice, 423–37
  - *Lycopus europaeus,* 421
  - *Prosopis juliflora,* 421
  - *Punica granatum* (pomegranate), 421–22
  - *Rauwolfia* spp., 421
  - *Rosemarinus officinalis,* 421
  - *Thymus vulgaris,* 421–22
- to treat resistant diseases, 47–48
- understanding plant synergists, 418–19

Syrups
- cough syrup, 550, **551–52**
- refrigeration of, 550

T

Tabebuia (pau d'arco), 568, 596
Tablespoon (measurement), 547
Tablets, herbal powder pressed into, 573
Tanacetum (feverfew), 596
Tannic acid, 176
Tannin, in sida, 220
Taraxacum (dandelion), 596
Teas
- Brigitte Mars's herbal tea for ear infections, **578–79**
- described, 544, 549
- Rosemary Gladstar's tea for diarrhea, **580**

Teasel root, 63, 587
Teaspoon (measurement), 547
Tehranolide, in artemisia, 252
Terminalia avicennoides, 178
Tetracycline, 21
Tetralogy of Fallot, 474
Thalictrum, 262
Thanking plants, 539
TheraMax, 351
Theramine, 173
Thrombomodulin, 115
Thuja (arbovitae, red or yellow cedar), 596

Thyme (*Thymus*)
  oil
    for Gram-negative bacterial diseases, 73–74
    inhalant for influenza, 128
  as synergist, 421–22
  tincture, 596
Thymus, functions of, 459
Tick-borne encephalitis (TBE), 130–32, 140–41, 146
  mechanisms of viral infection, 140–41
  natural treatments for, 146
  viruses of, 130–32
Tinctures. *See also specific ingredients*
  amount of alcohol in, 565
  combination for diarrhea, **580**
  combinations of plants, 186–87
  combination tincture formulas, 561, 563
  douches, 568
  dried plant, 560–61
  ear infection tincture combination, **579**
  fresh plant, 559
  how long they last, 562
  precipitation in, 562
  pressing herbal, 560
  vinegar, 566–67
Tinospora, 261, 267
Toddalia, 262
Togaviruses, 130
Toll-like receptors (TLRs), 106
Topoisomerase II, 198
Traditional Chinese medicine, herbs used in
  artemisia, 253–54
  astragalus, 473
  berberines, 274
  bidens, 238
  black pepper/piperine (*Piper* spp.), 452
  Chinese skullcap, 323
  cordyceps, 488–89
  cryptolepsis, 201
  elder, 347–49
  eleuthero, 514–15
  ginger (*Zingiber* spp.), 444
  houttuynia, 363–64
  isatis, 379–80
  juniper, 286–87
  licorice (*Glycyrrhiza* spp.), 434
  reishi, 522–23
  rhodiola, 530
  sida, 217–18
  usnea, 305
Transforming growth factor beta (TGF-β2), 110
Transposons, 20, 23
Trans-resveratrol, 150
Tribulus (puncture vine), 70–71, 596
Triclosan, 28
Trifolium pratense (red clover), 596
Trikatu, 448
Trillium (beth root), 596
Trypanosoma brucei, artemisia for, 247
Tryptanthrin, 185–86, 377
Tryptophan degradation, 138–39, 140
Tuberculosis
  spread of resistant disease, 25
  treating, 52–53
    juniper for, 288
    licorice for, 435
    sida for, 219
    usnea for, 306
Tumor necrosis factor alpha (TNF-α)
  influenza and, 107, 109, 111–12, 114
  La Crosse encephalitis virus (LCEV) and, 142
  tick-borne encephalitis and, 141
  West NIle encephalitis and, 136–38, 140
Turnera diffusa (damiana), 596

U

Ulcerated stomach, herbal regimen for, 573–74, **574**
Ulmus pumila (Siberian elm), 597
Umbellularia (California bay, Oregon myrtle), 597
Uncaria tomentosa (cat's claw), 147, 165–66, 597
Upper respiratory infections, steams for, 553, **553**
Ursolic acid, 350
Urtica (nettles), 597
Usnea (*Usnea*)
  actions of, 299
  active against, 299
  collection, 302–3
  common names, 297
  as douche, 568
  finding, 300
  habitat and appearance, 302
  heavy metal absorption by, 301
  herb/drug interactions, 302

lichen chemistry, 303–4
as localized antibacterial, 297–307, 299–300
parts used, 297
preparation and dosage, 297–98, 300–301
douche, 300
nasal spray, 300–301
tea, 301
tincture, 298, 300–301, 597
wash, 300–301
wound powder, 298
properties of, 299–300
scientific research, 305–7
side effects and contraindications, 301–2
species used, 297
toxicity, 301–2
traditional uses of, 304–5
Ayurveda, 305
traditional Chinese medicine, 305
Western botanic practice, 305
use to treat, 300
Gram-negative bacterial diseases, 59, 66
Gram-positive bacterial diseases, 50–53
Usnic acid, 301–3, 305–6

V

Vaccines, 82–83
chickenpox, 173
for encephalitis viruses, 130–32
for RNA virus *versus* DNA virus, 90
shingles, 173
Vaginal infections, douches for, 568
Valacyclovir, 158, 160–62
Valeriana (valerian), 597
Valganciclovir, for cytomegalovirus, 155
Varicella Zoster virus, 161–62, 173–76, **174**
Vascular cell adhesion molecule-1 (VCAM-1), 107, 136–37
Vegetalistas, 538
Velvet leaf (*Cissampelos pareira*), 146–47, 165–66
Verbascum (mullein), 597
Verbena (blue vervain), 597
Vibrio cholerae, treating, 74–75
Viburnum (cramp bark, black haw), 597
Vinca spp. (periwinkle), 597
Vinegar tinctures, 566–67
Viola odorata (violet), 597
Viruses, 87–95. *See also specific viruses*
antibiotic resistance and, 20
ecosystem functions of, 85–87
emerging, 79–95
encephalitis viruses, 130–54
gastrointestinal, 162–63, 176–78
genetic variability of, 90–91
infection process, 91–93
jumping of species by, 94
new paradigm for treating disease, 5–6
as nonliving particles, 88
number of, 88
properties of, 87–93
replication of, 89–90
resistance to antivirals, 115–16
sensing by, 89
structure of, 88–89
treatment
cytomegalovirus, 163–64
dengue fever virus, 164–66
encephalitis viruses, 132–33, 143–54
enterovirus 71, 167–69
Epstein-Barr virus, 169–70
gastrointestinal viruses, 176–78
medical, 132–33
neural herbs for, 147–54
Varicella Zoster virus, 173–76, **174**
types, 89–90
ubiquity of, 88
as vehicles for genetic change, 87
Vitamin B_{12}, 172, 175–76
Vitamin C effervescent salts, for constipation, 166
Vitamin U, 576
Vitamix, 561, 572
Vitex agnus-castus (chaste tree), 597
Volatiles, in hot infusions, 546
Vomiting and nausea, from elder, 331–34, 337

W

Washes, 552, **552**, 553
Water
hard, 194
quality, 543
as solvent, 543

Water extractions, 544–57
  decoctions, 548–52
    concentrated, 548–50, 550, **551**
    cough syrup, 550, **551–52**
    simple, 548, **549**
  evaporative concentrates, 553–54, **554–55**
  infusions, 544–48
    cold, 546–47
    equipment, 547–48
    hot, 545–46
    strength and weaknesses of, 545
    teas compared to, 544
  percolations, 555–57
  steams, 553, **553**
  washes, 552, **552**
Water softener, 194
Weight loss, usnea use for, 301–2
Western botanic practice
  changes in Western monotherapy, 416–17
  herbs used in
    artemisia, 254
    ashwagandha, 466
    astragalus, 473
    berberines, 275
    bidens, 238–39
    boneset, 405–6
    Chinese skullcap, 323
    cordyceps, 489
    echinacea, 500–501
    elder, 349–50
    eleuthero, 515
    ginger (*Zingiber* spp.), 444
    houttuynia, 364
    isatis, 380
    juniper, 287
    licorice (*Glycyrrhiza* spp.), 434–35
    lomatium, 395–97
    red root, 412
    reishi, 523
    rhodiola, 531
    sida, 218
    usnea, 305
West Nile virus, 81, 130–31
  cytokine/chemokine cascade, 136–40
  demographics of infection, 134
  infection progression, 135
  mechanisms of viral infection, 133–40
  medical interventions, 134
  natural treatments for, 146
  symptoms, 134
White blood cells, functions of, 459–60
Willow bark, 186
Withania spp. *See* Ashwagandha
Woad. *See* Isatis (*Isatis*)
Wogonin, 320, 321, 324–27
Wound powders, 572–73, **573**

X

Xanthoxylum (prickly ash), 598

Y

Yangonin, 185
Yarrow (*Achillea*)
  cold infusion, 546
  as diaphoretic adjunct, 124, 191
  for fever in influenza, 124
  hot infusion, 545
  for influenza, 124
  tincture, 581
Yerba mansa (*Anemopsis californica*), 353, 582
Yerba santa (*Eriodictyon* spp.), 120–22
Yogurt, for immune system, 460
Young's Rule, 578

Z

Zanamivir, 114
Zea mays (corn silk), 598
Zinc, 128, 172, 407
Zinc-containing foods, 461
Zinc sulfate cream, 172
Zingiber. *See* Ginger
Zuccagnia punctata, 57, 73